Biology
of
Sensory
Systems

Second Edition

C. U. M. SMITH

Vision Sciences, Aston University,
Birmingham, UK

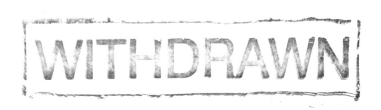

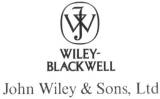

WILEY-
BLACKWELL

John Wiley & Sons, Ltd

Library of Congress Cataloguing-in-Publication Data

Smith, C. U. M. (Christopher Upham Murray)
  Biology of sensory systems / C.U.M. Smith. – 2nd ed.
    p. ; cm.
  Includes bibliographical references and index.
  ISBN 978-0-470-51862-5 (alk. paper) – ISBN 978-0-470-51863-2 (alk. paper)
  1. Senses and sensation. I. Title.
  [DNLM: 1. Sense Organs. 2. Evolution. 3. Molecular Biology.
4. Physiology, Comparative. WL 700 S644b 2008]
  QP431.S536 2008
  612.8–dc22   2008021435

ISBN: 978-0-470-51862-5

A catalogue record for this book is available from the British Library.

Set in 10/11.5pt Times by Aptara
Printed in Singapore by Markono Print Media Pte Ltd

First Impression 2008

Cover: Image of a horizontal section through the ommatidia of an insect's eye (Chrysopa; the green lacewing). Courtesy of Professor Adrian Horridge, Australian National University.

CONTENTS

PREFACE TO SECOND EDITION

Eight years have passed since the first edition of this text was published. Eight years in which the subject matter of sensory biology has seen huge developments. In particular, the molecular revolution of our times has continued apace and culminated in the publication of not only the human genome but also those of many other living forms. Although to the innocent eye the living world seems to be populated by an almost infinite variety of forms possessing an equally unimaginable variety of sensory systems, the explosive development of molecular biology shows that there is a deep underlying unity. In revising this book I have attempted to bring out this unity to an even greater extent than in the first edition. Not only has each chapter been thoroughly revised with this in mind but an additional chapter, Chapter 5, on genes and genomics has been inserted. Otherwise the overall organization of the book remains largely unchanged. The major themes remain as before: foundations in molecular biology and biophysics; a strong emphasis on evolutionary development and comparative anatomy; a focus on human systems; reference to the 'hard problem' of the relation of our sensory experience to the anatomy and physiology of sensory systems.

Although the overall structure of the volume remains much as it was in the first edition, each page has been subjected to detailed revision and updating and over forty new illustrations have been added. Several new sections have been inserted. Amongst these are sections on transient receptor potential channels (TRP channels), synaptic transmission, evolution of nervous systems, arachnid mechanosensitive sensilla and photoreceptors, electroreception in the Monotremata, language and the *FOXP2* gene;

the molecular biology of pain, mirror neurons and so on. One of the most interesting developments since the first edition was published has been the Nobel-Prize-winning work on olfaction in mammals and insects and the chapters on olfaction have been expanded to take this work into account. In addition a number of new Boxes have been incorporated into the text: on the genetics of hearing loss; on macular degeneration; on the nomenclature of genes and proteins; on the reality of cortical columns.

As I wrote in the preface to the first edition, the study of sensory systems can form a bridge between the worlds of biophysics, molecular biology and neurophysiology and the worlds of cognitive science and psychology. My hope remains that the overview presented in the pages of this second edition, as in the first, can form a basis on which special studies can be built. Although the book provides a wide sweep through the world of animal sensory systems the major focus remains on mammalian and especially on human systems. The ubiquity of the underlying molecular biology often means that the molecular disorders responsible for human disease and disability can be studied in infrahuman species. Wherever possible the opportunity is taken to bring out these connections and to outline the molecular bases of human sensory disorders and pathology. In spite of this focus on human sensory systems and their pathologies I hope that the wide coverage of other animals brings with it another message: that in studying sensory systems and their functioning we should bear in mind that human systems are but one among many.

In concluding, I can only reiterate the thanks offered in the preface to the first edition to all those who helped in the production of this book and, in particular, the many scientists and others who gave permission to reproduce their diagrams and illustrations. Finally, I cannot end without reference to the invaluable help and support of my wife, Jenny, who wanted to know, and to whom this book is dedicated.

C.U.M.S.
January 2008

PREFACE TO FIRST EDITION

'All men by nature desire to know. An indication of this is the delight we take in our senses; for even apart from their usefulness they are loved for themselves...' Aristotle, *Metaphysics*, Book 1, 980a

This book arises from the experience of teaching undergraduate classes in the biology of sensory systems over many years. It differs from the many other excellent texts in the subject in that, in addition to the neurobiology, it emphasises evolution, molecular biology and the wider philosophical implications of the subject. Humans are not the only beings with sensory systems on the surface of this planet. We are deeply interwoven with all the other biological forms which populate the biosphere. Some of these other forms, the other chordates, are related, albeit frequently quite distantly, by a common basic design plan; others, the mollusca, the arthropoda and so on have evolved separately for more than half a billion years. Comparisons between these forms often show how similar sensory problems have elicited sometimes different and sometimes remarkably similar solutions. At the basis of all these solutions are the sensory cells and the molecular mechanisms which make them especially sensitive to particular forms of environmental energy. One of the most interesting developments of recent years has been the dawning recognition that these molecular mechanisms are often much the same from nematode to man. Underlying the unimaginable variety of sensory systems in the biosphere is a remarkable unity. Finally, sensory systems provide each of us with our private subjective world. As we study sensory systems in ourselves and in the animals with which we share the planet

we should not lose sight of the problem posed by the mysterious transition (is it a transition?) between the world of molecules and cells and fibre tracts, with all its fascinating detail, and the very different world of scents and sounds and colours which all of us experience every day. This remains the major philosophical problem of modern times. It appears and reappears at intervals throughout the following pages.

The study of sensory systems forms a bridge between the world of biophysics, molecular biology, neurophysiology and the world of cognitive science and psychology. I hope that the overview provided in the following pages can form a basis upon which special studies can be built. The subject of sensory systems, like all aspects of contemporary science, is vast. All that has been attempted in the following pages is to present a basis, a framework, for further studies. In order to pursue these studies recourse has to be made to the libraries and to the various electronic databases nowadays available. To this end a reasonably full bibliography has been included. For ease of reading references have not been included in the text but are, instead, collected at the end of each the six parts of the book with short bibliographical introductions.

Finally, a number of self-assessment questions are also grouped at the end of each of the six parts. These questions are keyed into the text. After reading a chapter, a student should turn to these questions and make sure that answers spring readily to mind. If they do not, reference should be made to the relevant section of the text to refresh the memory.

No book, and certainly no book on so vast a subject as the biology of sensory systems, springs forth fully armed, as Athene is said to have sprung forth from the forehead of Zeus. All, as Isaac Newton said long ago, are founded on the work of countless predecessors and contemporaries. In this book the reference lists stretch back from mid 1999 to Aristotle and beyond, two and a half millennia ago. My thanks are accordingly due to innumerable workers, both past and present. In particular, those thanks must go to the many contemporary workers who have given permission to reproduce their diagrams and figures. It is said that one well-judged illustration is worth a thousand words and the books and papers of contemporary science abound with high-quality line drawings and half-tones. I am most grateful to the authors and their publishers for permission to reproduce them.

It is impossible in these acknowledgments to mention more than a very few of those who have helped me. In alphabetical order they would include Professor Allison for up to date information about face-sensitive regions in the human brain, Professor Paul Bach-y-Rita for help with the section on sensory substitution, Professor John E.Brugge for figures showing the positions of the auditory cortices in cat and monkey, Professor Alan J. Benson for a revised diagram of cochlear hair cells, Professor Oleg Orlov for valuable correspondence on visual systems and vision, Professor Adrian Horridge for information about arthropod eyes, Professor Jim Pickles for scanning electronmicrographs of cochlear hair cells. I would also like to thank the two anonymous reviewers of the first draft manuscript who provided expert feed-back. This has been incorporated where possible. The usual disclaimers are, of course, operative. All mistakes and misapprehensions are the author's own, not those of his advisors.

As indicated at the beginning of this preface, this book arises from the experience of teaching undergraduate students in biology and, latterly, in optometry at Aston University. My acknowledgements would not be complete without reference to their critical response to my courses: as is always the case in any teaching situation the teacher learns as much as (if not more than) the student. I would also like to thank my colleagues amongst the academic staff for support and discussion and for providing the time and facilities for carrying through this project. Technical assistance has also proved invaluable and I have not only benefited from the computer and IT expertise of others but also from the expert photographic talents of our visual aids technician, Mr Barry Brooks. Finally, in these acknowledgements, I cannot fail to include my publishers who, as with my previous books, have managed to put together illustrations, questions, bibliographies, tables, appendices, boxes and text to create a volume which (hopefully) will find favour amongst students and others at the beginning of our new century.

C.U.M.S.
November 1999

PART I: PRELIMINARIES

1

ELEMENTS

Origins: great antiquity - RNA and DNA - 'selfish' genes. **Allosteric effectors**: conformational change - co-operative allostery - protein kinases and phosphatases. **Membranes**: lipids - fluid-mosaic structure - proteins - mobility. **Receptor molecules**: 7TM conformation - molecular structure - G-protein binding - desensitisation. **Membrane signalling systems**: G-proteins - structure - collision-coupling biochemistry - various effectors - various second messengers. **Channels and gates**: TRPs, LGICs and VGICs - Na^+-channel, structure and functioning. **Concluding remarks**: ubiquity of molecular elements.

Three and a half thousand million years ago the first precursors of the prokaryocytes originated in already ancient oceans. Even before that time primitive self-replicating molecules had appeared in the primordial broth. It is likely that these earliest replicators were RNA rather than DNA. This is because some forms of RNA (the ribozymes) are known to have enzymic activity and replication proceeds more rapidly when enzyme-assisted. Although DNA replication is more efficient, it always depends on protein enzymes. These could hardly have been present in the primitive oceans. In consequence the more complex process of DNA replication must have evolved later. But whether with RNA or DNA, and *a fortiori* with the latter, effective replication depends on a multiplicity of molecules. It follows that these molecules must be kept in one another's vicinity. It may be that to begin with they were adsorbed on some common surface, perhaps a clay. But the most effective means of keeping a society of interacting molecules together is to enclose them in a tiny bag or vesicle.

The simplest contemporary prokaryocytes are the mycoplasmas. The smallest are only 0.3 μm in diameter and consist of no more than about 750 different types of protein. But even these tiny cells are more advanced than the protocells of three and a half billion years ago. For, in common with all contemporary cells, they use DNA rather than RNA as their hereditary material. But whether it is the simplest of living cells or their hypothetical ancestors that are being considered, one thing stands out: they stand out. They stand out from their surrounding environment. Their boundary membranes separate an 'internal' from an 'external' environment. Philosophically-inclined biologists trace the origins of the individual to this primordial period.

All organisms live in an environment. All organisms respond in one way or another to that environment. This is what distinguishes them from inanimate objects. It is clear that the boundary membrane between organism and environment must play a crucial role. It is here that specializations develop which are able to detect advantageous and disadvantageous changes. In other words, it is here that the simplest sensory systems originate. Informed of change in the external environment, the organism

---

Biology of Sensory Systems, Second Edition   C.U.M. Smith
© 2008 John Wiley & Sons, Ltd

can react to its own advantage. Advantageous, that is, for the prospects of that organism leaving viable representatives in the next generation. Ultimately this can be traced down to the replicating molecules. Those which replicate most efficiently, that is leave more replicants in the next generation, mop up the available resources and survive.

Let us begin at the beginning; let us look at the elements from which sensory systems are constructed.

1.1 ALLOSTERIC EFFECTORS

Textbooks of biochemistry and/or molecular biology show that enzymic proteins have a complex three-dimensional structure. The covalently-bonded primary structure consisting of one or more amino acid chains is twisted into intricate conformations, the so-called secondary & tertiary structures. These structures are stabilized by numerous 'weak' forces: hydrogen bonds, Van der Waals and hydrophobic forces and so on. It should be stressed that these forces are individually weak. Whereas single covalent bonds have energies of about 100 kcal/mole (double and triple bonds have correspondingly higher energies), hydrogen bonds have energies of only 1 to 5 kcal/mole whilst hydrophobic and the very short range van der Waals forces are weaker still at only some 1 kcal/mol. But although they are very weak compared with covalent bonds, they are often very numerous. Large numbers of these weak forces hold the complex weave of a protein molecule in place.

This does, however, mean that the 'higher' structure of enzymic proteins is very fragile and easily disrupted. It also means that the structure can often shift from one stable conformation to another. It is this feature which underlies the phenomenon of **allostery**. In essence this means that when a molecule (or **ligand**) binds to one site on a protein's surface, it causes a conformation change which unmasks an active site somewhere else on its surface. In a sense this can be seen as the most primitive of all sensory systems. The protein molecule alters its behaviour in response to some factor in its environment (Figure 1.1).

Allosteric transitions play such crucial roles that they have been said to underlie all cell biology. We shall meet them time after time in the following pages. Frequently such allosteric transitions occur in pro-

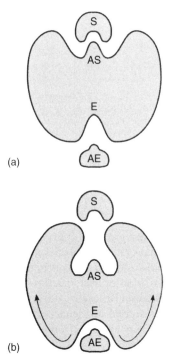

(a)

(b)

Figure 1.1 Conceptual diagram to show the effect of an allosteric effector on the activity of an enzyme. AE = allosteric effector; AS = active site; E = enzyme; S = substrate. When AE binds to the enzyme a change is induced in the latter's three-dimensional conformation (symbolized by arrows) so that AS is no longer accessible to the substrate molecule (S).

teins consisting of more than one subunit. In these cases when a ligand binds to the allosteric site on one subunit, it causes a change which facilitates binding of ligands to allosteric sites on all the other subunits. This is known as **cooperative allostery** and can create a much stronger alteration in the behaviour of the allosteric protein.

One of the most significant means of causing allosteric transitions is phosphorylation. We shall meet this mechanism again and again as we study the molecular bases of sensory systems, so it is worthwhile looking at it a little more closely here. The phosphorylation reaction is catalysed by a **protein kinase**. Protein kinases form a large family of several hundred members all of which share a 250 amino acid catalytic domain. The basic reaction is to transfer a phosphate group from ATP to a hydroxyl group on the side chain of an amino acid in the substrate

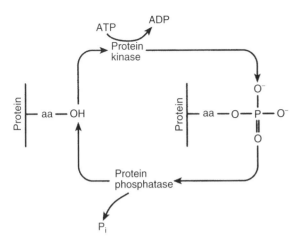

Figure 1.2 A protein chain is shown with an amino acid (serine, threonine or tyrosine) side chain: aa. Protein kinase uses a phosphate group from ATP to phosphorylate the side chain. Protein phosphatases later dephosphorylate the side chain.

protein. Only three amino acids – **serine, threonine and tyrosine** – present hydroxyl groups in their side chains, so only these amino acids are affected. The reaction is shown diagrammatically in Figure 1.2.

Whilst protein kinases in phosphorylating their substrate protein cause allosteric transitions, they are themselves subject to allosteric control. We need not in this book follow the biochemistry any further. The cascade of control mechanisms reaches deep into the biochemistry of the cell. But it is worth noting that other enzymes, the **protein phosphatases**, are present in the cytosol to undo the work which the kinases have done (Figure 1.2). These enzymes remove the phosphate from the substrate protein thus allowing it to relax back into its original conformation.

1.2 MEMBRANES

A second 'element' upon which all sensory systems are built is the biomembrane. Although the earliest membranes to form in primeval times may have been built of amino acids, all contemporary biological membranes (or biomembranes) consist of lipid bilayers with protein insertions. In addition, most membranes also contain carbohydrate. The lipids form a matrix or scaffolding in which the proteins

are embedded, whilst the carbohydrates (where they exist) are attached either to the lipids (glycolipids) or to the proteins (glycoproteins) (Figure 1.3).

1.2.1 Lipids

It can be seen (Figure 1.3) that lipids form a bimolecular sheet. They fall into three major groups: phospholipids, glycolipids and steroids (especially cholesterol). There is no need to discuss their detailed structure in this book (standard biochemistry texts all provide good accounts). It is worth noting, however, that they are all *amphipathic* molecules, that is they are partially soluble in water and partially in organic solvents. A typical membrane lipid will have one end bearing an electrostatic charge, so that it can enter the water structure, and the other end covalently bonded with no electrostatic charges, so that it is at home in organic solvents. As both the extracellular and intracellular media are overwhelmingly aqueous, it follows that membrane-forming lipids line up with their hydrophilic heads projecting into the aqueous environment and their hydrophobic 'tails' facing inwards toward each other away from the watery exterior or interior. Some typical membrane lipids are shown in Figure 1.4.

From what has been said, and from Figures 1.3 and 1.4, it is clear that biological membranes are very delicate structures. Their constituent lipids are held in position by hydrophobic forces and by occasional electrostatic attractions between their 'head' groups. The extremely tenuous nature of the phospholipid bilayer means that at room temperature the individual molecules are in continuous motion. Indeed, the hydrophobic fatty-acid tails of the molecules have been likened to a basketful of snakes, squirming about in perpetual motion. The interior of the membrane is thus, to all intents and purposes, an organic fluid. We shall see that the extreme fluidity of the lipid matrix of biomembranes is of considerable significance in sensory systems when we come to consider G-protein signal transduction.

Not all the lipid constituents of biomembranes are, however, as labile as the phospholipids. Cholesterol, in particular, is a very different type of molecule. As shown in Figure 1.4, it consists of three different regions: a hydrophilic 'head' consisting of the hydroxyl

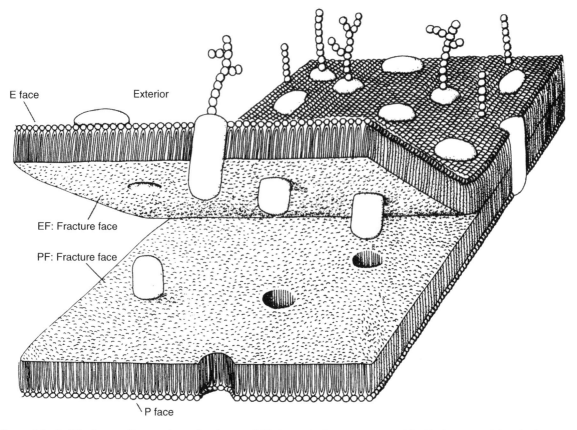

Figure 1.3 In this diagram the membrane has been quickly frozen to the temperature of liquid nitrogen and then broken open. The fracture plane runs along the centre of the lipid bilayer. The figure shows how proteins are embedded in the membrane and also the position of carbohydrate chain ('strings of sausages') projecting from the external face. Reproduced by permission of Executive of the Estate of Bunji Tagawa from Birgit Satir, 'The final steps of secretion', Scientific American, October 1975, p. 33.

group, a flat plate-like steroid ring and a flexible hydrophobic tail. The quantity of cholesterol present in biomembrane varies considerably. When it is present it stiffens the membrane and reduces its fluidity.

The fluidity of a membrane is, in fact, determined not only by the quantity of cholesterol that it contains but also by the length and saturation of the fatty acids that form its core. In artificial membranes formed of a single lipid species there is a sharp 'transition temperature', characteristic of the particular phospholipid, when the membrane changes from a fluid into a gel state. This temperature varies from place to place in a natural biomembrane depending on the amount of cholesterol and the saturation of the phospholipid 'tails'. A natural membrane can thus be envisaged as a mosaic of different fluidities.

1.2.2 Proteins

Embedded in this patchwork quilt of a membrane are the proteins. Although glycolipids (such as the cell adhesion molecules) are of great importance in intercellular recognition, the most important functional characteristics of biomembranes are conferred not by their lipids but by their proteins. The quantity of protein present varies from about 20% of the mass (myelin) to about 75% of the mass (mitochondrial inner membrane). Most membranes contain about 50% protein by mass.

The majority of proteins (as shown in Figure 1.4) are embedded in the membrane. They 'float' like icebergs in the variable phospholipid 'sea', or, to put it another way, they form a mosaic in the fluid

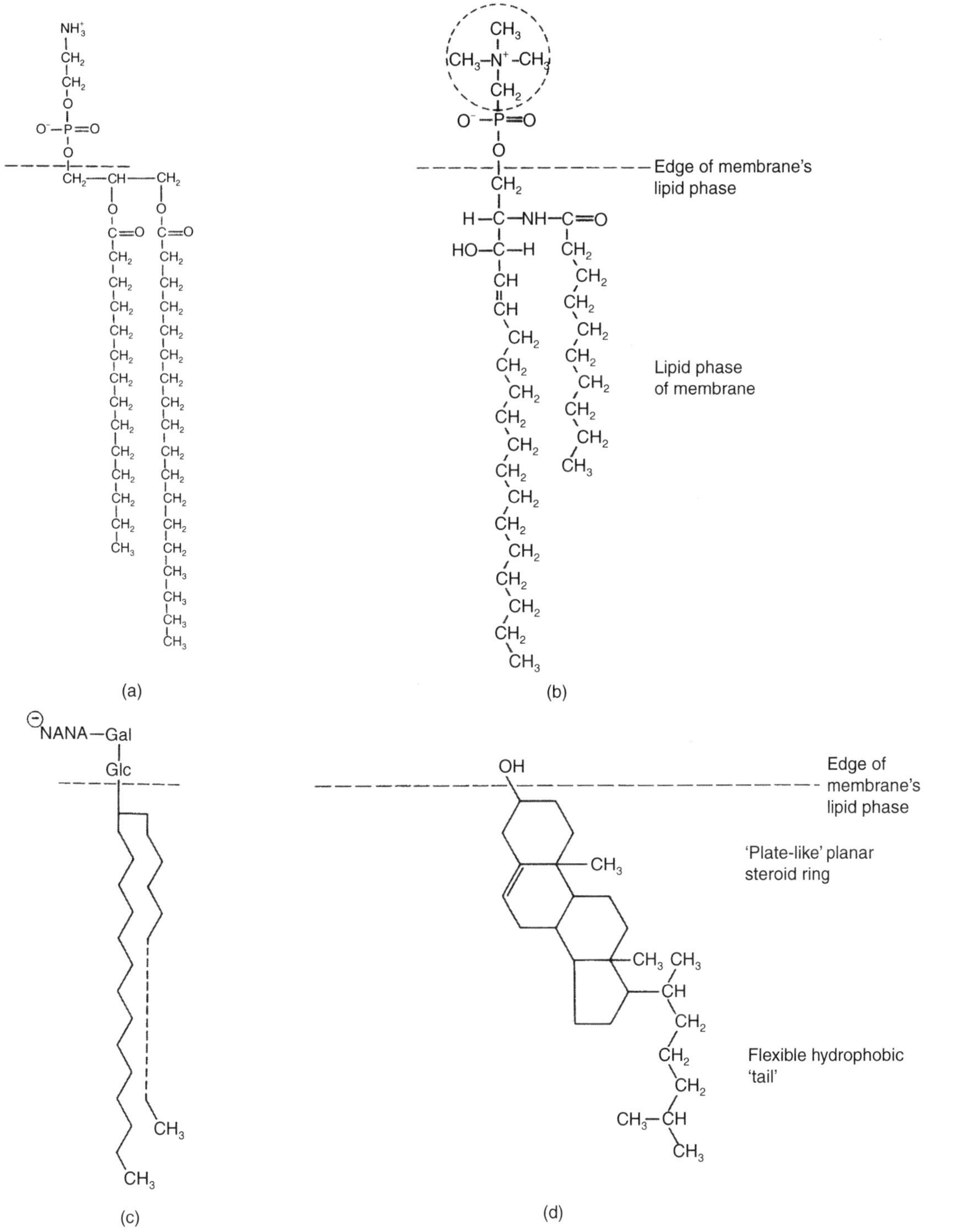

Figure 1.4 Some common membrane lipids. (a) Phosphatidyl choline (lecithin); (b) Sphingomyelin; (c) a ganglioside (the dashed line represents a lengthy CH_2 chain); (d) Cholesterol. Gal = galactose; Glc = glucose; NANA = *N*-acetylneuraminic acid.

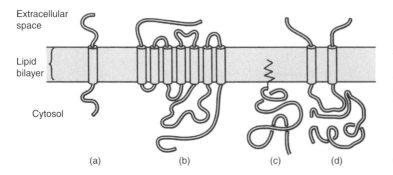

Extracellular space

Lipid bilayer

Cytosol

(a)   (b)   (c)   (d)

Figure 1.5 Some of the ways in which proteins are associated with membranes. The intramembranous cylinders represent alpha helices. (a) A single alpha helix passes through the membrane; (b) a number of alpha helices pass and repass the membrane; (c) the protein is held to the cytoplasmic leaflet of the bilayer by a fatty acid chain or prenyl group (significant examples of this are provided by G-proteins); (d) a membrane embedded protein is non-covalently attached to another protein in the cytosol.

phospholipid matrix. This concept is, for this reason, called the 'fluid-mosaic' model. In most cases the proteins project all the way through the bilayer and extend into both the intracellular and extracellular spaces. In other cases the proteins are attached to the membrane by a fatty acid chain, phospholipid or prenyl group. In these latter cases the protein itself is located in the cytosol. Some of these various means of attachment are shown in Figure 1.5. We shall see that membrane-bound proteins form the basic elements of all sensory receptors.

Transmembrane proteins are constructed in such a way that they have hydrophobic domains embedded in the membrane and hydrophilic domains projecting into the aqueous intracellular and/or extracellular compartments (Figure 1.5). In comparison with globular proteins of the aqueous cytosol the intramembranous domains of membrane proteins are, in a sense, inside out: their hydrophobic amino acid residues point outwards, their hydrophilic residues are tucked inside toward their cores. This ensures that the proteins stick in the membrane. Very commonly, as shown in Figure 1.5, the intramembranous domains consist of alpha-helical segments. Again, the vast majority of the amino acid residues making up these intramembranous alpha-helices are hydrophobic.

Studies which involve the incorporation of enzymatic proteins into artificial lipid bilayers show that the activity of such proteins is conditioned by their lipid environment. Features of the bilayer such as length of fatty acid chains, degree of saturation and the nature of the lipid 'heads' all influence the biological activity of the enzyme. Just as water-soluble enzymes are affected by features of the aqueous environment (pH, salt concentration, etc.), so lipid-embedded enzymes are affected by the precise nature of their lipids which surround them.

1.2.3 Mobility of Proteins

We have already likened membrane proteins to icebergs floating in a lipid sea. It is not surprising, then, to find that many have considerable lateral mobility. In the next section we shall see that this mobility has been pressed into service, with great effect, in the development of signalling systems based on proteins shuttling in the plane of the membrane. Protein diffusion coefficients range from about 10^{-9} cm^2/s for visual pigments in rod-cell outer-segments to about 10^{-11} cm^2/s for proteins in other membranes. In the first case a protein would travel about 0.1 μm (0.1 micron) per second, in the latter case 0.001 μm/s. There are a number of reasons for these great differences in mobility. First, it may be due to the differential lipid constitution of the membrane which, as indicated above, affects its fluidity. Or it may be that the protein is part of a large multiplex of other proteins and thus rendered too bulky to move easily. Alternatively, it may be impeded by structures external to the membrane, cell junctions, desmosomes, tight junctions and so on. Last, but far from least, it may be that the membrane protein is anchored to an element of the submembranous cytoskeleton.

1.3 MEMBRANE SIGNALLING SYSTEMS

The boundary membranes of cells, located as they are between the external environment and the internal environment of the cell's cytosol, have developed

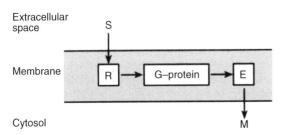

Figure 1.6 Schematic diagram to show G-protein signalling system. S = stimulus; R = membrane receptor; E = effector (enzyme, ion channel, etc.); M = second messenger.

many biochemical mechanisms which 'transduce' external events into 'messages' released into the cytosol. Most of these 'mechanisms' take the form of protein molecules embedded in the membrane. Some are ion channels which open directly in response to mechanical stimuli, others depend on the mobility of other proteins in the biomembrane. In essence the latter depend on the presence of a receptor molecule which can recognize an environmental stimulant and a means of transforming this recognition into a message which can diffuse into the receptor cell's cytosol.

As this type of receptor is of such importance and ubiquity, let us examine it in some detail. The system consists of three parts: the receptor molecule itself, a means of signalling its activation to a membrane-bound 'effector' and the effector itself. The system is shown schematically in Figure 1.6.

1.3.1 Receptor Molecules

The most important type of receptor molecule is the so-called '7TM' 'serpentine' receptor. It is called a 7TM receptor as it makes seven passes through the membrane or, in other words, has seven transmembrane domains (Figure 1.7). Its sinuous course through the membrane is also reminiscent of a serpent. 7TM receptors are found not only in receptor cells but also in the subsynaptic membranes of metabotropic synapses. Many, but not all, 7TM receptors are evolutionarily related. They form an extremely large superfamily of proteins, indeed it has been found that some 2% of the mamamalian genome codes for these proteins.

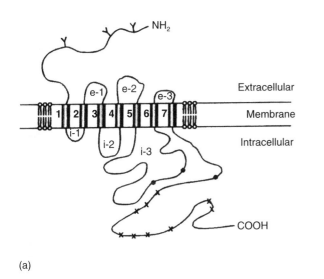

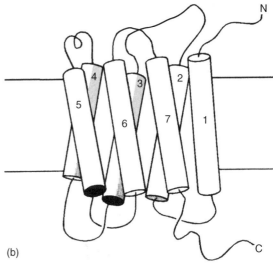

(a)   (b)

Figure 1.7 Architecture of a 7TM receptor. (a) Schematic view: the seven transmembrane (TM) helices are shown as columns in the membrane numbered 1–7. The N-terminal sequence is extracellular and normally has carbohydrate sequences attached (glycosylated). This is represented by Y's. The extracellular loops are labelled e-1, e-2, e-3 and these may also sometimes by glycosylated. The intracellular loops i-1, i-2, i-3 provide recognition surfaces for specific G-proteins. The dark spots signify phosphorylation sites for protein kinase and the crosses represent sites which specific desensitising protein kinases affect. (b) Three-dimensional conformation of the receptor in the membrane.

The plan view of Figure 1.7a shows how the seven transmembrane segments traverse the membrane. It also shows that there are also large extracellular and intracellular domains. Figure 1.7b shows that, when looked at in three dimensions, the seven transmembrane segments form the pillars of a hollow column, orientated rather like a 'barrel of staves'.

The 7TM receptors not only share a common architectural theme but also a common membrane-bound means of signal amplification. This mechanism (as we shall see in the next section) capitalizes on the lateral mobility of proteins, in this case G-proteins, in biomembranes and on the fact that the lipid bilayer holds such proteins in close proximity to each other so that they cannot diffuse away into the cytosol. Because 7TM receptors are almost always coupled to a G-protein system they are often known as G-protein coupled receptors (*GPCRs*). Careful structure–function analysis of the 7TM receptors shows that the first, second and third cytoplasmic loops (i-1, i-2 and i-3) and the carboxy-terminal tail (Figure 1.6a) are crucial to G-protein binding, with the third loop particularly involved in the recognition of particular G-proteins. Ultimately, when a receptor has been overexposed to its agonist, it becomes markedly less responsive. This is known as **desensitization**. We shall come across it many times in the following pages. Desensitization is brought about by specific protein kinases (Section 1.1) phosphorylating the hydroxyl groups of serine, threonine and tyrosine residues in the carboxyterminal tail of the receptor. These residues are symbolized by crosses in Figure 1.7a. They are additional to serine, threonine and tyrosine residues, which are affected by by nonspecific protein kinase (symbolized by spots). These phosphorylations, as we saw in Section 1.1, alter the three-dimensional conformation of the receptor. Sensitivity is restored by dephosphorylation by one of the many phosphatase enzymes that populate the cytosol.

1.3.2 G-proteins

When a 7TM receptor molecule located in the membrane of a sensory cell is activated by some change in the external environment it undergoes a **conformational change**. Recent successes in analysing the type-example of a GPCR, the β_2-adrenergic recep-

tor, at a 3.4/3.7 Å resolution has allowed molecular biologists the first detailed look into the precise chemical mechanisms which produce this change. The conformational change triggers an allosteric change in the associated **G-protein (Guanine-binding protein)** causing it to release its bound GDP which is quickly replaced by GTP. Once this has happened the G-protein complex splits into its constituent units (see below), which are released to travel in the membrane to activate an effector molecule also located in the membrane. This often (not always) leads to the release of a second messenger into the cytosol. The process is shown schematically in Figure 1.9.

The G-proteins involved in signal transduction are members of another large superfamily of proteins. They have been described as precisely engineered time-switches which can turn on and off the activity of other molecules. All the G-proteins are switched 'on' by binding to GTP and switched 'off' by the hydrolysis of GTP to GDP. This hydrolysis is catalysed by the GTPase activity of the G-protein itself. The process is comparatively slow, ranging from a few seconds to a few tens of seconds.

The G-proteins of biological membranes all have a heterotrimeric structure. They consist of a large alpha subunit (circa 45 kDa) and smaller beta and gamma subunits (Figure 1.8). The alpha subunit possesses the GTPase activity and in the inactive (or 'off') state it holds a GDP molecule in its active site. The smaller beta and gamma subunits are bound closely together; indeed it is impossible to separate them in physiological conditions. In the inactive state the beta–gamma complex is firmly attached

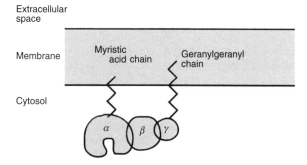

Figure 1.8 Conformation of a heterotrimeric membrane-bound G-protein. The α-subunit is shown with a cavity representing a site for GDP or GTP.

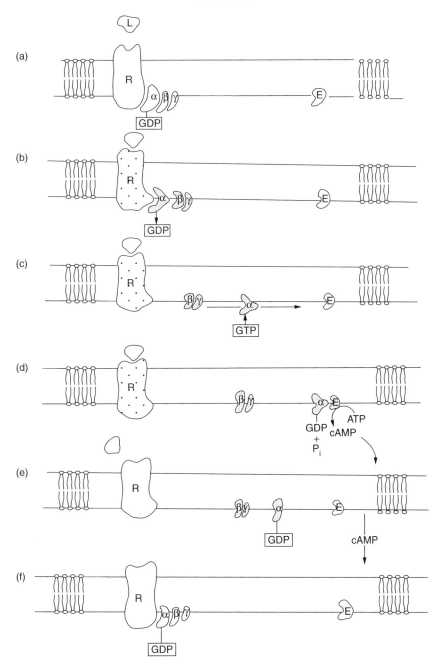

Figure 1.9 G-protein signalling system in a biological membrane. (a) Resting phase. (b) Ligand attaches and activates receptor. This causes a conformational change which releases the α-subunit of the G-protein. It also causes a conformation change in this subunit so that GDP is released from its binding site and the βγ-dyad set free. (c) The α-subunit is activated by accepting GTP and travels to the effector. (d) The α-subunit docks with and activates the effector which, in turn, catalyses the production of a second messenger, for instance cAMP, which diffuses into the cytosol. The α-subunit also catalyses the dephosphorylation of GTP to GDP and Pi. (e) Dephosphorylation of GTP deactivates the α-subunit which consequently detaches from the effector. (f) The receptor is deactivated by loss of its ligand and by other biochemical reactions (see text) and the receptor-G-protein complex is reformed. Stippling = activation; E = effector; L = ligand; R = GPCR.

to the alpha subunit. The gamma subunit is linked to the cytoplasmic leaflet of the biomembrane by a 20 carbon geranylgeranyl tail (related to cholesterol) and the alpha subunit is also linked into the membrane by a 14 carbon fatty-acid (myristic acid). These linkages ensure that the G-protein complex is both held in the plane of the membrane and is also able to move easily in that plane.

Alpha subunits are very variable. Those found in the olfactory system are, for example, distinctively different from those in the visual system. The beta and gamma subunits are less heterogeneous; even so, a number of different types are known. This molecular heterogeneity makes it possible to 'design' flexible and well-adapted signalling systems. We shall discuss this further when we meet with specific instances in later chapters.

When a GPCR is activated, it undergoes a conformational change which is transmitted to the alpha subunit of its attached G-protein complex. This, in turn, undergoes an allosteric transition releasing its GDP, separating from the receptor and from its beta and gamma subunits. As there is normally a plentiful supply of GTP in the cytosol, it diffuses in to occupy the vacant site on the alpha subunit. The beta–gamma complex goes its separate way. The alpha subunit with its attached GTP is now able to interact with an 'effector' in the membrane, an enzyme such as adenylyl cyclase, perhaps, or phospholipase C-β (PLC-β) or an ion channel such as TRP or mAChR. The enzyme may be switched on or off, the ion channel up or down regulated. Again we shall look at specific examples in later chapters. But this interaction only lasts so long as the alpha subunit retains its GTP. But, as we noted above, the alpha subunit is in fact a GTPase. So, very soon, the GTP attached to the alpha subunit is hydrolysed to GDP. When this happens, the alpha subunit changes its conformation once again and can no longer activate the effector. Soon the alpha-GDP meets up with the beta–gamma dyad, forms once again the timeric complex and reattaches to the deactivated receptor, thus completing the cycle (Figure 1.9).

Until recently it was believed that the beta–gamma complex played no real part in membrane signalling. That assumption is now being questioned. There is evidence that the complex may have an independent role. It is possible that it is able to inhibit the activity of free alpha subunits, or it may have an independent effect on membrane effectors.

1.3.3 Effectors and Second Messengers

There are various classes of effector molecule: cyclase enzymes, phospholipases, phosphodiesterases, membrane channels. We shall meet instances of all these effectors in this book. Similarly, there are various types of second messenger: cAMP, cGMP, inositol triphosphate (IP_3 or $InsP_3$), diacylglycerol (DAG) and the ubiquitous Ca^{2+} ion. In this section we examine only two classes of effector, the adenylyl cyclases (ACs) and phospholipase C-β (=PIP_2-phospholipase) both of which engender important 'second messengers'. We shall consider the role of phosphodiesterases and membrane channels and the other second messengers as appropriate in later parts of this book.

1.3.3.1 Adenylyl Cyclases

These enzymes catalyse the formation of cAMP: a ubiquitous and, perhaps, the most important 'second messenger' in animal cells. In turn, the most important role of cAMP is to activate the cAMP-dependent protein kinase (PKA). Once activated this multimeric enzyme phosphorylates (with the help of ATP) one or other of the many biologically active proteins present in the cell - enzymes, receptor and channel proteins, nuclear histones, transcription factors. The phosphorylation is normally of a serine, threonine or tyrosine residue, and the effect is either to inhibit (note the desensitization of G-coupled receptors already mentioned above) or activate the protein. Dephosphorylation back to the original status is by one of the many phosphatase enzymes with which the cytosol abounds.

Molecular biological techniques have shown there to be at least six different adenylyl cyclases in mammalian cells. All have a molecular weight of about 120–130 kDa and examination of hydrophobic sequences indicates that there are twelve transmembrane segments. The six cyclases differ in their sensitivity to the beta–gamma complex of G-proteins and to the calcium binding protein, calmodulin. Type 1 AC is, for instance, stimulated by Ca^{2+} calmodulin and inhibited by the beta–gamma dimer whilst Type 2 AC does not respond to the first and is stimulated by the second.

1.3.3.2 Phospholipase C-β (=PLC-β or PIP₂-phospholipase)

The activation of this second important effector results in the production of two second messengers: inositol triphosphate (IP₃) and diacylglycerol (DAG). Both these second messengers are derived by the cleavage by PLC-β of the phospholipid, phosphatidyl-inositol 4,5 biphosphate (PIP₂), which is predominantly located in the inner leaflet of the plasma membrane (Figure 1.10).

Figure 1.10 shows a membrane receptor picking up some external signal that leads via a G-protein mechanism to the activation of membrane-embedded PLC-β. This then reacts with PIP₂ to produce IP₃ and DAG. IP₃ is a water soluble molecule and hence it readily diffuses away into the cytosol. Here it may interact with receptors in the membranes of the endoplasmic reticulum (ER) leading to a release of Ca^{2+}. These ions have many and varied effects on cellular biochemistry. Ultimately IP₃ is inactivated by inositol triphosphatase. DAG, on the other hand, is hydrophobic and hence remains behind in the membrane.

We have not finished with the system yet. For the DAG left behind also has a job to do. It interacts with other membrane-bound proteins. There are two important cases: protein C kinase (PKC) and the transient receptor protein (TRP). These reactions are Ca^{2+}-dependent. Consequently, when the Ca^{2+} concentration of the cytosol rises (an effect, as we have just seen, of IP₃) DAG activates PKC and/or TRP. In the case of PKC, the activation requires the presence of phosphatidyl serine as well. This phospholipid is also located in the membrane's inner leaflet. The aroused PKC can now activate proteins that elicit specific biochemical responses. In neurons a number of effects have been demonstrated, including synthesis and secretion of neurotransmitters, alterations to the sensitivity of receptors and the functioning of the cytoskeleton. We shall outline the affect of DAG on TRP in the next section.

It can be seen from the above account that G-protein systems provide an extremely flexible means of transforming an external signal into a second messenger which can diffuse into the cytosol. The second messenger may take a number of forms (depending on the effector enzyme) but by far the most common is cyclic AMP (cAMP). Alternatively, as noted above, the alpha subunit may affect the operation of a membrane channel and this in its turn may alter the electrical polarity of the membrane.

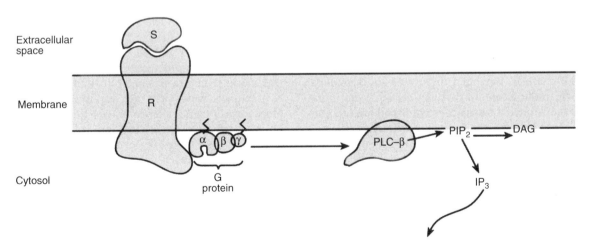

Figure 1.10 Second messenger formation via PLC-β. The activated receptor leads via the G-protein coupling system to activation of PLC-β. PLC-β catalyses the splitting of the membrane lipid PIP₂ into IP₃ and DAG. IP₃ diffuses into the cytosol; DAG remains in the membrane where it may exert further effects.

1.4 CHANNELS AND GATES

We saw above that biomembranes consist of proteins embedded in a lipid bilayer. The bilayer effectively prevents hydrophilic substances crossing the membrane. Embedded proteins act both as pumps and gated channels. We shall see in Chapter 2 that the pumps create a concentration gradient of small inorganic ions and hence a voltage gradient across the membrane. Other embedded proteins form hydrophilic channels through which inorganic ions and other water soluble materials can travel. Some of these channels, the so-called 'leak' channels, allow ions, such as potassium ions, to flow along their concentration gradients into or out of the cell; others play a more active role and act as gates controlling these flows. When these gates open, ions flow down their electrochemical gradients and the voltage across the membrane consequently drops. This change in voltage is known as **receptor potential** and in most cases is the first sign that an environmental change has been detected.

We shall meet many examples of these channels and gates in the following pages. There are several types: those directly affected by the environmental change, those activated by ligands (ligand-gated ion channels or *LGICs*) and those controlled by the voltage across the membrane (*VGICs*). The very large superfamily of TRP channels contains members which are responsive to all three types of stimuli.

1.4.1 TRP Channels

TRP channels were first discovered in *Drosophila,* where photoreceptors carrying certain gene mutations exhibited a **transient receptor potential** to continuous light, hence the acronym *TRP*. The channels responsible for this effect, the TRP channels, were isolated and their sequences analysed and used to search for similar channels in other organisms. It turns out that TRP channels are found throughout the living world, from Archaea to humans. Evolution has pressed them into many uses. In yeast TRP channels sense hypertonicity; in Nematode worms they sense noxious chemicals and touch; in mice they detect pheromones; in humans they are involved in sensing temperature, taste and are believed to play a crucial part in detecting sound These are just a

few of the rôles TRP channels play. We have already seen that they were first found playing a part in photoreception; they also have a fundamental rôle in mechanosensitivity. TRP channels are, moreover, not restricted to reacting to happenings in the external environment. They are deeply involved in responding to changes in the internal environment too. They are involved in detecting pH, osmolarity, vasodilation, growth cone guidance and numerous other aspects of the body's physiology.

Their very widespread distribution in the living world and the many uses to which they have been put indicates that they evolved very early in life's history. Indeed, they are believed to represent the most ancient of the cell's sensors. Metazoan TRPs have evolved into two major groups, Group 1 and Group 2 (Figure 1.11). Group 1 consists of five families (TRPC, TRPN, TRPM, TRPV and TRPA) while Group 2 consists of two families (TRPP and TRPML). Because their origin is so ancient and their common ancestor so far in the past, these families show rather little similarity in their amino acid sequence. That they are all members of the same superfamily of molecules is, however, shown by their sharing common tertiary and quaternary structures.

We have already noted that the tertiary structure involves six transmembrane domains (S1–S6) (Figure 1.12a). The so-called quaternary structure consists of four of these 6TM subunits, which may be similar or dissimilar, grouped around a central pore (Figure 1.12b). The architecture of this transmembrane pore is similar to that of the bacterial KcsA channel first worked out by MacKinnon and colleagues in *Streptomyces lividans*, and the total tetrameric structure is similar to that of the 6TM K^+-channels, which play such important roles in the biophysics of nerve cell membranes. Each of the subunits is orientated so that transmembrane segments S5 and S6 line the pore, forming a structure very much like an inverted wigwam, and between them provide a filter which selects cations, especially Ca^{2+} (Figure 1.12c).

It can be seen from Figure 1.12a that both N- and C-terminal ends of the polypeptide chain are located in the cytoplasm. These cytoplasmic domains are highly diverse and confer different properties on the different families. There is evidence (as yet not fully conclusive) that stretching forces in the membrane pull open the pore and that the selectivity filter

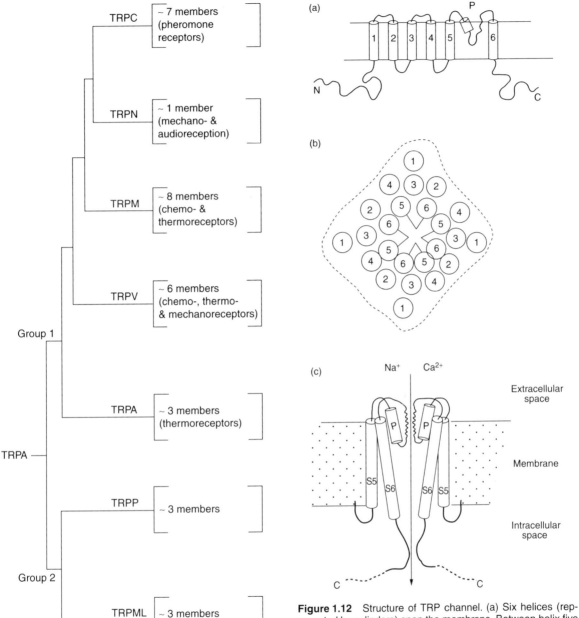

Figure 1.11 Schematic to show the evolutionary relationships of TRP channels. The number of members in each family as presently known is given and the involvement of the different TRP channels in sensory systems is indicated. Nomenclature: TRPA (ankyrin); TRPC (canonical); TRPM (melastatin), TRPML (mucolipin); TRPN (no mechanoreceptor potential C: NOMPC); TRPP (polycystin); TRPV (vanilloid)). Further explanation in text. Adapted from Venkatachalam and Montell (2007).

Figure 1.12 Structure of TRP channel. (a) Six helices (represented by cylinders) span the membrane. Between helix five and six there is a short helix followed by a series of amino acids (represented by zig-zag) which constitute the selectivity filter (P). (b) Plan view to show the disposition of the four subunits of the complete channel in the membrane. The pore (P) complex (represented by a 'hairpin') in each subunit faces inward to form the channel. (c) Detail of the channel. For simplicity only two of the subunits are shown and of these only the S5 and S6 transmembrane segments. The channel is a little over 5 Å in diameter and the selectivity filter consists of a group of amino acid residues represented by the 'saw-tooth' section between P and S6.

then ensures that Ca^{2+} and, to a lesser extent, Na^+ stream inward down their steep concentration gradients. This, as we shall see in Chapter 2, would depolarize the membrane (detectable as a receptor potential). Changes in ambient temperature also open TRP channels, although the biochemical mechanism is as yet not known. Thus TRP channels are directly involved in sensing **mechanical** and **thermal** stimuli.

Some TRP channels depend on 7TM receptors detecting other stimulus modalities – chemical or electromagnetic. Once a 7TM receptor is activated by an appropriate stimulus, a collision-coupling mechanism operates via PLC-β and DAG (as indicated in the previous section) to open TRP channels (Figure 1.10).

TRP channels are rapidly shut again by Ca^{2+}, which only exists in a free state for a few microseconds within the cytoplasm before being bound. Because TRP channels are responsive to many different types of stimuli, they are thought to play an integrative role in a cell's response to its environment. We shall meet TRP channels frequently in the following pages.

1.4.2 Ligand-Gated Ion Channels (LGICs)

There are many varieties of LGIC. The most intensively investigated is the nicotinic acetyl choline receptor (nAChR). This consists of a massive (268 kDa) pentameric protein embedded in the membrane. The five subunits consist of two (461 amino acid) α-subunits, one (493 amino-acid) β-subunit, one (506 amino acid) γ-subunit and one (522) δ-subunit. Each subunit makes four transmembrane passes (Figure 1.13a) and the five subunits are compactly assembled to surround a central ion pore (Figure 1.13b). When the ligand, in this case acetylcholine (ACh) attaches to binding sites on the two alpha subunits, the channel opens and univalent cations flow long their electrochemical gradients. Charged amino acids on TM2 (Figure 1.13) line the pore and select the ions that can pass through the channel.

Many other types of LGICs are known. These are activated by a variety of ligands (5HT, glycine, GABA, etc.) and all these major types are subdivided into numerous subtypes. So far as sensory systems are concerned, the most significant LGICs are those

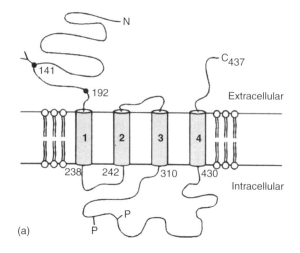

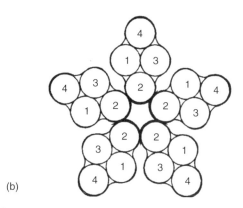

Figure 1.13 (a) Schematic view of the α-subunit of the nAChR. Four helices represented by cylinders span the membrane. Both C and N terminals are extracellular. (b) Plan view. The pentameric structure of the entire receptor is seen from above. It is believed that helix 2 of each subunit forms the lining of the pore.

found in olfactory and photoreceptor cells, which are activated by cyclic nucleotides (CNGs). They are similar to TRP channels and, like these channels, the subunit protein makes six passes through the membrane whilst the total channel consists of four of these subunits.

1.4.3 Voltage-Gated Ion Channels (VGICs)

There are also many types of VGIC. They are all activated by changes in membrane potential. They differ in the ion that they allow to pass. Thus there is

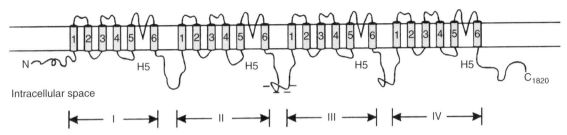

Figure 1.14 Schematic diagram of the disposition of the Na$^+$-channel protein in a membrane. The four domains are labelled I, II, III, IV. In life the four domains are clustered in the third dimension to form a huge protein with a central canal.

a large variety of voltage-sensitive K$^+$-channels and also various types of Cl$^-$, Ca^{2+} and Na$^+$ channel. In this section we shall confine ourselves to just one type of voltage-sensitive Na$^+$-channel. This is the channel that is responsible for the rising phase of the action potential and is thus the defining element of exciteable tissues such as nerve and striated muscle.

We shall see in the next chapter that the resting potential across most cell membranes is about 50 or 60 mV (inside negative to outside). This may not seem very much. It must be remembered, however, that biological membranes are very thin – no more than 6 or 7 nm. Hence the voltage drop is in fact very steep. A potential gradient of 60 mV in 6 nm works out as 10^5 V/cm. Voltage-sensitive proteins are very delicately poised in this intense electric field. Any change in the potential gradient will affect their conformation and thus the degree of opening or closure of any embedded ion channel.

The structure of the Na$^+$-channel has been the subject of intense research. It is nowadays well known. It is shown diagammatically in Figure 1.14. It consists of a single massive polypeptide (1820 amino acids) which, as the plan view in Figure 1.14 shows, consists of four successive domains. The domains are all homologous with each other and each has six membrane-spanning helices. The fourth helix (S4) in each domain contains a number of positively-charged amino acid residues (especially arginine and lysine) and it is consequently believed to form the 'voltage sensor' which is sensitive to any voltage change across the membrane. Between the fifth (S5) and sixth (S6) membrane-spanning helix in each domain the polypeptide chain is believed to form a 'hairpin' structure (H5) and to be inserted

into the membrane. When the protein forms up into its 3D form of a hollow cylinder, the hairpins line the pore and confer ion selectivity. Finally, the intracellular segment of polypeptide between homologous domains III and IV is responsible for inactivating the channel.

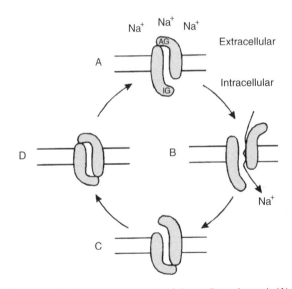

Figure 1.15 Conformation cycle of the sodium channel. (A) In the 'resting' membrane the sodium channel is closed. The activation gate (AG) is shut and the inactivation gate (IG) is open. (B) When the membrane is depolarized the voltage drop is sensed by a 'voltage sensor' and the activation gate opens. Sodium ions flow down their electrochemical gradient. They hop from one site in the channel to the next (as indicated) and hence proceed in single file. (C) After about 1 ms the inactivation gate closes. (D) As the membrane returns to its resting potential the activation gate closes and the inactivation gate reopens.

The physiology of the Na^+-channel has also been intensively studied. It can be shown that when the voltage across the membrane drops below some threshold value, the channel opens for about 1 ms and allows Na^+ ions carrying about 2 pA of current to pass. Once the 1 ms opening time has passed, the channel closes and will not open again while the membrane remains depolarized. This 'inactivation' is due, as we saw above, to the segment of polypeptide between domains III and IV blocking the channel. The channel protein thus exists in three major conformations: closed, open and inactivated. This cycle is shown in Figure 1.15.

The exact time of opening and closing of a channel is not strictly predictable: it is, in other words, stochastic. Furthermore, any patch of excitable membrane will have a large population of Na^+-channels and each individual channel will have a slightly different opening threshold. As an excitable membrane is depolarized more and more, Na^+-channels open. The influx of Na^+ ions depolarizes and ultimately repolarizes the membrane, a phenomenon which electrophysiologists record as the action potential. The biophysics of the action potential will be discussed in the next chapter (Section 2.6).

1.5 CONCLUDING REMARKS

In this chapter we have laid some of the groundwork. Biochemical detail has been deliberately omitted. Interested students should consult one or other of the many excellent texts on biochemistry and/or molecular biology. We shall see that the elements discussed above appear again and again at the core of the specialized and often highly elaborate sensory systems which have evolved in the animal kingdom. In particular we shall find that the biochemistry of biomembranes, receptors, G-protein systems and channels is linked to mechanisms controlling the electrical polarity of the membranes of sensory cells and endings. It is to this matter that we turn in the next chapter.

2

MEMBRANES, ACTION POTENTIALS, SYNAPSES

Ions and water: distribution across membranes. **Resting potentials (V_m)**: measurement - giant axons - the Nernst equation - the Goldman equation - examples. **Electrotonic potentials and cable conduction**: local circuits - electrotonic conduction - receptor potentials - generator potentials. **Sensory adaptation**: rapid and slow adaptation - biophysical causes. **Action potentials**: refractory period sets upper limit on frequency - myelination - rates of propagation - classes of axons. **Synapses** – outline of their biochemistry and molecular biology. **Concluding remarks**: ubiquity of molecular and biophysical elements - reductionism - mind-brain perplexity.

We saw in Chapter 1 that from the very beginning a lipid biomembrane demarcates the boundary between primordial cells and their environment. As contemporary eukaryocytes also contain many internal membranes (mitochondrial membranes, endoplasmic reticulum, lysosomes, etc.), it is useful to refer to the boundary membrane as the *plasma membrane*. We saw that protein elements of plasma membranes evolve to detect changes in the external environment and, in some cases, to signal those changes by a complex membrane-bound G-protein biochemistry. Plasma membranes also evolved means of controlling the movements of materials into and out of the cell. It will be remembered that the basis of all contemporary biomembranes is a lipid bilayer. Hydrophilic materials cannot (by definition) diffuse through the hydrophobic barrier of a lipid bilayer. This is no place to review the many mechanisms that have evolved to circumvent this difficulty but one such mechanism must be considered in some detail.

This is the mechanism (or rather group of mechanisms) which controls the movement of small inorganic ions across the membrane.

Inorganic ions are, of course, water soluble. Their electrostatic charges allow them to enter and mix with the water structure (Figure 2.1). On the other hand, they prevent them mixing with an organic phase such as that represented by a lipid bilayer. In order to pass through a biomembrane, hydrophilic 'pores' have to be present. Numerous such pores have evolved since the first prokaryocytes appeared three and half billion years ago. In all cases they are complex protein structures embedded in the membrane. As we shall see in later chapters, these channels are many and various. In general they are very specific, very choosy, about which ions they will select and allow to pass through.

The very fact that ions are charged particles means that their distribution across a membrane may bring with it electrical consequences. It has been known

Biology of Sensory Systems, Second Edition   C.U.M. Smith
© 2008 John Wiley & Sons, Ltd

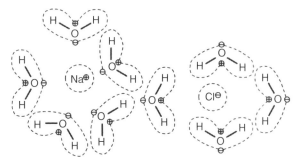

Figure 2.1 Ions in the water structure. Water molecules are electrically polarized. Because oxygen attracts hydrogen's electron, a fractional negative charge is associated with its end of the molecule. An equal and opposite fractional positive charge is associated with the other end. Hence, water molecules tend to cluster around positively and negatively charged ions such as Cl^- and Na^+ and keep them apart and thus in solution.

since the times of Galvani and Volta in the late eighteenth century that the functioning of nervous systems is associated with electrical phenomena. It was not, however, until the mid-twentieth century when the development of electrotechnology (especially electronics) was coupled with the recognition and use of appropriate biological preparations (giant axons) that a genuine understanding of 'animal electricity' was achieved.

In this chapter we shall look first at the origin of 'resting potentials' (V_m), which exist across all plasma membranes, and show how these change when a receptor cell is stimulated to give rise to so-called 'receptor potentials'. We shall then consider the passive flows of electrical current, the so-called 'cable' or 'electrotonic' conduction, which occur within cells and play an important role in all sensory and neurosensory cells. Finally, after a brief consideration of **receptor** and **generator potentials** and the nature of **sensory adaptation**, we shall end with a short account of **action potentials** and **synaptic transmission**.

2.1 THE MEASUREMENT OF RESTING POTENTIALS

It was stated above that resting potentials develop across all plasma membranes. Most cells, especially

neurons and sensory cells, are extremely small. Although methods have nowadays been developed to investigate their electrical characteristics, it was for a long time impossible to obtain reliable measurements. The recognition that certain large tubular (diameter 500–600 mm) structures in the squid, *Loligo*, were in fact giant axons was thus of enormous value to electrophysiologists. They were at last able to insert fine glass micropipettes filled with an electrolyte inside an axon and measure the electrical polarity of the membrane directly (Figure 2.2). They were also able to squeeze out the axoplasm (rather like toothpaste out of a toothpaste tube) and subject it to chemical analysis (Table 2.1). Most of the pioneering work which established the physical basis of the resting and action potentials was done on this convenient preparation.

Using a set up similar to that shown in Figure 2.2, it is found that the internal electrode records a voltage drop of some 50 mV across the membrane. This is defined as the resting potential, V_m. What causes this potential difference across the membrane?

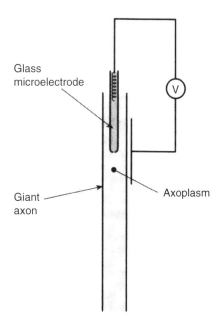

Figure 2.2 The diagram shows a glass microelectrode (filled with a potassium chloride solution) inserted into a giant axon. The circuit continues through a voltmeter to a plate electrode on the external surface of the axon.

Table 2.1 Ionic concentrations inside and outside some relevant cells

Ion	Intracellular concentration	Extracellular concentration
1. Squid giant axon		
	(mM/kg H_2O)	(mM/kg H_2O)
K^+	400	20
Na^+	50	440
Ca^{2+}	0.4	10
Mg^{2+}	10	54
Cl^-	100	560
Organic anions	$\cong 385$	—
2. Mammalian muscle cell		
	(mM)	(mM)
K^+	155	4
Na^+	12	145
Mg^{2+}	30	1–2
Ca^{2+}	1–2	2.5–5 (Only about 10^{-4} is free)
Cl^-	4	120
Organic anions	$\cong 150$	—
3. Cat motor neuron		
	(mM)	(mM)
K^+	150	5.5
Na^+	15	150
Cl^-	9	125

2.2 THE IONIC BASES OF RESTING POTENTIALS

We have just noted that the ionic constitution of the axoplasm can be determined (Table 2.1). There are important equations in physical chemistry which relate the electrical potential across a membrane to the distribution of the permeable ions across that membrane. The most well-known of these equations is the **Nernst equation**. It can be written as follows:

$$V_I = \frac{RT}{Z_I F} \quad \ln \frac{[I]_o}{[I]_i}. \qquad (2.1)$$

In Equation (2.1), V_I is the voltage across the membrane (in volts, though normally expressed in millivolts) due to the distribution of the ion, I; R is the gas constant; T the temperature in Kelvins; F

the Faraday (the quantity of electrical charge carried by one mole of univalent ions); Z_I is the valency of the ion under consideration ($+1$ for Na^+ and K^+; -1 for Cl^-); ln is $\log_e$; $[I]_o$ and $[I]_i$ the concentration of the ion, I, outside and inside the membrane. It is important to note that one of the premises from which the Nernst equation has been derived is that the membrane is fully permeable to the ion under consideration. If this condition holds, then if we know the equilibrium concentrations of the ion across the membrane, the equation will predict the countervailing electrical potential.

Let us test the equation by substituting some values for the K^+ concentration on both sides of the membrane. If we suppose, first of all, that the K^+ concentrations equal each other on both sides of the membrane, then substitution in the Nernst equation results in the logarithmic term becoming unity. As the log of 1 is zero, it follows that the equation predicts zero potential across the membrane. This, of course, is what is observed. When a cell dies, its membrane loses its integrity and its pumping mechanisms disappear. Ions flow along their concentration gradients until their concentrations become equal on each side of the membrane. The potential across the membrane vanishes.

Next let us test the equation by substituting the values for $[K^+]_o$ (i.e. 5.5 mM) and $[K^+]_i$ (i.e. 150 mM) shown in Table 2.1. Then:

$$V_K = \frac{RT}{Z_I F} \ln \frac{5.5}{150}$$
$$= 0.027 \ln 0.036$$
$$= -0.089 \text{ V}$$
$$\text{or} = -89 \text{ mV}$$

This is known as the **Nernst potassium potential**, V_K, or (alternatively) as the **potassium reversal potential**. The concept behind the latter term is that when the membrane has this potential gradient across it, no further net flow of K^+ ions occurs across it. Measurement of the actual resting potential, V_m, across cell membranes normally gives values of between -50 mV and -75 mV. V_K is evidently larger than this, but still of the right sign and order of magnitude. If, however, values for the concentration of the other significant ions (Cl^-, Na^+, etc.) are substituted in the Nernst equation, the predicted values

(V_{Cl}, V_{Na}, etc.) are very far from the observed V_m. This is especially the case when values for Na^+ are inserted.

The reasons for this failure are not difficult to find. Cell membranes are very complex structures. Their permeability to different ions varies dramatically and, as we noted above, the Nernst equation only works for ions for which the membrane is fully permeable. It is known, however, that both sodium and chloride ions have very low permeability coefficients in resting biomembranes.

Furthermore, and importantly, V_m does not depend on the transmembrane distribution of single ion species but on the distribution of whole 'teams' of ions. Thus, to gain a fuller understanding of the origins of resting potentials, we have to generalize the Nernst equation. We must derive an equation which takes into account the different permeability of the membrane to different ions and the fact that not just one ion species is in play but many.

The equation we need was developed by David Goldman and is consequently known as the Goldman equation. The equation is also sometimes known as the 'constant field equation', as it assumes that the electric field across the membrane (the electrical potential gradient, V_m) is unchanging. This, of course, is a large assumption to make. Nevertheless, the Goldman equation provides a useful first approximation to the biophysical situation. It is written as follows:

$$V = \frac{RT}{F} \ln \frac{P_K[K^+]_o + P_{Na}[Na^+]_o + P_{Cl}[Cl^-]_i}{P_K[K^+]_i + P_{Na}[Na^+]_i + P_{Cl}[Cl^-]_o},$$
(2.2)

where 'P' is the permeability constant of the ion, square brackets indicate (as usual) the concentration of the ion either inside (subscript 'i') or out (subscript 'o'), and R, T and F have their usual connotations.

Note that, whereas the external concentrations of the cations, K^+ and Na^+ are placed in the numerator of the equation, the external concentration of the anion, Cl^-, is placed in the denominator.

Let us try some test runs. First, if we make the permeability constants of Na^+ and Cl^- equal to zero (i.e. the membrane is completely impermeable to these ions) the equation reduces to the Nernst equation for potassium. Similarly, if we make $P_K = P_{Cl} = 0$ the equation reduces to the Nernst equation for Na^+ and predicts V_{Na} as the potential across the membrane (the Na^+ permeability terms cancelling out).

Now, as we observed at the beginning of this chapter, the lipid bilayer of plasma membranes is completely impermeable to inorganic ions. Their movement through the membrane is via a variety of channels constructed from membrane proteins. Many of these channels, the so-called 'leak' channels, are not well characterized. The permeability of plasma membranes to hydrophilic ions depends on these channels. How much these channels leak varies, moreover, form cell to cell. Neuroglial cells, for instance, seem to be much more permeable to K^+ than are neurons.

Most sensory cells, however, resemble neurons in being more permeable to K^+ than Cl^- or Na^+; that is $P_K \gg P_{Cl}, P_{Na}$. We can put some figures to these relative permeabilities from measurements of the flow of radiolabelled ions across plasma membranes:

$$P_K = 10^{-7}\,cm/s$$
$$P_{Cl} = 10^{-8}\,cm/s\,.$$
$$P_{Na} = 10^{-8}\,cm/s$$

Let us insert these permeability constants and the appropriate ionic concentrations (Table 2.1: cat motor neuron) into the Goldman equation:

$$V_m = 0.027 \ln \frac{(1 \times 10^{-7}\,[5.5]) + (1 \times 10^{-8}\,[150]) + (1 \times 10^{-8}\,[9])}{(1 \times 10^{-7}\,[150]) + (1 \times 10^{-8}\,[15]) + (1 \times 10^{-8}\,[125])}$$

$$= 0.027 \ln \frac{(55 \times 10^{-8} + 150 \times 10^{-8}) + (9 \times 10^{-8})}{(1500 \times 10^{-8}) + (15 \times 10^{-8}) + (125 \times 10^{-8})}$$

$$= -0.055\,V$$

$$= -55\,mV$$

This value for V_m is in fact very close to the value for the resting potential across cat motor neurons actually observed by microelectrode recording.

Next, let us see what happens if we increase the potassium permeability by an order of magnitude. If we insert $P_K = 1 \times 10^{-6}$ cm/s into the equation, keeping all the other permeability constants unchanged we find:

$$V_m = -83\,mV.$$

We have already remarked that the membranes of some glial cells are markedly more permeable to K^+ than the membranes of neurons. Hence we find that the V_m across these membranes is characteristically greater than the customary resting potential of neuronal membranes. In the retina (as we shall see in Chapter 17) large glial cells, known as Müller cells, have V_ms ranging from -70 to $-90\,\mathrm{mV}$. This larger than usual K^+ permeability is believed to be of considerable importance in mopping up excess K^+ generated in the nervous part of the retina in response to illumination. This excess K^+ is then discharged into the vitreous humour. Vice versa, if we increase the Na^+ permeability constant in the Goldman equation, a significant decrease in V_m is predicted. We shall find a very important instance of this when we come to consider the biophysics of retinal rod cells in Chapter 17.

Before completing this section it is worth noting that, as it is much easier to measure the relative rather than the absolute permeabilities of ions, the Goldman equation is often written in a slightly different form:

$$V = \frac{RT}{F} \ln \frac{[K]_o + b[Na]_o + c[Cl]_i}{[K]_i + b[Na]_i + c[Cl]_o}, \qquad (2.3)$$

where

$$b = P_{Na}/P_K,$$

and

$$c = P_{Cl}/P_K.$$

As the chloride ion plays only a minor part in many neurophysiological functions, the equation is sometimes simplified even further:

$$V = \frac{RT}{F} \ln \frac{[K]_o + b[Na]_i}{[K]_i + b[Na]_i}. \qquad (2.4)$$

We shall see, however, that although the chloride ion is unimportant in many areas of neurophysiology, it nevertheless plays a crucial role in hyperpolarizations such as those of inhibitory synapses and elsewhere. It is important to use the full form of

Goldman's equation in these and similar circumstances.

2.3 ELECTROTONIC POTENTIALS AND CABLE CONDUCTION

Consider Figure 2.3. A nonexcitable membrane is slightly depolarized. It has to be emphasized that the membrane we are considering is nonexciteable, so we are in no danger of initiating an action potential. Nevertheless, we are setting up the conditions for tiny so-called 'local circuits' to occur. The interior of the cell is in essence an ionic solution, as is the extracellular fluid. It follows that it can conduct electric currents. If we depolarize the boundary membrane at point 'x', we set up a voltage difference between it and the membrane a small distance away, at point 'y'. These distances are, of course, minute: seldom more than a micron or so. But tiny electric currents will flow between 'x' and 'y' until the voltage difference is eliminated. Hence the membrane at 'y' will be slightly depolarized. These minute potentials are known as **electrotonic potentials** and the local circuits are referred to as **electrotonic** or 'cable' **conduction**.

Electrotonic potentials are at least one order of magnitude and sometimes two or more orders of magnitude weaker than action potentials.

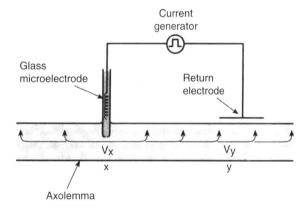

Figure 2.3 Electrotonic conduction. Current is injected at x to induce a voltage across the membrane of V_x. The return electrode at y measures the electrotonic potential V_y. The local circuits are represented by arrows. To retain simplicity the return current in the external solution is omitted.

Nonetheless, however small electrotonic potentials may be, they can have very considerable effect. To see that this is the case we need only recall the exquisite voltage sensitivity of voltage-gated ion channels such as the Na^+-channel discussed in Chapter 1. If local circuits spreading from a region where the membrane is depolarized should encounter a patch of membrane populated by Na^+-channels, the resulting depolarization may trigger an action potential which, propagated to the brain, may have incalculable consequences.

2.4 RECEPTOR AND GENERATOR POTENTIALS

Receptor and generator potentials are special cases of electrotonic potentials. When a receptor (= sensory) cell, such as a mechanoreceptive hair cell or a gustatory cell, is stimulated by an appropriate stimulus, a more or less complex set of events (we shall discuss them in detail in subsequent chapters) leads to change in the electrical polarity of a patch of its membrane. This is called a **receptor potential**. In most cases receptor potentials (as in the cases discussed in Section 2.3 above) are depolarizations. In some cases, however, notably in chordate retinal rod and cone cells, they are hyperpolarizations. But whether depolarizations or hyperpolarizations, the outcome is the same: local circuits are set up between the patch of membrane affected and other parts of the receptor cell's membrane (Figure 2.4). In the general case the change in electrical polarity (whether up or down) will influence the release of transmitter substance onto an underlying sensory neuron.

Not all sensory systems develop specialized sensory cells. Olfactory and some mechanoreceptive systems use neurosensory cells. In these instances the functions of detecting the appropriate environmental factor and conducting information to the brain are combined in one cell (Figure 2.5). The biophysical events are, however, analogous to those just described. When the sensitive ending of the neurosensory cell is stimulated, a more or less complex biochemistry leads to a change in its electrical potential. In the case of neurosensory cells this is always a depolarization. This depolarization spreads by a local circuit mechanism until it reaches a region of the membrane populated by voltage-sensitive Na^+-

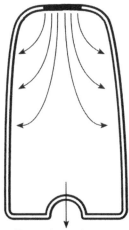

Transmitter substance

Figure 2.4 Figure showing local circuits spreading away from a depolarized patch of membrane (dark) on a receptor cell. In the general case this will lead to a depolarization of the cell and this, through a complex biochemical process, to the release of transmitter substance.

channels. If the depolarization is great enough the Na^+-channels are opened and an action potential is initiated which then propagates without decrement to the central nervous system. Because the initial depolarization does not occur in a separate receptor cell, it is often called a **generator potential**. Other scientists, however, refer to both cases as receptor potentials.

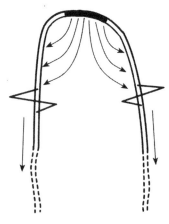

Figure 2.5 Depolarization of the ending of a neurosensory cell leads to local circuits which initiate action potentials.

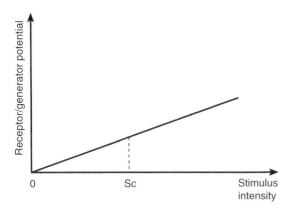

Figure 2.6 Stimulus intensity vs. receptor/generator potential. The graph shows the initial response to stimuli of different intensity. As indicated in the text, adaptation will generally occur and lower the magnitude of the receptor/generator potential if the stimulus is left on. Sc = critical intensity.

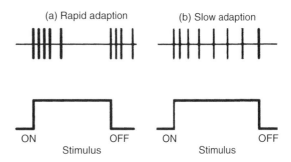

Figure 2.7 Sensory adaptation. (a) Rapidly adapting fibre. (b) Slowly adapting fibre.

The magnitude of generator and receptor potentials depends on the magnitude of the stimulus. Indeed, there is an approximately straight-line relationship between these potentials and stimulus intensity (Figure 2.6). Because of the necessity for the local circuits set up to be of sufficient magnitude to either trigger the release of transmitter (Figure 2.4) or to bring at least some of a population of voltage-sensitive Na^+-channels below threshold, the initiation of action potentials in a sensory nerve only occurs when the receptor/generator potential has reached a 'critical' magnitude (S_c in Figure 2.6).

2.5 SENSORY ADAPTATION

All sensory systems show adaptation. This means that the response (whatever it is) to a constant stimulus falls off over time. In metazoan systems it is the impulse frequency in a sensory nerve fibre which falls off with time. In these systems there are several different forms of adaptation. Two extremes are customarily identified: rapidly adapting and slowly adapting (Figure 2.7). In the first case there is a rapid burst of activity in the sensory fibre when the stimulus is turned on, which then quickly falls back toward zero until the stimulus is turned off. This is marked by another rapid burst of activity. In the second case there is once again a rapid burst of activity when the stimulus is turned on and, although this declines over

time, it never declines to zero. It remains at a 'plateau' until the stimulus is turned off, when it falls back to ground level. In both cases it is the frequency of the initial burst of impulses which signals the intensity of the stimulus.

The biophysical causes of sensory adaptation are many and various. We shall meet with many instances in the following pages. In some cases of bacterial chemosensitivity it is, for instance, due to methylation of 'receptor transducer' proteins. In many animal systems where receptor molecules are linked to G-protein systems it is partly due to inactivation of the receptor molecules by phosphorylation (Section 1.3.2). The presence Ca^{2+}-channels and calcium-dependent K^+-channels (K_{Ca}) amongst the Na^+-channels, where action potentials are initiated in sensory nerve endings, is also highly significant. When the membrane depolarizes in response to local circuits from the stimulated ending, the voltage-dependent Ca^{2+}-channels open and Ca^{2+} cascades down its concentration gradient into the neuron. The increased internal Ca^{2+} concentration opens the Ca^{2+}-dependent K^+-channels and excessive quantities of K^+ flow out of the neuron down its concentration gradient. In other words, the membrane becomes unusually permeable to K^+. If an increased permeability constant for K^+ is inserted into the Goldman equation, it will be seen that the equation predicts a hyperpolarization. In this condition it becomes much more difficult for the local circuits to open the voltage-dependent Na^+-gates and initiate an action potential. Hence the rate of impulse initiation is slowed. Hence sensory adaptation. This sequence of events is shown diagramatically in Figure 2.8.

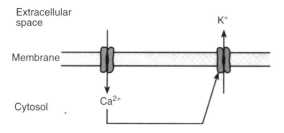

Figure 2.8 One mechanism which causes adaptation at sensory endings. Depolarization opens Ca^{2+}-gates; Ca^{2+} flows inwards and affects Ca^{2+}-dependent K^+-channels, leading to a countervailing increase in membrane polarity and a consequent decrease in the probability of impulse initiation.

The biophysical and molecular biological situation at the terminals of animal sensory fibres is undoubtedly highly complex. The preceding paragraph just scratches the surface. We shall encounter specific instances in later chapters.

2.6 ACTION POTENTIALS

This is not the place to develop a full account of the biophysics of action potentials. That is more properly done in texts of neurophysiology. However, as the output from animal sense organs is transmitted to the analytical apparatus of the central nervous system as action potentials in sensory nerve fibres, it will be sensible to give a bare outline here.

We noted above (and in Chapter 1) that when the membrane surrounding a population of Na^+-channel proteins is depolarized, the channels with the lowest thresholds begin to open and Na^+ begins to stream down its concentration gradient into the axon. This process has a positive feedback effect. As Na^+ streams inward the membrane becomes yet more depolarized and this opens neighbouring Na^+-channels with higher thresholds. More Na^+ flows in and the membrane depolarizes yet further and so on. The membrane reaches zero potential and then polarizes in the other sense (negative outside, positive within) until the Nernst Na^+ potential (V_{Na}) is approached. Because of the positive feedback effect the reversal of polarity happens very rapidly. In most cases V_{Na} is reached in about 0.5 ms. The Na^+-gates then begin to close.

Very soon after the Na^+-channels open, <0.5 ms, another set of gates, K^+-gates, begin to open, This allows K^+ to escape from inside the axon and, as the Na^+-gates close, the membrane returns to its original polarity, indeed somewhat overshoots that polarity and approaches the Nernst K^+ potential, V_K. The activity of the ATP-driven $Na^+ + K^+$ pump in the membrane now returns the membrane to its normal resting potential (V_m). These ionic events and the resulting changes in membrane polarity are shown in Figure 2.9.

This is all very well and good but the whole essence of the action potential, or nerve impulse, lies in its propagation. How is this dramatic change in membrane polarity propagated? Once again the answer lies in the action of local circuits. We saw in Section 2.3 that depolarization of a small section of membrane leads to tiny electrical circuits spreading away from that section to depolarize other parts of the membrane a small distance away. This is also the case, *a fortiori*, when the membrane dramatically reverses its polarity in an action potential. But, of course, these local circuits will, in depolarising other segments of membrane, open Na^+-channels in those segments and trigger the sequence of events responsible for the action potential described above. It has sometimes been said that the action potential may be likened to a flame shooting down a gunpowder trail. Each activated part triggers the next and leaves a trail of ash behind it. In the case of the nerve fibre the inactivation represented by the gunpowder ash represents the fact that the membrane is hyperpolarized behind the action potential (Figure 2.9). The analogy only works up to a point. For, unlike the inert gunpowder ash, the nerve fibre membrane quickly regains its original polarity by way of the $Na^+ + K^+$ pump. But it is important to note that this regenerative process takes time. The Na^+-gates remain closed, inactivated, for about 1.5 ms after their voltage-induced opening. The membrane is consequently said to be **refractory**.

This **refractory period** of about 1.5 to 2 ms is of considerable importance in sensory signalling. It restricts the frequency at which impulses can travel down a sensory nerve fibre. A refractory period of 2 ms means that, at the limit, a sensory fibre can only carry impulses at 500 Hz. This has significant implications for the detection of sound frequency and frequency discrimination by ears (Chapter 9).

Whilst the refractory period limits the frequency with which impulses can be conducted along a nerve

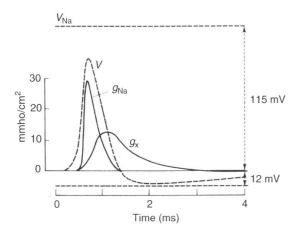

(a)

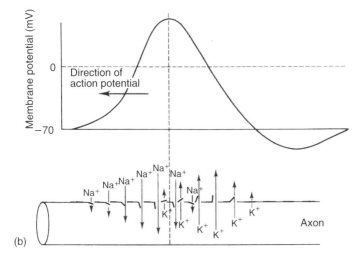

(b)

Figure 2.9 Principal ion channels and conductances responsible for action potentials. (a) Na^+ and K^+ conductances are shown by the curves labelled g_{Na} and g_K (the left-hand ordinate gives values in mmho/cm²). The dashed line shows the voltage across the membrane due to these conductances. The horizontal dashed lines at top and bottom of the figure represent V_{Na} and V_K respectively. From Hodgkin and Huxley (1952), *Journal of Physiology*, **117**, 500–544; reproduced by permission of the Physiological Society. (b) The time base of (a) has been greatly expanded. The upper part of the figure should be compared with the dashed line of (a). The lower part of the figure shows the flows of Na^+ and K^+. These flows, in turn, are due to the opening and closing of Na^+ and K^+-channels in the axonal membrane.

fibre, its diameter (other things being equal) determines rate of propagation (Table 2.2). This is because, as the diameter increases, local circuits can spread further along the axoplasm and hence open Na^+-gates further from the already active region. Hence in many invertebrates, annelid worms, for example, and cephalopod molluscs in particular, giant fibres are developed to allow the rapid conduction required for emergency reactions. The vertebrates, however, have evolved a different mechanism for increasing velocity of conduction: **myelination**.

Myelin consists of layers of Schwann cell membranes closely wrapped around an axon. These membranes provide a very effective electrical insulation. This prevents the internal elements of the local circuits leaking out of the axoplasm and hence, confined

within the fibre, they spread further. Action potentials consequently jump from one node of Ranvier to the next—a process known as 'saltatory' conduction. Invertebrates have not developed this particular and very effective means of increasing the rate of impulse conduction. However, we shall see, when we come to consider the operation of some insect sensilla in Chapter 13, that an alternative means of confining local circuits has been devised to ensure effective electrotonic conduction down the long outer segments of their gustatory cells.

The velocity of impulse propagation in mammalian **afferent** fibres is shown in Table 2.2. The afferent fibres from muscles consist of four overlapping classes (I–IV), whose conduction velocity ranges from about 120 m/s in the largest myelinated

.2 Some characteristics of mammalian afferent fibres

	Muscle afferent fibre	Cutaneous nerve afferent fibre	Fibre diameter (µm)	Conduction velocity (m/s)
Myelinated				
Large	I		13–20	80–120
Small	II	Aβ	6–12	35–75
Smallest	III	Aδ	1–5	5–30
Unmyelinated	IV	C	0.2–1.5	0.5–2

After Kandel *et al.* (1991).

fibres (circa 20 mm diameter) to about 0.5 m/s in the smallest unmyelinated fibres (circa 0.5 mm in diameter). Sensory nerves from the skin lack large high velocity class I (or Aα) fibres. Cutaneous nerve fibres are thus classified into three groups Aβ, Aδ and C, which correspond to class II, III and IV muscle afferents.

2.7 SYNAPSES AND SYNAPTIC TRANSMISSION

Synapses are many and various. They vary in size, position, molecular biology, pharmacology and biochemistry. Some operate directly by electrical transmission: an action potential in the presynaptic terminal directly exciting an action potential in the underlying postsynaptic cell. These are known as '*electrical*' synapses and we shall meet several instances in subsequent pages. Others, much more common in vertebrate nervous systems, are '*chemical*' synapses, where transmitter substances (neurotransmitters and neuromodulators) are released from a presynaptic terminal to diffuse across a synaptic gap to affect an underlying postsynaptic cell. Transmitter substances are themselves many and various: some excite the postsynaptic cell, others inhibit it, yet others act as modulators controlling its excitability or affecting the action of neurotransmitters. Some neurotransmitters or modulators, moreover, diffuse into the intercellular space and exert their effects some distance away, a process known as volume transmission. Finally, many neurotransmitters act back onto the presynaptic terminal in a positive or (more usually) negative feedback fashion to affect the release of further transmitters. We shall meet many of these

varieties later in this book. To grasp the basic nature of synaptic transmission, let us focus on an idealized chemical synapse (Figure 2.10).

Figure 2.10 shows that the biochemistry and molecular biology of synaptic transmission is extremely complex. It is as yet only imperfectly understood. Here only the briefest outline is appropriate. The whole process is initiated by the arrival of an action potential at the synaptic terminal (step 1). The depolarization of the presynaptic membrane opens Ca^{2+}-channels allowing Ca^{2+} to cascade into the terminal (step 2). The increased Ca^{2+} concentration causes the release of synaptic vesicles from their anchorages within the terminal. They are then free to migrate towards the presynaptic membrane (step 3). The increased Ca^{2+} concentration also helps to trigger the fusion of the vesicle membrane to the interior of this membrane (step 3). Other vesicles are already 'docked' on the presynaptic membrane. It has been shown that Ca^{2+}-channels are also present in their near vicinity (at a distance of about 20 nm). The influx of Ca^{2+} sets in train a very complex series of biochemical events involving whole teams of proteins, which leads to a complete fusion of the synaptic vesicle membrane with the presynaptic membrane (step 4). Once the two membranes are fused, a small 'fusion pore' develops between the interior of the vesicle and the synaptic cleft and this widens to allow the entire vesicle to open and void its contents (step 5). The remaining membrane of the vesicle mixes intimately with the presynaptic membrane (step 6) but, ultimately, small pits appear leading to an invagination of the 'mixed' membrane (step 7). The invaginated membrane is nipped off to form a vesicle and recycles to the interior of the terminal where it is refilled with transmitter substance (step 11). In the meantime

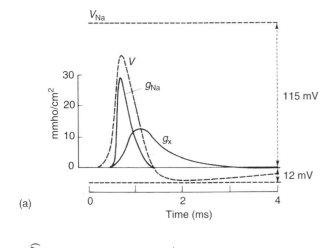

(a)

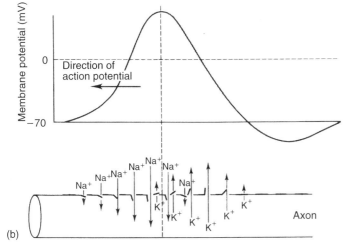

(b)

Figure 2.9 Principal ion channels and conductances responsible for action potentials. (a) Na$^+$ and K$^+$ conductances are shown by the curves labelled g_{Na} and g_K (the left-hand ordinate gives values in mmho/cm^2). The dashed line shows the voltage across the membrane due to these conductances. The horizontal dashed lines at top and bottom of the figure represent V_{Na} and V_K respectively. From Hodgkin and Huxley (1952), *Journal of Physiology*, **117**, 500–544; reproduced by permission of the Physiological Society. (b) The time base of (a) has been greatly expanded. The upper part of the figure should be compared with the dashed line of (a). The lower part of the figure shows the flows of Na$^+$ and K$^+$. These flows, in turn, are due to the opening and closing of Na$^+$ and K$^+$-channels in the axonal membrane.

fibre, its diameter (other things being equal) determines rate of propagation (Table 2.2). This is because, as the diameter increases, local circuits can spread further along the axoplasm and hence open Na$^+$-gates further from the already active region. Hence in many invertebrates, annelid worms, for example, and cephalopod molluscs in particular, giant fibres are developed to allow the rapid conduction required for emergency reactions. The vertebrates, however, have evolved a different mechanism for increasing velocity of conduction: **myelination**.

Myelin consists of layers of Schwann cell membranes closely wrapped around an axon. These membranes provide a very effective electrical insulation. This prevents the internal elements of the local circuits leaking out of the axoplasm and hence, confined

within the fibre, they spread further. Action potentials consequently jump from one node of Ranvier to the next—a process known as 'saltatory' conduction. Invertebrates have not developed this particular and very effective means of increasing the rate of impulse conduction. However, we shall see, when we come to consider the operation of some insect sensilla in Chapter 13, that an alternative means of confining local circuits has been devised to ensure effective electrotonic conduction down the long outer segments of their gustatory cells.

The velocity of impulse propagation in mammalian **afferent** fibres is shown in Table 2.2. The afferent fibres from muscles consist of four overlapping classes (I–IV), whose conduction velocity ranges from about 120 m/s in the largest myelinated

Table 2.2   Some characteristics of mammalian afferent fibres

	Muscle afferent fibre	Cutaneous nerve afferent fibre	Fibre diameter (μm)	Conduction velocity (m/s)
Myelinated				
Large	I		13–20	80–120
Small	II	Aβ	6–12	35–75
Smallest	III	Aδ	1–5	5–30
Unmyelinated	IV	C	0.2–1.5	0.5–2

After Kandel *et al.* (1991).

fibres (circa 20 mm diameter) to about 0.5 m/s in the smallest unmyelinated fibres (circa 0.5 mm in diameter). Sensory nerves from the skin lack large high velocity class I (or Aα) fibres. Cutaneous nerve fibres are thus classified into three groups Aβ, Aδ and C, which correspond to class II, III and IV muscle afferents.

2.7 SYNAPSES AND SYNAPTIC TRANSMISSION

Synapses are many and various. They vary in size, position, molecular biology, pharmacology and biochemistry. Some operate directly by electrical transmission: an action potential in the presynaptic terminal directly exciting an action potential in the underlying postsynaptic cell. These are known as '*electrical*' synapses and we shall meet several instances in subsequent pages. Others, much more common in vertebrate nervous systems, are '*chemical*' synapses, where transmitter substances (neurotransmitters and neuromodulators) are released from a presynaptic terminal to diffuse across a synaptic gap to affect an underlying postsynaptic cell. Transmitter substances are themselves many and various: some excite the postsynaptic cell, others inhibit it, yet others act as modulators controlling its excitability or affecting the action of neurotransmitters. Some neurotransmitters or modulators, moreover, diffuse into the intercellular space and exert their effects some distance away, a process known as volume transmission. Finally, many neurotransmitters act back onto the presynaptic terminal in a positive or (more usually) negative feedback fashion to affect the release of further transmitters. We shall meet many of these

varieties later in this book. To grasp the basic nature of synaptic transmission, let us focus on an idealized chemical synapse (Figure 2.10).

Figure 2.10 shows that the biochemistry and molecular biology of synaptic transmission is extremely complex. It is as yet only imperfectly understood. Here only the briefest outline is appropriate. The whole process is initiated by the arrival of an action potential at the synaptic terminal (step 1). The depolarization of the presynaptic membrane opens Ca^{2+}-channels allowing Ca^{2+} to cascade into the terminal (step 2). The increased Ca^{2+} concentration causes the release of synaptic vesicles from their anchorages within the terminal. They are then free to migrate towards the presynaptic membrane (step 3). The increased Ca^{2+} concentration also helps to trigger the fusion of the vesicle membrane to the interior of this membrane (step 3). Other vesicles are already 'docked' on the presynaptic membrane. It has been shown that Ca^{2+}-channels are also present in their near vicinity (at a distance of about 20 nm). The influx of Ca^{2+} sets in train a very complex series of biochemical events involving whole teams of proteins, which leads to a complete fusion of the synaptic vesicle membrane with the presynaptic membrane (step 4). Once the two membranes are fused, a small 'fusion pore' develops between the interior of the vesicle and the synaptic cleft and this widens to allow the entire vesicle to open and void its contents (step 5). The remaining membrane of the vesicle mixes intimately with the presynaptic membrane (step 6) but, ultimately, small pits appear leading to an invagination of the 'mixed' membrane (step 7). The invaginated membrane is nipped off to form a vesicle and recycles to the interior of the terminal where it is refilled with transmitter substance (step 11). In the meantime

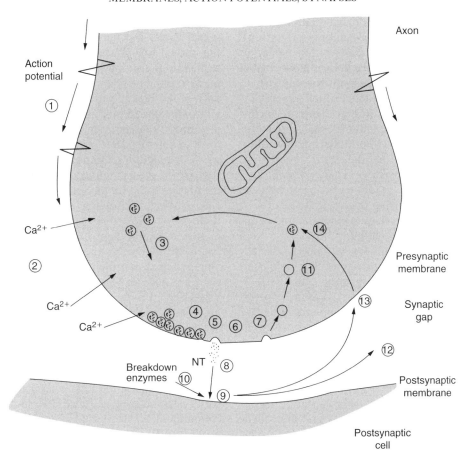

Figure 2.10   Schematic showing the molecular physiology of a 'chemical' synapse. Explanation in text.

the transmitter released into the cleft rapidly diffuses (step 8) across the synaptic gap or cleft to the post-synaptic membrane where precisely tailored receptor molecules await (step 9). Also awaiting on the post-synaptic membrane are enzymes designed to break down the neurotransmitters (step 10) so that their effects are extremely transient – a few milliseconds at most. The breakdown products either diffuse out of the cleft into the intercellular space (12) or are reabsorbed into the terminal (step 13) by specific transport systems. Once within the terminal they are resynthesized (if necessary) and moved back into a vesicle by, once again, specific vesicular neurotrans-mitter transporters (step 14).

We noted above that the response of the postsy-naptic neuron depends on the union of a neurotrans-mitter with a receptor molecule in the postsynaptic membrane. There are many different types of neu-rotransmitter (well over three dozen) and they all have postsynaptic receptor molecules specifically tai-lored to accept them. In general, however, we can say that these receptor molecules fall into two great classes: those which are coupled to G-protein col-lision biochemistry and those which are coupled to ion channels. Synapses are thus divided into those which give **metabotropic** responses and those which give **ionotropic** responses. Metabotropic responses depend ultimately on the nature and action of second messengers (Section 1.3.3 and Figure 1.6) and are thus many and various. Ionotropic responses, on the other hand, are of two main types: **excitatory** and **inhibitory**. Excitatory responses occur when the neurotransmitter causes ion channels to open allow-ing the flux of Na^+ and K^+ across the postsynaptic membrane, which (as the Goldman equation shows) leads to a **depolarization** of the membrane, thus initiating an action potential. The postsynaptic potential (PSP) is thus known as an **excitatory postsynaptic potential** (*EPSP*). Inhibitory responses occur when a neurotransmitter opens a channel which allows Cl^- to flow down its concentration gradient. If an increased permeability constant for Cl^- is inserted into the Goldman equation (without altering any other constant), it will be seen that the electrical potential across the membrane increases. This *hyperpolarization* makes it more difficult for an action potential to be initiated. The underlying postsynaptic neuron is thus inhibited. The postsynaptic potential is thus an *inhibitory* postsynaptic potential *or IPSP*.

Even this briefest of outlines will have indicated some of the biochemical and molecular biological complexity of synapses and synaptic transmission. There is obviously a far greater scope for control of the transmission process than is possible in 'electrical' synapses. We shall meet many variations on the above themes as we proceed through this book. We should not leave the topic, however, without noting that many presynaptic membranes develop specialized regions for accepting vesicles. These regions are often ordered to form a presynaptic grid and the points of attachment within this grid are called vesicle attachment sites (VASs). In some cases, especially the hair cells of the organ of Corti in the inner ear and the rod and cone cells of the retina, the organization of vesicle release assumes an even more specialized form. Here we find that vesicles line up alongside ribbon-like structures known (unsurprisingly) as synaptic ribbons (Chapters 9 and 17) awaiting release into the synaptic gap. With this forward look into later chapters we must leave our discussion of synapses and synaptic transmission. Interested readers will find further information on this complex and central topic in the references cited in the bibliography.

2.8 CONCLUDING REMARKS

In Chapter 1 we looked at some of the ubiquitous molecular elements responsible for the activity of sensory cells. In this chapter we have seen how these molecular elements are responsible for the equally ubiquitous biophysical characteristics of sensory cells and fibres. We have seen, once again, the central role played by biomembranes. We have seen how the biophysics of ion flows across these membranes engenders a resting potential, V_m. We have noted how electrotonic (or cable) conduction allows the spread of small variations in V_m for small distances along nerve cell membranes, and that this form of conduction is responsible for generator and receptor potentials. We noted in Chapter 1 that Although V_m seems minute, about 60 mV, because the membrane is so thin (about 7 nm), the voltage gradient is, in fact, exceedingly large, about 10^5 V/cm. It is clear that any voltage-sensitive protein embedded in such a membrane is exposed to a powerful electric field. And, of course, there are numerous such voltage-sensitive proteins, the most important being the Ca^{2+} and Na^+-channel proteins. Any change in the electrical polarity of the membrane has a major affect on the conformation of these channels. We noted the importance of these conformational changes in sensory adaptation and in the propagation of action potentials.

In the next chapter we stand back a little and refocus on some of the higher level features of sensory systems. Once again we shall find a number of commonalities. We should bear in mind that these properties can all, in principle, be traced back to the operation of the molecular elements and their biophysical outcomes discussed in these first two chapters. Indeed, as we go on through this book, we shall find that, although much detail needs to be filled in, there is no break in principle between the biochemistry and biophysics of these first two chapters and the far higher level phenomena of the visual, auditory and other sensory cortices discussed in later chapters. This is a first indication of the major unsolved perplexity of sensory science: how can the physics and chemistry at the root of the brain's functioning be responsible for the world of colours, scents and sounds that form the tissue of our subjective lives? This, of course, is merely a way of expressing the mind–brain problem. It is never far from the concerns of sensory science and, as such, it will appear at intervals in the following pages. Although attempts at a solution are often thought to be the subject matter of another discipline, philosophy, the student should not imagine the problem unimportant or simply best forgotten.

3

GENERAL FEATURES OF SENSORY SYSTEMS

Psychophysics/behaviour vs. sensory physiology: future unification? **Classification of the senses**: by adequate stimuli - by exterior or interior location. **Modality**: labelled lines - rerouting experiments. **Intensity**; frequency modulation - thresholds and psychometry - signal vs. noise - just noticeable differences (jnds) and Weber-Fechner law - Steven's psychophysical law. **Adaptation. Receptive fields (RFs)**: definition - organisation - variation in area **Mapping**: non-isomorphic sensory maps - 'binding problem'. **Hierarchic and parallel design. Feature extraction and trigger stimuli**: hierarchies - 'pontifical cells' . **Concluding remarks**: sensory systems and predator-prey arms races.

In the first two chapters we looked at some of the molecular and biophysical elements from which sensory systems are built. In this chapter we shall consider some of the larger scale features which sensory systems have in common. But before we begin, it is worthwhile to distinguish two different approaches to the study of sensory systems.

In the first approach a study is made of the correlation between the physical stimulus and the animal's (including human's) response. The sensory system is regarded as a 'black box'. The investigator analyses (often in great detail) what this 'black box' can and cannot do, what it can and cannot detect and discriminate. The investigator does not, however, reach inside the black box to find out what cogs and wheels and wires are responsible for its abilities. In the case of humans, the experimenter attempts to correlate the physical stimulus with the subject's report of his or her subjective experience. This undertaking is, for obvious reasons, called *psychophysics*. In the case

of nonhuman animals, the psychophysical approach is much more difficult. Here the correlation of the physical stimulus must be with some aspect of the animal's behavioural response. It is true that this behavioural response may be very subtle, the animal may be trained (conditioned) to give a response to a stimulus and the stimulus then varied in intensity to investigate whether it can be detected. It is also possible to argue, as some have, that the verbal response in human psychophysics is also no more than a behaviour. We are, as ever in our study of sensory systems, once more in the vicinity of the mind–brain problem. But putting all such complexities aside, it is clearly far easier to correlate stimulus and response in trained human subjects than it is in the other animals. Indeed, psychophysical study of humans has provided some of the most precise measures of what the central nervous system can and cannot do. This hope, as Box 3.1 indicates, motivated the work of Hermann von Helmholtz,

Biology of Sensory Systems, Second Edition   C.U.M. Smith
© 2008 John Wiley & Sons, Ltd

BOX 3.1   HERMANN VON HELMHOLTZ

Hermann Ludwig Ferdinand von Helmholtz was born in Potsdam on 31 August 1821, the eldest of four children. He inherited from his father a profound interest in music and painting and from his mother the equable temperament that served him well in later life. His father was deeply involved in the German Romantic movement of the early part of the nineteenth century and Fichte's son, Immanuel Hermann Fichte, was a frequent visitor to the house. Idealist philosophy, literature and science were constant topics of conversation within the household. It is not surprising that the philosophical aspects of science and especially of sensory physiology concerned Helmholtz throughout his scientific career.

The young Helmholtz was not an outstanding scholar but evinced an early interest in physics. His father, however, had not the wherewithal to send him to University and persuaded him to study medicine where he could obtain financial support from the State. Accordingly, in 1837, he accepted a five-year government grant to study at the Königlich Medizinische-chirurgische Friedrich-Wilhelms-Institut in Berlin. Whilst in Berlin he attended science courses at the University, including physiology under Johannes Müller. He grasped the opportunity of writing his dissertation under Müller's direction. Whilst working at the University, he met Ernst Brucke and Emil du Bois Reymond as fellow students and, together with Karl Ludwig, they initiated the '1847 school' of physiology which eschewed any explanation in terms of nonphysical or 'vital' forces.

After completing his medical degree in 1842 he entered the army as a surgeon. He did not, however, relinquish his connections with academic circles and in 1848 he was appointed professor of physiology at Konigsberg. It was here that he invented the ophthalmoscope (1851) and measured the velocity of the nerve impulse in frog sciatic nerve (1850), showing it to be about 90 feet/s, far slower than previous estimates. In 1855, with the help of Alexander von Humboldt, Helmholtz transferred to the chair of physiology at Bonn and it was here that he began to write and publish his ground-breaking three volume work on physiological optics: *Handbuch der physiologischen Optik* (vol. 1, 1856). His mechanistic approach to sensory physiology upset his idealistic father and the resulting coolness possibly prevented him continuing with the publication. His fame, however, continued to grow and in 1858 he was offered and accepted a chair at perhaps the pre-eminent centre for science in Germany, Heidelberg. Here he continued an interest in acoustics, culminating in the publication of *Die Lehre von den Tonenpfindungen als physiofische Grundlage fur die Theorie der Musik* (1863). It was in this treatise that he introduced his so-called place theory of frequency discrimination (Chapter 8, Section 9.3.2).

In 1858, Helmholtz' father died and this released him from any inhibitions about publishing the remaining volumes of his work on physiological optics. The final volume (vol. 3) of the *Handbuch* was, accordingly, published in 1867. The three volumes of the handbook contain much new research on colour vision, on lens accommodation (he had invented an ophthalmometer which allowed measurement of lens curvature), after-images and so on. In particular it built upon his teacher, Johannes Müller's, concept of 'specific nerve energies'. This concept implies that different sensory nerves are specialized to respond to 'specific' environmental energies (or stimuli), a concept which, as we have seen, is basic to our modern understanding in the form of 'adequate stimuli'. Helmholtz used the concept of specific nerve energies in his treatment of the trichromatic theory of colour vision and in his place theory of frequency discrimination. He was also much exercised by the controversy over how much of our sensory understanding was learnt through experience and how much inborn. Helmholtz, in contrast to the nativists, took a strongly empiricist line and argued that our knowledge of the external world was achieved through early and continued experience. Little or nothing was congenital (Chapter 24).

Helmholtz' work in sensory physiology thus led him close to the epistemological concerns of his early years in his father's house. He came to believe that sensory physiology was to some extent extending

(Continues)

(*Continued*)

and supporting the Kantian epistemology. He came to believe, in other words, that the sense organs, via Müller's law of specific nerve energies, impose structure on the world. However, he was far from uncritical of Kant. In the mid-1860s he showed that the axioms of Euclidean geometry, far from being synthetic *a priori* propositions, as Kant had proposed, were in fact built up from visual experience; they were, in short, *a posteriori* not *a priori*.

Helmholtz's work was far from confined to sensory physiology. He made basic contributions to several areas of physics, especially energetics, physical chemistry, electrodynamics and hydrodynamics. He was one of the last to be able to undertake seminal work across all the natural sciences. His motivation was the motivation he learnt from his father's friends at Potsdam – a burning desire to make out the great unifying principles which bound together and underlie the natural world. When he died at Charlottenburg on 8 September 1894, the scientific world was already becoming too large and diversified to allow any one man to make foundational contributions in more than one field. Helmholtz was the last who could have well have held Nobel prizes in all three of physics, medicine or physiology and chemistry.

REFERENCES

Cahan, D. (ed.) (1993) *Hermann von Helmholtz and the Foundation of Nineteenth-Century Science*, University of California Press, Berkeley.

Turner, R.S. (1972) Helmholtz, Hermann von, in *Dictionary of Scientific Biography* (ed. C.C. Gillispie), Scribner's, New York.

one of the most important founders of sensory physiology.

In the second approach the investigator attempts to reach inside the psyhcophysicist's black box. Attention is focused on the physiology of the sensory system including, in the case of mammals, the sensory cortices, rather than on the behavioural response. The reaction of this system to appropriate stimuli is investigated at various levels from the molecular and subcellular up to the sensory analysers in the brain. The investigator may be interested in the response of individual sensory cells to appropriate stimuli or, at the other end of the spectrum, he may devote himself to recording the physiological response of the cerebral cortex. Clearly the ultimate hope is that the two approaches, through sensory physiology and psychophysics/behaviour, will ultimately unify to give a complete understanding of the way in which humans and other animals detect and respond to their environments.

3.1 CLASSIFICATION OF THE SENSES

All organisms live in an environment full of changes, full, as it has been said, of 'happenings'. Some of these changes will be beneficial to the organism, others detrimental. Some will occur quite independently of the organism, others will be due to the organism's own activities. In order to survive, the organism requires the fullest possible information about what is going on. To this end it develops a panoply of sensory detectors. As ever, the job is done best by specialists. Sensory detectors specialize to respond to certain types of change. As we shall see, they become extraordinarily sensitive to their chosen type, in many cases reaching right down to the physical limit. The major categories of change in the environment (so far as the majority of organisms is concerned) may be grouped into the broad categories of mechanical, chemical, electromagnetic and thermal. In consequence we can classify the major sensory systems as **mechanoreceptors**, **chemoreceptors** and **photoreceptors**. Unlike these three major classes of receptor, **thermoreceptors**, although ubiquitous, never, in spite of beginnings in some snakes, develop into complex sense organs. In addition to these four types of receptor some animals develop **electroreceptors**, sensitive to electric fields, while **magnetoreceptors** are known in prokaryocytes and are suspected to exist in some animals, especially birds.

The type of stimulus to which a specific receptor is attuned is termed the *adequate stimulus*.

Classification of the sensory receptors according to the environmental energy to which they are most sensitive is one important and familiar way of grouping the sense organs. It is the classification we shall adopt in this book. An alternative classificatory scheme depends not on the type of energy detected but on whether the sensory ending looks inward at happenings in the internal environment or outwards at the external environment. This classification gives us **interoreceptors** and **exteroreceptors**. Whereas photoreceptors are exclusively exteroreceptors (there being no significant electromagnetic fields within the body which need monitoring) the other three sense modalities may be either exteroreceptors or enteroreceptors. Interoreceptors, although not so spectacularly highly evolved as many exteroreceptors, are equally important. In the 'higher' animals, especially the mammals and birds, monitoring the internal environment is essential for the homeostatic mechanisms upon which their continued life depends.

3.2 MODALITY

We noted in Chapter 2 (Section 2.6) that the biophysics of nerve impulses is identical from one nerve fibre to another. 'Evolution', once having hit upon an effective mechanism for transmitting information, has stayed with it and merely refined it over geological time. This, however, has the consequence that the information from the different sense organs is all transformed into identical signals to the central nervous system (CNS). It follows that the CNS has no way of telling whether the impulses cascading into it along the sensory nerve fibres tell of sound, light, temperature or odour, except by attending to precisely which fibre is active. It has been said that if these 'labelled' lines are surgically rerouted, if, for instance, the auditory fibres were directed into the visual cortex and the visual fibres into the auditory cortex, we should hear lightning as thunder and see thunder as lightning. This, of course, raises fascinating philosophical questions. For the auditory cortex and the visual cortex do not differ significantly at the cellular level, still less at the biophysical level, so why should activity in one cortex give the sensation of sound and the other the totally different sensation

of vision? Even more interesting, and perhaps going some way to answer the philosophical question, is the demonstration that, if precisely this rerouting is carried out in foetal mammals, the auditory cortex develops some of the physiological characteristics of the visual cortex and vice versa. The student is referred to the bibliography at the end of Part One for references to this fascinating work.

3.3 INTENSITY

The happenings in the world differ not only in their type but also in their intensity. Roughly speaking, stimulus intensity is signalled by the frequency of the action potentials in a sensory nerve fibre. The CNS thus needs to 'look' at *which* sensory nerves are active (which indicates the sensory **modality**) and the **frequency** of the impulse traffic in them (which indicates the **intensity** of that modality) to keep itself informed of the goings on in the external and internal environments.

The weakest stimulus that an organism can detect is known as the **threshold** stimulus (or sensory threshold). This is determined by presenting the organism (or in the case of humans, the subject) with a sequence of stimuli increasing from zero intensity and asked (either by conditioning, or verbally in the case of human subjects) when the stimulus is first detectable. The threshold is defined as that stimulus which is detected in half the presentations (Figure 3.1). The curve shown in Figure 3.1 is known as the **psychometric function or curve**.

Sensory thresholds are not constant. They depend on numerous factors, especially fatigue, context, practice and so on. This finding emphasizes the subtlety of the brain's physiology. Numerous feedforward and feedback loops are in play. We shall note, for example, when we come to consider pain in Chapter 22 that our sensitivity to this unpleasant sensory modality can vary greatly. In the heat of action we are frequently unaware of tissue damage, only afterwards are we incapacitated with pain. A shift in the psychometric function to the right also occurs in childbirth. It is also the case that thresholds for pain vary in different cultures. What is unacceptable in one is a matter of course in another.

Turning to the physiology underlying the psychophysics we should note first of all that, even when

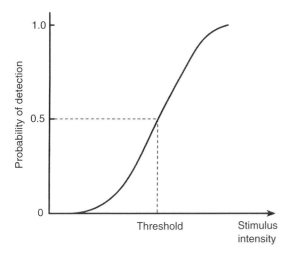

Figure 3.1 Psychometric curve. The threshold is defined as the intensity when half the responses are correct. The position of the curve on the apscissa is arbitrary. It will shift to the right or left according to circumstances.

there is no stimulus, sensory fibres transmit action potentials at a low frequency. This is known as the *maintained discharge*. It can vary (in different sensory fibres) from one or two impulses per second up to over 50 per second. When the adequate stimulus is present at sufficient intensity the impulse frequency increases. It is obviously important for the CNS to be able to distinguish between a signal showing the presence of the adequate stimulus (at a low intensity) and random fluctuation. It is, in other words, important to distinguish signal from noise.

Both the maintained discharge and the discharge due to the application of the adequate stimulus will vary about a mean. For example, the sustained discharge may be, say, $20 \pm 5\,Hz$ and the discharge due to a threshold stimulus may be, say, $25 \pm 6\,Hz$. Evidently the top of the maintained discharge overlaps the bottom of the discharge due to the threshold stimulus. The CNS cannot be certain whether a stimulus is there or not. Part of the time it would be right, part of the time wrong. This situation corresponds (approximately) to the sensory threshold defined above. As the stimulus intensity increases the signal is moved further and further out of the noise. At $30 \pm 7\,Hz$ there is little overlap with the maintained discharge and at $35 \pm 8\,Hz$ there can be no doubt that the adequate stimulus is present.

Note, however, in the hypothetical examples of the preceding paragraph, that the spread of impulse frequency around the mean increases as the stimulus is increased. This means that as the intensity of the stimulus increases, the magnitude of the physical change of the stimulus to generate a '*just noticeable difference (jnd)*' also increases. This relationship was captured by Weber in 1834 and is known as *Weber's law*:

$$\Delta\varphi = k \times \varphi,$$

where '$\Delta\varphi$' is the jnd, φ is the subjective experience of the original stimulus and k is a constant. The most frequently quoted example of the law has to do with the perception of mass. It is easy to sense the difference between 1 and 1.5 kg, very difficult if not impossible to detect the difference between 25 and 25.5 kg.

Later in the nineteenth century Fechner (1860) extended Weber's law to give a relationship between the subjectively-experienced threshold stimulus and suprathreshold stimuli. This relationship, known as the **Weber–Fechner law,** is as follows:

$$\varphi = k \log \phi/\phi_0,$$

where φ is the subjective magnitude of the stimulus compared to the threshold, ϕ is the physical magnitude of the stimulus, ϕ_0 is the threshold magnitude and k is a constant. Nearly a century later, in the 1950s, Stanley Stevens investigated a large number of sensory modalities and showed that the 'psychophysical law' followed a somewhat more complex relationship best expressed as a power function:

$$\varphi = k(\phi - \phi_0)^n$$
$$\text{or, } \log y = \log k + n \log(\phi - \phi_0)$$
$$\text{i.e. } \log y = K + n \log(\phi - \phi_0).$$

The exponent 'n' varies from one sense modality to another: $n \approx 1$ for perception of length; $n \approx 0.4$ for perception of brightness; $n \approx 3.5$ for electric shock. Some of these different relationships between stimulus and response are shown in Figure 3.2a. They are much easier to compare when the logarithmic form is used, as the expression then becomes that for a straight line (Figure 3.2b).

Although we have been assuming that the impulse traffic responsible for subjective experience is carried

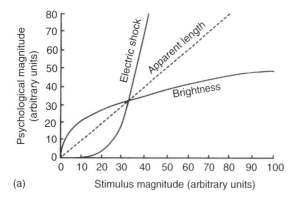

(a)

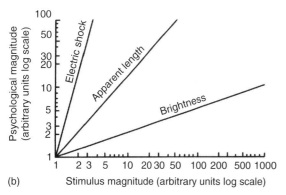

(b)

Figure 3.2 Psychophysical correlations. (a) When subjective magnitude is plotted against stimulus magnitude on linear coordinates the lines are frequently curved upwards or downwards. (b) When graphed against log–log coordinates, straight lines are obtained whose gradients depend on the value of the exponent, 'n'. From Stevens, S.S. (1957) On the psychophysical law. *Psychological Review*, **64**, 153–81. Copyright © 1957, American Psychological Association.

by a single sensory fibre in the preceding treatment, this is seldom, if ever, the case. In all naturally experienced suprathreshold stimuli more than one sensory fibre is involved. As the stimulus increases in intensity more and more sensory fibres are recruited.

3.4 ADAPTATION

We saw in Chapter 2 (Section 2.5) that all sensory fibres show adaptation. The response to a stimulus has an initial 'dynamic' stage, during which a comparatively large number of impulses flow down the sensory fibre, followed by a period when the impulse frequency drops to a much lower level. In some cases

there is a further burst of activity when the stimulus is turned off (Figure 2.7a).

There is no need to say more here. It is worth remarking, however, that in some cases adaptation may bring the impulse traffic in sensory fibres down to the threshold or below. Subjectively we become unaware of the stimulus. It is only when the stimulus is switched on and/or switched off that the impulse traffic varies sufficiently to engender conscious awareness. We have all experienced occasions when it is only when a constant stimulus abruptly ends that we remember that it was present at all.

3.5 RECEPTIVE FIELDS

Sensory nerve endings are generally sensitive to stimulation of a small patch of the surroundings. This patch is known as the **receptive field (RF)** of the sensory fibre. In many cases, as we shall see in later chapters, receptive fields have internal organization. It is often the case that stimulation of one part of a RF leads to excitation of the sensory neuron, whilst stimulation of another part leads to inhibition.

Receptive fields also vary markedly in area. In those parts of the sensory surface where it is important that any stimulus should be precisely localized, the RFs are small. Vice versa, where localization is not so important, RFs tend to be large. This was well shown by the classic **two-point threshold** experiments of Weber. Some parts of the body – the finger tips, the lips – are able to detect two closely-set punctate stimuli whereas other parts – the upper arm, the back – are only able to resolve much more widely spaced stimuli. In some cases there is a trade-off between sensitivity and precision of localization. If it is the case that only a certain fixed quantity of energy is interacting with the sensory surface, as is the case, for example, with the retina under constant illumination, then large receptive fields are able to collect far more of this energy than smaller ones. Other things being equal they will provide greater sensitivity. But, for the same reason, they cannot provide precise information concerning the exact part of the retina being stimulated.

Although sensory surfaces, such as the retina or the skin, may be considered as RF mosaics, it should not be thought that the RFs are sharply demarcated from one another, as are the tesserae which make up the decorative mosaics of classical or Islamic art. In fact, the RFs in a sensory surface show extensive overlapping and, moreover, especially in the retina, vary in size in different physiological conditions. This is just one more instance of the dynamic character of sensory systems; a character which, ultimately, is imposed on the comparatively 'hard-wired' network of neurons and sensory cells by their highly active biochemistry and molecular biology. They are very different from the unchanging inorganic components of our silicon-based electrotechnology.

3.6 MAPS OF SENSORY SURFACES

Sensory endings and their receptive fields are, with the exception of the olfactory system, arranged in two-dimensional arrays – maps. This is obviously the case with retinae, and it is the case with the touch receptors of the skin as well. Less obviously it is also the case with the basilar membrane of the cochlea. The spatial relations of these arrays are maintained into the CNS. In humans, as we shall see in subsequent chapters, there is a map of the body surface in the somatosensory cortex of the postcentral gyrus, a map of the retina in the primary visual cortex of the occipital lobe and a map of the basilar membrane in the primary auditory cortex of the temporal lobe. These maps are defined as **somatotopic, retinotopic** and **tonotopic** respectively.

It should not be thought, however, that these maps are isomorphic with the sensory surfaces. In all cases, those parts of the sensory surface which are of greatest biological importance, where greatest discrimination of the sensory input is required, are allocated disproportionately large areas of cortex. This *nonisomorphic mapping* is partly a reflection of the fact mentioned above that those parts of the sensory surface which are of greatest biological importance have smaller RFs and hence more sensory fibres per unit area. It is also due to an increased complexity of neuronal connectivity in these areas of the cortex. Although this nonisomorphic mapping is characteristic of all CNS maps of sensory surfaces, it is probably most widely known for the somatosensory cortex. The sensory 'homunculi' (Figure 8.20) of these cortices, with their huge lips, gigantic hands with outsize thumbs, tiny legs and feet, have attained almost iconic status.

In some sensory systems, especially the visual systems of primates, the map in the primary sensory area is projected onwards to secondary, tertiary and higher areas. Generally speaking, however, these higher level maps become topographically less precise. However, although these higher level maps may be topographically imprecise, they may well be organized to provide comparatively precise maps of other features of the stimulus. Again, taking the example of the primate (macaque) visual system, the best-known of all advanced sensory systems, we find that, in visual area 4, colour rather than spatial position on the sensory surface is mapped. The wavelength of light to which V4 cells respond varies in a regular way from cell to adjacent cell. Similarly, in visual area 5, which is concerned with movement of the visual stimulus, it is found that the direction of movement to which adjacent cells respond again varies regularly across the area.

But why maps? Why should sensory systems develop maps of the body's sensory surfaces at all? The short answer to this question is that nobody knows. There have been many speculations. We shall return to the question in Chapter 23 (Section 23.4). It may be, as argued there, that sensory fibres which normally fire together tend to group together. There is, as we shall see, considerable developmental evidence for this conclusion. Clearly sensory fibres originating from neighbouring parts of a sensory surface will be more likely than not to be activated together. There is also an argument which refers to economy of design. It is argued that sensory analysis, computation, is most efficiently done when similar parts of the sensory scene, either topographically or functionally, are kept close together. Unlike computers based on silicon and copper, brains do not work at the speed of light. The velocity of information exchange in the unmyelinated short axons and dendrites of grey matters is orders of magnitude slower than electrical conduction around the hardware of a computer. If large distances, centimetres rather than millimetres, had to be traversed, the coherence of the total 'percept' might be put in jeopardy. We are here in the vicinity of what is called the '**binding problem**'. This is the problem of how it is that our percepts are unified and coherent although the brain is highly heterogeneous and modular. We do not know the answer to the binding problem. We do not know the answer to the 'why' question about sensory maps.

It is not impossible that these two questions are as-pects of the same problem. When we begin to gain insight into one, we may begin to see the light with the other.

3.7 HIERARCHICAL AND PARALLEL DESIGN

The preceding section may have suggested that sen-sory systems are organized in an exclusively hierar-chical design. It may have suggested that the sensory surface projects to the primary sensory cortex, where it retains its topographical relationships, and then further projections, losing perhaps a little precision, transmit the information to further maps in other ar-eas of the cortex. Although this is true, it is only part of the truth. We shall see when we come to consider the major sensory systems, and especially the primate visual system, that there are multiple projections into the brain. There is not just one map projected for-ward in a hierarchical fashion, but several maps in parallel, interlinked and interacting with each other. Furthermore, the sequence of maps in the hierar-chical design is interlinked in both the 'forward' and 'backward' direction. The design of the sensory brain allows both parallel and sequential 'computing'; it might best be described, to use Hofstadter's term, as a 'tangled hierarchy'.

3.8 FEATURE EXTRACTION AND TRIGGER STIMULI

One final common feature of sensory systems must be mentioned before finishing. We shall see as we proceed through this book that, in highly evolved systems, such as those serving the auditory and visual senses, ever more specific features of the sen-sory world are 'extracted' as the sensory information streams upward through the brain. These features are aspects of the world which are of paramount impor-tance to the animal. Few cells in the auditory cortex respond to the continuous pure tones which are so effective in stimulating the basilar membrane of the cochlea. Instead, clicks, and crackles, as of predators creeping through the undergrowth, or frequency-modulated tones proceeding upwards or downwards

in pitch, prove far more effective. We shall see in Chapter 10 that these features are made use of in the highly specialized auditory cortices of humans (to build up speech sounds) and bats (for echoloca-tion). Similarly, in the visual system, the bright spots of light or continuous defocused illumination which are effective in stimulating the retina have little af-fect on cells in the visual cortices. Instead, edges at different orientation evoke strong responses in the primary visual cortex. Further up the system even more specific features trigger responses. In the upper reaches of the macaque visual system, the inferotem-poral cortex, for example, cells are present which only respond when specific features of monkey faces (full or profile) are in the visual field (Chapter 18, Section 18.4).

These specific features of the sensory world, fea-tures which as the preceding examples indicate are all of great significance in the animal's life, are known as **trigger stimuli**. Much research has been devoted to this category of stimuli. Early on the concept of a hierarchy of feature extractors became popular. It was suggested that ever more particular features of the visual scene were extracted until not only monkey face recognition cells were achieved but, in the case of ourselves, cells to recognize grandmother's face. The notion of **grandmother's face recognition cells**, or **pontifical cells**, gained wide currency, though it is to be suspected that it was always taken as a *reduc-tio ad absurdum* or, at least, with a very large pinch of salt. For could there be enough cells in the cor-tex to deal with grandmother in all her hairdoes and in all her moods, lightings and hats? Let alone all the other specific features of our visual experience? Would one be unable to recognize grandmother if the cell, for some reason, became defective or dis-eased? Furthermore, the philosophical problem ob-trudes once more. Is it really credible to suppose that activity in a single cell translates into visual con-sciousness of grandmother? It seems more likely, as we shall see in Chapter 18, that the recognition of grandmother depends on the activity of a popula-tion of cells throughout the visual cortices and in other parts of the brain including (and importantly) the emotional centres in the limbic system. This like-lihood is increased by the recognition (mentioned in the preceding section) of the great part that parallel processing plays in the visual system. The idea of a single hierarchical stream of information proceeding to ever higher 'centres' in the brain is falling into desuetude.

3.9 CONCLUDING REMARKS

'Evolution', Francois Jacob said, 'is a tinkerer'. In the case of sensory systems it has taken the biophysics and molecular biology reviewed in Chapters 1 and 2 and assembled it over a thousand million years into ever more remarkable and sensitive devices for detecting environmental events. Evolution may be a tinkerer but it is a tinkerer driven by the fear of death. Sensory systems are deeply involved in the struggle for existence, in what some have called evolutionary 'arms races'. As with the technological arms races with which we are all familiar as humans, information is all important. The battle of Britain and the battle of the Atlantic were won and lost by radar and cracking the codes of radio communications. Sensory systems have been exposed to the full merciless rigour of natural selection for a billion years. But as with the tinkerer of Jacob's metaphor, there has never been an opportunity to strip them down and start afresh. Tinkering is done on what already exists. The sensory systems of the most 'advanced' animals thus still bear the design traces of remote ancestors. In spite of this they have evolved, as we shall see in the remainder of this book, to a sensitivity which in many cases has yet to be reached by the artifices of human technology.

4

CLASSIFICATION AND PHYLOGENY

Systematics: evolutionary and cladistic classifications. **Six kingdoms**: the nature of animal phyla. **Unicellularity**: prokaryocytes (Archaebacteria and Eubacteria) - eukaryocytes (protista). **Multicellularity**: Fungi, Plantae and Animalia - Parazoa and Metazoa - invertebrates and vertebrates. **Protostomata and deuterostomata**: spiral and radial cleavage - schizocoely and enterocoely - formation of mouth - these profound embryological difffferences separate an annelid-arthropod-mollusc assemblage from an echinoderm-chordate assemblage - suggests independent evolution over more than half a billion years. **Classification of Metazoa**: Cnidaria - Platyhelminthes – Nematoda - Mollusca - Annelida - Arthropoda – Echinodermata - Chordata. **Evolution of neurosensory systems**: Cnidaria - Platyhelminthes – Nematoda - Annelida - Arthropoda – Mollusca Echinodermata – Chordata. **Concluding**: some animal designs more favoured than others - three great designs (Arthropods, Molluscs, Chordates) have proved outstandingly successful, they will consequently figure largely in this book.

In the following chapters we shall take a fairly wide sweep through the living world in our examination of sensory systems. Not all readers of this book will be familiar with the taxonomic and evolutionary position of the organisms mentioned, nor with the organization of their nervous systems. This chapter is designed to remedy that unfamiliarity.

4.1 SYSTEMATICS

Surprising as it may seem to the outsider, biological systematics is not a closed and fully agreed topic. Even the number of major groups (phyla) into which the animal kingdom may be subdivided remains a matter of controversy. Furthermore, with the intro-

duction by Hennig in 1950 of a non-evolutionary classificatory schema, known as '**cladistics**', systematics has found itself the subject of bitter polemics. Fortunately, we need not enter this minefield. Our interest in the classificatory position of organisms has a profoundly evolutionary basis. Our interest in the sense organs of animals other than ourselves is not only just because they're there, though that is indeed a thoroughly respectable motive, but mostly because of the light they throw on our own sensory systems and of the way in which they display alternative ways of solving the same problems. In some cases these solutions are radically different (insect and vertebrate eyes), in other cases they are surprisingly similar (cephalopod and vertebrate eyes). An understanding of the evolutionary relationships between animal groups is thus basic to a full understanding of animal sensory systems and, in particular, of those that we develop ourselves.

4.2 CLASSIFICATION INTO SIX KINGDOMS

In this book we shall use the conventional scheme of classifying organisms into six kingdoms: Archaebacteria, Eubacteria, Protista, Plantae, Fungi and Animalia. Within these six kingdoms organisms are further subdivided into great groups sharing a common body plan. These great groups are called *phyla* (botanists call them 'divisions'). This, as would be expected, is much more evident in the multicellular Fungi, Plantae and Animalia than in the three unicellular kingdoms. Indeed the subdivision into phyla is only fully accepted in the zoological world of the kingdom Animalia. In the study of sensory systems it is, of course, this kingdom which looms largest. In what follows our attention will consequently be largely concentrated on this kingdom.

4.3 UNICELLULARITY

The Archaebacteria and the Eubacteria (sometimes simply Archaea and Bacteria) are often grouped together as **Monera** (Gk: **Moneres**, single, solitary). Their biochemistry and molecular biology is, however, sufficiently different for systematists to place them in separate kingdoms. Well over 5000 species are known and they all consist of small cells lacking nuclei and organelles. Because these cells have no clearly demarcated nucleus (i.e. their nucleic acid is not partitioned off from the rest of the cell by a nuclear membrane), they are known as **prokaryocytes**. For nearly 2000 million years (from about 3600 million years BP to about 1600 million years BP) the Monera had the world to themselves. Their sensory systems are, of course, extremely simple. They are, however, of considerable interest to us in this book as they can often be shown to represent, at least at the biochemical level, primordia from which the almost infinitely complex systems of the Animalia have evolved.

After some 2000 million years had elapsed, the first larger and more complex cells, the **eukaryocytes**,

appeared. They are more closely related to the archaebacteria than to the eubacteria. All eukaryocytes have a definite nucleus (their genetic material is confined within a nuclear membrane) and organelles such as mitochondria, chloroplasts and so on are present outside the nuclear membrane in the cytoplasm. Earlier classifications grouped autotrophic unicellular eukaryocytes with the plants as *Protophyta* and the heterotrophic forms with the animals as *Protozoa*. An alternative and more modern analysis suggests that the unicellular eukaryocytes resemble each other more than they do the multicellular animals, plants and fungi and, moreover, that multicellularity may have evolved several times. It has consequently been proposed that they should be grouped into a separate kingdom the **Protista** or *Protoctista* (Gk *protos*, first; *ktistos,* established). The Protista are a highly diverse group of organisms, subdivided into anything up to thirty distinct phyla. They do not figure largely in this book. Perhaps they are most interesting, for our concerns, in showing the earliest photoreceptors – various types of eye spot. These are found in the phylum Eustigmatophyta, Chlorophyta and, especially, in the phylum Euglenophyta (*Euglena viridis*) and some members of the phylum Dinoflagellata (*Pouchetia sp., Erythropsidinium pavillardii*).

4.4 MULTICELLULARITY

Multicellularity probably originated some 1000 million years ago. Biologists recognize three kingdoms: Fungi, Plantae, Animalia. It is only the latter kingdom which is of interest in this book. Again there are several different methods of classification. In older texts the kingdom Animalia was subdivided into three subkingdoms: Protozoa, Parazoa (sponges) and Metazoa. More recently, as we have seen, the Protozoa have been grouped with other unicellular forms in the kingdom Protista. The Animalia are consequently subdivided into two subkingdoms, the **Parazoa** and **Metazoa**. The Parazoa are further subdivided into two phyla, the **Porifera** (sponges) and **Placozoa** (consisting of a single species, *Trichoplax adhaerens*, the size of large amoeba). All the other animals are grouped into the Metazoa. Very early in evolutionary history (Figure 4.3) **bilateral symmetry** emerged and this ancient stage is still represented by present-day Platyhelminthes. The next step on the evolutionary ladder was taken when a body cavity or **coelom** developed, separating the digestive tube from the rest of the body's musculature and thus allowing it to act independently. These developments are believed to have taken place deep in the Precambrian period perhaps a thousand million years ago.

4.5 PROTOSTOMES AND DEUTEROSTOMES

If we look deep into the early embryology of the coelomate metazoan, we find several fundamental features which suggest an ancient division into two great groups of animal forms: an annelid– arthropod–mollusc assemblage and an echinoderm– chordate assemblage (Figure 4.3). In the annelid–arthropod–mollusc assemblage the first divisions of the zygote (cleavage) take place in a **spiral** fashion (Figure 4.1A(a)). The daughter cells (**blastomeres**) arrange themselves between each other. Moreover, the fate of these cells is already **determined**. If one is removed, a particular part of the body which it was destined to form fails to develop. In contrast, in the chordate–echinoderm line, the zygote undergoes **radial** cleavage (Figure 4.1A(b)) and the daughter cells are arranged directly above and below each other. Moreover, the fates of the blastomeres are not at this stage determined. If one is removed, the others are able to compensate for the loss so that a normal embryo develops. It should be added here that there are a number of exceptions to this neat schematic. Not all protostomes show spiral cleavage and not all follow a totally determined development. Nature always seems to wriggle free from the neat compartments invented by biological bureaucrats.

Next, the two great assemblages of forms show deep-seated differences in the way in which the coelom, is formed. In the annelid–arthropod–mollusc assemblage it develops by a splitting of the mesoderm, a process known as **schizocoely**. In the chordate–echinoderm assemblage, on the other hand, it develops by an outpouching of the gut which is eventually nipped off, a process termed **enterocoely**.

Finally, there is an important difference in the way the mouth is formed. The ball of cells which results

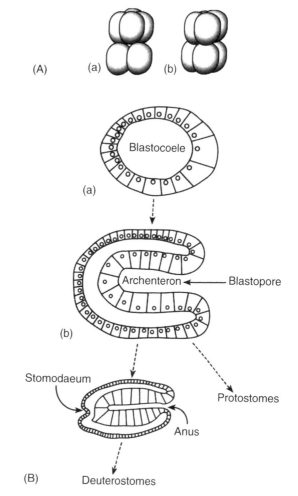

Figure 4.1 (A) (a) Spiral and (b) radial cleavage. After Caroll, R.L. (1988). (B) Protostomes and deuterostomes. (a) Blastula; (b) Invagination to form the gastrula. The blastocoele is largely obliterated and the new cavity forms the primitive gut or archenteron. Opening to the exterior is the blastopore. This develops into the mouth in the protostomes. In the deuterostomes a new invagination, at the opposite end from the blastopore, known as the stomodaeum, eventually appears and breaks through into the archenteron. This develops into the mouth; the blastopore becomes the anus.

from the first cell divisions of the fertilized egg – the **blastula** – ultimately invaginates to form a primitive gut – the **archenteron**. This process is known as gastrulation. In the annelid–arthropod–mollusc assemblage, the opening into this primitive gut, known as the **blastopore**, eventually develops into the adult's mouth. Animals in which the mouth originates in

.his way are called **protostomes**. In contrast, in the chordate–echinoderm assemblage the mouth develops in a different way. Here a new opening ultimately appears at the opposite end to the blastopore and the blastopore develops instead into the anus (Figure 4.1B(b)). Animals in which this type of development happens are called **deuterostomes** (because the mouth develops 'secondarily'). These two terms, 'protostomes' and 'deuterostomes', are commonly used to denote the two great assemblages of animal forms.

Although Haeckel's so-called 'biogenetic law' ('phylogeny recapitulates ontogeny') is nowadays regarded with some caution, it cannot be doubted that events early in embryology are fixed very early in evolutionary history. It follows that the crucial differences between the embryology of protostomes and deuterostomes arose very early in phylogeny. Molecular evidence suggests a common ancestor no later than about 670 million years ago (Figure 4.2). Indeed, recent work has pushed the date back yet further, to some 830 million years BP. The two great assemblages of animal forms have thus evolved independently for well over three quarters of a billion years. This makes a comparison between their sense organs a matter of considerable interest. We do not have to go to alien planets to gain insight into alternative evolutionary outcomes for carbon-based life-forms.

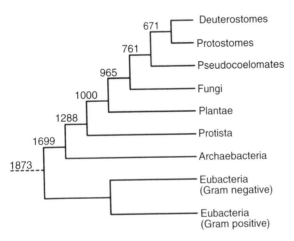

Figure 4.2 Evolutionary relationships between the major groups of organisms. The figures indicate approximate millions of years. The pseudocoelomates are represented by the nematode worms (e.g. *C. elegans*). Data from Doolittle *et al.*, 1996.

Finally, there is accumulating molecular evidence to suggest that the protostomata divided very early into two major groups. The first group, known as the Ecdysozoa, contains amongst others the nematodes and arthropods and is characterized by a tough external coat which requires periodic moulting (ecdysis) to allow growth. The other group, the Lophotrochozoa, is free of the constriction of a tough external layer (but by the same token less protected) and contains the annelid segmented worms, the molluscs and a number of other animal phyla.

4.6 CLASSIFICATION OF THE METAZOA

Let us now focus in on the major groups of animals within the animal kingdom. Systematists divide them into large groups known as phyla. A phylum, as mentioned above, consists of animals all sharing a common body plan. The study of the evolution of this body plan over geological time is known as **phylogeny**. Within a phylum zoologists classify organisms into subphyla, classes, orders, families, genera and, finally, species and subspecies. In some cases zoologists group orders together into superorders and families into superfamilies. Thus, for example, humans are classified as belonging to:

- *Kindom* Animalia
- *Phylum* Chordata
- *Subphylum* Gnathostomata
- *Class* Mammalia
- *Order* Primates
- *Family* Hominoidea
- *Genus* Homo
- *Species* sapiens
- *Subspecies* sapiens.

All animals, by definition, have to seek their food in a changeable environment and consequently all of the multitudinous forms grouped in the thirty or so phyla develop sense organs of one sort or another. The evolutionary relationships between the groups of animals that are significant in this book are shown in Figure 4.3. Prominent amongst these animals are the Arthropoda, the Mollusca and, of course, the Chordata.

Let us briefly review some of the phyla shown in Figure 4.3. The **Cnidaria** (formerly grouped with the

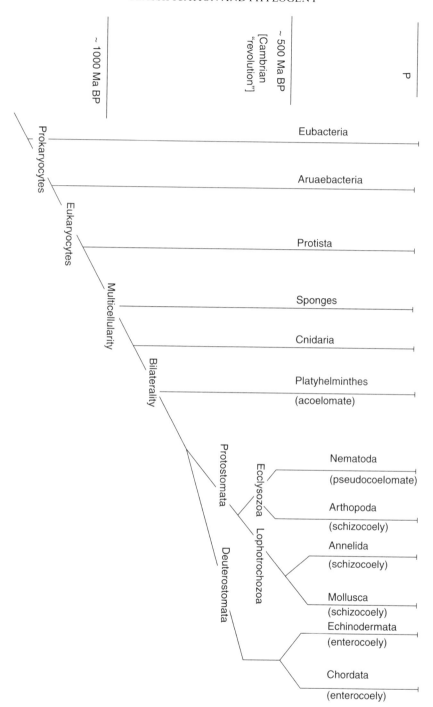

Figure 4.3 Evolutionary tree. There are, in fact, about thirty phyla. The figure shows just the phyla containing forms significant in the following pages of this book. Origin from the protista occurred some 1000 million years BP. The several major stages of body design are indicated in the diagram: multicellularity, bilateral symmetry (bilaterality); the development of mouth from blastopore (protostomata) or at the opposite end (deuterostomata); the formation of a coelom dividing the body and gut musculature either by schizocoely or enterocoely; the division of the protostomata into ecdysozoa and lophotrochozoa and so on. All these important developments occurred in Precambrian times.

Ctenophora as the **Coelenterata**) are the simplest of the Metazoa. They are also believed to lie at the evolutionary root of the Metazoa. An imprint of *Ediacara*, believed to be a hydrozoan, was found in South Australian sandstone dating back some 700 million years. The bodies of Cnidaria contain no cavity (coelom) and are constructed of just two layers of cells, ectoderm and endoderm. They develop no true central nervous system but make do with a diffuse nerve net. Well known members of this phylum are the jelly fish (class **Scyphozoa**), the hydroids, such as *Hydra*, *Obelia* and so on (class **Hydrozoa**) and the corals and sea anemones (class **Anthozoa**).

The *Platyhelminthes* (flatworms) show an evolutionary advance over the Cnidaria in that their bodies are built of three layers of cells: ectoderm, mesoderm and endoderm. There is still no body cavity but, unlike the Cnidaria, they are bilaterally symmetrical with a definite anterior and posterior extremity. The free-living forms develop ladder-like central nervous systems with an accumulation of nerve cells at the anterior end where a number of sense organs, including pigment-cup eye spots, are concentrated. There are three classes: class **Turbellaria** (free-living carnivorous flatworms, e.g. *Planaria*); class **Trematoda** (parasitic liver flukes); class **Cestoda** (tapeworms). Most zoologists believe that forms, such as present-day planaria, resemble the stem animals from which the rest of the Metazoa diversified some seven or eight hundred million years ago.

The phylum **Nematoda** (commonly known as '*roundworms*') consist of a large assemblage of forms (perhaps a million species) of which the best known are endoparasites, for example *Ascaris*, *Trichinella*. Roundworms have the beginnings of a body cavity but, as it does not form by a space originating within the mesoderm, it is known as a pseudocoelom rather than a true coelom. They possess very simple dorsal and ventral nerve cords connected by a nerve ring around the pharynx. Many nematodes are noted for their prodigious reproductive ability. Females sometimes contain tens of millions of eggs and may extrude them at a rate of over 100 000 a day. Because of this extraordinary fecundity and short generation time one of the free living roundworms, the small (0.5 mm long) free-living soil nematode, *Caenorhabditis elegans*, has been extensively studied by molecular biologists. At the molecular level it is probably the best known of all metazoan species. Striking similarities have been found between much of its fundamental molecular biology and that of 'higher' animals up to and including humans.

The phylum **Mollusca** consists of a great variety of different forms – over 100 000 species. They are all soft-bodied and unsegmented with a true body cavity or coelom. They range in size from a few millimeters up to the giant squid, *Architheutis*, the largest of all invertebrates, which may be over twenty meters in length from tip of tentacle to posterior extremity. The Mollusca have provided some of the most interesting and valuable preparations for neurobiological research. As Figure 4.3 shows they have evolved separately from the Chordates for seven or eight hundred million years. They might almost be considered a separate creation.

The Mollusca are divided into seven classes. The **Monoplacophora**, with one flat shell, live in subtropical and tropical deep waters. The **Aplacophora** include the worm-like solenogasters and also inhabit the depths of warm seas. The **Polyplacophora** include the common sea-shore, rock-clinging chitons. The **Pelycypoda** comprise perhaps the best-known of all the molluscs, the bivalves – oysters, muscles, scallops. We shall see in Chapter 14 that the scallops are known for their remarkable tentacular eyes. The **Gastropoda** consist of all those forms which crawl upon their stomachs – the snails, winkles, slugs and so on. The **Scaphopoda** possess conical shells and burrow into mud and sand. Finally, the most remarkable molluscs belong to the class **Cephalopoda**. The **Cephalopoda** are subdivided into three subclasses: the **Ammonoidea**, the ammonites, extinct, but frequently found as spectacular fossils; the **Nautiloidea** represented by the pearly Nautilus; and the **Belemnoidea** to which belong the squids, cuttlefish and octopi. We shall see that these remarkable marine predators, although the outcome of half a billion and more years of separate evolution and with totally different body plans, nevertheless show strikingly similar solutions to the problems presented in the design and operation of photoreceptors.

The phylum **Annelida** include the common terrestrial and aquatic (mostly marine) worms. Like the molluscs they are coelomate protostomes but, in strong contrast to the molluscs, they are distinctively segmented. There are four classes. class

Polychaeta consists of the mostly marine bristle worms, for example *Nereis*, the common sea-shore rag-worm. Polychaetes are often large, active forms with well-developed nervous systems and sense organs. Class **Oligochaeta**, with fewer 'bristles, includes the common earthworm, *Lumbricus*. Class **Hirudinea** is comprised of the ectoparasitic leeches, for example *Hirudo*. Finally the class **Myzostomaria** consists of a number of small parasites of the Echinoderms.

The phylum **Arthropoda** is perhaps the most successful of all the phyla in the animal kingdom. Many zoologists believe that, if all the species living today could be identified and enumerated, they would add up to something over ten million. Arthropods inhabit all the world's environments and range in size from microscopic mites to large spider crabs measuring well over a metre from outstretched leg to outstretched leg. Terrestrial arthropods, overwhelmingly represented by the insects, are, however, mostly small animals. This is because of their basic design principle. A hard chitinous exoskeleton does not permit continuous growth. Instead growth has to occur in spurts when the cuticle is shed during the process known as ecdysis. Without its cuticle, an arthropod, especially a terrestrial arthropod, is highly exposed and vulnerable. These soft-bodied periods must thus be kept short and minimized. Without this disastrous consequence of their design principle arthropods might well have become the monstrous land faunae of science fiction.

Arthropods, like annelids, are strongly segmented, coelomate protostomes. They differ from annelids in the possession of a hard, chitinous exoskeleton and jointed legs. It is from the latter character that they take their name. There are two large divisions which have been accorded subphylum status: the **Mandibulata** and the **Chelicerata**. The mandibulate arthropods have three body segments whilst in the Chelicerata the anterior two body parts are combined into a single cephalothorax.

The subphylum **Mandibulata** is subdivided into six classes. The class *Crustacea* consists of a large assemblage of aquatic, gill-breathing arthropods. The most significant order in this class, the order **Decapoda**, includes the lobsters, crayfish, crabs, prawns and shrimps. The **Crustacea** also include a number of smaller orders, the water fleas, copepods, barnacles and so on. The second class, the class **Diplopoda**, includes the millipedes. The class **Chilopoda** consists of the centipedes; the class **Pauropoda** contains centipede-like forms and the class **Symphyla** consists of yet another group of centipede-like animals. The last class in the subphylum is the class **Insecta,** which is by far the largest of all the arthropod classes. Insects are found in all the world's environments with the important exception of the sea. They are mostly highly active animals and hence develop an array of exquisitely designed sense organs. Because of their hard chitinous exoskeleton these sense organs are mostly based on cuticular sensilla. This design element is very different from that of soft bodied forms such as molluscs and vertebrates and hence insect sensory biology provides a valuable comparative study. We shall discuss numerous examples in the following pages.

The second arthropod subphylum, the subphylum **Chelicerata**, gains its name from the fact that the first pair of the normally six pairs of appendages develop grasping jaws known as chelicerae. There are three classes. The class **Pycnogonida** is represented by the sea-spiders which may be found at the bottom of the littoral zone; the class **Merostomata** includes the King or Horse-shoe 'crabs' (*Limulus*) whose simple compound eyes have provided very important preparations for sensory physiologists; finally a large and important class, the class **Arachnida**, contains the spiders, scorpions, harvestmen, mites and ticks. The sense organs of spiders (order *Araneae*), especially tactile hairs and, in some cases, ocellar eyes, have evolved to a very high sensitivity and we shall discuss them in some detail in Chapters 8 and 15.

The phylum **Echinodermata** (starfish, sea urchins, sea-cucumbers, etc.) are widely diverse, radially symmetrical and have a fascinating zoology but they do not provide any of the sense organs we discuss in this book. However, as Figure 4.3 shows, they are the closest evolutionary relatives of the Chordates and, when the genome of a sea urchin, *Strogylocentrus purpuratus*, was sequenced, fascinating biochemical similarities between the elementary sensory systems of their tube feet and our own hugely sophisticated sensory systems were discovered (Chapter 5). Let us, however, move directly to what is, for our purposes, the last significant phylum, the phylum **Chordata**. As this phylum includes *Homo sapiens* many will feel that it is the most significant phylum of them all. But as our rapid review has made clear it is in fact but one phylum of many, and, with some 45 000 species, one of the smallest. It includes all the mammals, reptiles, birds, amphibia and fish (i.e. all the vertebrates) and a few obscure groups of invertebrates commonly lumped together as protochordates. As we noted above, the chordates are deuterostomes and, as their vertebral columns clearly show, segmented. They may be defined by the possession (at some stage in their life history) of three features: (i) a **dorsal hollow nerve cord**; (ii) beneath the nerve cord but above the gut a stiff rod, the **notochord**, which in the vertebrates becomes transformed into a vertebral column; (iii) the presence of **gill clefts** at some stage in development, connecting the pharynx with the exterior.

The most widely accepted classification subdivides the chordates into four subphyla: two acraniate subphyla – the **Tunicata (=Urochordata)** and the **Cephalochordata**, and two craniate subphyla the **Agnatha** and the **Gnathostomata**. The latter two subphyla together constitute the 'vertebrates'. Most adult tunicates are sessile forms, many of which, such as the sea squirts, *Ciona intestinalis*, inhabit the littoral zone. Only the larval stage, which resembles a tadpole, develops a notochord, nerve cord and gill clefts. Members of one order, the Appendicularia, however, remains pelagic throughout their lives and resemble the ascidian 'tadpole'. The cephalochordates are represented by *Amphioxus lanceolatus*, the lancelet, a small (less than 5 cm long) slug-like form, tapered at each end, which lives, filter-feeding, half-buried in sea bed sediments. It shows many of the features which would be expected of a generalized primordial chordate possessing a dorsal nerve cord, notochord and gill slits throughout its adult life. The largely sessile life-style of *Amphioxus* suggests it may have 'degenerated' from a more free-swimming ancestor. Although there is no real anterior expansion of the anterior part of the nerve cord which deserves the name of brain, *Amphioxus* nevertheless develops, as we shall see, some interesting, if rudimentary, sense organs (Figure 4.10). The two craniate subphyla contain all the familiar vertebrate animals. Their probable evolutionary relationships are shown in Figure 4.4.

The subphylum **Agnatha** consists mainly of extinct fossil forms which lack both jaws and paired appendages. The only living representatives be-

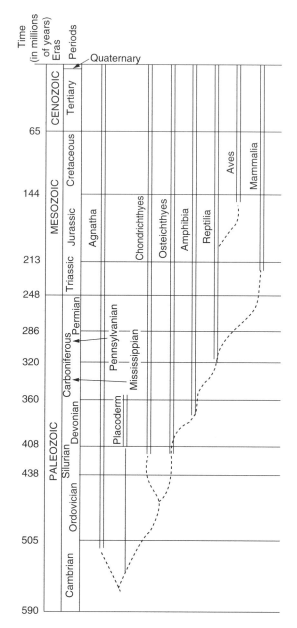

Figure 4.4 Probable evolutionary relationships amongst the vertebrates. After Caroll, R.L. (1988).

long to the class **Cyclostomata**, the lampreys and hagfish.

The subphylum **Gnathostomata**, possessing jaws and paired appendages, are subdivided into two superclasses – the superclass *Pisces* containing all the fish and the superclass **Tetrapoda**.

The living **Pisces** are subdivided into two great classes, the **Chondrichthyes** and the **Osteichthyes**. The class Chondrichthyes (=Elasmobranchii) consists of all the cartilaginous fish with rough dentinous placoid scales and is represented by the sharks, dogfish, skates, rays (including the electric ray, *Torpedo*) and saw fish. The class Osteichthyes contains all the bony fish. These develop bony scales known as cycloid or ctenoid depending on whether their edges are smooth or jagged. In numbers of species and variety of form the Osteichthyes are far more successful than the Chondrichthyes. Probably the most successful of all the orders of bony fish is the order **Teleostei**, the teleost fish, which includes herring, trout, salmon, carp, eels, flying fish, sticklebacks and so on.

The **Tetrapoda** are subdivided into four large classes: class **Amphibia**; class **Reptilia**; class **Aves** and class **Mammalia**. As shown in Figure 4.4, the **Amphibia** are the earliest of these four classes. Fossil forms can be traced back almost four hundred million years into the Devonian period. Contemporary amphibia belong to three distinctive subclasses: subclass **Urodela** (the newts, salamanders, etc.; subclass **Anura** (the frogs and toads); subclass **Apoda** (limbless, blind, burrowing, tropical forms).

The class **Reptilia** develop from eggs which, unlike those of the Amphibia, possess an amniotic membrane which adapts them to survive on land. The reptiles are thus the first fully terrestrial vertebrates. Zoologists sometimes use the term **amniotes** as a collective noun to describe the fully terrestrial vertebrates (reptiles, birds and mammals) in contrast to the **anamniotes** (amphibia and fish) which, lacking an amniotic membrane, necessarily spend part or all of their life cycle in water. There are many orders of extinct reptiles (including of course those terrible lizards, the Dinosaurs) but only four living orders: the **Crocodilia**, the **Chelonia** (tortoises and turtles) the **Rhychocephalia** (**Spenodon**) and the **Squamata**. (lizards, monitors, iguanas, snakes, etc.). The snakes, which are believed to have lost their limbs through a long period of subterranean living, have developed (in some cases redeveloped) some of the most interesting of vertebrate sense organs.

The class **Aves** are often regarded as feathered reptiles. There are over 9000 living species found in all parts of the world and in practically all habitats. As would be expected from their highly active lifestyles, the birds have evolved some of the most highly sophisticated sensory systems that the planet has known.

The class **Mammalia** is conventionally subdivided into three subclasses: the subclass **Prototheria** (**Monotremata**); the subclass **Allotheria** (all extinct) and the subclass **Theria** which is divided again into three infraclasses, the **Pantotheria** (extinct), the **Metatheria (Marsupialiana)** and the **Eutheria (Placentalia)**. The subclass **Prototheria** includes the egg-laying mammals of Australasia – the duck-billed platypus (*Ornithorhynchus*) and the spiny ant-eater (*Tachyglossus*). The subclass **Metatheria** are again largely confined to Australasia but there are some North and South American species. They are distinguished by possessing an exterior pouch for nurturing the young, which are born very immature. The subclass **Eutheria** consists of all the modern mammalian orders – the Insectivora (hedgehogs, shrews, moles, tree shrews, etc.), the Chiroptera (bats), the Rodentia (rats, mice, etc.), the Lagomorpha (rabbits and hares), the Carnivora (cats, dogs, bears, weasels, seals), the Cetacea (whales, dolphins, porpoises), the Perissodactyla (horses) and Artiodactyla (cattle, pigs, etc.), to name just a few, and, of course, the Primates to which we, together with the lemurs, tarsiers, bush-babies, new and old world monkeys and the apes, belong.

4.7 EVOLUTION OF NERVOUS SYSTEMS

The evolution of animal nervous systems is a vast topic. All that is intended (and all that can be achieved in the space available) is a brief introduction for those who have not had the benefit of an introductory course in biology or zoology. The origin of animal nervous systems is likely to remain speculative, as soft tissues, although they may leave impressions in sedimentary rocks, leave no fossils and **a fortiori** no information about cellular function. Examination of the most primitive motile forms may, however, yield a clue. The reproductive medusae of the hydrozoa show that depolarizing potentials spread through large sheets of epithelial tissue, helping to coordinate the pulsatile movements of the bell. Thus it is suggested that nervous systems originated from epithelial tissues whose cells intercommuncate by tight junctions or **electrical synapses** (Section 2.7). This suggests that electrical synapses preceded the chemical variety which are so much more prominent in the nervous systems of the 'higher' animals, especially the vertebrates.

4.7.1 Cnidaria

In addition to the passage of depolarizing potentials directly through epithelial sheets the Cnidaria have developed a reticulated nervous system known as a **nerve net**. This is developed not only in the bells of jelly fish but also in sessile bodies of sea anemones and fresh water polyps such as *Hydra* (Figure 4.5a). Here neurons conduct impulses in both directions making 'en passant' synapses with each other (Figure 4.5b). In consequence, impulses spread in every direction from a stimulated point and the body contracts in a unified manner.

4.7.2 Platyhelminthes

As indicated in Section 4.4, the next major step in animal evolution was the development of bilateral symmetry. Nothing in biology is simple and clear cut. Genetic evidence indicates that genes involved in the production of bilateral symmetry exist in the Cnidaria. Indeed, molecular analysis has recently shown that an active, muscular, parasitic worm, *Buddenbrockia plumatellae*, is in fact a Cnidarian. This suggests that bilaterality may have arisen by selection for efficient internal circulation rather than, or perhaps as well as, for locomotion. Did bilateral symmetry exist in the Cnidaria during Precambrian times only to be lost in the vast majority of modern forms? We do not know. At present, however, the most primitive bilateral forms are represented by **platyhelminth turbellaria** (flatworms) where one end faces forward during locomotion. Clusters of sense organs (including eye spots) develop on this forward end as it is generally the first part of the worm to encounter new environments. Associated with the sense organs a bilateral cerebral ganglion or primitive brain develops to analyse the information picked up by the senses; from this, one, or usually two or more, nerve trunks run back along the rest of the worm's body. Numerous transverse fibres run between the two nerve cords giving a ladder-like appearance (Figure 4.6).

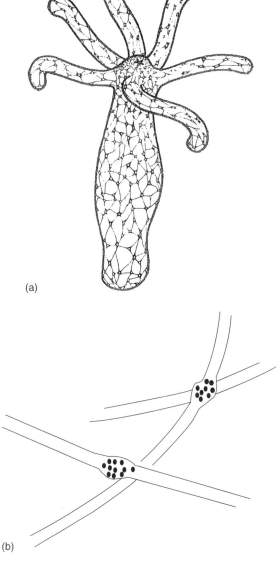

(a)

(b)

Figure 4.5 Nerve net and 'en passant' synapses. (a): Hydra to show nerve net. Note the concentration around the mouth. (b) 'en passant' synapses in nerve net. The synaptic varicosities contain numerous dense-cored vesicles.

4.7.3 Nematoda

Nematodes, of which the best known is the exhaustively studied *Caenorhabditis elegans*, also have exceedingly simple nervous systems. There is no

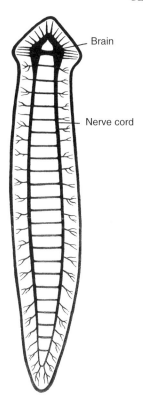

Figure 4.6 Turbellarian (flatworm) 'ladder' nervous system. From Buchsbaum, R. (1948) *Animals without Backbones*. Copyright © 1948 University of Chicago Press.

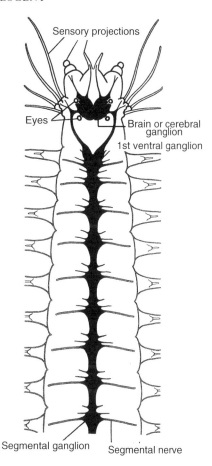

Figure 4.7 Nervous system of the polychaete worm, Nereis. From Buchsbaum, R. (1948) *Animals without Backbones*. Copyright © 1948 University of Chicago Press.

defined cerebral ganglion or 'brain', only a circumoesophageal commissure or 'nerve ring' made up of four ganglia surrounding the oesophagous from which six posterior nerves and six anterior nerve cords spring. Like the nervous system the sensory system is also very simple. The most obvious features are a pair of 'amphids' near the mouth and, a pair of 'phasmids' situated in a lateral position. Both these structures are believed to be chemosensory. Tactile cilia are developed at the anterior end of the body.

4.7.4 Annelida

In contrast to the nematodes, the free-living annelids (segmented worms) develop much more complex nervous systems. They all share an underlying design in which a cerebral ganglion is located at the anterior end. This is connected to a ventral

nerve cord by circumpharyngeal connectives that run round each side of the pharynx (Figure 4.7). The ventral nerve cord consists, primitively, of two pairs of nerve tracts which run the length of the body. In more advanced members of the phylum, these two cords become fused to form a single longitudinal tract. The cord expands in each segment to form a ganglion from which segmental nerves run to innervate the body musculature and intestine. Sensory organs are, as usual, concentrated at the anterior end of the body. The polychaetes often possess quite well developed eyes; statocysts are also found in association with the cerebral ganglion; touch sensivity is spread over the body surface and in some cases concentrated in so-called 'lateral organs'.

Polychaetes also develop chemosensory nuchal organs, innervated from the posterior part of the cerebral ganglion. The nervous systems of oligochaetes such as earthworms are nowhere near as well developed as that of the polychaetes but, nevertheless, are still recognizably of fundamentally the same design, whilst those of the Hirudinea (leeches) are much reduced and specialized for their ectoparasitic life style.

4.7.5 Arthropoda

The arthropods are a highly diverse group of organisms yet their nervous systems are all built on a basic underlying plan. This plan is, in essence, similar to that of the annelids to which they are believed to be evolutionarily related. A dorsal brain, or cerebral ganglion, is connected to a ventral nerve cord by a pair of circumoesophageal commissures. The nerve cord is developed into ganglia in each segment and segmental nerves run out to the body musculature and intestine.

Clearly this plan is much modified in different members of this largest of all phyla. Thus, although decapod crustaceans such as prawns, shrimps and lobsters have typical arthropod nervous systems as described above, their close relatives, the crabs, have condensed the system into two large ganglia: a cerebral ganglion between the eyes and an even larger thoracic ganglion located in the middle of the body. Centipedes and millipedes, on the other hand, although developing relatively large surpraoesophageal ganglia, retain a characteristic ganglionated ventral nerve cord connected to the supraoesophageal ganglia by a pair of circumoesophageal commissures. In the spiders the ganglia are concentrated once again, this time into the cephalothorax, where two major ganglia develop – the supra and suboesophageal ganglia. The supraoesaphageal ganglion is generally regarded as the most important as sense organs throughout the body are connected to it.

Lastly the insects show a great number of variations on the underlying theme. In the general case this theme is quite evident (Figure 4.8a). The brain is

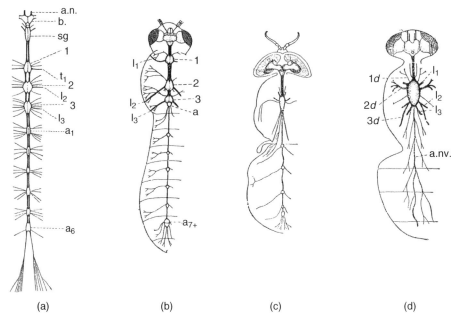

Figure 4.8   Insect nervous systems to show increasing 'concentration'. (a) *Forficula* (earwig); (b) *Chironomus* (midge); *Stratiomya* (fly); (d) *Musca* (tachinid housefly). 1, 2, 3 = thoracic ganglia; 1d, 2d, 3d = dorsal thoracic nerves; $a_1 \ldots a_6$ abdominal ganglia; a.n = antennary nerve; a.nv = abdominal nerve cord; b = brain (surpra-oesophageal ganglion); l_1, l_2, l_3 = nerves to legs; sg = suboesophageal ganglion. Modified from Imms, (1946).

composed of three paired ganglia fused together, the protocerebrum, the deuterocerebrum and the tritocerebrum. The protocerebrum is largely concerned with vision. It is also believed to be involved with higher cognitive functions, such as memory. From it spring a couple of indented structures which, because of their shape, are known as 'mushroom bodies' or corpora pedunculata. The deuterocerebrum is concerned with information collected by the antennae whilst the tritocerebrum integrates sensory inputs from the other two parts of the brain. The tritocerebrum also links the brain with another complex of fused ganglia, the suboesophageal ganglion, and the rest of the nervous system by (as usual) a pair of circumoesophageal commissures. The suboesophageal ganglion, which is believed to consist of three fused ganglia, controls the insect's mouth parts, salivary glands and neck muscles. Behind the suboesophageal ganglion a ganglionated, paired nerve cord runs through the thorax and abdomen to terminate in a pair of abdominal ganglia which often fuse to give a single caudal ganglion. This ganglion innervates the anus, genitalia and sensory receptors, such as cerci, found at the insect's posterior end.

In some insects, for instance *Musca domestica*, the housefly, the nervous system becomes yet more concentrated (Figure 4.8d). The primitive chain of three thoracic ganglia become fused to form a single large ganglion which controls both flight and walking movements and many other functions of the thoracic and abdominal regions, for there are no abdominal ganglia.

All arthropods, and especially insects, are provided with a wide range of sensory systems and many of these will be discussed in later chapters. These include not only exquisitely sensitive touch and chemical senses but also intricate photoreceptors which are not only sensitive to light of wavelengths which humans and most other animals cannot detect but in some cases are also able to detect the plane of polarization.

4.7.6 Mollusca

The molluscs, like the arthropods, are also an extremely diverse and extremely large phylum (perhaps over 100 000 species), ranging from simple chitons to highly complex and active squids and octopi. Their nervous and sensory systems are in consequence highly diverse. Nevertheless, an underlying design is discernable. This underlying design is not too dissimilar to that of the turbellarian flatworms. Indeed, the chiton nervous system is hardly an advance on that of the flatworms (Figure 4.9a). A nerve ring surrounds the oesophagus and two nerve chords run down each side of the body from which numerous nerves run out to innervate the foot muscle. Many chitons develop primitive eyes, indeed in some species several thousand minute eyes are found, detectable as black spots on their shells.

The gastropod nervous system still shows traces of the chiton ladder-like design. It is shown in Figure 4.9b. Although it is complicated by the spiral form of the shell, which twists it into a figure of eight, it can still be seen to be basically a ladder-like structure. As the figure shows, it is distinctly ganglionated with cerebral, pleural and pedal ganglia surrounding the oesophagus, a parietal ganglia controlling the posterior part of the foot and visceral ganglia controlling the intestine. In many gastropods, for instance the pulmonates, which include the snails and slugs, several of these ganglia have fused together, creating a more unified system. Gastropods are well supplied with sense organs and often have well developed eyes. Their most characteristic sense organ, which they share with other mollusks, is however the osphradium. This is an olfactory organ consisting of elongated sensory cells associated with the mollusc's gills and thus able to sample the water currents passing over the gills during respiration.

The bivalve nervous system is simpler that that found in the gastropods, as it does not have to contend with the torsion of the body. It still retains the foundational bilateral architecture. There are three pairs of ganglia and two pairs of lengthy nerve cords or commissures (Figure 4.9c). The cerebropleural ganglia are placed on both sides of the oesophagus, a pair of visceral ganglia are located close to the posterior adductor muscle and a pair of pedal ganglia are located in the foot. Bivalves are well supplied with sense organs. An osphradium is located in the exhalant siphon close to the posterior adductor muscle, a statocyst (gravity sensor) develops close to the pedal ganglion and simple eyes are usually found lining the edge of the mantle or on the siphons. These eyes become quite well developed in the Pectinidae and they will be discussed further in Section 15.2.3.

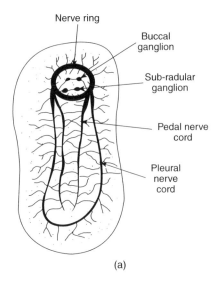

(a)

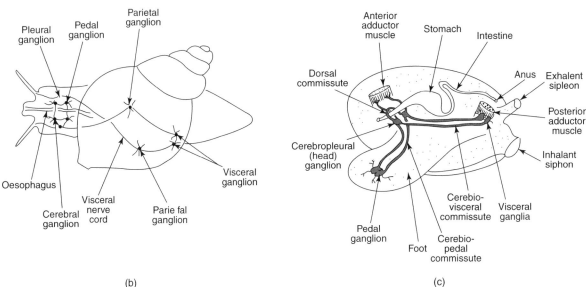

(b)   (c)

Figure 4.9   Mollusc nervous systems: (a) Chiton. A nerve ring surrounds the oesophagus and is thickened anteriorly but not differentiated into ganglia. Connectives run from the ring to buccal and subradular ganglia. Posteriorly there are two sets of nerve cords, the pedal and pleural cords. From these cords numerous connectives and other fibres branch to the body's musculature. (b) Gastropod. A ganglionated nerve ring surrounds the oesophagus. The cerebral and pleural ganglia are in the dorsal position and nerve fibres run from the cerebral ganglia to the eyes and tentacles. Beneath the oesophagus a pair of pedal ganglia control the musculature in the anterior part of the foot. From the pleural ganglia nerve cords, or connectives, run back to parietal ganglia controlling the posterior part of the foot and to visceral ganglia which innervate the intestine. Gastropods are many and various and the system described here has many variations. (c) Bivalve. A pair of cerebropleural ganglia are connected above the gut by a dorsal commissure. A pair of cerebro-pedal commissures run to the pedal ganglia, which are normally fused. These control the foot. Another pair of commissures, the cerebro-visceral commissure, run to the paired visceral ganglia located on the posterior adductor muscle. These ganglia are, again, often fused together.

The cephalopods are the most highly evolved and active of all the molluscs and, indeed, are often regarded as the peak of invertebrate evolution. They have a cartilaginous brain case and well developed brains and central nervous systems. Their sensory systems are similarly highly evolved. We shall discuss their well developed eyes in Chapter 15. They possess large gravity-detecting statocysts on each side of the brain case. Their sense of touch is also highly evolved, being most acute at the rim of each tentacular sucker.

4.7.7 Echinodermata

The Echinoderms, like the Cnidaria, exhibit radial symmetry. Although, like the Cnidaria, they do not possess a central nervous system or anything resembling a brain (although small ganglia are found in some species), they nevertheless have evolved an intricate radial nervous system which lies in and just below the skin. The oesophagus is surrounded by one or more nerve rings from which run radial nerves that, in the case of star fish and brittle stars, innervate the arms. This system allows coordinated body movement (righting when flipped over) and also integrates the action of the multitudinous tube feet when crawling over a substratum. As noted earlier, when the genome of a sea urchin (*Strongylocentrotus purpuratus*) was deciphered it was found that it contained a number of genes coding for neurosensory circuits in the tube feet. These genes showed striking similarities to some of those coding for sensory functions in humans. Echinoderms, like chordates, are deuterostomes and are hence believed to be (very) distant cousins (Figure 4.3).

4.7.8 Chordata

The design of the chordate nervous system is radically different from that of the other bilateral forms we have reviewed. Firstly, instead of consisting of one or more solid nerve cords with an anterior cerebral ganglion or brain, it consists of a single hollow nerve tube which is expanded at its anterior end to form a vesicular brain. There is no trace of a ladder-like origin. Secondly, and most importantly, instead

of running along the ventral surface of the animal beneath the gut, it is positioned in the mid-dorsal position above the gut and above the notochord. There has been much controversy over whether a chordate (a deuterostome in contrast to the protostome nature of the other major animal groups) can be regarded as an invertebrate rotated 180° on its long axis. This idea first surfaced in the nineteenth century and has received significant support from twenty-first century studies of developmental genetics. These twenty-first century studies indeed suggest that all central nervous systems share a common origin in the Precambrian period.

This is no place to enter a detailed discussion of the evolution of the chordate central nervous system. There is good evidence that *Amphioxus* and the ascidian larvae of tunicates provide reliable pointers to the ancestral neurosensory systems of all chordates. Both possess primordia of a dorsal hollow nerve cord and the beginnings of an anterior vesicular brain. So far as sensory systems are concerned, both the ascidian 'tadpole' and amphioxus develop eye spots, statocysts and olfactory tissue. The eye spot, or ocellus, of *Ciona intestinalis* consists of a group of ciliary-type photoreceptor cells surrounded by a large pigment-containing cell. The 'lamellar body' of *Amphioxus* is thought to be a homologue of the vertebrate pineal body, whilst its 'frontal eye' (also associated with a pigmented eye spot) is related to the paired eyes of vertebrates (Figure 4.10). The recent sequencing of the genome of *Ciona intestinalis*, an ascidian, has thus been particularly valuable for those interested in chordate origins (Chapter 5) and the *Amphioxus* genome is eagerly awaited.

From these simple beginnings the hugely complex brains and sensory systems of humans and other vertebrates have evolved. They will be discussed at length in the following chapters.

4.8 CONCLUDING REMARKS

At the conclusion of this rapid survey is it possible to make any generalizations? Some have thought that the array of living forms which presently populate the planet's surface are the result of pure happenstance. They *could* have been very different from what they in fact are, both in form and function. Stephen Gould has popularized this view with his account

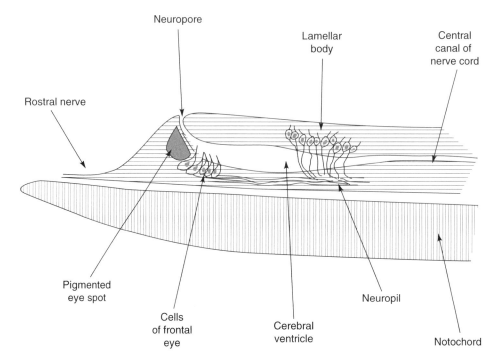

Figure 4.10 Anterior nerve cord of *Amphioxus* larva to show the organization of the photoreceptor apparatus. Both the frontal eye and the lamellar body consist of ciliated cells. The neuropore closes in the adult. After Holland and Holland (1999) and Lacalli (2007).

of the weird and wonderful fossils to be found in the Burgess Shale deposits of 525 million years ago. Others, especially Conway Morris, have pointed to the fact that only a few great groups of animal forms have successfully won through to the present day. Our review has shown that three major designs have proved overwhelmingly successful: the Mollusca, the Arthropoda (especially the insects) and the Chordata. No doubt there is nothing preordained about detail, or that any particular species should emerge, including that most interesting of all species, *Homo*

sapiens, but perhaps the perpetual sifting of natural selection finds that only certain basic body plans provide starting points from which to develop forms able to persist through a billion year time span. In the following pages, although due deference is given to our own self-absorption by devoting most space to mammalian, indeed human, sensory systems, comparisons will frequently be made with those other two great solutions to the problems of surviving the billion year period of animal life on earth: the Mollusca and the Arthropoda.

5

GENES, GENOMICS AND NEUROSENSORY SYSTEMS

Definitions – chromosome nomenclature – genes – point mutations – nomenclature – completed genomes – genomes and neurosensory systems – genomes on the path to mankind – concluding remarks

5.1 INTRODUCTION

A **genome** is defined as the entire hereditary information carried by an organism. So far as the animal kingdom is concerned this information is carried in the DNA sequence of one set of chromosomes. Some organelles – mitochondria, chloroplasts – have their own non-chromosomal DNA. Thus it is possible to speak of mitochondrial and/or chloroplast genomes. The study of this totality is called **genomics** to distinguish it from genetics which, in contrast, largely studies single genes and their interactions.

The structure of DNA and the various techniques for determining the sequence of nucleotide bases from which it is built are outside the remit of this book. The student is referred to the many excellent texts on biochemistry and molecular biology for information on this topic. It is worth, however, noting a few salient features of the human genome. It consists of 22 pairs of autosomal chromosomes and a pair of sex chromosomes, XX in females, XY in males. Each chromosome constricts to a **centromere** more or less half way along its length. During cell division spindle fibres attach to the centromere so that the two chromatids can be drawn to opposite poles

of the cell before the cytoplasm divides. The ends of the chromosome also have specialized structures and functions and are called **telomeres**.

As the centromere is only more or less in the middle, it divides the chromosome into a short arm called '**p**' and a long arm called '**q**', Chromosomes are not normally visible in the nuclei of eukaryotic cells. They only condense just before cell division. When this happens, they can be stained with a dye such as the Giemsa stain, which brings out a specific pattern of bands that can be seen in the optical microscope (Figure 5.1). The bands, known as **G-bands** for the Giemsa stain, are numbered on each arm from the centromere towards the telomere. The rough position of each gene on a chromosome is given with respect to one or other of these numbered bands. Thus the gene which in humans is responsible (when mutated) for the most common form of Usher syndrome (hereditary deaf–blindness) is located on the long arm of chromosome 1 on band 41, that is 1q41, whilst that for the congenital deafness presenting as Jervell and Lange–Nielsen syndrome (JLNS1) is found on the long arm of chromosome 21 between bands 22.1 and 22.2, that is 21q22.1-q22.2.

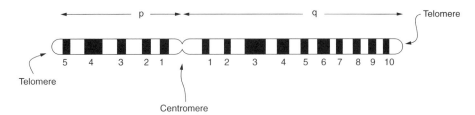

Figure 5.1 Chromosome nomenclature. Each Giemsa band is numbered from the centromere outward towards the telomere. In reality a human chromosome would have far more bands than those shown in the figure. Further explanation in text.

But what is a gene? A quick search of the world-wide web reveals a multitude of definitions. They range from a DNA sequence which carries information from one generation to the next, to the name of an English rock group which became prominent in the mid-1990s. Here we shall restrict ourselves to the first definition. Most genes encode proteins. Each amino acid in a protein is specified by a triplet of nucleotides (or **codon**) and the sequence of nucleotides making up the coding strand of DNA is 'read' continuously from 'left' (5′) to 'right' (3′). As proteins often consist of many hundred amino acid residues the nucleotide sequence is often over well over a thousand units in length. Even so there is much so-called 'junk' DNA between one gene and the next (but see Section 5.2). Although the human genome consists of 3.2 thousand million base-pairs (3.2 Gb) there are only about 22 000 genes (Table 5.1) . Simple arithmetic shows that only about 10% of the DNA strand consists of genes.

Each coding sequence that makes up a gene consists of stretches (**exons**) which potentially code for the amino acid sequence of a protein, interrupted by stretches (**introns**) which have no such function (Figure 5.2). The first step in the process by which the sequence information held in DNA is used to specify an amino acid sequence is known as **transcription**. In this process the nucleotide sequence (base sequence), including both introns and exons, is transcribed into a matching sequence in **messenger RNA (mRNA)**. This is known as the **primary transcript**. When this has occurred the introns are excised and the exons spliced together. The resultant mRNA (and there is much scope for differential resplicing) travels to a ribosome for **translation** into protein. The first and last exons also contain 'start' and 'stop' sequences and are not translated into protein (Figure 5.2).

Although most of the proteins synthesized at the ribosome are enzymes and other components of a cell, some act back on the DNA controlling the

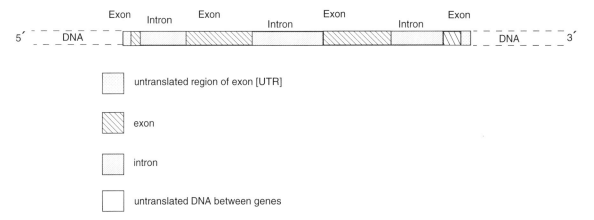

Figure 5.2 Gene structure. The gene is transcribed from the 5′ to the 3′ end into mRNA. Introns are excised and exons respliced before translation into the amino acid primary structure of a protein at a ribosome. The untranslated regions (UTRs) act as start and termination signals and also control the rate at which translation occurs.

BOX 5.1 NOMENCLATURE OF GENES AND PROTEINS

Molecular biology is a huge and diverse subject. As in all areas of science it has developed its own vocabulary and conventions. This is of vital importance if scientists and others are to understand each other. This Box outlines some of the vocabulary used in this book.

Proteins, as we have noted, are, in essence, long chains whose links are amino acid residues. The chain may have over a thousand links though, more usually, only several hundred. The amino acid links are **numbered** from the N-terminal to the C-terminal end of the chain.

There are twenty different amino acids each with its own biochemical characteristics and name. These names are usually abbreviated to three letters: Glycine → gly; Threonine → thr; Tyrosine → tyr; Proline → pro; Phenylalanine → phe and so on. In addition, for yet further compactness, each amino acid is also assigned an uppercase letter symbol: Glycine → G; Threonine → T; Tyrosine → Y; Proline → P; Phenylalanine → F. Complete lists can be found in all good biochemistry texts.

The names of genes are also abbreviated into a two, three or four letter code. Thus, for example, the genes which control mechanosensitivity in *C. elegans* (Chapter 8) are abbreviated as *mec* genes. As there are a number of these genes they are given suffixes, – *mec-1*, *mec-2* and so on. The convention is to **italicize genes** and to write their protein products in Roman type. Thus the *mec-1* gene codes for a mec-1 protein. It is customary, also, to write vertebrate genes with an initial capital and human genes in capital letters throughout. Thus one of the genes important in the development of eyes (Box 15.2) is written as *pax-6* in *Drosophila*, *Pax-6* in *Mus* and *PAX-6* in *Homo*. It is not always possible to adhere to these conventions but where it is they should be employed.

activity of the genes. This they do by attaching themselves to **regulatory regions – promoters** of various types, **enhancers** and **silencers** – which switch on or off, or up- or down-regulate transcription of a gene. The molecular biology is highly complex and students should consult one or other of the biochemistry/molecular biology texts recommended in the Bibliography.

Genes are subject to mutation. There are various types but the most common are '*point*' mutations where one nucleotide base is changed for another. As each triplet of nucleotides codes for an amino acid, any change can lead to a different amino acid being specified. There are two cases. If the substituted amino acid is the same as the original it is called a **synonymous mutation**. If it differs from the original it is called a **non-synonymous mutation**.

The difference between the two types of mutation arises from the degeneracy of the genetic code. In many cases, two or more codons code for the same amino acid. GGU, GGC, GGA and GGG, for instance, all code for Glycine. It follows that if the third place U mutates to C, A or G, Glycine will still be specified thus giving a synonymous mutation. If,

however, second place G mutates to A giving GAU then Aspartic acid is specified, and if second place G mutates to A giving GAG then Glutamic acid is specified – both non-synonymous mutations.

Non-synonymous point mutations, along with gene duplications, are the stuff of evolutionary change. We shall meet many cases as we go through this book. If we can make plausible estimates of the rate at which these mutations occur, we can calculate the time which has elapsed from the duplication event (see glossary) which generated a pair of homologues.

Molecular biologists have developed a convenient shorthand to indicate where a non-synonymous point mutation has occurred in a polypeptide chain. For instance, **gly$_{234}$→asp**, or **G234A**, signifies that glycine has been replaced by aspartic acid at position 234 in the chain. Note that the symbolism is read from left to right: the original amino acid is on the left, the substitution on the right. We shall come across many examples of this shorthand in the following chapters, especially when we discuss some of the molecular causes of sensory pathologies.

A final type of point mutation occurs when a nucleotide base is deleted altogether. The base sequence to the 'right' of the mutation (remember the sequence is continuously read, as if with a reading frame, from left to right in groups of three) is consequently altered. It follows that all the amino acids to the right of the mutation are also altered and the protein, far more likely than not, will be functionless. This type of mutation is known as a '**frame shift**' mutation.

5.2 COMPARATIVE GENOMICS

After these preliminaries let us look at what the sequencing of genomes has told us about the molecular bases of sensory systems. In a short chapter it is impossible to do more than scratch the surface. It is, nevertheless, worth remarking that the sequencing of genomes is one of the brilliancies of twenty-first century biology. It is a huge technical accomplishment, involving not only highly sophisticated molecular biology but also cutting-edge computer science. It is a multi-million dollar enterprise, involving huge teams of highly qualified researchers.

The first genomes were sequenced in the 1980s. At first small organisms and organelles – viruses, archaebacteria, eubacteria, mitochondria – were analysed. Subsequently, the far larger genomes of eukaryotic organisms, including many members of the animal kingdom, were sequenced. In a sense the enterprise culminated in 2003 with the final draft of the human genome, exactly fifty years after Watson and Crick published their ground-breaking paper. This final draft is stated to be 99.9% accurate, in other words less than one error in 10 000 base pairs. This is, of course, a remarkable achievement. The human genome consists of 3.2 Gb (3.2 thousand million base pairs), so that just to read off the sequence at one base pair a second without break for food or sleep would take rather more than a hundred years. Sequencing did not, however, stop in 2003. Quite the opposite. New methods, new techniques, new equipment have ensured that the flow of genomes completed and published has tended to increase rather than decrease. Table 5.1 shows the metazoan genomes published up to but not including 2008.

The completed genomes shown in Table 5.1 are no more than the tip of an iceberg. Literally hundred of genomes are in process of being sequenced including dozens of vertebrates. By the time this second edition is published many more will be in the public domain and many more insights into the evolutionary process gained.

Even the sparse data given in Table 5.1 hold some surprises. It has been found, for instance, that there is extensive genomic similarity between *Nematostella*, the tiny starlet anemone, and modern vertebrates. Indeed, because insects and nematodes have lost many genes and jumbled others together, the anemone genome resembles those of the vertebrates more than it does those of these other 'lowlier' forms. This emphasizes once again the astonishing antiquity of our genetic foundation and points up the huge evolutionary developments that must have occurred during the 2000 Megayear 'dark ages' of the Precambrian. Only after this immense period had elapsed was a base genome available from which the animal kingdom could evolve. The genes of the Cnidaria appear to be at the root of whole families of genes in more recently evolved organisms. As Figure 4.3 shows, the last common ancestor of the vertebrates and the Cnidaria is believed to have lived before bilaterality had been 'invented'. Indeed, as we saw in Section 4.6, some of the earliest fossil remains are those of these stem cnidarians.

When a comparison is made with Protistan genomes, it is satisfactory to find that many of the novel genes in the sea anemone have to do with communication between cells and the development and functioning of the neuromuscular system. Thus we find genes coding for various aspects of synaptic transmission and muscular contraction – nicotinic acetylcholine receptors (nAChRs), calcium ion channels and so on – are either new developments, having no known homologues in Protistan genomes, or modifications of earlier Protistan genes by the addition of so-called 'animal only' domains. Full details of these profound developments may be found in the papers cited in the bibliography.

Although, as we noted above, insects have lost many of the genes in the original metazoan blueprint as represented by *Nematostella*, they nevertheless still share a major portion of their genomes with vertebrates. Fruit flies, for instance, share about 60% of their genomes with humans. Once again we can only marvel at the stability of the genome: fruit flies and humans have gone their own separate ways for well over 500 million years (Figure 4.3). The core genome, once 'invented', persists; it is merely modified and elaborated over vast periods. The members

Table 5.1 Metazoan genomes

Organism predicted	Genome	No. of genes
Phylum Cnidaria		
Class Anthozoa		
Nematostella vectensis (starlet sea anemone)	450 Mb	18 000
Phylum Nematoda		
Class Secernetea		
Caenorhabditis elegans	97 Mb	19 000
Caenorhabdidtis briggsae (for comparison with *C. elegans*)	104 Mb	19 500
Phylum Arthropoda		
Class Insecta		
Aedes aegypti (Yellow fever mosquito)	1376.0 Mb	15 419
Anopheles gambiae (Malaria mosquito)	272.9 Mb	13 111
Apis mellifera (Honeybee)	236 Mb	10 157
Bombyx mori (Moth)	530 Mb	18 500
Drosophila melanogaster (Fruit fly)[a]	117 Mb	13 718
Phylum Echinodermata		
Class Echinoidea		
Strongylocentrotus purpuratus (sea urchin)	814 Mb	23 300
Phylum Chordata		
Subphylum Tunicata		
Class Ascidiacea		
Ciona intestinalis	116.7 Mb	16 000
Subphylum Gnathostomata		
Class Osteichthyes		
Danio rerio (Zebra fish)	1.7 Gb	—
Takifugu rubripes (Puffer fish)	390 Mb	22–29 000
Tetraodon nigroviridis (Puffer fish)	385 Mb	—
Class Aves		
Gallus gallus (Chicken)	1 Gb	20–23 000
Class Mammalia		
Subclass Metatheria		
Mondodelphus domestica (Opossum)	3.475 Gb	18–20 000
Subclass Eutheria		
Mus musculus (Mouse)	2.5 Gb	24 174
Rattus norvegicus (Rat)	2.75 Gb	21 166
Canis familiaris (Dog)	2.4 Gb	19 300
Macaca mulatto (Rhesus monkey)	2.87 Gb	20 000
Pan troglodytes (Chimpanzee)	3.1 Gb	—
Homo sapiens (Human)	3.2 Gb	22 000

Further detail is given in the papers cited in the Bibliography.
[a]The genomes of 12 other species of Drosophila have been sequenced ranging from *D. grimshawi* with six chromosomes and 201 Mb of DNA to *D. pseudoobscura* with four chromosomes (the more usual complement) and 156 Mb of DNA.

of the living world, wrote Darwin in the nineteenth century, 'may all be netted together': genomics has confirmed his vision at a deeper level than even he could have imagined.

Another surprise presented by genomic research is the finding that although the human genome is the lengthiest in the list (indeed one of the lengthiest presently known) the number of genes it encodes is no larger than that of several other genomes. This was unexpected. It had been assumed that with increasing biological complexity the number of genes would necessarily increase. Before the publication of the human genome, estimates often suggested it would be found to contain some 100 000 genes. To find that the number of genes scarcely exceeded that presented by the lowly nematode worm and, in fact, falls far short of the 60 000 or so in the Japanese rice plant (*Oryza sativa japonica*) came as something of a shock. However, it needs to be borne in mind that genes are not the end of the story. Genes have many different roles to play in biology. Even the information encoded in the so-called 'structural' genes which code for the body's structural elements, the proteins, undergoes complex manipulation before the protein is synthesized. The primary transcript is cut and respliced, introns are removed, exons shuffled and rejoined, so that, on average, each human gene is responsible for three different mRNAs being presented to the ribosomes for translation into protein. Quite recently it has also been shown that the 'dark matter' of the human genome, the 90% of the DNA sequence that is not translated into protein, that in other words does not form genes, and which has accordingly often been referred to as 'junk DNA', may have an important part to play in the body's economy, especially in switching the genes on and off. It may be, therefore, that the comparatively small number of genes in the human genome is not so surprising after all. The noncoding part of the human nucleotide sequence, which at 3.2 Gb is the longest so far sequenced, may not be 'junk' at all, but play a vital role in human genetics.

How has this great flood of knowledge affected our understanding of sensory systems? Again some interesting and unexpected insights have emerged. There is, as noted above, an unlooked for homogeneity in genomes from bacteria and yeast through Cnidaria to humans. Only 94 of the 1278 protein families encoded by our genomes are specific to vertebrates. All the rest are found throughout the living world. These ubiquitous genes code for the enzymes involved in DNA replication and transcription, for ribosomes and the translation of mRNA into protein, for the 'housekeeping' functions of intermediate metabolism and protein transport and so on. It seems that once the biochemistry of these core processes had been put together in the early history of the biosphere, they became universally incorporated and like the **qwerty** keyboards of typewriters and computers became too familiar to shift.

Building on these core processes it appears that the major developments in the transition from Protista to Metazoa are those that have to do with the neuromuscular system and intercellular communication; this process is continued in the Primate line leading to humans where genes concerned with the immune response, with the nervous system and its development and with intercellular and intracellular signalling pathways, show particularly rapid evolutionary development. Even here, however, comparative genomics does not show dramatic change. In other cases dramatic developments are evident. When, for instance, the honeybee genome is compared with those of *Drosophila* and *Anopheles* a remarkable expansion of genes coding for olfactory receptors is found. In contrast, genes for gustatory receptors have been lost. We shall return to some of these very recent genome discoveries in later chapters. Here let us end this chapter with a brief review of some of the recent results of genome sequencing in the vertebrate line leading to *Homo sapiens,* with neurosensory systems principally in mind.

5.3 GENOMES AND NEUROSENSORY SYSTEMS

In Chapter 4 we noted that the closest invertebrate relatives of the vertebrates were the echinoderms and that the two groups together have been called, on the basis of their embryology, the deuterostomes. The common ancestor of the echinoderms and the chordates lies far back in the past, long before the Cambrian age began some 600 million years ago. Until the first echinoderm genome, that of the sea urchin *Strongylocentrotus purpuratus*, was published in 2006 it was thought that echinoderms held little interest to those interested in sensory systems, as they had few obvious sense organs. The genome has shown that we were wrong. Well over 7000 sea urchin genes are shared with the vertebrates and amongst these are to be found genes homologous to those which in mammals code for the chemosenses (over 600 genes), for balance, for sound and, surprisingly, a number of different photorhodopsins and other proteins concerned with vision. Many of these genes are expressed in the tube feet, suggesting that they have a previously unrecognized sensory sophistication. The thousands of tube feet each have their own reflex apparatus of sensory neurons, ganglia and motor neurons. Each can thus be looked at as an independent neurosensory module. It is interesting, also, to find that although genes encoding chemical neurotransmitters (with the exception of melatonin and epinephrine) are well represented, those which in the rest of the animal kingdom code for the components of gap junctions (electrical synapses) seem to be altogether lacking. Finally, it has been found that the sea urchin genome contains many genes homologous to those which in humans are implicated in neurological disorders such as Huntington's chorea, muscular dystrophy and, of particular interest in the context of this book, the Usher syndromes (Box 9.2) which affect hearing and balance and are involved in retinitis pigmentosa. In humans the latter genes encode a set of membrane and cytoskeletal proteins that form a network controlling the organization of stereocilia in the hair cells of the inner ear; they also play a role in the organization and/or development of photoreceptors. Modern genomics emphasizes the immense antiquity of these biochemical systems. They remain at work in each and every one of us.

Ciona intestinalis, the sea squirt, is even closer to the ancestral line leading to the verterbates and ultimately mankind. As noted in Chapter 4, its larval stage, adapted for dispersal, develops a notochord, nerve cord and gill clefts. The adult has lost all this motility and resembles nothing so much as a bag of jelly attached to a rock or other firm substratum in the littoral zone. The genome of *Ciona* is compact and contains a core of protostome genes that presumably originate from ancestral bilateralia. In addition to these ancestral genes, the genome also exhibits genes which code for neural crest and the ectodermal placodes which presage the paired sense organs. The nervous system of the ascidian 'tadpole' is one of the smallest known: the cerebral ganglion consists of just 300 or so cells and the hollow dorsal nerve tube is merely four cells in circumference. Genes coding for the formation and maintenance of myelin are missing. Myelin is probably superfluous

in a nerve cord extending only a few millimeters. Similarly, genes for the synthesis of epinephrine are lacking, as are those for melatonin and histamine. One of the most interesting findings, however, has to do with photoreception. The three rhodopsins found in *Ciona* are closely related to the pineal opsin of vertebrates, suggesting that the ocular system is derived from the pineal complex. Many homologues of the vertebrate phototransduction cascade are also found in the *Ciona* genome. When we come to examine vertebrate photoreception in Section 17.2.1 we shall find that exposure to light shuts off a so-called 'dark current' carried by Na^+. It is thus fascinating to find a similar mechanism obtains in *Ciona* and that the genes coding for components of the phototransduction cascade are homologous to those of the vertebrates. We shall find in Chapter 15 that *Ciona* is not the only invertebrate to resemble vertebrates in the molecular biology of phototransduction (Section 15.2.3), but that it does so is nevertheless interesting. It provides support for the belief that the tunicates are indeed related to the ancestral chordates.

Monodelphus domestica (an opossum) is very much further up the evolutionary tree leading to humanity. Because the opossum is a marsupial, the common ancestor lies at the divergence of the eutherian and metatherian branches of the mammalia, some 180 million years ago. Nevertheless, the vast majority of its 18 000–20 000 genes have orthologues in the eutheria. It is interesting to find that some of the most rapidly evolving of these homologous gene families are those which have to do with sensory perception. In particular, genes encoding the γ-crystallin family of lens proteins and the olfactory, gustatory and pheromonal receptors show particularly rapid evolutionary developments, especially by duplication events.

The mouse (*Mus musculus*), in addition to being one of the commonest laboratory animals and consequently an animal whose biology is very well worked out, is also far closer to us than the opossum. In contrast to the marsupials, the point of divergence between the evolutionary lines leading to mice and humans is 'only' some 75–65 million years in the past. In consequence about 40% of the nucleotide sequence of mice and men are held in common and 99% of mouse genes have homologues in the human genome. So far as sensory systems are concerned, the major evolutionary developments seem to be concentrated in the olfactory system. Duplication of olfactory genes and independent evolution of the duplicants appears to have happened frequently. Olfactory genes are important not only in dietary selection but also in reproductive success. Defects in pheromone responses reduce chances of successful mating and hence the production of offspring for the next generation. We shall return to these developments in Part 3.

Finally we come to the primates themselves. At the time of writing the genomes of three primate species have been sequenced: rhesus monkey (*Macaca mulatto*), chimpanzee (*Pan troglodytes*) and human (*Homo sapiens*). The monkey line diverged from that leading to humans some 25 million years ago and the chimpanzee six million years ago. The nucleotide sequence of macaque and human shows between 90.76% and 93.54% similarity and 97.5% of the genes are orthologous. Compared with humans, the macaque genome shows a significantly larger number of olfactory genes. An interesting and so far unexplained finding is that the monkey genome presents genes whose amino acid sequences are mutated forms of several human genes which when mutated in humans are associated with disease. An instance of this is provided by human Stargardt disease, a form of early onset macular degeneration (Box 17.2). This is associated with a point mutation in the *ABCR* gene on chromosome 1 that leads to a lysine residue being replaced by glutamine at position 223 (K223Q) in the human ABC retinoid transporter protein. This, it turns out, is the **normal** sequence found in the monkey and, indeed, as far back as *Xenopus*, the clawed toad.

The closest of human relatives is of course the chimpanzee, *Pan troglodytes*, sharing a common ancestor with us a mere six million years ago. The chimpanzee genome was published in 2005 and showed, as expected, a very close relationship to our own. It turned out that typical human and chimp homologous proteins differed on average by only two amino acids, with 30% of our proteins having exactly the same sequence as the chimpanzee's. About 600 genes were identified as having been subjected to strong positive selective pressure. Many of these, as in the other mammalian genomes discussed above, had to do with the immune system and defence against pathogens.

So far as sensory systems are concerned, it emerged that olfactory receptors are rapidly evolving, as in the other mammals, and the chimpanzee

and human complements are rapidly diverging. Of particular interest, however, was the finding that, compared with the chimpanzee, a region in chromosome seven which contains the Forkhead-box P2 transcription factor, or *FOXP2* gene, which is associated with speech development (Section 10.8) has undergone rapid evolution. Even so the human FOXP2 protein only differs from that expressed in chimpanzee and gorilla by two amino acid residues and from that expressed in the orang-outan and mouse by three and four respectively. There is, moreover, no evidence, so far, to suggest that the two residues found in the human protein have any dramatic functional importance. Nonetheless, it is satisfactory to find that the two specifically human residues have become fixed in the genome only in the last 200 000 years – a period consistent with the emergence of *Homo sapiens*. Several genes involved in hearing were also shown to have evolved rapidly in humans compared with chimps. This points to the importance of auditory communication – language – in human prehistory. Taken together with the fact that the greatest acceleration in the evolution of the *FOXP2* gene occurred in the last 200 000 years, these findings make for a satisfactory tie up with the palaeontological evidence of human evolution.

5.4 CONCLUDING REMARKS

This very rapid survey of a very rapidly developing field has concentrated on the evolutionary line leading out of the Precambrian period to humans. It has focused largely on that part of the evolving genome devoted to sensory systems. We have noted, throughout our survey, that it is olfactory systems (i.e. olfactory receptor genes) which have been subjected to the greatest selective pressures. This reflects its crucial role in life's two great interests – food and sex. But we have also noted how ancient are many of the genes controlling the structure and functioning of sensory systems. The senses by which we find our way through our life-worlds are built upon elaborations of systems whose primordia reach far back into the Precambrian period. We shall return to these genomic insights as we proceed through this book. The molecular approach is changing our understanding of ourselves and at the same time providing us with a multitude of insights into the causes of the disorders and diseases which blight so many lives.

PART I: SELF ASSESSMENT

The following questions are designed both to help you assess your understanding of the topics covered in the text and to direct your attention to significant aspects of the subject matter. The sequence of questions follows the sequence in which the subject matter is presented in the text. It is thus easy to refer back to the appropriate page or pages. After reading each chapter and/or each section you should look through these questions and make sure you know the answers and the issues involved.

CHAPTER 1: ELEMENTS

1.1   Why is it believed that DNA was *not* the original genetic molecule? life?

1.2   Give approximate dates for the earliest prokaryocytes and the earliest eukaryocytes.

1.3   Distinguish between the primary, secondary, tertiary and quaternary structures of proteins (consult glossary if in doubt).

1.4   Explain what is meant by the terms 'allostery' and 'allosteric effector'. What is cooperative allostery?

1.5   What are protein kinases and how are they involved in allosteric transitions? What role do protein phosphatases play?

1.6   Why is it important that membrane lipids are amphipathic molecules?

1.7   Is the interior of a biological membrane hydrophilic or hydrophobic? Why?

1.8   Biomembranes are said to have a 'fluid-mosaic' structure. What is meant by this?

1.9   What structural characteristic holds proteins in biomembranes? Describe one important structural motif shown by many receptor proteins.

1.10 How far and how fast can proteins move in biomembranes? Why is this mobility important in many sensory cells?

1.11 What does the *three dimensional* conformation of a 7TM protein resemble?

1.12 What does the acronym 'GPCR' stand for?

1.13 How are protein kinases involved in the desensitization of receptor proteins?

1.14 What does the 'G' in G-proteins stand for?

1.15 Explain how G-proteins can be likened to 'time switches'.

1.16 Name three types of membrane bound 'effector'.

1.17 Name three second messengers.

1.18 In a few sentences and (preferably) with a diagram explain how G-protein-based second-messenger systems provide a very flexible stimulus–response mechanism.

1.19 What do the acronyms 'LGIC' and 'VGIC' stand for? Give examples.

1.20 What does the acronym 'TRP' stand for?

1.21 Which ions flow through open TRP channels and what is their effect on membrane potential?

1.22 Draw a diagram showing the conformational cycle of the Na^+-channel.

1.23 Do all the Na^+-channels on a patch of excitable membrane have the same voltage thresholds for opening? Why is the answer to this question important?

CHAPTER 2: MEMBRANE, ACTION POTENTIALS, SYNAPSES

2.1 What is the approximate value of V_m? Why were cephalopod molluscs important in its estimation?

2.2 Write down the Nernst equation. Determine V_I when $[I^+]_o = 150$ mM and $[I^+]_i = 15$ mM; when $[I^+]_o = 5.5$ mM and $[I^+]_i = 150$ mM; and when $[I^-]_o = 125$ mM and $[I^-]_i = 9$ mM.

2.3 Using the Goldman equation and the values for the exterior and interior concentrations of K^+, Cl^- and Na^+ and for P_K, P_{Cl} and P_{Na} given in the text, determine V_m across the membrane of a squid giant axon and a cat motor neuron.

2.4 Using the values of K^+, Cl^- and Na^+ which you used in question 2.3 find the value of V_m across a cat motor neuron (i) if P_{Na} becomes 5×10^{-7} cm/s; (ii) if P_{Na} becomes 1×10^{-6} cm/s and (iii) P_K becomes 5×10^{-6} cm/s.

2.5 Use the simplified form of the Goldman equation (Equation 2.4) and the concentrations of K^+ and Na^+ given in Table 2.1 to determine V_m of the squid giant axon.

2.6 With the aid of a figure explain the nature of electrotonic (=cable) conduction.

2.7 Distinguish between a receptor and a generator potential.

2.8 Why is it that, although receptor potentials are linearly related to stimulus intensity, sensory and neurosensory cells only respond when a certain critical threshold stimulus (S_c) is reached?

2.9 Define 'sensory adaptation'. What is the difference between 'fast' and 'slow' adaptation?

2.10 Explain the role which calcium-dependent K^+-channels (K_{Ca}-channels) play in some cases of sensory adaptation.

2.11 What is the first event in an action potential?

2.12 Describe the sequence of changes through which Na^+-channels cycle during an action potential.

2.13 What ionic mechanisms repolarize an excite-able membrane after the peak of an action potential?

2.14 What is the afterhyperpolarization (AHP) and how long does it last?

2.15 Approximately how long does a refractory period last? What is its physiological significance? If the refractory period on a nerve fibre lasts 3 ms, what is the maximum frequency of impulses that that fibre can conduct?

2.16 How is the velocity of impulse propagation related to fibre diameter, and why? In what way does this account for the presence of 'giant fibres' in many invertebrates?

2.17 What alternative have vertebrates evolved in place of giant fibres? What advantages does this alternative have over invertebrate giant fibres?

2.18 Does fibre diameter influence propagation rate in vertebrate fibres? Name one other factor which has an influence on impulse conduction rate.

2.19 There are two major types of synapse: what are they?

2.20 Draw a diagram showing the most important steps in transmission at a 'chemical' synapse.

2.21 What is the rôle of Ca^{2+} in synaptic transmission?

2.22 Describe the difference between the two major types of 'chemical' synapse.

2.23 What does the acronym 'IPSP' stand for? Does the electrical potential across the membrane increase or decrease during an IPSP?

2.24 What are synaptic ribbons, where are they found and what rôle are they believed to play in synaptic transmission?

CHAPTER 3: GENERAL FEATURES OF SENSORY SYSTEMS

3.1 Distinguish, with examples, between the two major approaches to the study of sensory systems.

3.2 Describe two ways of classifying sensory receptors and explain what is meant by the term 'adequate stimulus'.

3.3 Explain why experiments involving the rerouting of sensory fibres in foetal ferrets raise intriguing questions of the relation of sensation to brain.

3.4 Define 'sensory threshold'. Does the sensory threshold of a given stimulus modality vary, or is it constant?

3.5   Say what is meant by 'just noticeable difference' (jnd). How is the jnd related to stimulus intensity?

3.6   Quote Stevens' 'psychophysical law' and give some examples of stimuli with different exponents in Stevens' law.

3.7   Define a receptive field (RF). Explain why there is generally a 'trade-off' between sensitivity and localization.

3.8   What is meant by the term 'nonisomorphic'? Why are sensory maps generally 'nonisomorphic'?

3.9   What did Johannes Müller mean by 'specific nerve energies'? What term do we use nowadays for Müller's concept?

3.10   Referring also to Chapter 23 (Section 23.4) consider why sensory information delivered to the brain should be arrayed in maps.

3.11   What is the 'binding problem'?

3.12   Distinguish between 'hierarchical' and 'parallel' designs. Are sensory systems organized according to one or other or both of these principles?

3.13   What is meant by 'trigger feature'? Give an example from the visual system.

3.14   Define what is meant by 'grandmother's face recogniton cell' or 'pontifical cell'. Do you think such cells are credible?

3.15   Explain the concept of an evolutionary 'arms race'.

CHAPTER 4: CLASSIFICATION AND PHYLOGENY

4.1   List three significant differences between the prokaryocytes and the eukaryocytes. At what approximate date did the eukaryocytes originate from the prokaryocytes?

4.2   Name the three kingdoms into which multicellular organisms are divided.

4.3   Describe three differences between the protostomes and the deuterostomes. Why do zoologists believe that this division marks a very early evolutionary divergence between these two groups of animals?

4.4   Describe the characteristic which divides the two major groups of protostomate animals.

4.5   What is meant by the term 'phylogeny'? Explain what is meant by the phrase 'ontogeny recapitulates phlogeny'.

4.6   Why is the division of the animal kingdom into vertebrates and invertebrates regarded as 'anthropocentric'?

4.7   Using the classificatory scheme of Section 4.6, classify (i) the macaque, (ii) the domestic cat; (iii) the fruit fly, (iv) the squid. According to this scheme, which of the four animals is most closely related to humans?

4.8   To which phylum does *Caenorhabditis elegans* belong? Why is this animal important in molecular neurobiology?

4.9   To which phylum do snails, winkles, cockles, mussels, squids and octopi belong?

4.10   Which charactertistic of arthropods prevents their growing to an excessive size?

4.11   Name the two subphyla into which arthropods are divided.

4.12   Does the possession of a hard exoskeleton affect the nature of the sense organs which arthropods can evolve? If so, how?

4.13   About how many species of chordates are there believed to be? How many species of molluscs? How many species of arthropods?

4.14   Which phylum is most closely related to the Chordata?

4.15   To which subphylum does the lancelet, *Amphioxus*, belong?

4.16   Distinguish, with examples, between the Chondrichthyes (Elasmobranchii) and the Osteichthyes.

4.17   Of the classes of vertebrates, which are anamniotes and which amniotes? To what structure do the latter two terms refer?

4.18   For what evolutionary reason do snakes lack limbs?

4.19   To which order of mammals do the bats belong? To which order the mice and rats? To which order the macaques and humans?

4.20   How is the nervous system organized in the Cnidaria?

4.21   Which animals show the most primitive form of central nervous system? What form does it take?

4.22 Draw a labelled diagram to show the structure of the central nervous system in a generalized insect. Which ganglia do the circumoesophageal commissures connect?

4.23 What are 'mushroom bodies' and where are they found?

4.24 Why is the snail's nervous system twisted into a figure of eight?

4.25 Explain the major differences between the 'plan' of chordate and nonchordate central nervous systems. Why do some authorities believe that a chordate is a nonchordate rotated 180° on its long axis?

4.26 Of which vertebrate organ is the lamellar body of *Amphioxus* believed to be a primordium?

4.27 Do you think that animal forms could have been very different from how they are today, or do you think that the evidence suggests that natural selection causes morphologies to converge on a certain small number of optimal designs? Provide evidence for your argument and answer.

CHAPTER 5: GENES, GENOMICS AND NEUROSENSORY SYSTEMS

5.1 Define the term 'genome'.

5.2 How many chromosomes make up the human genome?

5.3 What is meant by the term 'autosomal'?

5.4 Distinguish the 'p' and 'q' arms of a chromosome and explain the nomenclature that defines a gene's position.

5.5 What is a codon? Distinguish between an 'exon' and an 'intron'. Is it possible for one gene to encode several different polypeptides?

5.6 Explain the difference between 'synonymous' and 'non-synonymous' point mutations.

5.7 Explain what is meant by a 'frame shift' mutation and why do they normally lead to a functionless protein?

5.8 Give the size of the human genome in nucleotide base-pairs. Approximately how many genes does it contain?

5.9 Which is the most primitive metazoan genome yet sequenced and what are the most significant developments when compared with protistan genomes?

5.10 Do sea urchin genomes possess photoreceptor genes? If so, why is this surprising?

5.11 In what way can sea urchin genomes assist our understanding of certain disorders of the human neurosensory system?

5.12 How does the phototransduction cascade in the sea squirt, *Ciona intestinalis*, resemble that found in vertebrate eyes?

5.13 How similar are the genomes of mice and men?

5.14 What is meant by the term 'orthologous' in the phrase 'orthologous genes'?

5.15 How do genes responsible for Stargardt disease in humans resemble those in the macaque?

5.16 How does a comparison of chimpanzee and human genomes throw light on the evolution of speech?

5.17 Which of the various senses appears to be subject to the greatest selective pressures?

PART I: NOTES, REFERENCES AND BIBLIOGRAPHY

CHAPTER 1: ELEMENTS

The premise of the first sections of this chapter is that of the 'selfish gene' which Richard Dawkins (1976, 1995) has done so much to popularize. Detail of the structure and functioning of ribozymes is given by Narliker and Hereschlag (1997) and Herschlag (1998). An exhaustive account of molecular biology may be found in, for example, Alberts *et al.* (2002) and discussions of membrane structure, receptor proteins and channels in Smith (2002). The ubiquity of 7TM receptors is stressed by Shepherd *et al.* (1998) and G-protein signalling systems are discussed in Birnbaumer *et al.* (1990) and Bourne, Sanders and McCormick (1991) whilst an overview is given by Smith (1995). A detailed account of the X-ray diffraction analysis of the structure of the β_2-adrenergic receptor (the type-example of a GPCR) is given by Sprang (2007). The significance and molecular biology of TRP channels is well described by Clapham (2003), Owsianik, D'Hoet, Voets and Nilius (2006), Christensen and Corey (2007), Venkatachalam and Montell (2007) and in great detail in three papers in the *Annual Review of Physiology* (2006). A discussion of the molecular anatomy and physiology of ion channels may be found in Smith (2002). Shepherd *et al.* (1998) describe the 'human brain project' which was initiated in the early 1990s and funded by a number of funding agencies in the United States. By making use of state-of-the-art internet informatics it is intended to archive the vast quantity of neuroscience data, at many different levels, from molecule to whole brain, that pours from the research laboratories. In this respect it is comparable with, though far more complex than, the hugely successful human genome project in molecular biology.

Alberts, B., Johnson, A. and, Lewis, J. *et al.* (2002), *Molecular Biology of the Cell*, 4th edn, Garland Press, New York.

Birnbaumer, L. *et al.* (1990) Roles of G-proteins in coupling receptors to ion channels, in *Transmembrane Signalling: Intracellular Messengers and Implications for Drug Development* (ed. S.R. Nahorski), John Wiley & Sons, Ltd, Chichester.

Bourne, H.R., Sanders, D.A. and McCormick, F. (1991) The GTPase superfamily: conserved structure and molecular mechanism. *Nature*, **349**, 117–27.

Christensen, A.P. and Corey, D.P. (2007) TRP channels in mechanosensation: direct or indirect activation? *Nature Reviews Neuroscience*, **8**, 510–21.

Clapham, D.E. (2003) TRP channels as cellular sensors. *Nature*, **426**, 517–24.

Dawkins, R. (1976) *The Selfish Gene*, Oxford University Press, Oxford.

Dawkins, R. (1995) *River Out of Eden*, Weidenfeld and Nicholson, London.

Herschlag, D. (1998) Ribozyme crevices and catalysis. *Nature*, **395**, 548–9.

Narliker, G.J. and Hereschlag, D. (1997) Mechanistic aspects of enzyme catalysis: Lessons from comparison of RNA and Protein enzymes. *Annual Review of Biochemistry*, **66**, 14–59.

Owsianik, G., D'Hoet, D., Voets, T. and Nilius, B. (2006) Structure-function relationships of the TRP channel superfamily. *Reviews in Physiology Biochemistry and Pharmacology*, **156**, 61–90.

Shepherd, G.M. *et al.* (1998) The Human Brain Project: neuroinformatics tools for integrating, searching and modelling multidisciplinary neuroscientific data. *Trends in Neurosciences*, **21**, 460–8.

Smith, C.U.M. (1995) Membrane signalling systems, in *Biomembranes: General Principles*, Vol. **1** (ed. A.G. Lee), JAI Press, Greenwich, Ct., pp. 245–70.

Smith, C.U.M. (2002) *Elements of Molecular Neurobiology*, 3rd edn, John Wiley & Sons, Ltd, Chichester.

Sprang, S.R. (2007) A receptor unlocked. *Nature*, **450**, 355–6.

Venkatachalam, K. and Montell, C. (2007) TRP channels. *Annual Review of Biochemistry*, **76**, 387–417.

CHAPTER 2: MEMBRANE AND ACTION POTENTIALS

Accounts of the resting potentials and action potentials across excitable membranes are to be found in all textbooks of neurophysiology. Aidley (1989) provides a more advanced treatment and Hille (2001) provides probably the best account currently available of the biophysics and molecular biology of ion channels. The classical account of electrotonic conduction is given by Rall (1977) and less mathematical introductions may be found in Shepherd (2003) and Smith (2002). An up-to-date account of synaptic transmission may be found in Lisman, Raghavachari and Tsien (2007).

Aidley, D.J. (1989) The Physiology of Exciteable Cells, 3rd edn, Cambridge University Press, Cambridge.

Hille, B. (2001) *Ionic Channels of Exciteable Membranes*, 3rd edn, Sinauer, Sunderland, MA.

Kandel, E.R., Schwartz, J.H. and Jessel, T.M. (eds) (1991) *Principles of Neuroscience*, Elsevier, New York.

Lisman, J.E., Raghavachari, S. and Tsien, R.W. (2007) The sequence of events that underlie quantal transmission at central gluatminergic synapses. *Nature Reviews Neuroscience*, **8**, 597–609 and on-line at doi: 10.1038/nrn2191.

Rall, W. (1977) Core conductor theory and cable properties of neurons, in *Handbook of Neurophysiology*, Vol. **1**, section 1, American Physiological Society, Bethesda, Md., pp. 39–97.

Shepherd, G.M. (2003) *The Synaptic Organisation of the Brain*, 5th edn, Oxford University Press, Oxford.

Smith, C.U.M. (2002) *Elements of Molecular Neurobiology*, 3rd edn, John Wiley & Sons, Ltd, Chichester.

CHAPTER 3: GENERAL FEATURES OF SENSORY SYSTEMS

The pioneering experiments in which sensory fibres were re-routed in foetal mammals are described in Metin and Frost (1989) and in Sur, Garraghty and Roe (1989). Stevens (1957) is the classical paper on the relation between physical and subjective intensity. Material on the 'binding problem' is to be found in Crick (1994). Felleman and van Essen (1991) provide a seminal account of the 'tangled hierarchy' of the visual cortices where both sequential and parallel processing occur and where information travels both 'upwards' and 'downwards'. Jacob (1977) discusses the 'bricoleur' nature of the evolutionary process.

Crick, F.H.C. (1994) *The Astonishing Hypothesis*, Simon and Schuster, London.

Fechner, G.T. (1860) *Elemente der Psychophysik*, Breitkopf and Hartel, Leipzig; reprinted, 1999, Thoemmess Press, Bristol. First volume (translated into English: H.E. Adler and eds D.H. Howes and E.G. Boring), 1966, *Elements of Psychophysics*, Holt, Rinehart and Winston, New York.

Felleman, D.J. and van Essen, D. (1991) Distributed hierarchical processing in the Primate cerebral cortex. *Cerebral Cortex*, **1**, 1–47.

Hofstadter, D.R. (1979) *Godel, Escher, Bach: an Eternal Golden Braid*, Harvester Press, Hassocks.

Jacob, F. (1977) Evolution and tinkering. *Science*, **196**, 1161–6.

Metin, C. and Frost, D. (1989) Visual responses of neurons in somatosensory cortex of hamsters with experimentally-induced retinal projections to somatosensory thalamus. *PNAS (USA)*, **86**, 357–61.

Stevens, S.S. (1957) On the psychophysical law. *Psychological Review*, **64**, 153–81.

Sur, M., Garraghty, P.E. and Roe, A.W. (1989) Experimentally-induced visual projections into auditory thalamus and cortex. *Science*, **242**, 1437–41.

CHAPTER 4: CLASSIFICATION AND PHYLOGENY

The two publications by Hennig (1950, 1966) are the foundation works of the method of zoological classification known as 'cladistics'. Students interested in this alternative to the more conventional evolution-based classifications may also be interested to read Nelson and Platnick (1984) and the book by Wiley (1981). The distinction between Archaebacteria and Eubacteria was first introduced by Woese and Fox (1977); see also Woese (1981). The Archaebacteria (or Archaea) are now mostly confined to extreme conditions: hot springs, anaerobic methane-rich conditions and so on. It may be that these conditions resemble those found early in Earth's history. The Archaebacteria are thus regarded as a relict group of the most ancient of the globe's inhabitants. They differ in several points of biochemistry and molecular biology from their successors, the Eubacteria. They are, nevertheless, more closely related to the eukaryocytes than are the Eubacteria. The molecular evidence for the relatedness of the major groups of organisms is provided by Doolittle *et al.* (1996) and by Gu (1998). Balavoine and Adoutte (1998) discuss the evidence for a fundamental division within the protostomia. The pitfalls and uncertainties of molecular methods of determining phylogenies are succinctly reviewed by Lake and Moore (1998). Conway Morris (1998b) discusses recent palaeontological work on the origin of the Metazoa and provides an annotated bibliography. A comprehensive, easily-read overview of the classification of the living world may be found in Margulis and Schwartz (1998). Jiménez-Guri *et al.* (2007) describes the work which indicates that the parasitic worm, *Buddenbrockia plumatellae*, is a Cnidarian.

Stephen Gould (1989) gives a fascinating account of the discovery and implications of the weird and wonderful Precambrian fossils of the Burgess Shale, high in the Canadian Rocky Mountains and Conway Morris (1998a) provides an equally exciting account of these and other fossil locations, coming to different and equally interesting conclusions. Telford (2007) provides evidence for the common origin of annelid and chordate central nervous systems and modern reviews of the origin of vertebrate brains and sensory systems in the protochordates is given by Holland and Holland (1999) and Lacalli (2001, 2007). For an up-to-date comprehensive review of the evolution of animal nervous systems (somewhat biased towards the vertebrates) advanced students can do no better than consult the four volumes of Kaas (2007).

Balavoine, G. and Adoutte, A. (1998) One or three Cambrian radiations? *Science*, **280**, 397–8.

Caroll, R.L. (1988) *Vertebrate Palaeontology and Evolution*, Freeman, New York.

Doolittle, R.F. *et al.* (1996) Determining the divergence times of the major kingdoms of living organisms with a protein clock. *Science*, **271**, 470–77.

Gould, S.J. (1989) *Wonderful Life*, Norton, New York.

Gu, X. (1998) Early metazoan divergence was about 830 million years ago. *Journal of Molecular Evolution*, **47**, 369–71.

Hennig, W. (1950) *Grundzüge einer Theorie der Phylogentischen Systematik*, Deutscher Zentralverlag, Berlin.

Hennig, W. (1966) *Phylogenetic Systematics*, University of Illinois Press, Urbana.

Holland, L.Z. and Holland, N.D. (1999) Chordate origins of the vertebrate central nervous system. *Current Opinion in Neurobiology*, **9**, 596–602.

Imms, A.D. (1946) *A General Textbook of Entomology*, 6th edn, Methuen, London.

Jiménez-Guri, E. *et al.* (2007) *Buddenbockia* is a Cnidarian worm. *Science*, **317**, 116–8.

Kass, J.H. (editor in chief) (2007) *Evolution of Nervous Systems: A Comprehensive Reference*, Vol. **4**, Elsevier, Amsterdam.

Lacalli, T.C. (2001) New perspectives on the evolution of protochordate sensory and locomotory systems, and the origin of brains and heads. *Phil. Trans. Roy. Soc. B*, **356**, 1565–72.

Lacalli, T.C. (2007) Basic features of the ancestral chordate brain: a protochordate perspective. *Brain Research Bulletin* **75**, 319–23.

Lake, J.A. and Moore, J.E. (1998) Phylogenetic analysis and comparative genomics, in *Trends in Bioinformatics*, Elsevier, Cambridge, pp. 22–4.

Nelson, G. and Platnick, N. (1984) Systematics and evolution, in *Beyond Neo-Darwinism* (eds Mae-Wan Ho and Peter Saunders), Academic Press, London.

Margulis, L. and Schwartz, K.V. (1998) *The Five Kingdoms: An Illustrated Guide to the Phyla of Life on Earth*, 3rd edn, W.H. Freeman, San Francisco.

Morris, S.C. (1998a) *The Crucible of Creation*, Oxford University Press, Oxford.

Morris, S.C. (1998b) Metazoan phylogenies: falling into place or falling to pieces? A palaeontological perspective. *Current Opinion in Genetics and Development*, **8**, 662–67.

Telford, M.J. (2007) A single origin of the central nervous system? *Cell*, **129**, 237–9.

Wiley, E.O. (1981) *Phylogenetics: The Theory and Practice of Phylogenetic Systems*, John Wiley & Sons, Inc., New York.

Woese, C.R. (1981) Archaebacteria. *Scientific American*, **244** (6), 98–122.

Woese, C.R. and Fox, G.E. (1977) The concept of cellular evolution. *Journal of Molecular Evolution*, **10**, 16.

CHAPTER 5: GENES, GENOMICS AND NEUROSENSORY SYSTEMS

The sequencing of animal genomes is proceeding rapidly and on a very broad scale and promises considerable insight into the evolutionary relationships in the animal kingdom. This chapter should thus be read in conjunction with Chapter 4. It is early days yet but genomics is already providing fascinating insights into the development and inter-relationships of neurosensory systems. Interested students can do no better than go to the original papers, mostly published in *Nature* or *Science*, and they will often be directed to web sites featuring videos and podcasts as well as editorial comment.

The earliest eumaetazoan genome to be sequenced, that of the starlet anemone, *Nematostella vectensis*, was published by a large group headed by Putnam (2007); the honeybee genome (*Apis mellifera*) was sequenced by another large group, the *Honeybee Sequencing Consortium* (2006) and the *Nature* honeybee web site has a video and podcast giving further detail and interviews with scientists of the bee *Consortium*. The full sequence of the sea urchin, *S. purpuratus*, was published by another Consortium, the *Sea Urchin Sequencing Consortium* (2006), and further detail about sea urchins and their genome may be found at http://sugp.caltech.edu/intro/index.php. A sequence for *Ciona intestinalis* was published by Dehal *et al.* (2003) and further detail is at http://genome.jgi-psf.org/Cioin2.home.html. Other large groups of investigators have sequenced various insects (the mosquito, moth and fruit fly), fish (zebra fish and two species of puffer fish), birds (chicken) and mammals (ranging from the opossum through rodents to a number of primates. The comparative genomics of twelve species of *Drosophila* is described and discussed by Gunter *et al.* (2007), Ledford (2007) and in detail in subsequent articles of the same volume of *Nature*. The final draft of the human genome was published in *Science 300:* 197–376 and Collins *et al.* (2003) give an expert discussion. Further detail may be found at the *National Human Genome Research Institute* web site http://genome.gov/HGP/. Carroll (2003) gives a recent review of the genetics of human evolution and, finally, the *Encode Consortium* (2007) reports the recent unexpected finding that far more of the human genome is involved in the coding process than previously thought. In their concluding paragraphs the *Consortium* write that the traditional view that the genome contains a 'defined set of isolated loci transcribed independently does not seem to be accurate' (p. 812).

Canestro, C., Bassham, S. and Postlethwait, J.H. (2003) Seeing chordate evolution through the *Ciona* genome sequence. *Genome Biology*, **4**, 208–11.

Carroll, S.B. (2003) Genetics and the making of *Homo sapiens*. *Nature*, **422**, 849–57.

Chimpanzee Sequencing and Analysis Consortium (2005) Initial sequence of the chimpanzee genome and comparison with the human genome. *Nature*, **437**, 69–87.

Collins, F.S. *et al.* (2003) A vision of the future of genomics research. *Nature*, **422**, 835–47.

Dehal, P. *et al.* (2003) The draft Genome of *Ciona intestinalis*: Insights into chordate and Vertebrate origins. *Science*, **298**, 2157–67.

Encode (Encyclopaedia of DNA elements) Consortium (2007) Identification and analysis of functional elements in 1% of the human genome by the ENCODE pilot project. *Nature*, **447**, 799–816.

Gunter, C. *et al.* (2007) Genome labours bear fruit. *Nature*, **450**, 183.

Ledford, H. (2007) Attack of the genomes. *Nature*, **450**, 142–3.

Mouse Genome Sequencing Consortium (2002) Initial sequencing and comparative analysis of the mouse genome. *Nature*, **420**, 520–62.

Nene, V. *et al.* (2007) Genome sequence of *Aedes aegypti*, a Major Arbovirus Vector. *Science* **316**, 1718–22.

Putnam, N.H. *et al.* (2007) Sea Anemone Genome Reveals Ancestral Eumetazoan Gene Repertoire and Genomic Organisation. *Science*, **317**, 86–94.

Rhesus Macaque Genome Sequencing and Analysis Consortium (2007) Evolutionary and Biomedical Insights from the Rhesus Macaque Genome. *Science*, **316**, 222–34.

Sea Urchin Genome Sequencing Consortium (2006) The Genome of the Sea Urchin *Strongylocentrotus purpuratus*. *Science*, **314**, 942–52.

Tarjei, S. *et al.* (2007) Genome of the marsupial *Monodelphis domestica* reveals innovation in the non-coding sequences. *Nature*, **447**, 167–77.

The Honeybee Genome Sequencing Consortium (2006) Insights into social insects from the genome of the honeybee *Apis mellifera*. *Nature*, **443**, 931–49.

PART II: MECHANOSENSITIVITY

Without touch it is impossible for an animal to exist . . . . . the loss of this one sense alone must bring death

Aristotle, *de Anima*, (435b4-5).

Of all the senses touch has often been regarded as the most basic. Aristotle, greatest of biologists, saw this two and half millennia ago in Greek antiquity. As the introductory quotation makes plain, he regarded it as the fundamental sense of all animal life. In the same treatise he also insists that 'It is the only sense that all animals without exception possess' (*de Anima*, 414b3). That opinion has hardly changed down the ages. We shall see at the end of this book (Chapter 24) how crucial it has seemed to many of the empiricist philosophers. Although we may be blind or deaf, and in some tragic circumstances both blind *and* deaf, the sense of touch remains, and as the famous case of Helen Keller showed, enables life to be lived.

The tactile sense, the response to mechanical distortion, is evolutionarily very ancient, as we shall see in this Part. It can be traced back to the earliest prokaryocytes which needed, like all contemporary cells, to detect the integrity of their boundary membranes. Swelling due to osmotic forces needed counteraction, swelling due to increase in size prior to cell division also needed to be sensed. We shall see in the chapters of this Part that mechanosensors are built around stretch-sensitive channels in the plasma membrane. We shall see, also, that this means that the detection is immediate and the response rapid. There is no need to involve a complex G-protein membrane biochemistry such as is involved in receptors for the other senses.

Mechanoreceptors play many roles in the animal kingdom. Not only are they basic to the detection of tension and touch but they are also essential in sensing vibrations, accelerations, sounds, body movements and positions and so on. As already indicated, these many roles are based ultimately on stretch-sensitive channels in plasma membranes. The only such channels which are known in molecular detail are (to date) those expressed in *E. coli* and *C. elegans*. Accordingly we shall start, in Chapter 6, by reviewing the *E. coli* stretch detector. It will also be appropriate to discuss some of the stretch receptors that detect volume change and tension in eukaryotic cells. In particular, we shall look in detail at the cells in the mammalian hypothalamus which detect and, in detecting, set in train homeostatic control of the osmolarity of the blood.

In Chapter 7 we shall pass to the complex systems in which stretch receptors are involved in the 'higher' animals. All animals need to know the relative positions of the parts of their own bodies. In animals with stiff, rigid, exoskeletons, such as the arthropods, this can be largely (but not entirely) achieved by detecting the movements and positions of the different segments and articulations of their bodies. In soft bodied forms supported by endoskeletons, such as vertebrates, kinaesthesia depends on detecting the movement and state of tension in the body's muscles and joints.

Biology of Sensory Systems, Second Edition   C.U.M. Smith
© 2008 John Wiley & Sons, Ltd

Next, in Chapter 8, we shall turn to the sense of touch itself and look at the well characterized touch detectors of *C. elegans* before going on to review some of the many other types of touch receptors in the animal kingdom. We shall consider two major cases: arthropods and vertebrates. Again the great difference in design of these two groups of animals ensures that the means of tactile sensitivity are vastly different. The spiders and insects, with their hardened exoskeletons, make use of tactile hairs, slit sensilla, chordotonal organs and so on. We shall follow the development of these types of tactile receptor until, in the insects, they evolve into those most delicate of sense organs, those which detect the gentle touch of sound. We shall, in other words, end by giving some consideration to insect 'ears' and especially the ears of moths, which have evolved to detect the ultrasonic sonar of marauding bats. Turning to the vertebrates we shall concentrate our attention on the several types of tactile receptors in the mammalian skin. The skin, unlike the hard carapace of the arthropods, can be considered a sensory surface in its own right and we shall follow the information it collects to its destination in the somaesthetic cortex. We leave a discussion of the vertebrate ear until the next chapter.

In Chapter 9, we discuss the vertebrate hair cell. These are some of the most remarkable of all the sensory cells developed in the animal kingdom. We shall follow the ways in which they have been put to use as mechanoreceptors, from the echolocation devices of fish lateral line canals, to the equilibrium detectors of the membranous labyrinth and the sound detectors of the mammalian cochlea. It is not difficult to argue that in this latter organ mechanoreception reaches its evolutionary climax. We shall look at how the cochlea has been elaborated in insectivorous bats to detect the faint echoes returned from manoeuvring insects, thus continuing the remarkable story of the arms race between moth and microchiropteran which we began in Chapter 8.

We shall end Part Two by considering, in Chapter 10, what happens to the information picked up by the vertebrate ear when it reaches the central nervous system. We shall look at the way in which the input from the membranous labyrinth is used to maintain posture and equilibrium. We shall examine the auditory pathway to the primary auditory cortex in the temporal lobe of the brain, noting how significant features for an animal's life are extracted. In the insectivorous bats these significant features are the echoes returned from their ultrasonic sonar. We shall thus complete the story broached in Chapters 8 and 9 by discussing the analysis of these ultrasonic echoes in the microchiropteran cortex. In *Homo sapiens* the most significant features of the auditory input are the sounds basic to language. We shall close the section with a look at the nature of these sounds and how they are processed.

From this brief resumé it can be seen that mechanoreceptors are many and various. Although there may be unity of design at the molecular level – ion channels sensitive to stretch – the multitude of different macroscopic designs suggest several different evolutionary pathways. Mechanoreceptors differ in this respect from chemoreceptors and photoreceptors, which show a greater homogeneity in design across the animal kingdom. In the atmospheric blanket that surrounds planet Earth, and to a lesser extent in the hydrosphere, mechanoreceptors have evolved to provide astonishingly sensitive and sophisticated means of communicating between one individual animal and another.

6

MECHANOSENSITIVITY OF CELL MEMBRANES

E. coli: formation of giant cells - patch clamping - two mechanosensitive channels (MscL and MscS) - isolation of MscL: structure, biophysics, biological significance as osmoreceptor - other bacteria. **Mammalian osmoreceptors**: magnocellular neurons (MCNs) in hypothalmus - neurosecretion of vasopressin, oxytocin - patch clamping of MCNs - biophysics - stretch inactivated (SI) channels - feedback loops controlling water loss or retention in response to hyper or hyptonicity of ECF. **Concluding remarks**: molecular structure of most mechanosensitive channels still unknown - possible commonalities - at the centre of intricate neuroendocrine loops.

Mechanoreceptors are evolutionarily very ancient. They are ubiquitous. They have been pressed into service in many different ways to detect stretch and touch, even the gentle touch of water and sound waves. It may be that they all share a rather similar molecular basis. In this chapter we shall look first at the only mechanoreceptors which (at the time of writing) are known in molecular detail. These are the mechanosensitive channels which develop in the plasma membrane of *E. coli*. Then we shall turn our attention to the detection of stretch by eukaryotic cells in higher organisms. In both cases stretch receptors are particularly important in detecting osmotic swelling. In consequence they are employed as such by osmoreceptors in the mammalian hypothalamus.

We shall see in later chapters that a great deal is known about the molecular structure and function of chemoreceptors and photoreceptors. Our knowledge of the molecular structure and function of mechanoreceptors is, in contrast, rather lim-ited. The fact that only one mechanosensitive receptor has been analysed in molecular detail is largely due to the lack of highly enriched sources such as are available for the other types of receptor. However, advances in molecular genetics provide hope for the future. A member of the TRPV family (Chapter 1) is believed to confer mechanosensitivity on *C. elegans* nose cilia, a gene coding for a member of the TRPN channel family (*Tprn1*, also known as *nompC*) has been identified as essential for mechanoreception in *Drosophila*. Subsequently, two other TRP genes have been shown to be involved in hearing in flies and recent reports suggest that yet another TRP gene, coding for Trpa1, is implicated in vertebrate hair cell transduction and the mammalian auditory sense. Finally, it has been shown that TRPV and TRPC channels act as stretch receptors in mammalian skeletal muscle fibres. Commonalities at the molecular level are thus beginning to emerge. We shall return to these developments in

Biology of Sensory Systems, Second Edition   C.U.M. Smith
© 2008 John Wiley & Sons, Ltd

Chapters 8 and 9. In this chapter, however, we shall concentrate on the fully understood **stretch-activated** channels of bacteria and, in particular, those of *E. coli* and then pass to the less wellknown **stretch-inactivated** channels of mammalian osmoreceptors.

6.1 MECHANOSENSITIVE CHANNELS IN *E. COLI*

Why choose *E. coli*? Simply because it is perhaps the best known of all organisms. Its rapid generation time and ease of culture ensures that large masses can be accumulated rapidly. Its genetics and molecular biology are very well understood. *E. coli* is a gram negative archaebacterium and, like other such bacteria, has a complex boundary consisting of an outer lipopolysaccharide membrane, a peptidoglycan cell wall and an inner plasma membrane. The latter membrane is a characteristic phospholipid bilayer, containing embedded proteins such as we discussed in Chapter 1. Many of these proteins have been cloned and subjected to analysis using the techniques of molecular biology.

To determine a membrane's biophysical response to mechanical stretch it is necessary to use the technique of patch clamping. This technique is outlined in Appendix A, but in essence it involves placing a glass micropipette (tip diameter $0.5\,\mu m$) on to the membrane of interest. A very high resistance seal (some $10\,G\Omega$) develops between the tip and the membrane and this allows tiny currents in the pico-ampere range to be detected. The micropipette is filled with an electrolyte and connected to appropriate electronics so that flows of current across the membrane can be detected. The membrane may be left *in situ* or, by the application of gentle suction, detached and examined in isolation. In either case it is possible to record the flows of current through single membrane channels.

Unfortunately for patch clampers, the majority of bacteria are too small to allow them to practise their art. *E. coli*, for instance, is only about $2\,\mu m$ long and $1\,\mu m$ in diameter – too small to be patch clamped with presently available techniques. It would seem then that the small size of prokaryocytes protects them from the prying investigations of the physiologist. However, physiologists are not easily discouraged and a way around the problem was ultimately

worked out. If *E. coli* was too small for the physiologist then it must be made bigger!

Fortunately, there are various methods for generating 'giant' *E. coli* cells by means of antibiotics. If, for instance, *E.coli* is cultured in cephalexin, an analogue of penicillin, DNA replication and cell elongation occur without cell division. As a result, long string-like filaments are formed, maybe over $100\,\mu m$ in length and these, when subjected to EDTA–lysozyme treatment, transform into spheres up to $10\,\mu m$ in diameter known as **spheroplasts**. This is a practicable size for patch clamping and, sure enough, patch clamping techniques proved successful. The only question remaining was whether the patch clamp seal was formed with the outer or the inner membrane. Further investigation confirmed that the seal was indeed made with the inner cell membrane. It seems that during the suction phase of the patch clamp technique, the pipette tip breaks through the outer membrane and the cell wall and seals into the inner membrane. This technique is shown diagrammatically in Figure 6.1.

Two types of mechanosensitive channel (Msc) were detected: a large-conductance channel (MscL) with a conductance of about $3000\,pS$ and a small-conductance channel (MscS) with a conductance of about $1000\,pS$. If the lateral tension on the patch clamped membrane is increased by gentle suction, the channels are caused to open. That the MscS and MscL conductances are due to two separate channels and are not merely different states of the same can be shown by 'knocking out' the gene for MscL. The conductance characteristic of the MscS channel can still be detected in these 'knock-out' bacteria. The tension required to open this smaller channel is about 70% of that which is required to open the large channel. There is also evidence to show that other, smaller, mechanosensitive channels exist in the membrane.

The analysis of the MscL channel has been taken further by the sophisticated techniques of modern molecular biology. These techniques involve the incorporation of *E. coli* membrane fragments into liposomes composed of foreign phospholipids and testing again with the patch clamp technique to confirm the presence of the mechanosensitive channels. The proteins can be extracted from these liposomes by the use of mild detergents and refined by biochemical techniques, all the time patch clamp testing for

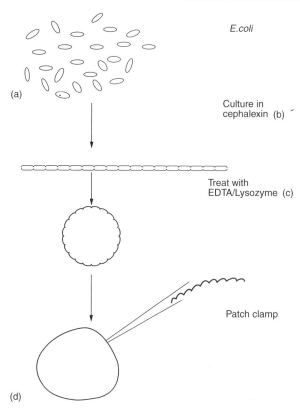

E.coli

Culture in
cephalexin (b)

Treat with
EDTA/Lysozyme (c)

Patch clamp

(a)

(d)

Figure 6.1   Patch clamping *E. coli*. (a) *E. coli* cell. (b) Cultured in medium containing cephalexin and forms lengthy filaments. (c) Filament treated with EDTA–Lysozyme transforms to form large spheroplast. (d) Microelectrode (tip diameter about 0.5 μm) inserted to form a patch clamp. Further explanation in text.

detail. Like most membrane channels it shows multiple conducting states (Figure 6.2). It also shows strong dependence on lateral tension in the membrane. There is, in fact, a steep sigmoid curve relating the probability of being open with the tension. There is no evidence of ion selectivity and this, along with its large conductivity, suggests a wide water-filled pore.

The isolation of the MscL protein and the identification of its gene allows the molecular biologist to determine its molecular structure. It turns out to be a relatively small protein consisting of some 136 amino acid residues. Examination of the sequence shows that the N-terminal is followed by a section of hydrophilic residues and then by a segment of strongly hydrophobic amino acids (19–49) followed by another hydrophilic region (50–69), then a second hydrophobic segment (72–100) and, finally, a hydrophilic sequence to the C-terminal. Careful examination of the physico-chemical characteristics of the polypeptide indicates that the two hydrophobic segments form alpha helices (M1 and M2) spanning the membrane. Both the N-terminal and C-terminals are located inside the cell and there is reason to believe that there is another short helical region (S3) in the extracellular segment between M1 and M2 (Figure 6.3a).

A single MscL protein could not form a gated channel with the biophysical characteristics of the native MscL channel. The operational channel must be a multimeric complex. This is consistent with the structure of many other channel proteins. X-ray analysis (see below) shows that the MscL channel consists of five MscL subunits grouped around a central water-filled channel (Figure 6.3b). The response of this complex structure to mechanical stretch of the membrane in which it is embedded is described below.

The isolation of the MscL channel protein and its gene, *mscl,* opens the possibility for genetic investigation of structure–function relationships. This investigation is, of course, greatly helped by the intimate understanding of *E. coli* genetics built up over the years. Research is continuing at the time of writing and a number of interesting relationships have been teased out. One amino acid residue at the 'bottom' of the S3 periplasmic helix seems particularly critical. This is the Glutamine residue in position 56 (Q56) (Figure 6.3a). A number of amino acid

MscL activity, until a pure preparation of channel protein is obtained. This turns out to have M_r of about 17 kDa. The N-terminal amino acid sequence of this 17 kDa protein was sequenced and then the very full database of the *E. coli* genome searched for a gene containing a corresponding nucleotide sequence. Such a sequence was found in a gene whose function was previously unknown. Through complex molecular biological procedures the gene was caused to express itself and the resulting protein incorporated into phospholipid liposomes which, on being patch clamped, showed the presence of the mechanosensitive channels.

Once the MscL channel had been isolated and incorporated into artificial phospholipid liposomes, its biophysical characteristics could be examined in

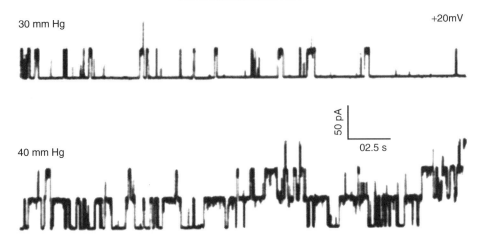

Figure 6.2 Biophysical characteristics of the MscL channel. The channel protein was purified and incorporated into phosphatidyl choline/phosphatidyl serine liposomes. The liposomes were patch clamped and the membrane subjected to different degrees of suction in the patch clamp pipette (30 and 40 mm Hg). The upward excursions indicate ion flows carrying a depolarizing current. It can be seen that the open probability is significantly increased when suction is increased. From Blount, P. *et al*. (1996), *EMBO J.*, **18**, 4798–805, Copyright ©1996, Nature Publishing Group.

substitutions at this point significantly lengthen the time for which the channel stays open under a given stretch. Indeed, some of these substitutions, in particular the substitution of Proline for Glutamine at this position (in the shorthand of molecular biolo-

gists: Q56P) makes the channel sensitive to stretching forces far below those normally required, indeed below those necessary to open the MscS channel. Substitutions in other parts of the channel protein, though not so dramatic in their effects, nevertheless

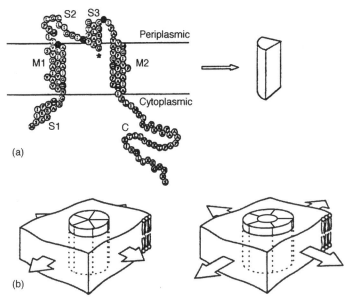

Figure 6.3 Structure and membrane topology of the MscL channel. (a) Orientation of the MscL channel protein in the membrane. Further explanation in text. The critical glutamine residue at position 56 in the amino acid chain is indicated by an asterisk. (b) Five MscL subunits are grouped form a compact cylinder through the membrane. When the membrane is stretched, a hydrophilic pore opens in the centre of the cylinder. (Modified from Sukharev *et al.*, 1997).

alter function in interesting and thought-provoking ways. Clearly this continuing genetic research into structure–function relationships will ultimately lead to an understanding of this mechanosensitive channel in full molecular, indeed atomic, detail.

Do similar channels develop in the plasma membranes of other bacteria? Once the nucleotide sequence for the *mscl* gene had been determined, it became possible to prepare matching oligonucleotide probes to search for homologous genes in other bacteria. Such genes have been shown to exist in a number of other bacteria, for instance *Mycobacterium tuberculosis*, *Haemophilus influenzae*, *Pseudomonas fluorescens*, *Clostridium perfringens* and *Staphylococcus aureus*.

The MscL in *M. tuberculosis* (TbMscL) has proved particularly valuable. It shows a 37% sequence identity with *E. coli* MscL (EcoMscL) and of all the MscL channels cloned it proved the easiest to crystallize. When the crystals were subjected to X-ray analysis, a fascinating structure was revealed. TbMscL turned out, like the EcoMscL channel, to be a homopentamer – five identical subunits arranged around a central pore. Each subunit consists, as expected, of two transmembrane helices (M1 and M2) and both N-terminal and C-terminal ends continue into the cytoplasm. The M1 and M2 helices line the pore, which is funnel-shaped with the rim at the periplasmic end and a constriction at the cytoplasmic end. The C-terminal domains of the five subunits surround a cytoplasmic continuation of the pore. The MscL channel thus has a double structure, part in the lipid bilayer, part in the cytoplasm immediately beneath (Figure 6.3).

In contrast, when the McsS channel from *E.coli* (EcoMscS) was eventually isolated, crystallized and analysed it turned out to be homoheptamer – seven identical subunits arranged around a central pore. Each subunit consists of three transmembrane helices with a tertiary structure entirely different from that of the MscL subunit; the whole heptameric structure is considerably bigger and more complex than MscL. Once again each subunit has a cytoplasmic domain and, together, these domains form an intricate cage-like structure in the cytoplasm.

Highly sophisticated biophysical techniques have been employed to find how these complex structures respond to membrane stretch. It can be shown that the stretching forces are delivered by the lipid bilayer and not by any elements of the cytoskeleton or extracellular matrix. When the membrane is stretched, both the MscL and MscS channels open by a twisting motion similar to that of a camera's iris diaphragm. The transmembrane helices surrounding the central pore take up more diagonal positions. In the case of MscL, the cytoplasmic ring, free from these membrane forces, remains closed and plugs the exit from the pore. Further stretching opens this ring to produce a wide canal up to 30Å in diameter.

What role do these mechanosensitive channels play in the life of bacteria? Perhaps somewhat surprisingly there is no generally accepted answer to this question. The most likely reason for their existence probably has to do with osmoregulation. When exposed to fresh water, perhaps downpours from the sky, bacteria experience considerable osmotic stress. Water molecules flow down their concentration gradients into the cell. The consequent swelling would certainly be sensed by the mechanosensitive channels in the plasma membrane. It may be that in letting solutes (other than macromolecules) flow out they counteract the osmotic stress by making the water concentration gradient less steep. In addition to a function in detecting osmotic swelling, stretch receptors have also been thought to play a part in detecting swelling due to growth and thus signalling the onset of a period when cell division should occur.

Finally, do similar channels exist in eukaryotic cells? Searches using the nucleotide sequences of bacterial mechanosensitive channels to pull out homologues in eukaryotic cells have so far proved disappointingly negative. However, the yeast genome has yielded a mechanosensitive channel located in vacuolar membranes that, although not related to the mechanosensitive channels of prokaryocytes, has many of the same biophysical characteristics – responding to mechanical or osmotically induced stretch in the membrane. This channel is a member of one of the TRPV family of channel proteins. We shall find that TRP channels are at the centre of several mechanosensitive channels in the animal kingdom. Thus it may well turn out that bacterial channels, although not directly relevant to those in eukaryotic cells, nevertheless provide valuable models for similar channels underlying the mechanosenses present in the vertebrates, including ourselves.

6.2 DETECTION OF OSMOTIC SWELLING BY HYPOTHALAMIC CELLS IN MAMMALS

Osmotic stress is just as significant for the eukaryotic cells of animals as it is for the prokaryotic cells of the Monera. The majority of animals are poikilo-osmotic: the osmolarity of their 'internal environment' quickly comes into equilibrium with the osmolarity of the external environment. A few animals, amongst which we may count the mammals, are able to control the osmolarity of their internal environments. These are defined as being 'homeo-osmotic' (or, homoio-osmotic). The reflex mechanisms which exert this control depend on sensing changes in the osmolarity of the internal environment, that is the extracellular fluid (ECF). This sensing is carried out by stretch receptors in the membranes of '**osmoreceptor**' cells. These cells may thus be regarded as entero-mechanoreceptors.

In mammalian bodies osmoreceptors take the form of large ('**magnocellular**') neurons located in nuclei in the anterior part of the hypothalamus. The most important of these nuclei are the **paraventricular nucleus** at the anterior extremity of the hypothalamus and the **supraoptic nucleus** positioned just above the optic chiasma (Figure 6.4). The magnocellular neurons (*MCNs*) of the paraventricular nucleus send some of their axons to the supraoptic nucleus and others directly down the infundibular stalk to the posterior pituitary. Axons of the MCNs of the supraoptic nucleus also project through the infundibular stalk to terminate in the posterior pituitary. In both cases the axons end in richly branching telodendria full of neurosecretions. These secretions are mostly small peptides. The neurosecretions of most interest in the present context are the 9-amino acid peptide hormones **vasopressin** and **oxytocin**. Both hormones are released into the hypophyseal vessels from whence they are carried into the general circulation. In humans, oxytocin causes uterine contraction and milk secretion from the mammary glands during lactation but in the rat (where the experimental manipulations are carried out) it is **natriuretic** (i.e. causes excretion of Na^+). Vasopressin in both humans and rats is **antidiuretic** (i.e. causes the retention of water).

The capillary beds of the supraoptic nucleus are extremely well developed. Careful quantitative studies with the microscope have shown that their density, volume fraction and surface area is four times greater than in nonmagnocellular hypothalamic nuclei. The capillaries, although exceedingly numerous, have, however, an unusually small calibre. This, in impeding plasma throughput, suggests that water and other small molecules have an unusually good chance of escaping through the capillary endothelium into the intercellular space. The paraventricular nucleus is even more exposed to the plasma. There is no blood–brain barrier and the endothelial walls of the dense capillary beds are extensively fenestrated. The MCNs in this nucleus are thus even more exposed to changes in the constitution of the plasma than those in the supraoptic nucleus.

Electrophysiological recording from MCNs in both hypothalamic nuclei shows that impulse frequency varies with osmolarity. At the set point of about 280 mosmol/kg the firing rate is rather irregular at around 2–3 Hz. Intraperitoneal injection of water (leading to a hypotonic ECF) reduces the firing rate, whereas injection of hypertonic solutions increases the rate. The analysis has been taken further by investigating MCNs in thin hypothalamic slices. Here it can be shown that the cells depolarize in response to hypertonic solutions. Ultimately, microelectrode recording of isolated single MCNs showed that hypertonic solutions produced membrane depolarization whereas hypotonic solutions induced the opposite, a hyperopolarization.

Is it possible to relate these electrophysiological responses to osmotically-induced volume change in the MCNs? There is now good evidence to show that this is indeed what is happening. The very delicate task of correlating changes in volume of MCNs with cation conduction rates through the cell membrane in response to hypertonic stimuli has been achieved. The technique involved using confocal laser scanning microscopy and whole cell patch clamping. It was shown that a decrease in size of the cell due to the hypertonic stimulus was correlated with **increased** membrane permeability to Na^+ and K^+.

Can we go further and show that this response is due to mechanosensitivity of the cell membrane? The alternative would be that the electrophysiological response was simply due to changes in solute concentration in different osmotic conditions. Fortunately, it is reasonably easy to answer this question. In whole cell patch clamping it is possible to alter the pressure

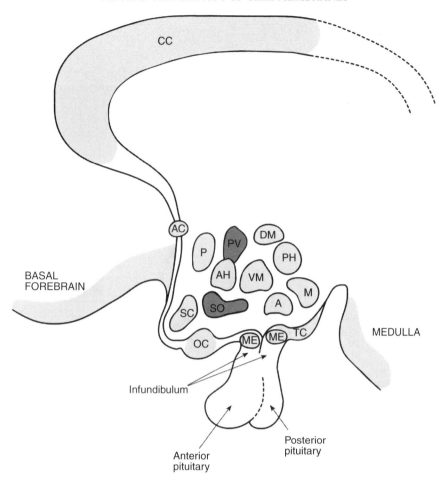

Figure 6.4 Parasagittal section through the hypothalamus to show positions of nuclei. The hypothalamus contains a great number of nuclei, most of which are concerned with regulation of the internal environment. As indicated in the text, the paraventricular (PV) and supraoptic (SO) nuclei (both shaded) are the two most intimately concerned with osmoregulation. A = arcuate nucleus; AC = anterior commissure; AH = anterior hypothalamic nucleus; CC = corpus callosum; DM = dorsomedial nucleus; M = mammillary body; ME = median eminence; OC = optic chiasma; P = preoptic nucleus; PH = posterior hypothalamic nucleus; PV = paraventricular nucleus; SC = suprachiasmatic nucleus; SO = supraoptic nucleus; TC = tuber cinereum; VM = ventromedial nucleus.

on the cell membrane by altering the pipette suction. It was readily shown that decreases and increases in cell volume due to pipette pressure were correlated in the expected way with depolarizations and hyperpolarizations respectively.

When a membrane is patch clamped, suction causes it to bow upwards into the pipette (concave, as seen from inside); as the suction is reduced the membrane returns to an unstrained position (approximately horizontal) and then bows downwards (con-

vex) (Figure 6.5A). It is found that the opening probability (P_o) of the mechanosensitive channels is maximal at the mid position and **decreases** when the membrane is strained into a convex or a concave formation. This suggests that the cation channels are, like *E. coli*'s MscL channels, sensitive to lateral stretch of the membrane (Figure 6.5B). It should be noted, however, that the MCN mechanosensitive channels respond to stretch in the opposite way to that characteristic of the *E. coli* MscL channels. Instead of

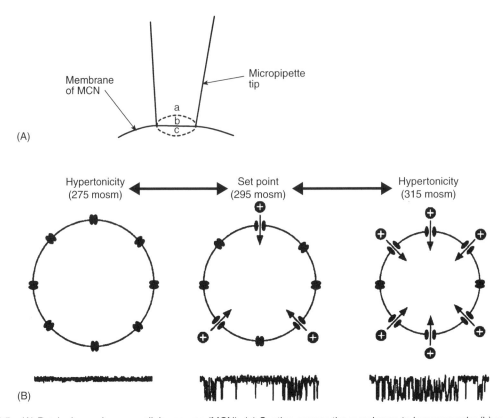

Figure 6.5 (A) Patch clamped magnocellular neuron (MCN). (a) Suction causes the membrane to bow upwards; (b) reduction in suction allows the membrane to return to it normal position; (c) when suction is reduced still further the membrane bows downwards. The opening probability of the mechanosensitive channels is maximal at (b). (B) Response of stretch inactivated (SI) channels to tonicity of surrounding medium. In isotonic conditions a few cationic channels are open and allow some influx of positive charge to maintain normal values of resting potential. Hypotonic solutions cause the cell to swell and the channels are switched off and the cell hyperpolarizes. Hypertonic solutions cause the cell to lose water and shrink, the opening probability of the cationic channels increases and the cell depolarizes. Further explanation in text. (From Bourque and Oliet, 1997: with permission, from the *Annual Review of Physiology*, Volume 59, © 1997, by Annual Reviews http://www.AnnualReviews.org).

opening in response to stretch, they close. They are, in other words, **stretch inactivated** (SI) channels.

At the time of writing the molecular structure of SI channels is not known. They are not restricted to magnocellular osmoreceptors but have been found in several other tissues, including skeletal muscle fibres and narrow diameter pain fibres. Although they have been isolated and cloned from mytotubes their structure has yet to be fully determined. Only when this has it been accomplished will it be possible to give a complete account, at the same level as that for *E. coli* stretch activated receptors, of how stretch-

ing induced, in the case of osmoreceptors, by the inflow of osmotic water can cause them to close. But we can already see how decreases in the osmolarity of the blood leads, via a removal of water from the MCN cells, to an inactivation and thus reduction in release of vasopressin and oxytocin. These hormones act on the kidney tubules to decrease loss of water (antidiuresis) and increase loss of Na^+ (natriuresis). Reduction in secretion of these hormones due to hypotonic inactivation of the MCNs thus leads to an increase in blood osmolarity until the MCN set point is once again reached.

6.3 CONCLUDING REMARKS

We are clearly just at the beginning of an understanding of the nature of mechanosensitive channels in cell membranes. Although the channels in *E. coli* seem at present very different from those present in the membranes of hypothalamic magnocellular neurosecretory neurons, it may be that, as research continues, molecular commonalities will become apparent. As we shall see in later chapters, it is often the case that molecular mechanisms hit upon very early in life's evolution are retained at the core of the highly complex and highly evolved sensory systems of 'higher' animals. We can see that this may well be the case with the MCN osmoreceptors discussed above. The molecular mechanisms in the membranes of these cells are fundamental to the elaborate neuroendocrine feedback loops which control the osmolarity of the mammal's 'internal environment'. We noted, also, that stretch sensitive and stretch insensitive channels are now known to exist in mammalian nociceptive and striped muscle fibres. Thus it may be that a deeper understanding of these channels will have medical applications in pain control and in treating the devastating condition of muscular dystrophy.

7

KINAESTHESIA

Kinaesthetic sense vital for active animals. **Kinaesthesia in arthropods: crustacea** – stretch receptors; **insects**: hair plates - campaniform sensilla - chordotonal organs; flight equilibrium - dipteran halteres. **Kinaesthesia in mammals**: muscle spindles: motor units - extrafusal and intrafusal fibres - bag and nuclear chain fibres - coactivation - fusimotor set; Golgi tendon organs: structure - function - reflexes to homonymous, antagonistic and synergistic muscles; joint receptors; cerebral representation. **Concluding remarks**: the kinaesthetic control of behavioural movements compared to the clumsiness of contemporary robotics.

Active animals need some way of sensing and controlling the dynamic position and orientation of their bodies. To do this the central nervous system needs to know (amongst other things) the state of contraction and/or tension of the body's multitudinous muscles and the positions of its various joints. In animals with a hard exoskeleton, such as the arthropods, this can largely be done with external sensors detecting the movements and positions of the jointed carapace and appendages. In soft-bodied forms with an endoskeleton, such as the vertebrates, much more emphasis is placed on the ongoing state of tension or relaxation of the body's musculature. This information is vital to active vertebrates and is thus *a fortiori* vital for ourselves: think of the miracles of balance and control displayed by the ice dancer or the Olympic gymnast, not to speak of our everyday experience of walking, running down stairs or carrying a tray laden with drinks. The control of posture and behavioural movements requires the continuous monitoring of muscle length and tension and the position of the joints. This so-called kinaesthetic sense is in large part unconscious; nevertheless, we all possess a 'body image', we all are aware when we stop to think, of the position of our limbs and so on. The kinaesthetic sense has thus sometimes been called the 'sixth' sense and for most of us it is just as important as the other five.

This kinaesthetic information is, of course, combined with information from the equilibrium sensors in the membranous labyrinth and visual information from the eyes. These inputs will be considered in Chapters 10 and 18, respectively. In the insects analogous information is also provided by the eyes and by sensory detectors at the bases of the wings, at the neck and in the Diptera, spectacularly, by the halteres. We shall discuss these latter mechanisms in Section 7.1.3.

7.1 KINAESTHETIC MECHANISMS IN ARTHROPODS

Arthropods differ radically from other animals in that their skeleton is external (exoskeleton) rather

Biology of Sensory Systems, Second Edition   C.U.M. Smith
© 2008 John Wiley & Sons, Ltd

than internal (endoskeleton). This fact has many large consequences. Perhaps the largest of all is that arthropods are, in general, restricted in size. Most are to be measured in millimeters and centimeters rather than meters. It also has large consequences for their sense organs. A hard, chitinous exoskeleton is not appropriate for the development of sense organs sensitive to depression or stretch of the surface. Nevertheless, as we noted in Chapter 4, arthropods, especially insects, are perhaps the most successful of all animal phyla and most are highly active forms. The kinaesthetic sense is well developed. Sense endings develop not only in the muscles but also in exoskeletal joints of the appendages and other parts of the body.

7.1.1 Stretch Receptors in Crustacean Muscle

The large abdominal muscles of long-bodied decapod and similar crustacea are of great importance in the biology of these animals. Contraction of the ventral muscles flexes the abdomen and this, with the help of the telson, causes the animal to shoot backwards out of danger. The proper management of these muscles is thus of considerable importance. In particular, it is important for the CNS to be kept informed of their state of tension and contraction.

Stretch receptors in the large muscles of the dorsal abdomen of decapod and other crustacea were studied in classical experiments carried out by Alexandrowicz in the 1950s. In long-bodied decapod crustacea such as the lobster, *Homarus gammarus*, and the crayfish, *Astacus fluviatilis*, a pair of modified muscle fibres known as **receptor muscles**, RM1 and RM2, are to be found on each side of the six abdominal segments and also in the extensor muscles of the seventh and eighth thoracic segments. Half way along the length of each of these muscle fibres the contractile machinery fails to develop and instead it is replaced by a clear region, over which the dendrites of a large multipolar neurosensory neuron ramifies (Figure 7.1) (compare the mammalian muscle spindle described below).

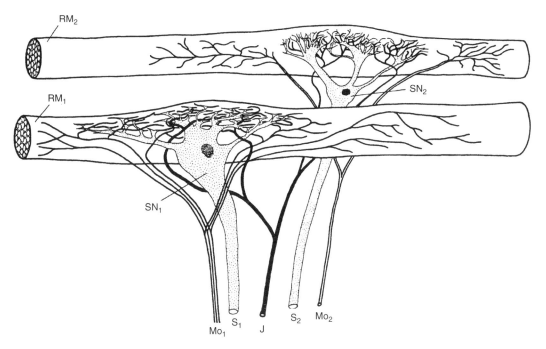

Figure 7.1 Schematic drawing of the stretch receptors in the abdominal segments of the crayfish, *Astacus fluviatilis*. RM1, RM2 = receptor muscles 1 and 2. SN1 = slow-adapting sensory neuron; SN2 = fast-adapting sensory neuron; S1, S2 = sensory fibres; Mo1 = three thin motor fibres to RM1; Mo2 = thick motor fibre to RM2; J = inhibitory fibre. From *Handbook of Physiology, Section 1, volume 1, Neurophysiology* (1959), p. 378. Reproduced by permission of The American Physiological Society.

Figure 7.1 shows that, in addition to the large neurosensory cells, motoneurons also supply the RMs. These motor fibres bifurcate and run along the surface of the RMs before forming myoneural junctions with their contractile extremities. In addition, one or more accessory fibres run to the neurosensory cell and either terminate on its perikaryon and dendrites and/or ramify over the clear central region of the RM.

Intracellular recordings show that in the relaxed condition the sensory cell has a V_m of about 70 mV. Stretch depolarizes the dendrites and the greater the stretch, the greater the depolarization. When the depolarization brings the membrane of the neurosensory cell innervating RM2 to about 20 mV (i.e. a depolarization of some 50 mV), an action potential is initiated in its axon. The neurosensory cell innervating RM1 requires a greater depolarization (some 60 mV) before it, in turn, fires. In the case of the RM2 neurosensory cell, the impulses adapt out in about a minute in response to a steady stretching force. It is consequently known as the **fast adapting** cell. In contrast, the neurosensory cell innervating RM1 hardly adapts at all and returns a steady stream of impulses for several hours in response to a steady stretch. It is known as the **slow adapting** cell. The frequency of impulses in both fast and slow adapting neurosensory axons is directly related to the intensity of stretch to which their respective RMs are subjected.

The central nervous system is able to set the sensitivity of these stretch receptors by means of accessory fibres. These fibres are of two types: inhibitory and excitatory. Stimulation of the inhibitory fibres inhibits discharge along the neurosensory cell axons in response to stretch. This is because the inhibitory discharge reduces the depolarization induced in the neurosensory cell by moderate stretch. The excitatory fibres, like the gamma fibres running to mammalian intrafusal fibres (see below), cause the RMs to contract in unison with the normal extensor muscle fibres of the crustacean abdomen. If the much more powerful normal fibres do not contract sufficiently far, this leaves the RM fibres under tension as they attempt to contract further. A reflex feedback then ensures that the normal fibres contract further until this tension is released and the neurosensory cells no longer detect stretch. These reflexes are very similar to those found in mammalian systems, where they have been much more intensively researched and

are, in consequence, better understood. Mammalian systems will be described in detail in Section 7.2.

7.1.2 Insect Sensilla

Because of their small size, the stretch receptors of insect muscle are not so well known as their crustacean counterparts. Multipolar neurons are, however, associated with many muscles and their free dendritic terminals, ramifying over the sarcolemmae, act as stretch detectors. In other cases the dendritic terminals ramify beneath the epidermis and respond to movement of the cuticle. There is evidence that they share a common origin, along with the far better known cuticular sensilla, from sensilla progenitor cells (SOPs).

Cuticular sensilla take a great and bewildering variety of forms (Figure 7.2). Fortunately, they all have a fundamentally similar plan, whichever sense modality they serve. We shall examine their structure more fully in Chapter 8 (Section 8.3) and there we shall note that they all contain one or more neurosensory cells within a cuticular housing. So far as

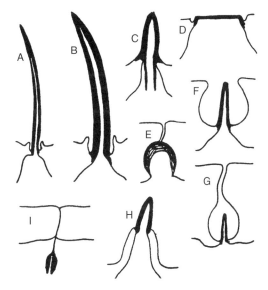

Figure 7.2 Various types of insect sensilla. A = trichoidea; B = chaetica; C = basiconica; D = placodea; E = campaniformia; F = coeloconica; G = ampullacea; H = styloconica; I = scolopophora. From Zacharuk, R.Y. (1985) in Gilbert, L.L. & Kerkut, G.A. (eds), *Comprehensive Insect Physiology, Biochemistry and Pharmacology, Vol. 6*, with permission from Elsevier Science.

kinaesthesia is concerned, sensilla may either be designed to detect the movements of cuticular joints of the exoskeleton and/or appendages, or may be positioned to respond to the relative movements of structures within the body cavity. In this section we shall focus on campaniform sensilla and chordotonal organs. Before turning to these kinaesthetic organs, however, it is worth noting that in some cases hair sensilla also play significant roles in sensing exoskeletal movements.

Hair sensilla are, for instance, strongly represented at joints in the body and appendages. Here they sometimes form' hair plates' consisting of dense brushworks (Figure 7.3a). The distribution of these

mechanosensitive sensilla on the body of a worker ant belonging to the species *Formica polyctena* is shown in Figure 7.3b. It can be seen that the ant's central nervous system is provided with a stream of information regarding the position, movement and direction of movement of the various parts of the anatomy. We shall see in the next section that vertebrates, in particular mammals, lacking an exoskeleton have evolved an equally elaborate system for detecting the movement and positions of their muscles and endoskeleton.

In contrast to the externally projecting hair of tactile sensilla, the hair in **campaniform sensilla** has been reduced to a simple dome or cupola, which is either circular or elliptical at its base (Figure 7.4). The dendrite from which a **tubular body** springs is usually located centrally. Deformations of the exoskeleton depress the dome and thus compress the tubular body. An inward movement of the dome by as little as 0.1 nm has been shown to be sufficient to stimulate the neurosensory cell. Elliptical domes are most sensitive to compression along their short axis. In this way directional selectivity is achieved. Campaniform

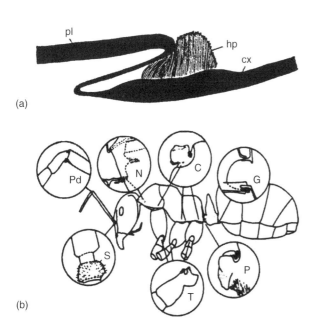

(a)

(b)

Figure 7.3 (a) The figure shows the brushwork of sensilla at the articulation of the second leg of the cockroach, *Periplaneta americana*. The thick cuticle of the pleuron (pl) thins to a delicate articular membrane and then thickens again to form the cuticle surrounding the coxa (cx), the first segment of the leg. The brush of sensilla forms a hairplate (hp). From Pringle J.W.S. (1938) *Journal of Experimental Biology*, **15**, 467–73, Copyright © 1938, The Company of Biologists Ltd. (b) Worker ant of the species *Formica polyctena* to show the distribution of some of the hair plates. C = coxal joints; G = gaster; N = neck; P = petiole (narrow connection between thorax and abdomen); Pd = joint between first and second antennal segments; S = joint between antenna and head; T = joint between coxa and trochanter (second leg segment). From Markl, H. and Tautz, J. (1975), *Journal of Comparative Physiology*, **99**, 79–87, Copyright © 1975, Springer.

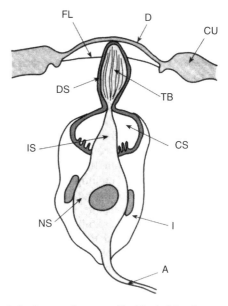

Figure 7.4 Campaniform sensilla. The hair has been reduced to a dome or cupola into which the tubular body is inserted. A = sensory axon; CS = ciliary sinus; Cu = cuticle; D = dome; DS = dendritic sheath; FL = fibrous layer; I = inner sheath cell; IS = inner segment; NS = neurosensory cell; TB = tubular body.

sensilla are often found in the vicinity of joints and articulations and at the bases of tactile hairs.

Other types of mechanosensitive sensilla develop within the body cavity. The best known and most widely distributed of these are the **chordotonal organs**. They are composed of specialized sensilla known as **scolopidia** (Figure 7.5). A scolopidium consists of one or more neurosensory cells from whose dendrite, as in other mechanoreceptive sensilla, a sensory cilium springs. A tubular body is never found. A distinguishing feature is the presence of scolopale cells which surround the cilium and secrete a dense intracellular sheath, the **scolopale**. This sheath consists of a barrel-shaped sleeve of fibrous scolapale rods. The sensory ending of the scolopidium is enclosed within an envelope or attachment cell

and the whole attached to a cap cell. The cap cell, in turn, connects, sometimes through accessory cells, with internal structures such as tracheae, muscles, gut and so on.

Chordotonal organs form one of the principal proprioceptor types within the insect body. They are present in nearly every exoskeletal joint and between body segments. They vary in complexity from consisting of a few scolopidia to several thousand. Many of them are also very sensitive to vibration. A well known example of this function is provided by the **subgenual** organ located in the prothoracic leg of many insect species. Here twenty to fifty scolopidia are massed together within the tibia and attached to its cuticle. In the cockroach, *Periplaneta americana,* the subgenual organ is sensitive to vibrations within

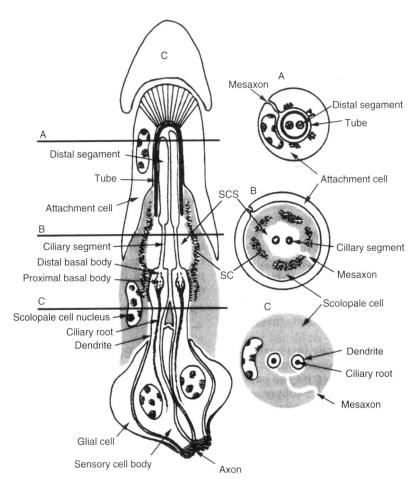

Figure 7.5 Diagrammatic longitudinal section through a scolopidium with transverse sections at various levels. C = cap cell; sc = scolopale; scs = scolopale space. Modified from Moulins, 1976.

the range 1000–5000 Hz with a threshold amplitude of between 1 and 100 nm. Detection of vibration is not only important as a danger signal but is also used by many social insects as a means of communication. This brings us towards the topic of sound detection. This topic will, however, be left until Chapter 8, when the detection of acoustic stimuli by insects will be considered.

7.1.3 Maintenance of Equilibrium in Flight

Anyone who has contemplated the flying skills of the humble housefly must have marvelled at its ability to retain its orientation and sense of direction. Insect flight is reflexly controlled. It may be initiated by interrupting the contact of tarsal mechanoreceptors with the substratum. It is maintained through stimulation of pads of mechanosensitive sensilla at the bases of the wings by air currents. Deviation from correct orientation in flight may be described as rotations about the three spatial axes: **pitching** – rotation anteroposteriorly about a horizontal axis at right angles to the body's long axis; **yawing** – rotation of the body's long axis around a vertical axis; **rolling** – rotation about the longitudinal axis (Figure 7.6).

Orientation is maintained partly by visual input from the eyes, partly by sense organs at the bases of the wings (especially in insects with two pairs of wings), partly by sense organs at the connection of the head to the thorax and, in Dipteran insects, partly by the **halteres**. Large dragonflies are some of the most expert fliers in the insect world, hunting and catching other insects on the wing. They possess three pads of hair sensilla on each side of the neck which can detect angular accelerations. In flight the head is held in position by visual input from the eyes. If the body twists out of position this is signalled by the hair pads. The two pairs of wings act reflexly to bring the body back in line with the head. This mechanism is also at work in most other flying insects. In the dipteran insects the hind wings are modified to form dumb-bell shaped halteres with numerous campaniform sensilla at their bases (Figure 7.7). The halteres oscillate through 180° at frequencies of 100 Hz to well over 500 Hz in synchrony with the beat of the wings. The campaniform sensilla sense differing forces on the haltere–thorax articulation as the insect pitches, yaws or rolls. Removal of the halteres adversely affects the reflex compensations of the wing muscles to these incipient rotations.

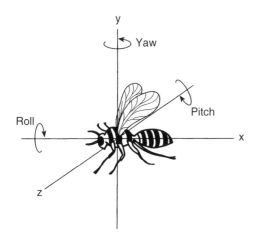

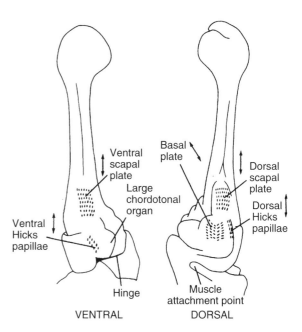

Figure 7.6　Pitching, yawing and rolling. Rolling occurs when the body rotates on its long axis (the *x*-axis); yawing occurs when the body rotates on the *y*-axis; pitching occurs when the body rotates on its *z*-axis.

Figure 7.7　Dorsal and ventral aspects of Dipteran halteres. The orientation of the various groups of campaniform sensilla are indicated by double-headed arrows. Adapted from Pringle (1938).

7.2 KINAESTHETIC MECHANISMS IN MAMMALS

Lacking a rigid exoskeleton, the kinaesthetic mechanisms in mammals (including ourselves) are of necessity restricted to sense endings in muscles, tendons and internal joints. These work together to provide the central nervous system with a continuously updated 'picture' of the state of tension or relaxation of the body's musculature and the position of the joints. In this section, we shall consider each of these sense endings in turn, starting with **spindles**, going on to **tendon organs** and ending with **joint mechanoreceptors**.

7.2.1 Intrafusal Spindle Endings

Skeletal (voluntary) muscles consist of many thousand multinucleate striated fibres. In humans each muscle fibre is innervated by a single motoneuron. The motoneuron, however, branches as it enters the muscle and hence will innervate a number of fibres. This is known as multiterminal innervation and the group of muscle fibres plus the single motoneuron is defined as a **motor unit**. It is the smallest functional unit of the muscular system. The number of muscle fibres constituting a motor unit varies from muscle to muscle. Where fine control is required, as, for instance, in the finger or extrinsic eye muscles, the motor unit is small, perhaps no more than five to ten muscle fibres; where fine control is unnecessary, as, for example, in the muscles of the back or thigh, the motor unit is far larger consisting of perhaps more than a thousand fibres.

Mammalian muscle fibres are divided into two major types: **extrafusal fibres**, which do all the work, and **intrafusal fibres**, which are specialized to detect stretch. Both sets of fibres originate in much the same way during embryological development but, whereas the extrafusal fibres develop a full complement of actin, myosin and other contractile proteins, the intrafusal fibres only develop this contractile machinery at their extremities. Instead, the intrafusal fibres are associated with the spiral endings of 1a and group II sensory nerve fibres to form **spindle stretch receptors**. There are, in fact, three types of intrafusal fibre: two types of **nuclear bag fibre** and one type of **nuclear chain fibre**. Typically, two bag fibres and a number of chain fibres are associated together and surrounded by a loose-fitting connective tissue capsule to form the spindle ending (Figure 7.8).

The nuclear chain fibres, as their name indicates, are short and slender and contain a long row of nuclei. They respond to steady stretching forces. The nuclear bag fibres, in contrast, are larger and longer and contain a group of nuclei in a swelling (or bag) towards their centre. One type of nuclear bag fibre (dynamic) responds to the onset or release of a stretching force while the other (static) responds, like the nuclear chain fibres, to a steady state stretch. The spindle is innervated by four sets of nerve fibres (Figure 7.8) which all enter the capsule at its slightly enlarged middle section. Two of these four sets of fibres are sensory and two motor. The sensory fibres are of two types: group 1a axons (large diameter) and group II axons (small diameter). The group 1a fibres normally end by spiralling around all the intrafusal fibres in the spindle. The group II axons, however, terminate only on the nuclear chain fibres and the static nuclear bag fibre. The motor fibres are all small calibre, slowly conducting, **gamma fibres**. But, as Figure 7.8b shows, they can be divided into two sets: dynamic and static depending on which type of intrafusal fibre they innervate. In both cases they run to the extremities of the intrafusal fibres, where some contractile machinery still exists, and terminate in myoneural junctions.

The spiral endings of the sensory fibres are very closely adposed to the intrafusal fibres. If the latter are subjected to stretch, the endings of the sensory fibres will also be stretched. This, as in the other cases considered in this chapter, is the adequate stimulus and leads, via the opening of ion channels, to a generator potential. This, in turn, sets off an action potential at the initiating site in the sensory fibre. Group 1a sensory fibres are rapidly conducting (circa 120 m/s) and group II fibres also conduct relatively rapidly (circa 75 m/s) (Section 2.6, Table 2.2). The signal is conducted to the spinal cord via the posterior (= dorsal roots) of the spinal nerves (Figure 7.9).

Whilst the innervation of the intrafusal fibres is by gamma motoneurons, the innervation of the surrounding extrafusal fibres is by large diameter rapidly conducting **alpha motoneurons**. These two systems of motoneurons are thus quite distinct and have been termed the **fusimotor** and **skeletomotor** systems, respectively. Unfortunately, as so often happens in

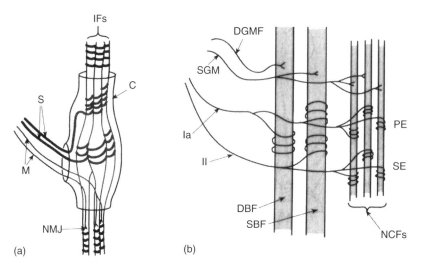

Figure 7.8 Mammalian muscle spindle. (a) A group of three intrafusal fibres is shown. *In vivo* these would be surrounded by extrafusal fibres. Their extremities retain actinomyosin contractile machinery and are hence cross striated. The central region of the intrafusal fibre is somewhat swollen and surrounded by a connective tissue capsule. It is innervated by two types of gamma motor fibre. These fibres enter the capsule and run to the extremities where they make junctions with the intrafusal fibres. M = gamma motor fibres; C = capsule; S = 1a and II sensory fibres; IFs = intrafusal fibres; NMJ = neuromuscular junction. (b) Schematic figure to show the five types of intrafusal fibre which are found in the mammalian muscle spindle. DBF = dynamic bag fibre; DGMF = dynamic gamma motor fibre; NCFs = nuclear chain fibres; PE = primary ending; SBF = static bag fibre; SE = static ending; SGMF = static gamma motor fibre. Further explanation in text. Adapted from Kandel, E.R., Schwartz, J.H. and Jessel, T.M. (eds) (1991).

biology, the situation is not quite clear-cut. It has been shown that some alpha motoneurons send branches into the spindle to innervate the intrafusal fibres. These fibres are said to constitute a skeleto-fusimotor system and appear to be present in all mammalian spindle preparations. It is worth noting that there is no clear-cut distinction between fusimotor and skeletomotor systems in anamniote vertebrates.

How does all this work? The spindles, as we have seen, are located in parallel with the extrafusal fibres. When a signal is sent down the spinal cord from higher centres commanding a muscle movement, both alpha and gamma motoneurons are activated (Figure 7.9a). This is known (for obvious reasons) as **coactivation**. Alpha motoneurons conduct action potentials very rapidly (up to 120 m/s) and consequently will reach and activate the extrafusal fibres long before a message coming slowly down the gamma fibres reaches the intrafusal fibres. The muscle will consequently contract and release any tension on the intrafusal fibres. Any activity in the sensory fibres will cease. However, as soon as the gamma fibre input reaches the intrafusal fibres they

will also contract. If the gamma fibre input demands a greater contraction of the intrafusal fibres than was achieved by the surrounding extrafusal fibres, then they (i.e. intrafusal fibres) in attempting, unsuccessfully, to contract will be tensed. This tension will be detected by the spiral endings of the sensory neurons, which will consequently transmit a tattoo of impulses back to the central nervous system.

What effect does this have? To answer this question we have to consider the reflex circuits controlling muscular contraction. These are, in fact, highly intricate but for our present purposes we can consider just one element (Figure 7.9a). The cell bodies of the alpha and gamma motoneurons are located in the anterior (=ventral) horn of the grey matter. As Figure 7.9a shows, the 1a sensory fibres from the spindles make excitatory synapses with these alpha motoneurons. The diagram is, of necessity, simplified. The 1a fibres not only excite alpha motoneurons to the homonymous (i.e. same) muscle but also those running to synergistic muscles. These are muscles that move the joint in a similar way to the homonymous muscle. In addition, as Figure 7.9b shows, a branch of the 1a fibre runs to an inhibitory interneuron in

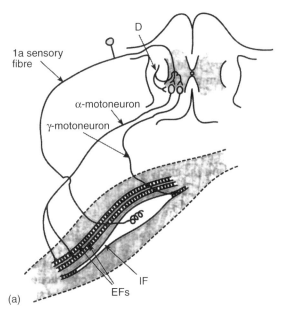

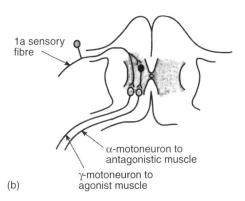

Figure 7.9 (a) Coactivation. The figure shows a transverse section of the spinal cord and a simplified version of the nerve fibre connections to the intra- and extrafusal fibres of a skeletal muscle. D = fibre descending in the cord's white matter from higher centres; EFs = extrafusal fibres; IF = intrafusal fibre. (b) Inhibition of antagonistic muscle(s). Inhibitory neuron is black. Further explanation in text.

This reflex circuitry ensures that, when the intrafusal fibre experiences tension, it is quickly released by further contraction of the extrafusal fibres. In essence, the central nervous system has only to set the length of the intrafusal fibres and the reflex servomechanism in the spinal cord ensures that the extrafusal fibres arrive at and maintain that length. The joint is moved to the required position.

But why the complex organization of the spindle? Why the differentiation into nuclear bag fibres and nuclear chain fibres and so on? The answer to these questions emerges from the different physiological properties of the bag and chain fibres. We noted above that whereas the chain fibres responded to maintained stretch, one of the nuclear bag fibres, the dynamic fibre, responded best to onset and release of stretch. The activity in the two sets of sensory fibres innervating the spindle ending thus differs. The 1a fibres signal onset and release of tension, the group II fibres signal maintained tension (Figure 7.10). In addition the 1a fibres are maximally

the grey matter of the spinal cord. This inhibitory neuron synapses on the cell bodies of motoneurons running to antagonistic muscles. These muscles are thus prevented from contracting at the same time as the agonist. This latter mechanism can be overridden by messages from higher centres so that we can, as we all know, balance the contraction of one muscle against another.

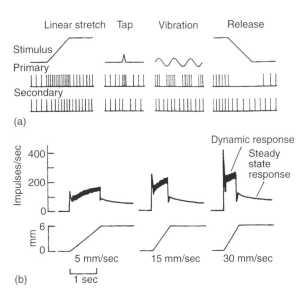

Figure 7.10 Responses of primary and secondary endings of muscle spindles (see Figure 7.8). (a): The 1a fibres from primary spindle endings signal onset of stretch by a burst of activity and release of tension by a temporary silence. The group II fibres from secondary spindle endings signal steady stretch. (b): The primary endings are responsive to different velocities of stretch. The figure shows that the 1a fibres respond more vigorously the more rapid the onset of stretch. Further explanation in text. From Kandel, E.R., Schwartz, J.H. and Jessel, T.M. (eds) (1991), *Principles of Neuroscience*, Copyright © 1991, Elsevier.

sensitive to small changes in length (<1 mm) and also, and importantly, to rate of change. 1a fibres, in other words, are **velocity sensitive**. Hence discharge from the 1a and group II sensory fibres encodes not only steady state stretch (group II fibres) but also the velocity of contraction (group 1a).

It can be shown that there is separate gamma control of dynamic bag fibres and static bag and chain fibres. One set of gamma motoneurons controls the static fibres and another set of gamma motoneurons controls the dynamic fibres. This differential innervation is due to the different structure and physiology of the two types of intrafusal fibre. In the case of the dynamic fibre, the central region is specialized to respond quickly to onset and release of tension. Activation of the dynamic gamma motoneurons enhances the sensitivity of this central region. In the static fibres, on the other hand, the whole extent of the fibre responds in a more sustained way to stretching forces. Activation of the static gamma motoneurons causes the contractile extremities to contract (as described above), stretching the whole of the central region.

The delicate control of muscle contraction is obviously of paramount importance to all animals and, in particular, to active animals such as mammals. So it is, perhaps, not surprising to find that, superimposed on the highly evolved feedback and feedforward system described in the preceding paragraphs, there is a higher control known as **fusimotor set**. When a mammal, such as a cat, is resting, very little if any impulse traffic can be detected in the either the static or dynamic gamma motoneurons. When the animal gets up and stretches itself and pads slowly away, a low level of activity in the static gamma motoneurons is present. Very little if any activity is present in the dynamic gamma system. As activity increases, as the animal undertakes difficult and demanding manoeuvres, activity in the static system decreases and activity in the dynamic system cuts in and becomes increasingly vigorous. The central nervous system is thus able to adjust the sensitivity of its control to suit the circumstances in which its owner finds itself.

7.2.2 Golgi Tendon Organs

Golgi tendon organs work in conjunction with the muscle spindles to signal the state of contraction and tension of the skeletal muscles. Whereas the spindles signal changes in muscle length, the tendon organs signal tension. Whereas spindles work 'in parallel' with extrafusal muscle fibres, tendon organs operate 'in series'. This complementarity is reflected in the fact that tendon organs are often anatomically associated with spindles. In some muscles of the cat's leg (soleus, medial gastrocnemius, etc.) 25% of tendon organs were found in 'dyad' association with spindles, and in jaw muscles virtually all tendon organs were paired with spindles.

Although their name suggests that they are located in tendons and/or aponeuroses, this is not wholly correct. In fact, the vast majority of tendon organs are located at the junctions between tendons (or aponeuroses) and muscles. Furthermore, it used to be thought that it was immaterial how the tension was generated – by active contraction of 'their' muscle or passive stretch. It has, however, been shown more recently that passive stretch is not a very effective means of stimulation: the 'adequate stimulus' is muscular contraction. The association between tendon organs and motor units is often quite precise. Individual tendon organs monitor the tension induced by single motor units.

The sensory endings of a tendon organ are housed within a lamellar capsule which is continuous with the perineural sheath of a fast-conducting Ib sensory axon (Figure 7.11). The capsule varies greatly in magnitude (from 242 to 1045 μm in length (mean 521 μm)) and diameter (from 66 to 220 μm (mean 125 μm)). The capsule is divided internally into a number of compartments filled with braided collagen fibres. Once within the capsule the Ib sensory fibre divides many times, losing its myelin sheath and weaving between the braided collagen fibres, eventually forming terminals on them. These terminals are filled with mitochondria and closely invest the collagen fibres.

When the muscle fibre contracts, the resulting alteration to the disposition of the attached collagen fibres deforms the sensory endings, thus inducing conductance changes across their membranes. The resulting generator potential spreads electrotonically to an impulse-initiating site where an action potential is engendered. In experiments using cat dorsolateral tail muscle fibres it was shown that, when the collagen fibres were subjected to a steady stretching force, the generator potential was linearly related to

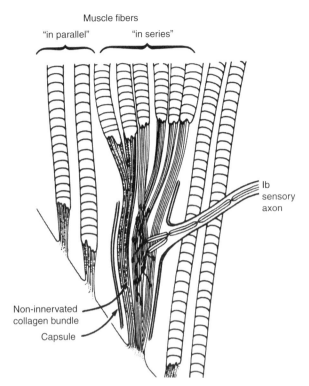

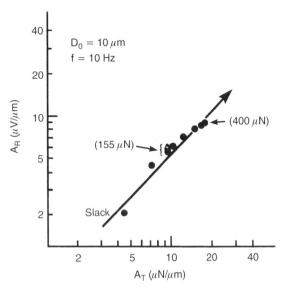

Figure 7.12 Relation between receptor potential (A_R) and tension (A_T) in response to a 10 Hz, 10 μm, sinusoidal stretch delivered at different initial tensions (T_I). The initial tensions varied from zero (slack) to 400 μN. D_0 = stretch amplitude; f = frequency. From Wilkinson and Fukami (1983) *Journal of Physiology*, **49**, p. 984, Figure 16, by permission of the American Physiological Society.

Figure 7.11 Schematic figure of a tendon organ. The capsule is shown cut in section. The figure shows that the muscle fibres 'in series' with the tendon organ are surrounded by larger number of fibres, 'in parallel', which are inserted into the same tendon or aponeurosis. From Jami, 1992: From *Physiological Reviews*, **72**, 623–66, by permission of the American Physiological Society.

the tension. Using the more dynamic conditions of an oscillating stretching force it was shown that for very small stretches (0.5–5 μm) the gain was constant (circa 10 μV/μm stretch at 10 Hz). The magnitude of the receptor potential could also be shown to depend on the initial tension (Figure 7.12). Finally, it could be shown that the gain depended on the frequency of stimulation: the higher the frequency, up to about 20 Hz, the greater the gain. When larger stretches were applied or higher frequencies, nonlinearities appeared and, as mentioned above, the situation may be yet more complex *in vivo*.

The precise position where the action potential is initiated remains in doubt. It may be at the first node of Ranvier but other possibilites exist. In experiments with oscillating stimuli the impulse frequency in the Ib sensory fibre was locked to the stimulus frequency

rather than its amplitude. The CNS, however, needs to 'know' the magnitude of the stretching force experienced by the tendon. It thus appears that it is the pooled discharge of all the tendon organs which provides this information. Even this, however, is not fully borne out by experiment. It appears that what is signalled to the CNS is not so much the level of tensile force at any given moment but the dynamic events in the development of that force. This information is, itself, obscured by the nonlinear character of the muscle fibres and sheaths and the properties of tendons. As we shall see in other cases, the working of sensory systems is slow to yield to simple mechanistic analyses. The CNS has to deal with and make sense of a flood of incoming impulses. It is probably the overall pattern of this gigantic traffic which is significant rather than any particular element.

Action potentials in Ib sensory nerve fibres run into the spinal cord and (for the most part) make synapses with inhibitory interneurons which synapse on homonymous motor neurons (Figure 7.13). Inhibitory interneurons also inhibit motor neurons to synergistic muscles (not shown in Figure 7.13).

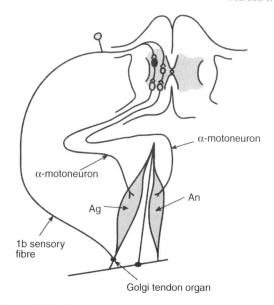

α-motoneuron

α-motoneuron

Ag

An

1b sensory
fibre

Golgi tendon organ

Figure 7.13 'Wiring diagram' for the negative feedback control provided by Golgi tendon organs. Compare with the wiring diagram for spindle control shown in Figure 6.9. Note that there is no monosynaptic pathway in the tendon organ reflex and that the whole system works in the opposite sense to the spindle reflexes. Ag = agonist muscle; An = antagonist muscle. Further explanation in text.

Finally, the Ib sensory fibre also synapses with an excitatory interneuron which, in turn, makes synapses on motor neurons to antagonistic muscles.

What is the upshot of this complex system? Although the details are still being researched and although we are far from understanding the full complexity of the system, the outlines seem clear. Tendon organs remain quiet when the muscle is quiet. When it starts to contract they begin to discharge. They signal changes in the build up of contractile force. The impulse traffic in the Ib sensory fibres damps down the activity of homonymous motor neurons and restrains the recruitment of new units. It also restricts activity in motor neurons to synergistic muscles and excites the activity in motor neurons to antagonistic muscles. In this way it ensures that the contraction is smooth and closely related to the task required. Working together with the muscle spindle system it ensures that when we pick up an object, the muscular power is closely suited to its mass. It ensures that when we touch a surface or palpate a texture,

we do so with a delicacy which allow our cutaneous touch receptors (Chapter 8) to report its smoothness, dryness or tackiness.

7.2.3 Joint Receptors

Three types of sensory ending exist in most joints: Ruffini-type endings (Chapter 8) located in the joint capsule; Golgi-type endings present in the ligaments of the joint; and Pacinian corpuscle type endings (Chapter 8) found near the attachment of ligaments to the periosteum. When the joint is in a median position, very little impulse traffic can be detected in the afferent fibres leading away from these receptors. However, as the joint flexes or extends towards its extreme positions, the impulse traffic dramatically increases.

Studies of single Ruffini-type units show that they are, for the most part, slowly adapting and that each has an 'excitatory angle': an arc of maximal sensitivity covering a few degrees of angular movement of the joint. This angle differs for different units. The discharge of each unit is related to the rate of angular displacement and, furthermore, increases as it reaches the limit of its 'excitatory angle'. Whereas there are few units monitoring movement of the joint to each side of its central position, there are many units sensitive to movement at its extremes. This nicely accounts for the observation noted in the previous paragraph that impulse traffic in afferent nerve fibres rises to a maximum as the joint moves to its extreme positions.

The situation is complicated by the finding that rotation of a joint, such as the much-studied knee or elbow joint, about its long axis affects the discharge from the Ruffini-type endings. Where such movement occurs, the Ruffini discharge will not signal completely unambiguous information about joint position or rate of movement to the CNS. The other types of sense ending around a joint, particularly the Golgi and Pacinian endings, are likely to signal information about the tension of the activating muscles rather than the exact position of the joint. Nevertheless, the location of these latter sensory endings in and around the joint capsule ensures that maximal activity will occur when the joint moves to its extreme positions or rotates out of true.

7.3 CONCLUDING REMARKS

We have only to look at the clumsy creations of robotic engineers to recognize the suppleness and subtlety of an animal's 'sixth sense'. Robotics has, of course, developed hugely since the primitive contraptions of earlier times. The hydraulically powered automata of St Germaine en Laye, which so impressed René Descartes in the early seventeenth century, or the mechanical prostheses invented by the French military surgeon, Ambroise Paré, in the late sixteenth century, or even the mechanical flute player of Vaucanson in the eighteenth century, seem crude indeed compared with the devices engineered for modern industry and the military. Yet even these modern devices, able, like the Mars Rover, to clamber over difficult terrain and sample the subsoil or, like the universally jointed arms of automated welding machines in modern automobile factories, to reach into and spot-weld awkward and obscure seams, fall far short of their biological counterparts. Partly this is due to their rigid construction and lack (up to now) of sufficient miniaturization. But mostly it is due to their huge deficiency, when compared with their animal exemplars, in the multitudinous sense organs and endings we have been considering in this chapter. The sensory input raining in on the CNS from this multitudinous array ensures the suppleness and adaptedness of the motor output to the behavioural muscles. Over evolutionary time this sensory inflow, this sixth sense, has been honed to provide the fluidity and sensitivity of response that we take for granted as part of what it is to be alive. But, as we have seen in this chapter, it depends on the integration of innumerable feedback and feedforward loops. Researchers are still uncovering the full subtlety of these mechanisms which, as we have again noted, reach right down to the molecular level. This, too, is a point of contrast with the robot, which is ultimately constructed of amorphous parts: metals, ceramics, silicon.

The feedback and feedforward loops of the animal's sixth sense all pass through the central nervous system, either the spinal cord (as we saw in this chapter when discussing the spinal reflexes) or higher, into and through the brain, especially the brain stem, pons, cerebellum and motor cortices. There we shall not follow them in this book. The interested student must consult one or other of the texts in neurophysiology listed in the bibliography. Suffice it to say that the sensory input from the muscles, joints and tendons is (in the case of mammals) integrated with input from the vestibular system, the eyes and elsewhere, so that the brain computes output to the muscular system appropriate to the animal's ever-changing circumstances. It will be many years, if ever, before the robotics engineer can compete.

8

TOUCH

Touch sensitivity in *C. elegans*: mec mutations - touch receptor neurons - genetic analysis - MEC proteins - resemblance to mammalian ENaCs - other mec genes and their protein products - possible molecular structure of *C. elegans* tactile receptor – TRP channels on nose rays. **Touch sensitivity in spiders**: tactile hairs – trichobothria – slit sensilla – lyriform organs. **Touch sensitivity in insects**: tactile sensilla – TRP channels - subgenual organs - detection of water ripples by pond skaters and water-boatmen - acoustic sensilla – Drosphila: Aristae - Johnston's organ - sensitivity to wing-beat frequencies - tympanal organs (ears): stucture and function - communication - prey detection - detection of insectivorous bats by lacewings and moths - structure of Noctuid ear - Noctuid countermeasures against bats. **Touch sensitivity in mammalian skin**: fast adapting receptors: Pacinian corpuscles, Meissner's corpuscles, Krause's end bulbs, hair follicle receptors; slow adapting receptors: Merkel cells, Ruffini organs, C-mechanoreceptors. **Central pathways in mammals**: tracts in spinal cord - somaesthetic cortices - columnar structure - receptive fields - somaesthetic homunculus. **Plasticity of the cortex**: mice whisker barrels - monkey fingers - cello players - Braille readers. **Concluding rremarks**: a universal sense - social grooming - communication and bonding.

It can be argued, as we noted in the introduction to Part Two, that touch is the indispensable sense. It is difficult to imagine what it would be like without this sense modality. Indeed, it is difficult to imagine how the world would appear to a being lacking the sense of touch. Our very notions of solidity, resistance, of objectivity itself, would hardly have developed in the absence of this all-pervading sense. Yet, compared with our intimate knowledge of the molecular biology of olfactory and visual receptors, our understanding of the precise mechanisms by which our tactile receptors work is as yet sparse and unsatisfying. This, however, is slowly beginning to change with advances in molecular biology and the use of simple 'model organisms', such as the tiny soil-dwelling roundworm, *Caenorhabditis elegans*.

8.1 MECHANORECEPTION IN *CAENORHABDITIS ELEGANS*

We noted in Chapter 5 that *C. elegans* has been intensively studied by molecular biologists. In essence, when geneticists felt that the major outlines of prokaryocyte biology had been established with work on *E. coli* and that protistan biology was well advanced in the type–example of yeast, *Saccharomyces cervisiae*, the next and final frontier

Biology of Sensory Systems, Second Edition   C.U.M. Smith
© 2008 John Wiley & Sons, Ltd

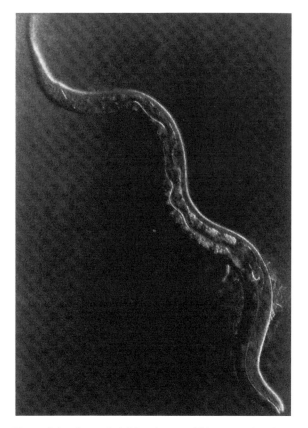

Figure 8.1 *Caenorhabditis elegans*. This worm is about 200 mm in length. *C. elegans* consists of 959 somatic cells of which 302 constitute the nervous system. The body is translucent and many of its cells can be distinguished in the living animal. From White, J. G. (1985), Neuronal connectivity in Caenorhabditis elegans, *Trends In Neurosciences*, **8**, 277–283, © 1985 with permission from Elsevier Science.

beckoned in the Metazoa. Geneticists consequently looked for an animal that was easily cultured and had a rapid generation time, so that the powerful methods used in microbial genetics could be adapted and applied. The organism chosen was the small (circa 0.5 mm long) free-living soil nematode *Caenorhabditis elegans* (Figure 8.1). Over some forty years of intensive investigation this organism has yielded up the secrets of its genetics, its physiology, its anatomy and its behaviour. The precise number of nerve cells in its central nervous system is known (302), the synaptic structure of the nervous system and each of its neurons has been totally elucidated in the electron microscope and its genome was determined in 1998.

Like all animals *C. elegans* is sensitive to touch. There are two systems. Touch to the body wall is detected by a group of six neurons, whilst that to the nose is detected by three neurons in the mechanosensitive rays, or 'cilia'. Let us consider each in turn.

Mechanosensitivity of the lateral body wall has been investigated using two touch stimuli: a gentle touch on the body with an eyelash glued to a cocktail stick and a more vigorous prod with a thin wire. The most interesting results have come from investigations of the response to the gentle stimulation.

When *C. elegans* is placed in a petri dish it moves forward with a sinusoidal motion until it encounters a tactile stimulus. If it is given a gentle touch on the anterior part of its body the movement reverses and the worm squirms backward across the dish; if the gentle touch is applied to the posterior it will move forward. A large number of mutations (over 440) affecting 15 genes have been shown to interfere with these responses. That the worms were still capable of movement was confirmed by using the vigorous wire prod. Most of these mutations were classified as *mec* mutants because the phenotype they generate is described as mechanosensitive abnormal (mec). In consequence, the genes are called *mec* genes and the proteins which they designate MEC proteins.

It can be shown that touch is detected by six touch detector neurons. There are: two anterior lateral microtubule cells (left and right) – ALML and ALMR; two posterior lateral microtubule cells (left and right) – PLML and PLMR; one anterior ventral microtubule cell – AVM. One further neuron seems to be involved although, unlike the others, it is unable to mediate touch avoidance on its own. This is the posterior ventral microtubule cell – PVM. The anatomical location of these touch detector neurons is shown in Figure 8.2.

The touch receptor neurons, as their names indicate, are filled with a bundle of extra large microtubules. Electron microscopy suggests that the individual microtubules in the bundle are linked together and they all have the peculiarity of consisting of 15 protofilaments (rather than the 11 protofilament ultrastructure of other *C. elegans* microtubules or the 13 protofilaments found in microtubules elsewhere in the animal kingdom). These extra-large and ultrastructurally rather odd microtubules are much shorter than the neuron (no more than about 5% of the latter's length) and seem to run obliquely to the

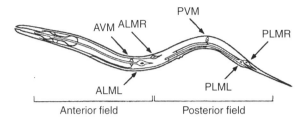

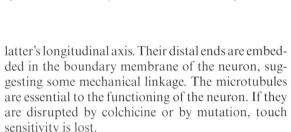

Figure 8.2 *C. elegans* touch receptor neurons. Note that there are two fields of touch sensitivity determined by the disposition of the neurons in the nematode's body. ALML = anterior lateral microtubule cell left; ALMR = anterior lateral microtubule cell right; PLML = posterior lateral microtubule cell left; PLMR = posterior lateral microtubule cell right; AVM = anterior ventral microtubule cell. From Tavernarakis and Driscoll, 1997: with permission, from the *Annual Review of Physiology*, Volume 59, by Annual Reviews, http://www.Annual Reviews.org.

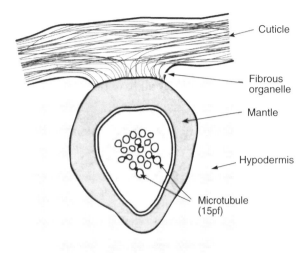

Figure 8.3 Ultrastructure of *C. elegans* touch receptor neuron in transverse section. The neuron is surrounded by a connective tissue mantle and is attached to the cuticle by a 'fibrous organelle'. It contains a bundle of microtubles (each composed of 15 protofilaments (pf)). Adapted from Tavernarakis, N. and Driscoll, M. (1997).

latter's longitudinal axis. Their distal ends are embedded in the boundary membrane of the neuron, suggesting some mechanical linkage. The microtubules are essential to the functioning of the neuron. If they are disrupted by colchicine or by mutation, touch sensitivity is lost.

The touch receptor neurons themselves run just beneath the cuticle ('skin') of the worm to which they are attached by an extracellular 'mantle' of fibrous material (Figure 8.3). The ultrastructure suggests that there is mechanical continuity between the cuticle and the microtubules within the touch neurons. It is worth recalling that the tubular body of insect mechanosensitive hairs is also composed of close-packed microtubules, in this case bridging the neurosensory cell and the cuticle (Sections 7.1.2 and 8.2.1).

Genetic analysis proceeded by generating mutations in the worm and examining their progeny for loss of response to gentle touch. When such a loss was detected, molecular biological techniques were employed to determine what structure the mutated gene normally designated. In some cases the genes were found to be responsible for factors necessary for the development of the touch cells themselves, in other cases for controlling the action of other *mec* genes. In more interesting cases genes were discovered which designated channel proteins and accessory elements connecting the channels to the cuticle on the one hand and to the neuronal microtubules on the other.

Mec-4 and *mec-10* are the two genes which designate the channel proteins – MEC-4 and MEC-10. These genes have also been called 'degenerins' because mutations in them, leading to defective MEC-4 and MEC-10, cause the cells in which they are expressed to swell and die. Both MEC-4 and MEC-10 belong to a superfamily of proteins which includes the three subunits of the mammalian epithelial Na^+-channel protein (ENaC). There are two transmembrane segments; both C-terminal and N-terminal are intracellular and there is a large extracellular loop (Figure 8.4). Although the precise structure of the MEC channel has yet to be determined, analogy with other channels, especially the mammalian ENaC channel, suggests an assembly of six subunits, possibly a mixture of MEC-4s and MEC-10s. There is some evidence that *mec-6* encodes another channel subunit, MEC-6, in which case the channel would consist of a heteromultimer of MEC-4, MEC-6 and MEC-10 subunits.

As mentioned above, far more than merely two *mec* genes are known. The roles played by the proteins these other *mec* genes encode has in many cases been elucidated. Mutations in *mec-7* and *mec-12*

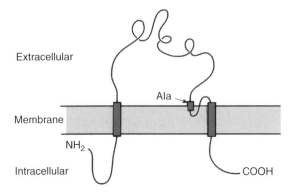

Figure 8.4 Transmembrane topology of the MEC-4 protein. There are two transmembrane domains and a small membrane insertion just before the second transmembrane helix. The bulk of the 768 residue protein is, as indicated, in the extracellular space . When Alanine$_{713}$ (Ala) is replaced by a bulkier amino acid cell death ensues. Adapted from Tavernarakis, N. and Driscoll, M. (1997).

disrupt the 15 protofilament microtubules which are so characteristic of the touch receptor neurons. Another gene, *mec-2*, has been shown to designate a 481 amino acid protein (similar to the stomatin of mammalian red blood cell cytoskeleton) that is believed to act as a link between the MEC channel and the microtubules (Figure 8.5). Yet other genes, *mec-1, mec-5, mec-9* code for proteins (MEC-1, MEC-5, MEC-9) which are found outside the plasma membrane in the mantle.

An interesting, though so far somewhat speculative, model has been proposed to link all these el-

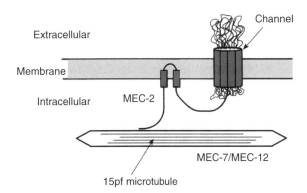

Figure 8.5 Proposed linkage provided by MEC-2 to one of the 15 pf microtubules of a touch receptor neuron. It is suggested that the N-terminal of MEC-2 interacts with a microtubule and the C-terminal with the channel. Adapted from Tavernarakis, N. and Driscoll, M. (1997).

ements together into a functioning tactile receptor. This model is shown diagrammatically in Figure 8.6. MEC-1, MEC-5 and MEC-9 are organized to transmit pressure on the cuticle to the MEC-4 subunit and open the channel. When the channel opens, Na$^+$ ions flow down their concentration gradients and the neuron is depolarized. This mechanical transmission works if the channel is stabilized by attachment to an internal microtubule. This attachment, as we have seen, is provided by MEC-2. Alternatively, the mechanical deformation might displace the microtubule network which, as it is attached to the membrane (see above), might increase the tension on the plasma membrane and thus open the channel. The number of 'mights' in the preceding sentence shows that here we are at the frontier of research. Only further careful experiment will eliminate false hypotheses where they exist.

Although, as indicated, much remains speculative, the *C. elegans* body-wall touch receptor is much the best known animal mechanoreceptor at the molecular level. Before moving on, it is worth looking forward to Chapter 9, where we shall be concerned with vertebrate hair cells. It has been suggested that the molecular mechanism worked out for the *C. elegans* mechanoreceptor may help elucidate the operation of these very different sense organs. We shall consider this interesting comparison in more detail in Section 9.3.2 and Box 9.1.

The second type of touch receptor in *C. elegans* is much less well known. These receptors are located on three sensory neurons in the nose 'rays' of the worm. A member of the TRPV family, OSM-9, is expressed at the tip of each neuron. Loss of function mutations of the OSM-9 gene (*osm-9*) leads not only to loss of sensitivity to nose touch but also to hyperosmolar solutions and the normally attractive odorant, diacetyl. The finding that OSM-9 is involved in several other sense modalities suggests that, although it may form a crucial link in the detection of mechanical distortion of the anterior rays, it may not itself be involved in the gating mechanism. It is interesting and perhaps significant to note that the mammalian homologue of OSM-9 known as TPRV4 (or OTRPC4) is a selective Ca^{2+}-channel. Quite recently it has been discovered that another TRP channel, TRPA1, is involved in nose touch and foraging responses. Mutations of *trpa-1* lead to defects in nose touch responses and this, and other evidence, points to the presence of this cation channel which, in this case, can be

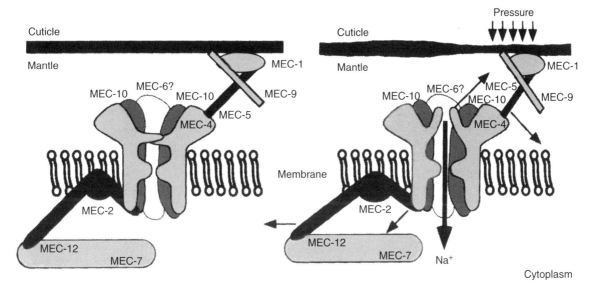

Figure 8.6   Conceptual model of *C. elegans* touch receptor. Explanation and nomenclature in text. From the *Annual Review of Physiology*, Volume 59, © 1997, with permission from Annual Reviews, http://www.Annual Reviews.org.

activated by mechanical pressure. These findings are of considerable interest, as members of the TRPA subfamily have not only been implicated in *Drosophila* thermosensitivity but also in mammalian cold sensitivity and mechanoreception.

8.2 SPIDERS

We looked at the cuticular sensilla of insects in Section 7.1.2, and we shall discuss them in more detail in the next section. In this section we shall examine the mechanoreceptors of those insect predators – the spiders. Spiders resemble insects and other arthropods in the possession of a hard exoskeleton, so their mechanoreceptors bear many resemblances to those found in insects although the common insect–arachnid ancestor is many hundred million years in the past. These resemblances thus show a remarkable evolutionary parallelism and indicate that the sensory problems presented to terrestrial animals living within a hard exoskeleton have only a few optimal solutions. Because of their age-old warfare with the insects, evolutionary forces have tuned spider sensory systems to respond to tiny changes in the environment with extreme rapidity. In order to catch their prey, their eyes and mechanoreceptors have achieved remarkable levels of sensitivity.

The most important external mechanoreceptors are tactile hairs, trichobothria and slit sensilla.

8.2.1 Tactile Hairs

Spiders are notoriously hairy. Indeed, this may account for some of the distaste they engender. But the hairs are not merely for decoration or defence: most of them are innervated and respond to tactile stimuli. Careful examination shows that they consist of a lengthy cuticular shaft springing from a shallow socket in which it can move (Figure 8.7). Three dendritic nerve endings are attached to the bottom of the shaft and electrophysiological recording shows that, when the shaft moves, action potentials are generated in the sensory fibres. The response is very rapid (less than 10 ms) and also rapidly adapting.

8.2.2 Trichobothria

Trichobothria are extremely slender hairs which spring from highly specialized sockets (Figure 8.8). They are some 0.1–1.4 mm in length and no more than about 10 μm in diameter. They are far less common than tactile hairs and are often arranged in regular rows. Indeed the arrangement of trichobothria is often used by systematists to classify spider species, a

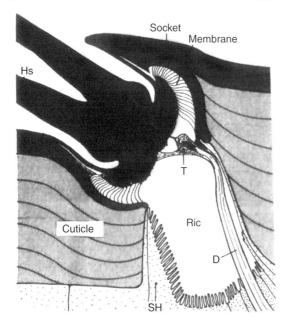

Figure 8.7 Arachnid tactile hair. The hair is inserted into a socket in the cuticle and three dendritic terminals attach to its base. D = dendrites; Hs = hair shaft; Rlc = receptor lymph cavity; SH = sheath cell; T = terminals of dendrites. From Harris, D. J. P. and Mill, P. J. (1977) *J Comp Physiol A Sens Neural Beh*, **119**, 37, with kind permission of Springer Science and Business Media.

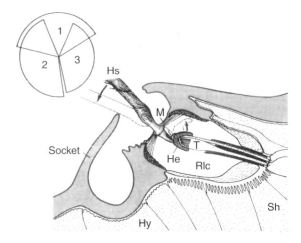

Figure 8.8 Trichobothrium. The long slender hair shaft (Hs) is inserted through a very thin cuticle (M) into a helmet shaped structure (He). The potential movement of this structure is shown by the arrow. The terminals (T) of four sensory neurons make contact with this helmet and three of the four have directional selectivity (see inset figure). Hy = hypodermis; Rlc = receptor lymph cavity; Sh = sheath cells. From Foelix (1982) *Biology of Spiders*, Copyright © 1982, Harvard University Press.

procedure known as trichobothriotaxy. Trichobothria are extraordinarily sensitive. The base of the hair is embedded in an extremely thin (0.5 μm) cuticular membrane and is continued as a 'helmet' into the socket (Figure 8.8). The dendrites of four sensory nerves are inserted in the helmet and three of these have been shown to have a directional sensitivity. The normal stimuli are changing air currents and low frequency pressure changes in the atmosphere. Trichobothria never respond to continuous static deflection.

Biophysical investigations have shown that spider thrichobothria are among the most sensitive of all mechanoeceptors, only rivalled by the rather similar filiform hairs of crickets. It has been calculated that the energy required to reach response threshold is between 2.5×10^{-20} J and 1.5×10^{-19} J, a fraction of the energy present in a single photon of green light and very near the limit imposed by Brownian motion. This extreme sensitivity is believed to be the outcome of a phenomenon called stochastic resonance (SR).

In this process, interestingly enough first applied on a global scale to account for the periodicity of the ice ages, an oscillating subthreshold stimulus is assisted at random (stochastic) intervals to reach threshold by an unrelated underlying set of fluctuations. In the trichobothrian case, the principal stimuli are fluctuating air flows, perhaps due to the beat of nearby insect wings and the random underlying fluctuations are provided by Brownian motion.

It can be shown that the optimal frequency response of the trichobothrium hair is related to its length. Short hairs are most sensitive to low frequencies and long hairs to higher frequencies. Thus the regular rows of trichobothria mentioned above contain hairs of many different lengths and thus cover a whole range of frequencies. They are, in consequence, well adapted to detecting air turbulence created by nearby insects, especially flying insects, at distances up to 25 cm.

8.2.3 Slit Sensilla and Lyriform Organs

We have already noted (Chapter 7) that insects develop a number of mechanoreceptors to detect stress and strain on the exoskeleton. This is also the case with spiders. The best known of these are the so-called 'slit' sensilla. These sensilla detect not only movement of the body but also vibrations produced by mates, prey and predators and haemolymph pressure. These receptors are embedded in the exoskeleton and distributed over the entire body surface, al-though the greatest density is found in the legs. In many cases slit sensilla line up to form parallel rows which, because of their resemblance to the musical instrument, are called **lyriform organs**.

Each slit sensillum, as Figure 8.9a shows, consists of a trench some 8 to 200 μm long and 1–2 μm wide

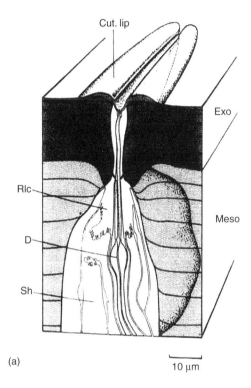

(a)

10 μm

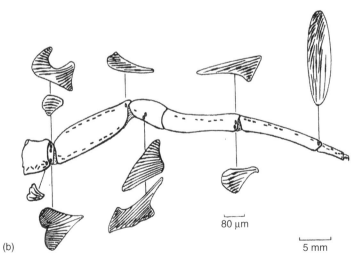

(b)

80 μm

5 mm

Figure 8.9 (a) Slit sensillum. The slit runs through the exocuticle into the mesocuticle where a large receptor lymph cavity holds the dendrites (D) of two sensory neurons. One of these dendrites reaches up to the very delicate cuticle covering the slit and the other reaches the bottom of the slit. Rlc = receptor lympn cavity; Sh = sheath cells. (b) Lyriform organs on the posterior side of the first leg of the wolf spider *Cupenius salei* of Central America. The black dots indicate the positions of the lyriform organs on the legs and the enlargements show the direction of the slit sensilla in the organs. From Foelix (1982) *Biology of Spiders*, Copyright © 1982, Harvard University Press.

bordered by prominent lips and covered by a thin cuticular membrane. Beneath this membrane the slit reaches down through the exocuticle to an underlying chamber where two sensory dendrites are located, one of which attaches to the covering cuticular membrane. In the tip of this dendrite is found a typical 'tubular body', such as is found in insect mechanoreceptor sensilla (Section 7.1.2). Stimulation of slit sensilla is by mechanical deformation. Downward pressure on the slit pushes the lips together and the cuticle connecting them bows inwards. This stimulates the underlying dendrite. It has been found that only compression not dilation elicits impulses in the sensory fibre. Groups of slit sensilla arranged parallel to each other (Figure 8.6b) are known as lyriform organs. It is found that the peripheral slits of lyriform organs are deformed more easily than those at the centre, so this may provide some information about the degree of exoskeletal stress.

What role do slit sensilla and lyriform organs play in a spider's life? It is clear that they provide feedback on the spider's own movements, but they also have a significant role to play in detecting pressure waves in the atmosphere – sound – and other external stimuli. The tarsal slit sensilla of a number of spiders show maximum sensitivity to atmospheric pressure waves in the frequency range between 300 and 700 Hz. It can be no coincidence that the wing beats of many insects fall within this range. The metatarsal lyriform organs of web spiders belonging to the order Aranaidae act as highly sensitive vibration detectors. A displacement of the leg tip by as little as 1–2.5 nm at 2–5 kHz is sufficient to elicit a response in these spiders. Any vibration of the web is thus instantly sensed. Tibial and femoral lyriform organs provide kinaesthetic orientation in wandering spiders (order Lycosidae). When these organs are intact, these spiders can retrace an earlier run without the aid of external cues by 'replaying' their earlier motility pattern. If the lyrifom organs are destroyed, this ability is also destroyed.

8.3 INSECTS

We looked at the role of sensilla in insect kinaesthesia in Chapter 7 (campaniform sensilla and chordotonal organs). Here we shall look in more detail at tactile

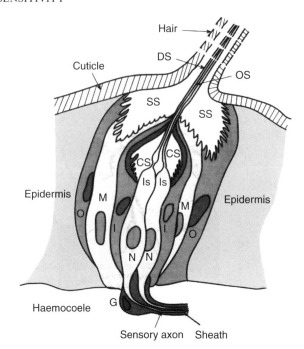

Figure 8.10 Typical insect sensillum. CS = ciliary sinus; DS = dendritic sheath; G = basal glial sheath cell; M = intermediate or trichogen cell; N = neurosensory cell; IS = inner segment; O = outer or tormogen cell; OS = outer segment (cilium); SS = sensillar sinus After Gilbert, L. L. & Kerkut, G. A. (1985).

sensilla. Figure 8.10 shows a typical hair sensillum. It consists of a cuticular projection enclosing one or more neurosensory cells and several sheath cells. The neurosensory cells have large nuclei and send a lengthy dendrite into the cuticular projection. This dendrite is differentiated into two distinct regions, often at about the middle of its length. The proximal segment (**inner segment**) resembles the rest of the perikaryon; the distal segment (**outer segment**) is, however, a modified cilium. It is often referred to simply as the cilium and possesses the characteristic internal 9×2 ultrastructure of microtubules. This ultrastructure is continued to the tip, unless the dendrite branches. In these latter cases the microtubules become distributed among the branches. The sensory axon springing from the base of the cell travels directly back to the CNS in a sensory nerve.

The number of sheath cells varies greatly from one sensilla to another but typically there are three types: **inner sheath cell** (= **thecogen cell**) which are homologous to the scolopale cell of scolopidia (see Section

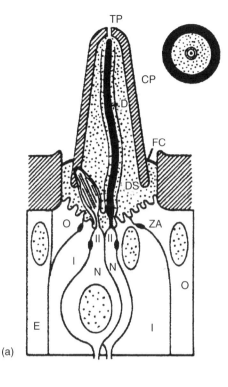

(a)

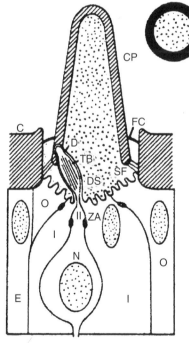

(b)

7.1.2), the **intermediate** or **trichogen cell** and outermost of all, the **outer** or **tormogen cell**. The inner sheath cells secrete the dendritic sheath. Proximally they enclose a small fluid-filled sinus, the **ciliary sinus** (Figure 8.10). The intermediate and outer cells form the **sensilla sinus** beneath the cuticle and around the dendritic sheath. The proximal ends of the intermediate and outer cells abut the haemolymph in the haemocoele and their distal ends send large numbers of microvilli into the sensillar sinus. They are thought to have an important function in both nutrition and in the formation of the fluid in the sensillar sinus. Their strategic position between the haemocoele and the latter sinus makes them well adapted to this function. In addition to the sheath cells, intermediate and basal cells are often present. The latter are sometimes referred to as glial cells as they wrap around the sensory axons, insulating them from each other and from the haemolymph.

Far from all sensilla are mechanosensory. In other parts of this book we shall meet gustatory, olfactory, hygroscopic and thermal sensilla. The sense modality is determined by the dendrite of the neurosensory cell contained within the sensillum. In many cases, where there is more than one neurosensory cell, there may be dual or even more modalities. For instance, mechanosensitive and chemosensitive neurosensory cells may inhabit the same sensillum. Partly for this reason, the classification and terminology applied to insect sensilla has been complicated and confusing. Whereas olfactory and gustatory sensilla (for obvious reasons) develop terminal pores (Figure 8.11a), many mechanosensitive sensilla are without pores (aporous) (Figure 8.11b).

Mechanosensitive hair sensilla sometimes spring directly from the cuticle but more often are attached

Figure 8.11 (a) Uniporous bimodal sensillum. In addition to the mechanosensory neuron with its tubular body there are one or more other neurosensory cells whose dendritres extend up towards the terminal pore. CP = cuticular process; D = dendrite outersegment; DS = dendritic sheath; E = epidermal cell; FC = flexible cuticle; I = inner sheath cell; N = neurosensory cell; O = outer sheath cell; OS = outersegment of dendrite; TP = terminal pore; ZA = zonula adherens intercellular junction. (b) Mechanosensory sensillum in a flexible socket. The dendrite is attached to a tubular body which is inserted into the cuticle of the hair. D = attachment of tubular body to cuticle of hair; SF = suspensory filaments. Other labels as in (a). (After Blum, 1985: with permission).

by flexible sockets to the exoskeleton. Movement of the sensory hair provides the adequate stimulus to depolarize dendrite. Movement in one direction causes depolarization, movement in the other hyperpolarization. In many cases the sensillary hairs are, constrained by their points of insertion into the exoskeleton to move most freely in one plane: they are, in other words, strongly direction selective.

In Figure 8.11b the hair sensillum is represented as containing a single neurosensory cell whose dendrite is attached to the interior of the hair by a **tubular body**. Electron microscopy shows that this body consists of from 50 to 100 closely packed microtubules. These microtubules are exquisitely sensitive to distortion induced by movement of the sensillum. It can be shown that their lower threshold is a distortion of 3–5 nm. Can we make a connection with the microtubules which pack the neurosensory cells of *C. elegans*? Deflection of the sensillary hair in one direction causes a depolarization; deflection in the other direction leads to a hyperpolarization. These voltage changes across the membrane occur within 100 μs of the onset of the deflecting stimulus. This implies that they are due to opening and shutting of ion gates in the membrane. We shall see, in Chapter 9, that vertebrate hair cells have a similar biophysics. On this analogy it is concluded that the opening and closing of ion gates is stretch activated. Suspensory filaments which attach the base of the sensillary hair to the cuticle, together with the cuticular embedment and the attachment of the tubular body, ensure that there is an optimal plane through which the sensillum can move. This directional sensitivity is obviously of considerable importance in detecting in which way body parts, air or substrate are moving.

Is anything known about the 'ion gates' underlying the voltage changes across the membrane of the tubular body ? In fairly recent times there has been a great deal of evidence that members of the ubiquitous TRP superfamily of cation channels are involved. A gene encoding a *Drosophila* hair cell mechanotransduction channel has been identified. When this gene, *nompC* (*no m*echanoreceptor *p*otential C), mutates, the fly loses its mechanosensitivity. It is left with practically no sense of balance and often almost falls over itself when it attempts to walk. Analysis of the gene shows it to be a member of the TRPN family of TRP channels. It is thus suggested that, when the sensillary hair moves in a specific direction, it stretches the

tubular and/or dendritic membrane, opening TRP channels and the consequent influx of cations depolarizes the membrane. The response to stretch may be by a bilayer mechanism similar to that we discussed for the MscL channel in *E. coli* (Chapter 6). Movement of the hair in the opposite direction has an opposite effect: the channels are closed and the membranes hyperpolarize. It may be that the hair cells in the mammalian (including human) inner ear also use members of this superfamily of channels in their rather similar microphysiology. We shall look at this microphysiology in the next chapter.

Not all insect sensilla, as we have already noted, are mechanosensory. Thus in many cases, as Figure 8.11a shows, the tip of the sensillum is penetrated by a pore and contains at least two neurosensory cells only one of which is mechanosensitive. The sensillum is thus bimodal. The other sensory cells may be olfactory or gustatory. The dendrite of the mechanosensitive neurosensory cell is, as in the previous case, attached to the interior of the sensillary hair by a tubular body. The other neurosensory cells develop single long, often branched, 'dendrites' extending the full length of the sensillum, terminating just beneath the pore. These 'dendrite(s)' are in fact modified cilia and are often called 'outersegments'. We shall meet well studied examples of chemosensitive cilia when we come to examine vertebrate gustatory cells (Chapter 13) and olfactory cells (Chapter 14), where we shall also discuss insect chemoreception.

Returning, however, to mechanosensory sensilla, it will be remembered from Chapter 7 that extensive brushworks of mechanosensitive sensilla develop at the joints between insect segments and appendages, thus providing the animal with a wealth of kinaesthetic information. Mechanosensitive sensilla are also, of course, employed as tactile hairs all over the body, particularly the head, and are richly developed in the antennae, especially the antennae of nocturnal, crepuscular and cave dwelling and/or underground forms. The cerci of cockroaches, for instance, have an abundance of lengthy filiform sensilla.

Mechanosensitive sensilla also play important roles in the detection of vibration. The subgenual organ of many insects is particularly significant in detecting vibrations in the 10–50 Hz range. In the American cockroach, *Periplaneta*, the range is much higher (as we saw in Section 7.1.2) and encroaches on that which we would define as the acoustic domain. In addition to vibration detection by the subgenual organ, a number of insects develop vibration detecting scolopidia in their tarsi. Several species of aquatic Hemiptera and Coleoptera make use of these vibration sensors to detect the radiating ripple engendered by prey which has just dropped into their pond. The hemipteran pond-skater, *Gerris*, touches the water surface with its tarsi from above, whilst the water-boatman, *Notonecta*, swims on its back with its tarsi palpating the surface film of the water from below. A wave amplitude of no more than 0.5–4 μm provides an adequate threshold and the optimal frequency ranges from 20–200 Hz. Time differences of 1–4 ms combined with amplitude differences between the outspread tarsi are used to determine the direction of the source of disturbance. In these cases the sense organs involved consist of a small number, less than ten, scolopidia in the tarsi. It is no great step from these vibration detectors to mechanoreceptors which, like those of the vertebrates (Chapter 9), have evolved to detect the gentle atmospheric vibrations that we subjectively know as sound. Indeed it is not easy to separate insect vibration detectors from acoustic detectors for, unlike vertebrates, the same receptors are often activated by oscillations in the ground, in water and in air.

8.3.1 Acoustic Sensilla and Tympanic Organs

Insects develop two basic types of specialized sound detector: hairs and tympanic organs. Hairs are only significant sound detectors very near the sound source. They depend on distortion by the lateral movement of the air. Thus sensory hairs on the cercae of cockroaches and orthopteran insects, such as the locust, are able to detect acoustic stimuli emitted at a distance of a few centimeters, whilst sensory hairs on the bodies of some moth caterpillars respond to the wing beat frequencies of approaching predatory wasps. The fruit fly, *Drosophila*, develops feathery 'aristae' on the third antennal segment (Figure 8.12b); these are tuned to detect at close range the wing vibration which acts as the mating call of the species. In many insects **Johnston's organ** also acts as a vibration detector. This organ is, in fact, found in the second antennal segment, or pedicel,

of nearly all insects. It consists of a large number of closely packed scolopidia. In different insects it has different functions, ranging from flight speed indicator (bees) to gravity detector (*Dytiscus*, the water beetle). In the mosquitoes and chironomid midges it is greatly developed and consists of many thousands of scolopidia attached to an intricate internal structure. In these insects it functions to detect the wing beat frequencies (a few hundred Hz) of conspecifics, especially prospective mating partners, at distances of up to a meter.

The other type of sound detector evolved in the insects – tympanic organs, or ears – respond not so much to lateral movement of the surrounding air (as is produced by the flapping of wings) but to pressure waves. Like the ears of vertebrates, they are thus able to detect sound sources at considerable distances and are sensitive to frequencies ranging up to and beyond 100 kHz. Tympanal organs are developed in at least seven insect orders including Neuroptera, Lepidoptera, Coleoptera, Hemiptera, Orthoptera, Diptera and so on. They are used in communication, attack and defense.

In essence, the insect tympanal organ consists of three elements (Figure 8.12e): a much thinned area of cuticle which often has a silvery appearance known as the **tympanum** or **tympanic membrane**; beneath the tympanum is an **air filled cavity** derived from the tracheal spaces; connected to the tympanum are the **chordotonal organs** which sense any vibration. This basic design is elaborated into a wide variety of different structures so that insects have a great diversity of auditory mechanisms. Tympanal organs are, moreover, found in many different parts of the insect's anatomy. The locations where tympanal organs have been found in different insects are shown in Figure 8.13. Insect 'ears' are by no means as anatomically restricted as those of vertebrates.

Acoustic communication is well developed in the Orthoptera (grasshoppers, crickets) and Hemiptera (suborder Homoptera: cicadas). Usually it is the male which emits a loud calling song and the female is induced to fly or walk towards him. Cicada calls are often of high intensity; indeed, they are audible to the human ear at distances of over a mile in the tropical forest. Selection pressure has also ensured that they are very distinctively different from one species to the next. Mole crickets (Gryllotalpidae) are also highly vociferous. The male constructs

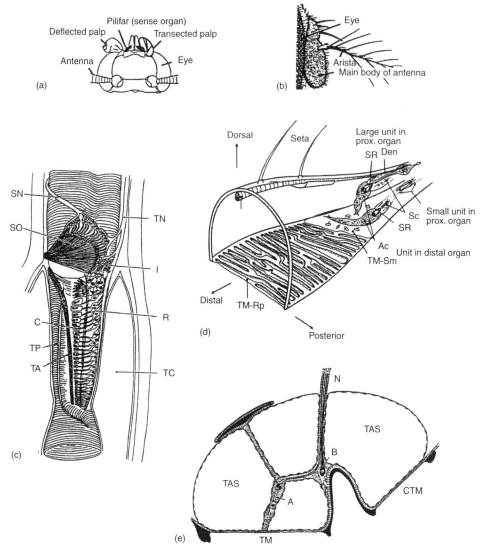

Figure 8.12   Various types of insect acoustic sensilla. (a) The *Hawkmoth* has two major types of acoustic sensilla: tympanal organs in the palps and pilifer organs. The tympanal organs in the palps are filled with air sacs crossed by delicate membranes (right hand palp transected). They act as pressure detectors and in combination with the pilifer organs can detect the ultrasonic emissions of insectivorous bats. (b) The *Fruit fly* (*Drosophila*) arista springs sideways from the third antennal segment. It is tuned to respond to viscous movement amongst the gases making up air in response to the wing beat of conspecifics. B from Frazier, J.L. (1985) with permission from John Wiley & Sons. (c) Tibial ear of the *long-horned* (*Tettigoniid*) *grasshopper*. These insects (also crickets) develop ears in the tibia of their forelegs (C = cap cell; I = intermediate organ; R = receptor cell; SO = subgenual organs; SN = subgenual nerve; TA = anterior trachea; TC = tracheal cavity; TN = tympanic nerve, TP = posterior trachea). (d) *Lacewings* develop acoustic receptors in the form of swellings in the veins of the anterior pair of wings. The swelling is bounded laterally and dorsally by a thick cuticle but ventrally by a thin rippled cuticle. Two chordotonal organs consisting of altogether about 25 scolopidia (only two shown in figure) are attached to this thin tympanal cuticle. The organ responds to high frequency bat echolocation calls (Ac = attachment cell; Den = dendrite; Sc = scolopale cells; SR = scolopale rod; TM-Rp and TM-Sm = rippled and smooth parts of tympanic membrane; Tr = trachea). (e) *Noctuid moth* ear. This is found in the metathoracic segment and consists of extensive segments of tympanal membrane covering an air-filled space. Two receptor cells (A) respond to vibration of the tympanic membrane (B = nonauditory neuron; CTM = counter-tympanic membrane; N = tympanic nerve; TAS = tympanic air sac; TM = tympanic membrane. A, C, D and E from Michelsen A. (1974) *Handbook of Sensory Physiology, Vol V/1* p.395, fig 5; p. 396, fig 6, © 1974, by permission of Springer-Verlag.

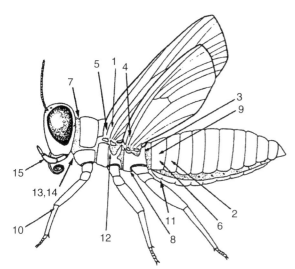

Figure 8.13 Distribution of tympanal organs on insects. The figure shows a 'generalized' insect giving the position of tympanal organs. *Lepidoptera*: 1 = wingbase (*Chrysopa*), 2 = abdomen (noctuid moths, etc.), 3 = metathorax (noctuids) 4 = base of fore or hind wing (Papilionoidea); 5 = forewing base (Hedyloidea), 15 = pilifer organ (hawk moths); *Coleoptera*: 6 = abdomen (Cicindelidae (beetle)), 7 = cervical membranes (Scarabaeidae (beetle); *Dictyoptera*: 8 = ventral metathorax (Mantodea (*Mantis*) and Blattoidea (cockroaches)); *Orthoptera*: 9 = first abdomenal segment (Acridida (locusts)), 10 = prothoracic leg (Gryllidae (*Gryllus*)); *Hemiptera*: 11 = abdomen (Cicadidae (*Cystosoma*), 12 = mesothorax (Corixidae (*Corixa*); *Diptera*: 13 = ventral prosternum (Tachinidae (*Ormia*)), 14 = ventral prosternum (Sarcophagidae (*Colcondamyia*). From Hoy and Robert, 1996: with permission, from the Annual review of Entomology, Vol 41, © 1996, by Annual reviews (http://www.Annual Reviews.org).

a horn-shaped burrow which acts as a megaphone. The male's great cry attracts females flying high in the air. In some grasshoppers the male's song elicits a replying call from the female so that a duet is set up between them.

Detection of prey by acoustic means is practiced by some tachinid flies. *Ormia ochracea*, for instance, listens for the mating call of male field crickets, *Gryllus integer*, and homes in to deposit its parasitic larvae. The ears of these flies can be shown to have adapted so that they are most sensitive to the dominant frequency (4.8 kHz) of the male cricket's song. But, perhaps the most interesting use of insect tympanal organs is that developed by nocturnal and crespuscular lacewings and moths to detect and avoid predatory bats.

Green lacewings (*Chrysopa carnea*) possess a tympanal organ near the base of each anterior pair of wings (Figures 8.12d and 8.13). They comprise two chordotonal organs consisting of a total of about twenty five scolopidia. These tympanal organs are able to detect bat cries in the range 13–120 kHz. Bats, as we shall see in the next chapter, emit from 7 to 30 search pulses per second. When prey is located and the bat homes in for the kill, the pulses increase in frequency. The lacewing tympanal organs detect the search pulses and the insects reflexly fold their wings and nosedive out of the sky before the bat sonar locks on.

In most moths tympanal organs develop bilaterally in the metathorax. In some cases they are also to be found in first, second and seventh abdominal segments and, in the case of hawk moths, in balloon-shaped palps on the head (Figure 8.12a). Their anatomy varies very little from one moth species to another (Figure 8.12e). They consist of a tympanum (about 1 μm thick) behind which is a tracheal air sac connected to the exterior via a spiracle. Vibration of the tympanum is detected by one, two or four neurosensory cells supended in a connective tissue strand that runs between the centre of the tympanum and a cuticular support.

In moths of the very large superfamily Noctuoidea each tympanic organ has two neurosensory cells, A1 and A2, whilst four are present in the abdominal ears of members of the superfamily Geometridae. Noctuid moths are sensitive to airborne sound over the range 3–150 kHz. It is interesting to note that both the range and peak sensitivities vary in island faunae that are exposed to particular populations of bat predators. In other words, noctuid hearing is tuned to the intensities and frequencies of indigenous bats. The two neurosensory cells of the noctuid ear respond to different intensity ranges. The A1 cell responds to a lower intensity range (peak sensitivity, in some species, at 40 dB) and the A2 is tuned to respond at a higher intensity (e.g. 60 dB). There is no evidence at present that frequency can be discriminated and, indeed, it is difficult to imagine a physiological mechanism (with a two cell system) that could achieve this function. Direction of the sound source can, however, be detected. This depends on the presence of bilateral ears. If one ear is inactivated, experimentally or by infestation with the ear mite, *Dirocheles phalenodectes*, the ability to locate the sound source is lost. Another mite, *D. scedastes*, infests both of the noctuid's ears but does not destroy the tympanum or acoustic nerve. In this case the ability to localize a sound source remains and the moth is better able to avoid marauding bats. In this particular 'arms race' with the three players, mite, moth and bat, *D. scalestes* is better adapted to survive than *D. phalenodectes*.

The A1 cell of noctuid moths can normally detect the ultrasonic search pulses of an insectivorous bat at a distance of 30–40m. If the bat is flying at about 8m/s this gives the moth four or five seconds to take defensive action. Because of its ability to detect the direction of the sound source, the moth normally turns and flies directly away from the bat. The bat, in turn, will probably not be aware of the moth until it is within 5 m or so. Its call will then increase in intensity and pulse repetition rate and will consequently activate the A2 cell. The moth has now less than a second to avoid capture. It undertakes a series of desperate avoidance manoeuvres. These consist of zig-zags, loops, spirals, power dives or passive falls into cluttering foliage. Some moths are also able, during these last desperate fractions of a second, to emit sound in a final attempt to escape the sharp, oncoming teeth.

There remains some controversy over the exact function of these moth sound emissions. It may be that it is to warn the attacking bat that the moth is obnoxious or poisonous. In this sense the warning sound may be analogous to the bright warning colouration that warns birds off distasteful daytime insects. If this is the case, it would be interesting to determine whether moth acoustics show instances of Batesian mimicry. Other investigations have, however, suggested that moth clicks are attempts to jam the bat's echolocation. It has been shown that they are almost identical to the echoes which bats would expect to pick up from their own emissions. It may be, therefore, that these sounds confuse the bat's analysis (Chapter 10) making it 'see' an obstruction where there is none and, in veering to avoid it, miss its mark on the moth.

Let us turn now from the remarkable sophistications of insect mechanoreceptors to the seemingly more prosaic topic of the sense of touch in the mammalian skin. We shall see that it too can be regarded as a sensory surface. It is responsive not only to mechanical stimuli but also to thermal stimuli and to

those which cause pain. These latter stimuli we shall consider in Chapters 20 and 22. In the next section of this chapter only sensitivity to mechanical stimulation will be considered. In Chapter 9, where we consider vertebrate 'hair cells', we shall return to the extraordinary sensitivities of devices evolved to detect the gentle touch of acoustic vibrations and the huge opportunities thereby opened for communication across distance. We shall also return to the continuing crepuscular contest between moth and microchiropteran.

8.4 TACTILE RECEPTORS IN MAMMALIAN SKIN

The mammalian skin is home to a great array of mechanoreceptors. In this chapter we only consider those found in the skin of the eutheria, in particular in the skin of *Homo sapiens*. In Chapter 21 we discuss all-too-briefly the remarkable push-rod mechanoreceptors found in prototherian mammals, the platypus and spiny anteater.

There are several ways to classify the sensory endings in the skin of euthrian mammals. One commonly used classification is into fast and slow adapting receptors. The first respond only during initial indentation of the skin and remain silent during steady pressure; the latter respond both during onset of the stimulus and during constant displacement.

8.4.1 Fast Adapting Receptors

Fast adapting receptors include **Pacinian corpuscles**, **Meissner's corpuscles**, **Krause's end bulbs** and **hair follicle sense endings**. Pacinian corpuscles are found in both glabrous (i.e. non-hairy, such as the palms of the hand and the soles of the feet) and in hairy skin; hair follicle endings (by definition) only in hairy skin; Meissner's corpuscles only in primate glabrous skin; and Krause's end bulbs only in non-primate glabrous skin.

8.4.1.1 Pacinian Corpuscles

These are oval structures ranging from 0.5–2 mm in length. They are to be found in the deeper layers of the dermis of the skin. In section, an onion-like structure is revealed. They consist of layers of connective

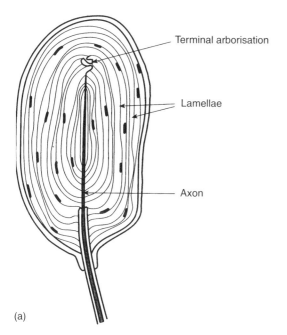

(a)

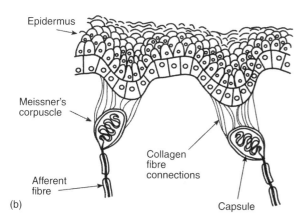

(b)

Figure 8.14   (a) Pacinian corpuscle. (b) Meissner's corpuscle.

A generator potential (depolarization) can be detected in the unmyelinated ending, when the corpuscle is compressed. This results in a short burst of impulses in the sensory fibre, which adapts in one or two seconds to zero or a very low frequency. As their physiology suggests, the principle function of Pacinian corpuscles in the skin is to detect vibration. The frequency to which they respond ranges from as low as 70 Hz to as high as 1000 Hz. They are, however, most sensitive in the middle of the range (200–400 Hz), where a deformation of no more than 1 μm is a sufficient stimulus.

8.4.1.2 Meissner's Corpuscles

These are also found in the dermis of glabrous skin. The nerve endings are surrounded by a connective tissue capsule that is connected to the overlying stratified epithelium by collagen fibres (Figure 8.14b). This provides an effective mechanical linkage between the surface of the skin and the sense organ. The nerve endings themselves form a spiral within the capsule, the helices of which are separated by sheets of Schwann cells. The endings are stimulated by movement of the skin and, in particular, by vibration. The frequency range of the vibratory stimuli is lower than that characteristic of Pacinian corpuscles, ranging from 10–200 Hz.

8.4.1.3 Krause's End Bulbs

These are rather similar to Meissner's corpuscles. They are, however, mainly restricted to non-primate mammals where they are, once again, found in glabrous skin. They have a lamellated capsule surrounding either a rod-like or a spiral nerve ending. Like Meissner's corpuscles they respond to vibrations in the low frequency range, 10–100 Hz.

8.4.1.4 Hair Follicle Receptors

Sensory nerve endings form a complex meshwork around a hair follicle just beneath the sebaceous glands (Figure 8.15). Each ending forms an enlargement filled with mitochondria and tightly enclosed by Schwann cells. The endings are distributed around the follicle, some in the outer vascular layer, others penetrating to a position between the outer and inner root sheath cells. Some branches run vertically up along the hair follicle, others circle around it. Yet

tissue surrounding an unmyelinated nerve fibre (Figure 8.14a). It is believed that the layered structure has the function of transforming a steady indentation of the skin into a transient stimulus. This is accomplished by the indentation causing a momentary slippage of the layers over each other until, rapidly, a new equilibrium is reached, when the pressure on the sensory nerve ending is relieved. Hence Pacinian corpuscles are able to detect vibration even when subjected to steady pressure.

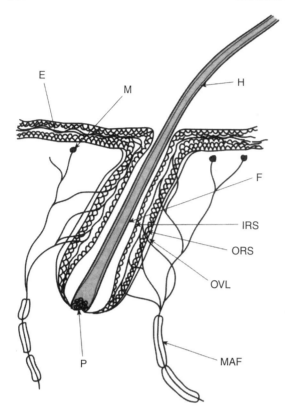

Figure 8.15 Sensory innervation of hair follicle. E = epidermins, F = follicle; H = hair; IRS = inner root sheath; M = Merkel disc; MAF = myelinated afferent fibre; ORS = outer root sheath; OVL = outer vascular layer; P = papilla.

other branches terminate in Merkel discs beneath the epidermis. The hair follicle receptors are classified into at least three different types (D,G,T) according to their sensitivity and rate of discharge. They respond to any movement of the hair. In many mammalian species the hairs in the vicinity of the mouth are extended to form elongated whiskers (vibrissae) and tactile hairs. The receptors associated with these hairs include both fast and slow adapting types. We shall give further consideration to vibrissae when we come to consider the central analysis of tactile information later in this chapter.

8.4.2 Slow Adapting Receptors

In contrast to the fast adapting receptors of the previous section, these receptors respond to the dis-

placement of the skin but sustain their discharge when the skin is held in its new position. There are three types: **Merkel cells**, **Ruffini endings** and **C-mechanoreceptors**. It is conventional to group these slowly adapting receptors into two categories. Type I receptors respond if the skin is stroked rapidly, type II receptors respond to a constant displacement of the skin, particularly when it is stretched.

8.4.2.1 Merkel Cells

These fall into the type I category. They lie just beneath the epidermis and possess large, irregularly formed nuclei and microvilli which project into the epidermal cells (Figure 8.16a). At their bases are disc-like expansions of the ends of sensory axons (Merkel discs). A group of ten to twenty Merkel cells make synaptic contact with the ending of a single sensory axon. They respond to sudden displacements of the skin, as in stroking.

8.4.2.2 Ruffini Endings

This is a type II ending and responds to steady displacement of the skin. They are found in the deep layers of the dermis. As shown in Figure 8.16b, the termination of the sensory axon breaks up into a network of fine processes which ramify in the interior of the connective tissue capsule.

8.4.2.3 C-mechanoreceptors

Large numbers of unmyelinated C-fibres take their origin in the dermis of the skin, many of them starting close to the dermo–epidermal junction. There are no differentiated sense endings associated with these fibres. They respond with a slowly adapting discharge to steady indentation of the skin. C-fibres also respond to other sensory modalities: temperature (Chapter 20), tissue damage (pain) (Chapter 22).

8.5 CEREBRAL ANALYSIS OF TOUCH

The vast majority of sensory fibres from the skin's sensory receptors enter the spinal cord via the dorsal (= posterior) roots and terminate in the dorsal horn of the grey matter. The mechanoreceptive afferents, which are generally large diameter fibres (except, of

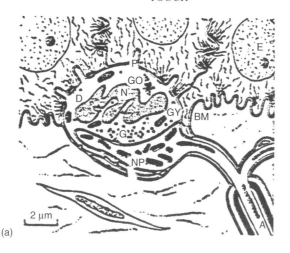

(a)

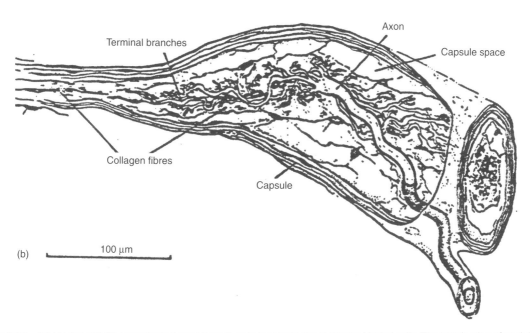

(b)

Figure 8.16 (a) Merkel cell. The myelinated axon branches to innervate ten to twenty Merkel cells. The termination of each branch is expanded to form a disc (Merkel disc). A = afferent axon; BM = basement membrane of epidermal cells; D = desmosomes; E = epidermal cell; GO = Golgi bodies; N = nucleus of Merkel cell; NP = Merkel disc. (b) Ruffini ending. The sensory axon breaks up within the connective tissue capsule to form an interweaving complex of terminals. A and B from Iggo, 1982: by permission of Cambridge University Press.

course, the C-fibre mechanoreceptors), usually take a central position in the dorsal root, surrounded by finer fibres from pain and thermoreceptor endings. The cytons of all the fibres are located in the dorsal root ganglia. A fair proportion of the small diameter unmyelinated fibres (about 30%) travel back down a portion of the dorsal root and then turn into the ventral roots to terminate in the ventral horn of the grey matter (Figure 8.17). Most of these fibres originate in the viscera. The area of skin sending input into each dorsal root is termed a dermatome (Figure 22.5). Adjacent dermatomes overlap.

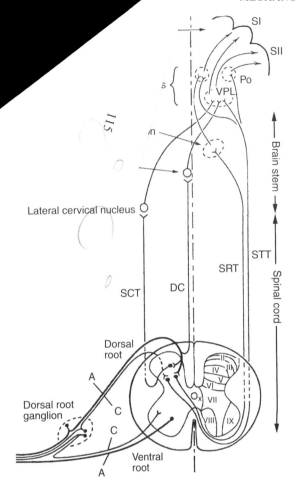

Lateral cervical nucleus

Dorsal root
ganglion

SCT   DC

Dorsal
root

A

C

C

Ventral
root

A

SI

SII

Po

VPL

n

s

115

STT

SRT

Brain stem

Spinal cord

Figure 8.17 Afferent pathways in spinal cord. The A and C fibres are shown entering the spinal cord through the dorsal (= posterior) root. A proportion (circa 30%) of the C-fibres turn back and find their way to the ventral horn of the grey matter via the ventral (= anterior) root. All the sensory fibres have their cell bodies in the dorsal root ganglia. The pathways in the CNS to the somatosensory cortices are shown. Further explanation in text. DC = dorsal column fibres; IL = Intralaminar nucleus; Po = posterior thalamic nucleus; S1 = primary somaesthetic area; SII = secondary somaesthetic area; SCT = spinocervical tract; SRT = spinoreticular tract; STT = spinothalamic tract; VPL = ventroposterior thalamic nucleus. From Iggo, 1982: by permission of Cambridge University Press.

Once in the spinal cord, the fibres take a number of routes to the cerebral cortex. Four major routes are recognized (Figure 8.17) although they do not form anatomically distinct tracts. The spinocervical tract (SCT) and dorsal column fibres (DC) travel up the ipsilateral side of the spinal cord to end in the lateral cervical and dorsal column nuclei, respectively. From there a further relay crosses over, in the region of the medulla, to terminate in the ventro-posterior nucleus of the thalamus. A final neuron then runs on to terminate in the primary or secondary somaesthetic areas of the cerebral cortex. The other two routes, as shown in Figure 8.17, involve a cross-over at the level of the spinal cord (within two segments of the point of entry) to form the spino-reticular tract (SRT) and spino-thalamic tract (STT). Fibres in the SRT run up in the ventro-lateral quadrant of the spinal cord to nuclei in the midbrain and thalamus. From there the input is directed to the cortical somaesthetic areas. Finally, the STT consists of fibres in the antero-lateral quadrant of the spinal cord, ending in three thalamic nuclei (Figure 8.17). A significant number of nociceptive fibres track towards the cerebrum in this tract. Once again a final fibre leads upwards into the cerebral somaesthetic areas.

These pathways and nuclei ensure that a certain amount of information processing occurs before the somaesthetic input reaches the cortex. Although it is believed that individual dorsal horn neurons have a one-to-one relationship with their input fibres, there is little doubt that interneurons within the dorsal horn are also influential. We shall meet a significant instance of this synaptic interaction when we come to consider nociceptive fibres and the sensation of pain in Chapter 22. More extensive interaction between different types of mechanosensory input occurs in the thalamic nuclei.

The first destination of the somaesthetic fibres in the cerebral cortes are the two somaesthetic (or somatosensory) cortices. The primary somaesthetic cortex is located in the postcentral gyrus, just behind the Rolandic fissure, and the secondary cortex is located (in primates) on the superior wall of the Sylvian fissure.

The primary somaesthetic cortex is subdivided into three cytoarchitectonic areas: Brodmann areas 1, 2, 3a and 3b (Figure 8.18). Somaesthetic fibres from the thalamic nuclei terminate in areas 3a and 3b and the cells in those areas then project to areas 1 and 2. The thalamic nuclei also send a sparse projection to the secondary somaesthetic cortex but most fibres to this region originate from all four subdivisions of the primary somaesthetic cortex. Indeed, this cortex is very dependent on the primary cortex.

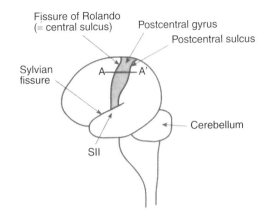

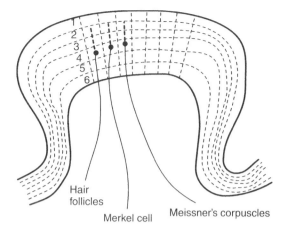

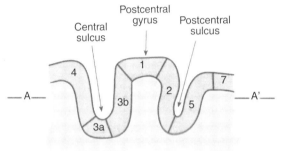

Figure 8.19 Schematic section through somaesthetic cortex to show its horizontal stratification into six layers and its vertical subdivision into columns. As indicated in the text each column is dedicated to one submodality. Although each BA receives a full set of somaesthetic input there is some specialization. BA3a is dominated by input from muscle spindles; BA3b by cutaneous receptors; BA2 by deep pressure receptors and BA1 by rapidly adapting cutaneous receptors.

Figure 8.18 Upper part of figure shows lateral view of cerebrum to show the position of the somaesthetic cortices. SII = secondary somaesthetic cortex. The bottom part of the figure shows a section through the cortex (labelled AA′ in upper figure). The Brodmann cytoarchitectonic areas (BA areas) are labelled.

If the connections from the primary cortex are severed, the neurons in the secondary cortex fall silent. In contrast, removal of parts of the secondary cortex has no effect on the primary cortex.

If we turn to the histological structure of the primary somaesthetic cortex, we find that it, like all other regions of the mammalian neocortex, displays a six-layered stratification (Figure 8.19). The input fibres from the thalamic nuclei terminate in layer 4. The other layers contain cells whose axons run out of the cortex to other parts of the brain. Layers 2 and 3 project to other cortical regions, especially Brodmann areas 5 and 7. Layer 5 projects to subcortical nuclei and Layer 6 projects back to the thalamus.

Less obvious to the microscopist is a columnar structure running orthogonal to this stratification (Figure 8.19). These columns were first discovered

during microelectrode analysis by Vernon Mountcastle. Although special staining techniques reveal them to have histological reality, they are perhaps best regarded as units or modules of physiological activity. The columns are 300–500 μm in diameter and run vertically through the cortex and thus include cells from all six histologically distinguishable layers. Microelectrode recording has shown that all the cells in a given column respond to the same type or subtype of stimulus. Indeed, Mountcastle found that the specificity was even greater: all the cells in a given column respond to the same type of receptor. For example, all the cells in one column may respond to movement of the hairs on a particular part of the body's surface; all the cells in another may respond to rapidly adapting Meissner corpuscles in the same or different part; in yet another column the cells will respond only to slowly adapting Merkel receptors and so on. A cortical column is thus a very specific computing module. It receives precise information about one sense submodality from one small area of the body's surface. It will also receive input information from other columns in the somaesthetic cortex and (via the corpus callosum) from equivalent columns on the other side of the brain.

Microelectrode recording shows, furthermore, that not only does each columnar cell respond to a very particular sense modality but it is also very specific about where the stimulus is coming from. Cells in the primary somaesthetic cortex can thus be said to have 'receptive fields (RFs)' (Chapter 3). The receptive fields of neighbouring cells will often overlap and there is a certain dynamic shifting of boundaries. The size of the RFs in different parts of the anatomy varies widely. RFs for cells receiving input from the finger tips are about 3–4 mm in diameter. In contrast, RFs for cortical cells receiving input from the trunk are over one hundred times larger. In other words the system is arranged so that it makes biological sense. Those parts of the body from which fine discrimination is demanded are 'scrutinized' in minute detail by cells in the somaesthetic cortex. Parts that do not normally need such attention have correspondingly few cells devoted to them.

Cortical cells whose receptive fields are located in the same part of the body's surface are grouped together in the cortex. This leads to a representation of the contralateral body surface developing in the primary somaesthetic cortex that can be mapped by the physiologist's microelectrode. This is sometimes called the **somaesthetic homunculus** (Figure 8.20). It was, in fact, first detected by the Canadian neurosurgeon, Wilder Penfield, during brain operations carried out under local anaesthetic. To be sure that any excisions did not lead to disastrous outcomes, Penfield would stimulate the cortex at various points and ask the patients to report what they felt. Because the magnitude of the RFs of the cortical cells varies so widely, the resulting map is strikingly nonisomorphous. It should be noted, moreover, that the somaesthetic cortex contains not just one homunculus but four: one in each subregion, that is Brodmann areas 1, 2, 3a and 3b. These maps are all in rough alignment with each other. Finally, it can be shown that the homunculus varies in a biologically appropriate manner from one mammal to another.

We noted above that the RF areas of cells in the somaesthetic cortex were not fixed and rigid but able to expand and contract in response to different circumstances. Similarly the quantity of cortex devoted to particular parts of the body can also change in response to experience. Perhaps the best known experimental examination of this lability was carried out on the vibrissae of mice.

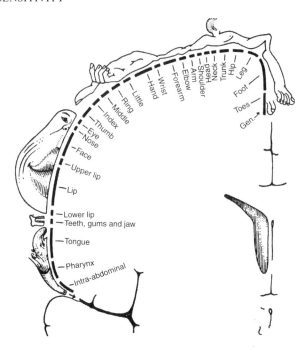

Figure 8.20 Somaesthetic homunculus. The figure shows a coronal section through the postcentral gyrus. Note the large areas devoted to the hand and to the face and lips.

8.6 PLASTICITY OF THE SOMAESTHETIC CORTEX

We saw above that rapidly adapting mechanosensory fibres invest the lower parts of hair follicles and detect any movement of the hair. In many mammals this sense is greatly enhanced by the development of vibrissae (whiskers) in the region surrounding the mouth. In the mouse the quantity of cortex devoted to the whiskers is greater than that devoted to the paws. Each whisker sends about 100 myelinated fibres via the trigeminal nerve ultimately to the primary somaesthetic cortex. The fibres terminate in layer IV of the cortex in specialized structures called 'barrels' (Figure 8.21). Each barrel consists of between 1500 and 2500 neurons and is from 100 to 300 μm in diameter. The number of barrels corresponds exactly to the number of vibrissae on the contralateral side of the face and, furthermore, they are arranged in the same way as the whiskers are arranged.

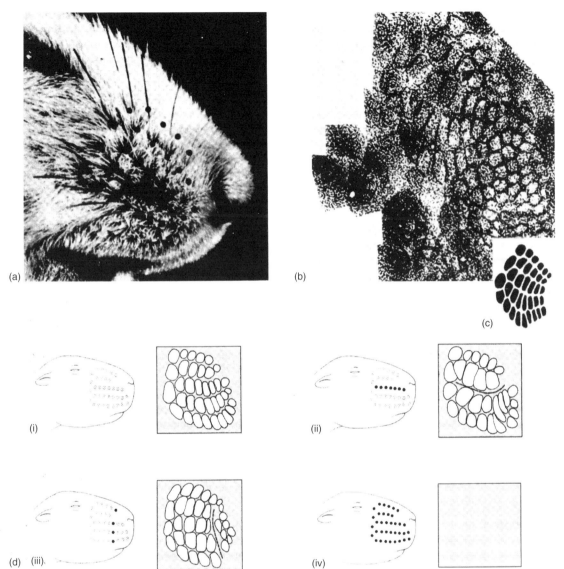

Figure 8.21 Mouse whisker barrels. (a) Head showing five rows of vibrissae. (b) Section of cortex showing 'barrels', each corresponding to one whisker. (c) Diagram to show the organization of the whisker barrels. (d) Diagrams to show the effect of removing whiskers. (i) Full set of whiskers, full set of barrels; (ii) one row of whiskers removed, unaffected barrels grow into territory of unused barrels; (iii) one column of whiskers removed; again unaffected barrels colonize space left by missing barrels; (iv) total removal of whiskers; loss of all barrels. From Woolsey and Van Der Loos, 1970, *Brain Research*, **17**, 205–42, Copyright © 1970, Elsevier.

Woolsey and Van Der Loos carried out some very instructive experiments on this well characterized system. If mice were bred with extra whiskers, extra barrels appeared in the somaesthetic cortex. However, the entire barrel field did not increase in extent but the extra barrels were squeezed in between the usual array. It is as if the vibrissal input is competing for limited cortical space. Similarly, if vibrissae were removed, the corresponding barrels atrophied and their space was taken over by the remaining barrels.

The exact biochemical mechanisms by which this remarkable lability of the cortex in response to peripheral input is achieved is still the subject of much research. We shall see a similar plasticity when we come to consider the primary visual cortex.

Experiments with monkeys trained to carry out a task involving two finger tips touching a revolving wheel revealed a similar plasticity in the somatosensory cortex. Maps of the finger area (obtained by microelectrode recording) before and after the training showed a several-fold increase in the cortical representation. Furthermore, although the total area of finger representation in the somaesthetic cortex increased, the areas of the receptive field of the cells penetrated by the microelectrode were significantly smaller than in the untrained cortex. Similar results have been shown in monkeys that have lost digits, although in these cases, of course, the cortical representation of the missing digit shrinks whilst that of the remaining digits increases.

The advent of sophisticated techniques of neuroimaging, especially functional magnetic resonance imaging (fMRI) and magnetoencephalography (MEG), has enabled analogous investigations to be carried out on humans. MEG studies have shown that the somatosensory representation of the fingers of the left hand is significantly expanded in string players (violin, viola, cello, double base, etc.) when compared with the representation of the digits of the right hand or with the representation of the left hand digits of non-string orchestral players.

Another interesting investigation has been carried out with patients adjusting to blindness by acquiring Braille reading skills. The use of fMRI and the location of somatosensory evoked potentials (SEPs) by EEG techniques have shown that there is an enlargement of the area of somatosensory cortex dedicated to the Braille-reading finger. It appears that there is at first an 'unmasking' of pre-existing neural connections and later these are made permanent by structural changes. In those afflicted with blindness early in life, the occipital cortex is also drawn into the response to the Braille-reading finger. This is interesting as it is well known (Chapter 18) that the occipital cortex is normally concerned with vision. fMRI and SEP scans again show that in these individuals cortico-cortical connections are established (or confirmed) between the somatosensory/

motor cortices, which normally process information relating to touch and movement of the Braille-reading finger, and visual cortices 1 and 2. These connections seem to be important for reading accuracy. We shall see when we come to Chapter 18 that the primary visual cortex also (at least in the sensitive period) adapts to sensory (in this case visual) input. The maps in the sensory cortices are by no means fixed and unchangeable: like other parts of the anatomy, they respond to use and disuse.

8.7 CONCLUDING REMARKS

Aristotle, as we noted in the introductory quotation to Part Two, believed that 'touch' was the defining characteristic of an animal. He also believed it was the most fundamental of all the senses. We can see what he meant. In this chapter we have gone, where the Stagirite had no means of going, beneath the skin and looked at the various sense organs and endings responsible for the sense of touch. We have seen how right the philosopher was in his estimate of its universality and antiquity. We have remarked how touch sensitivity in the tiny nematode, *C. elegans*, promises to throw light on mechanisms at work even in ourselves. We noted also how touch receptors had been developed by the insects to detect ripples on the surface of water and the atmospheric pressure changes we know as sound. We shall look at analogous developments in the vertebrates in the next chapter, where we consider the vertebrate ear.

But our examination of the sense of touch took us further into the life of animals than 'mere' detection of atmospheric vibration. We saw how insect 'ears' are used (amongst other things) for interindividual communication. We noted how moths and lacewings are able to detect the onrush of predatory bats. But, more than this, touch has become deeply enmeshed in the social life of many animals. Anyone who has watched the interaction of social insects, such as ants and bees, will know that the sense of touch is vital: they continuously subject each other to sessions of intense palpation. This use of the sense of touch is also of crucial importance in some of the social mammals, particularly some primates. The processes of mutual grooming, although originally evolved to clear monkey pelts of ectoparasites, has transferred to social bonding. Some monkey troops (depending on size) spend up to 20% of their time in this activity. Such tactile interaction has profound effects on the neuroendocrine system, enabling often exciteable and aggressive animals to live calmly in close proximity to each other. Some have said that humans have substituted vocal gossip to generate the same effect as this tactile bonding. But touch remains profoundly significant in our own species. From shaking hands to more intimate contact, the touch of two skins plays an indispensable role in communication between human individuals.

9

EQUILIBRIUM AND HEARING: THE USES OF HAIR CELLS

Structure and functioning of hair cells: structure of hair cells - stereocilia and kinocilia - tip-links - directionality - gated ion-channels - gating-spring model - comparison with *C. elegans* MEC touch receptor - adaptation. **Lateral line canals**: neuromasts - echolocation - adaptation of canals to different aquatic environments. **Evolution of ear**: early relation to lateral line system - outline structure. **Equilibrium**: membranous labyrinth: structure and function - utricular and saccular maculae and otoliths - cupule-capped cristae in ampullae of semi-circular canals. **Phonoreception**: fish (Weberian ossicles) - amphibia - reptiles (development of lagena) - birds (cochlea, organ of Corti) - mammals (cochlea, organ of Corti). **Anatomy and physiology of mammalian cochlea**: basilar membrane - inner and outer hair cells – genetics - sensitivity control - microphonic potentials - volley and place mechanisms of frequency discrimination - tuning of hair cells - high frequency sensitivity in dogs, rodents, cetacea, and bats - bat echolocation: specialisations for different habitats - independent evolution in mega- and microchiroptera - the sensory world of the insectivorous bat. **Concluding remarks**: the ubiquity of immobile cilia.

Of all the delicate arrays of sense organs developed by the vertebrates, hair cells are perhaps the most remarkable. They are found throughout the phylum and appear to differ little from fish to philosopher. It has been computed that, at the limit of sensitivity in the mammalian ear, hair cells are stimulated by a tip movement of only a tenth of a nanometer. Hudspeth has provided a powerful analogy. He likens the adequate stimulus at the tip of a hair cell's stereocilium to the movement of a thumb's breadth at the top of the Eiffel Tower. Indeed the sensitivity of hair cells is only limited by the random roar of Brownian motion.

9.1 ANATOMY AND PHYSIOLOGY OF HAIR CELLS

The structure of hair cells is shown (very diagrammatically) in Figure 9.1. From a cuticular plate at the distal end of the cell springs a group of up to 60 'hairs'. These 'hairs' are of two types: fifty or sixty **stereocilia** and a single **kinocilium**. It should be noted that the kinocilium is not always present. Indeed, mature mammalian cochlear hair cells lack this structure. The fifty or sixty stereocilia are membrane-ensheathed bundles of actin microfilaments whilst the single tall kinocilium is a true, immobile, cilium,

Biology of Sensory Systems, Second Edition   C.U.M. Smith
© 2008 John Wiley & Sons, Ltd

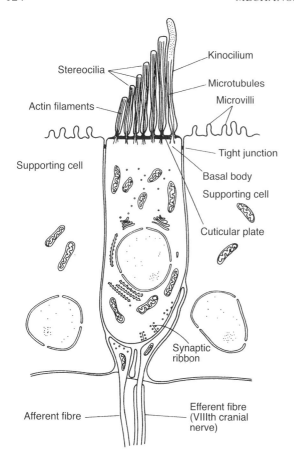

Figure 9.1 Hair cell. This schematic diagram shows the main elements of a typical vertebrate hair cell. Normally there are many more stereocilia (up to sixty) than shown, but there is always only one kinocilium.

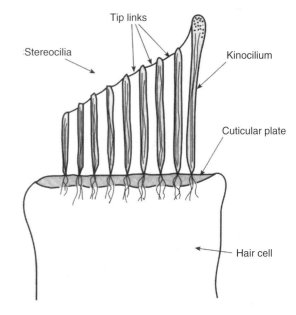

Figure 9.2 Tip links. The tips of the stereocilia are linked together and ultimately to the kinocilium by fine threads.

often with a bulbous tip. The figure shows that all the hairs narrow to a slender 'neck' where they are inserted into the cuticular plate and that they increase in length toward the kinocilium end of the group.

If we examine the stereocilia at higher magnification, we find that they are, in fact, much longer than most cilia, perhaps 5 μm and in, for example, the lizard some 30 μm. They also have a greater diameter, up to 900 nm, though the base tapers to less than 100 nm. In addition to actin mocrifilaments, stereocilia contain appreciable quantities of myosin and calmodulin. Finally, and importantly, careful electron microscopy shows that the tips of the stereocilia are linked together by fine polypeptide threads. Further analysis suggests that the polypeptide is cad-

herin 23. These cadherin links originate in a tangle from the shorter stereocilium and then run singly towards the taller neighbour. The linking fibres are under a certain degree of tension for, if they are severed, the somewhat 'tented' membrane of the lower stereocilium from which they originate subsides (Figure 9.2).

The extraordinary sensitivity to mechanical stimuli has already been mentioned. This can be tested by moving the stereocilia this way and that with a fine microprobe. The stereocilia are found to move in a rigid manner, pivoting on their tapered bases. Threshold movements induce receptor potentials of about 100 μV across the hair cell's membrane. The sign of this potential depends on which way the stereocilium is moved (Figure 9.3). If the stereocilia bundle is moved towards the kinocilium a depolarization occurs; on the other hand, if it is moved away from the kinocilium, a hyperpolarization ensues. Movement at right angles to this axis induces no change in the membrane potential at all. These receptor potentials saturate at movements above about 100 nm.

The transduction process is extremely rapid. Many mammals, members of the cetacea and the chiroptera, for example, respond to sound frequencies

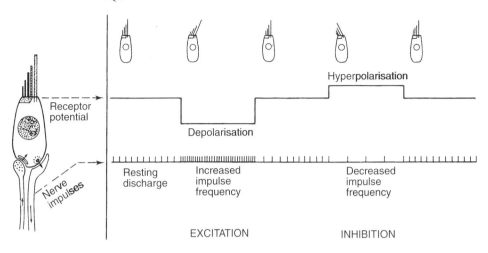

Figure 9.3 Electrical response of hair cell to movement of stereocilia. Movement of the stereocilia in one direction causes depolarization of the hair cell; movement in the opposite direction causes hyperpolarization. These variations in polarity are translated into increased or decreased activity in the sensory nerve fibre. From Flock, "Transducing Mechanisms in the lateral Line Canal Organ Receptors", Cold Spring Harbor Symp. Quant. Biology 30 (1965) Figure 14, p. 142, with permission from Coldspring Harbor Laboratory Press.

up to at least 100 kHz. There is no time for the elaborate biochemistry of 'collision coupling' and second messengers which is at work in chemo- and photoreception. Gated channels in the hair cell membrane must open and shut very rapidly indeed. The electrical response must be due to near-instantaneous flows of ions down their concentration gradients. Where are these gates located?

Again careful experiments have gone far to answer this question. It is probable that the maximum ionic flows in response to movement occur near the tips of the stereocilia. The response, moreover, is found to be extremely rapid: beginning within a few microseconds of stimulus onset and saturating within about 100 μs. The currents (about 50 pS at 30 °C) are mostly carried by K^+ ions which, as we shall see, are present in high concentration in the endolymph in which mammalian stereocilia are bathed. The fact that experiment shows that other cations, including Ca^{2+} and even some small organic cations, for example choline, can pass shows that the channel is fairly wide – perhaps 0.7 nm in diameter. It is estimated that there are about four such channels in each stereocilium.

A model for the biophysics of stereocilia has been put forward by Hudspeth and others. We have already noted that stereocilia are connected near their tips by cadherin threads (tip links) to the next tallest neighbour (Figure 9.2). Experimental evidence shows that these threads are, in fact, attached to ion channels. It is believed that, when the stereocilium is at rest, the channels are somewhat leaky. This is represented in Figure 9.4 by giving an 'open probability' of about 0.1. When a mechanical stimulus moves the assembly of stereocilia towards the kinocilium at the taller end of the group, the 'open probability' of the channels is shifted towards unity. Because, as we noted above, the hairs project into a K^+-rich medium (the endolymph), K^+ is the principal ion to flow into the cilium. This, combined with a parallel influx of Ca^{2+} ions, induces a membrane depolarization. When the movement is in the opposite direction, the 'open probability' is decreased towards zero. The K^+/Ca^{2+} flux is shut off and the membrane hyperpolarizes.

Identification of the ion channels has proved difficult, as there are only three or four in each stereocilium. The amount of protein is thus vanishingly small (a few attomoles). Is it possible, however, to use a comparative approach? One of the striking outcomes of modern molecular biology has been the demonstration of a remarkable unity across the living world

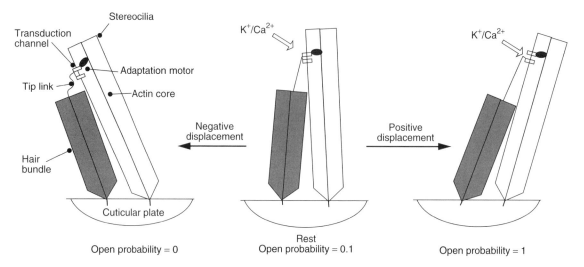

Figure 9.4 Gating-spring model of hair cell stimulation. Explanation in text. From Gillespie, P. G. (1995) *Current Opinion in Neurobiology*, **5**, 449–55, Copyright © 1995 Elsevier.

at the molecular level. In Chapter 8 we looked at the touch receptors in *Caenorhabditis elegans*. We saw that there was evidence that they were related to vertebrate epithelial Na^+-channels (ENaCs). Could the ion channels in stereocilia belong to the same family? Suggestive evidence in support comes from studies of channel blockers. ENaCs are very sensitive to amiloride. The renal Na^+-channel is blocked by nanomolar concentrations of this agent. It is found that amiloride also blocks the channels in stereocilia. It may be, therefore, that the *C. elegans* channel and that of vertebrate hair cells are related. If this is so, some of the elegant molecular biology carried out on the nematode may have relevance to the operation of the human ear. But there are other candidates. In addition to the ENaCs, there is evidence that members of the TRP superfamily of cation channels may be implicated. Interestingly, both the NompC channel (TRPN), which we met when discussing *Drosophila* mechanosensitive sensilla, and the TRPA1 channel are found in nonmammalian vertebrates. The NompC channel is present in the **kinocilia** of lateral line and vestibular hair cells of *Xenopus*, and TRPA1 localizes to the tips of bullfrog stereocilia. In mammals there is evidence that TRPA1 channels are located in kinocilia but the evidence for their presence in stereocilia is as yet controversial. Thus, at the time of writing,, although there are a number of candidates, the precise nature of the cation channels

responsible for cochlea stereocilia microphysiology is still under investigation.

Whichever channel carries inward flows of cations, the mechanotransductive mechanism outlined above ensures that the response to mechanical stimulation is almost instantaneous – as it is observed to be. It is also known that most hair cells adapt very rapidly (at most a few tens of milliseconds). In other words, when the deflection of the stereocilia is maintained for more than about a millisecond, the influx of K^+/Ca^{2+} and the consequent depolarization ceases. How is this brought about? Recent investigations have revealed a remarkable mechanism within the stereocilium. A schematic of the ultrastructure is shown in Figure 9.5. In addition to external tip links, the figure shows that channel protein is attached via a myosin 'motor' to the internal actin microfilaments. This attachment provides a platform to stabilize the position of the channel in the membrane so that increased tension on the tip links does not simply pull the whole channel protein down the stereocilium in the plane of the membrane. Again an interesting comparison can be made with the way in which the *C.elegans* touch receptor is attached to tubulin molecules with the neurosensory cell (Figures 8.5 and 8.6).

The mechanism responsible for adaptation depends on the influx of Ca^{2+} when the ion channel is opened. One theory suggests that this leads to a

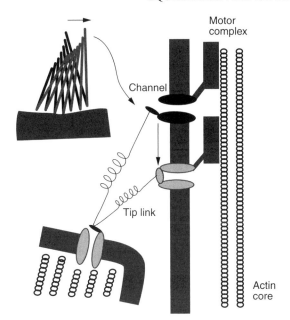

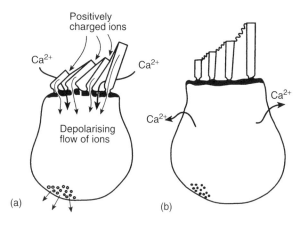

Figure 9.5 Adaptation in hair cells. When the hair is deflected the channel is opened and the 'motor complex' detaches from the actin filaments. The channel complex slips down the stereocilium and the tension on the gate is released. It closes. Later, when the stereocilium returns to its upright position, the 'motor complex' climbs back up the actin filament dragging the channel back to its resting position. Further explanation in text. From Gillespie, P. G. and Corey, D. P. (1997), *Neuron*, **19**, 955–58, Copyright © 1997 Elsevier.

Figure 9.6 Mechanoelectrochemical transduction in hair cells. (a): the stereocilia are all pulled towards the right and the K^+/Ca^{2+}-channels are opened. The influx of cations causes a depolarization which opens further Ca^{2+}-channels in the cuticular plate and elswhere. The influx of Ca^{2+} leads to the release of transmitter substance on to the dendrite of an underlying neuron. (b): the stereocilia return to their resting position. The ion channels close and the cell repolarizes. Ca^{2+} is pumped out of the cytosol and the release of transmitter ceases.

loosening of the linkage between the myosin 'motor' and the actin microfilaments within the stereocilium. This, in turn, allows the ion channel to slip down the stereocilium's membrane, thus releasing tension on the tip link. The 'open probability' of the channel then decreases and the membrane polarity returns to its resting value. When the stereocilium returns to its normal near upright position, the channel protein – now under no internal tension – moves toward an 'open probability' of zero. In the absence of Ca^{2+} influx, the motor climbs back up the actin filament, pulling the channel with it, thus returning the tension on the tip link to its original value and the open probability to about 0.1. A word of caution: although the hypothetical mechanism of adaptation is very appealing, much more research is needed to establish its reality beyond a peradventure.

In addition to Ca^{2+} influx through the stereociliary transduction channels, further Ca^{2+} ions will enter through voltage-dependent channels located in the cuticular plate. These channels open when the membrane depolarizes which, as we have seen, occurs as a consequence of stereociliary displacement. The influx of Ca^{2+} ions leads in turn (through a complex series of events outlined in texts on molecular neurobiology) to the release of transmitter substance from the base of the hair cell (Figure 9.6). Depending on the nature of the transmitter and the nature of the underlying dendrite, this will either initiate or inhibit a generator potential. In the first case an action potential will be triggered which will be propagated along a sensory nerve into the central nervous system.

Although the ground-breaking investigations of the biophysics of the vertebrate hair cell have been carried out on the hair cells of the inner ear, there is little doubt that the mechanisms there discovered can be generalized to apply to the working of hair cells in other parts of the subphylum Vertebrata. Hair cells are, in fact, evolutionarily very ancient and develop in all classes of the vertebrates from the ancient Agnathan fish to the mammals. In the Cyclostomata, which include the only living representatives of the Agnatha (the hagfish, *Myxine,* and the lamprey, *Lampetra*), hair cells are developed in both the lateral line canals and in the ears.

9.2 LATERAL LINE CANALS

Bony fish (Osteichthyes), cartilaginous fish (Chondrichthyes) and aquatic amphibia (and the aquatic larvae of terrestrial amphibia) develop canals along the sides of their bodies and especially over the head (Figure 9.7a). The object of this system is to detect vibrations in the surrounding water. These vibrations may be due to disturbances in the water caused by other aquatic organisms or they may be reflections from neighbouring objects of the disturbances produced by the fish itself. The system can thus be regarded as a primitive form of echolocation. We shall meet, towards the end of this chapter, a more highly evolved form of echolocation when we consider the flight and feeding habits of the Chiroptera.

The receptors in the lateral line system are groups of hair cells, called **neuromasts**, surrounded by epithelial cells and surmounted by a gelatinous cupule. The tips of the hairs are embedded in this cupule (Figure 9.7b). The group of neuromasts and epithelial cells are often grouped together on a small hillock. The neuromasts may form clusters isolated in the skin (as in the cyclostomes and amphibia) but more usually they are to be found at intervals in a series of grooves or canals in the head and body. These canals may be sunk in the dermis of the skin and completely enclosed or take the form of open grooves. The more stormy the water in which the fish customarily lives, the more protected is the lateral line system. The system is particularly well developed in deep sea fish. The neuromasts are innervated by the lateral line nerve (a branch of the Xth cranial nerve, the vagus nerve) and, in the head region, by the VIIth and IXth cranial nerves.

Lateral line nerves show a spontaneous activity which originates from the neuromasts. This frequency of discharge is much increased when the water in the vicinity of the canal is disturbed. Recording from lateral line fibres in a Japanese eel showed that narrow diameter fibres give slowly adapting responses, whilst large diameter fibres provided high frequency rapidly adapting responses. Although in some fish the lateral line nerve fibres fire in synchrony with vibrations up to about 200 Hz, there is no evidence that fish can discriminate different frequencies by this system. It is, perhaps, best thought of as a form of 'distant touch', a 'water touch', although it may turn out to have other functions as well, perhaps in temperature detection. The evolutionary

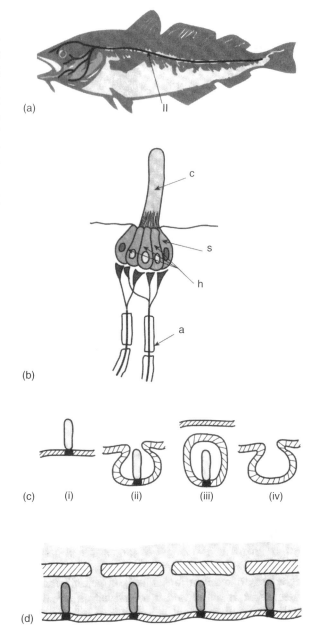

Figure 9.7 (a): Generalized bony fish to show the position of the lateral line system. ll = lateral line. (b): Neuromast: a = sensory fibre; c = cupule; h = hair cell; s = supporting epithelial cell. (c): Relationship between superficial neuromasts and canal organs: (i) isolated neuromast; (ii) neuromast in 'gutter'; (iii) neurmast in enclosed canal; (iv) region of enclosed canal which opens to the exterior by a pore. (d): Longitudinal section through lateral line to show relation between neuromasts and pores. Cupule, stippled; neurmast cells, black; epithelial cells, cross hatched. After Sand, O. (1984).

possibilities inherent in lateral line systems are brought out in Chapter 21, where we shall see that in a number of Chondrichthyan and Osteichthyan fish it is supplemented by a highly evolved system of electroreceptors. This system has evolved from the same primordia as the mechanosensitive lateral line system.

Although, as mentioned above, the lateral line system is still to be found in aquatic amphibia and aquatic amphibian larvae, it is completely missing in their evolutionary successors, the reptiles, birds and mammals. In spite of the fact that many of these forms have returned to an aquatic lifestyle, a lateral line system never reappears.

9.3 EVOLUTION OF THE VERTEBRATE EAR

There is little doubt that lateral line systems and ears are closely related. In the lampreys an inpushing in the surface of the head region quickly becomes closed off from the exterior and develops into two fluid-filled tubes, set at right angles to each other, and two other fluid-filled chambers. The tubes are the **semicircular canals** and the chambers, the **utriculus** and the **sacculus**. The three chambers together constitute the **membranous vestibule**. The chambers of the membranous vestibule are regarded by some as specialized regions of the lateral line system in the head and this early design remains, as Figure 9.8 shows, to form the core of the ear throughout the vertebrates. Only in the crocodylid reptiles, birds and mammals does the inconspicuous **lagena** of the fish (an outgrowth from the sacculus) undergo spectacular development to form the **cochlea**. The semicircular canals, the utriculus, sacculus and and lagena (or cochlea where it exists) are together defined as constituting the **membranous labyrinth**.

9.3.1 Equilibrium

The ear was at first an organ of balance and equilibrium. The detection of sound, which looms so large in the mammalian and human worlds, is a more recent addition. The membranous vestibule remains remarkably unchanged throughout the half billion or so years since the origin of the vertebrates

(Figure 9.8). In all the jawed vertebrates an extra semicircular canal, orthogonal to the two present in the lamprey, is present. The whole system is filled with an aqueous fluid, the **endolymph**, and is suspended in the otic cavity, where it floats free in another aqueous fluid, the **perilymph**. The two fluids differ radically in their ionic constitution. Whereas perilymph resembles other extracellular fluids in having a high Na^+ concentration (150 mM/l) and a low K^+ concentration (3–4 mM/l), endolymph is much more like an intracellular fluid in being rich in K^+ (150 mM/l) and poor in Na^+ (1–2.5 mM/l). We noted above, when discussing the biophysics of hair cells, that the ion flows into stereocilia are largely comprised of K^+. We shall see below that the stereocilia project into the endolymph. Hence, endolymph's anomalous ionic constitution is an indispensable part of the ear's physiology. Finally, we should note that, although the labyrinth floats free in the otic cavity, it is tethered to the walls of the cavity by collagen fibres. In most cases a slender tube, the **ductus endolymphaticus**, extends from the sacculus to terminate within the cranial cavity as the endolymphatic sac.

In the walls of both the utriculus and the sacculus, spots consisting of sensory hair cells develop. These are known as the utricular and saccular *maculae*. The utricular macula lies on the floor of that compartment and the saccular macula is usually in the vertical plane, on the wall of that chamber (Figure 9.9a). The maculae are innervated by fibres belonging to the vestibular nerve. In fish a small elongation of the sacculus, called the lagena, also contains a sensory macula. The hair cells of the maculae are very similar to the neuromasts of the lateral line canals. But here two types can be distinguished: amphora-like Type I cells and cylindrical Type II cells (Figure 9.9b). Like neuromasts, groups of hair cells are surmounted by a gelatinous cupule. In the utriculus, sacculus and lagena this gelatinous cupule usually becomes impregnated with crystals of $CaCO_3$ (calcium carbonate) to form an **otolith** or 'ear stone'. The saccular otolith normally shows the greatest development and in many teleost fish almost fills that chamber. Indeed, so characteristic is the shape of this 'stone' in the bony fish that it can often be used to identify its one-time owner.

The functions of the utriculus and sacculus are quite simply to detect linear acceleration of the head in space. There are two cases. In the first case, when

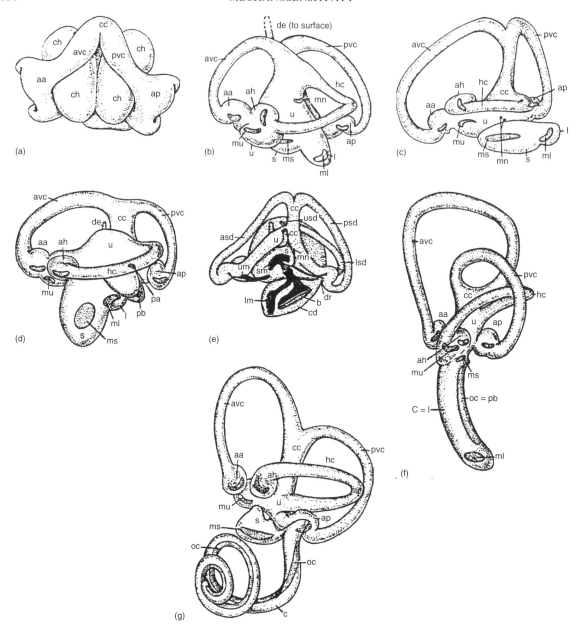

Figure 9.8 Evolution of the membranous labyrinth. (a): *Petromyzon* (Lamprey); (b): *Scyllium* (Dogfish); (c): *Scomber* (Mackerel); (d): *Rana* (Frog); (e): *Lacerta* (Lizard); (f): *Columba* (Pigeon); (g): *Cavia* (Guinea pig). For figures (a), (b), (c), (d), (f), (g): aa = ampulla of anterior canal; ah = ampulla of horizontal canal; ap = ampulla of posterior canal; avc = anterior vertical canal; c = cochlear duct; cc = crus commune; ch = chambers lined with ciliated epithelium; de = ductus endolymphaticus; hc = horizontal canal; l = lagena; ml = macula of lagena; mn = macula neglecta; ms = macula of sacculus; mu = macula of utriculus; oc = organ of Corti; pa = papilla amphibiorum; pb = papilla basilaris (i.e. basilar papilla); pvc = posterior vertical canal; s = sacculus; u = utriculus. Figure (e): asd = anterior semicircular canal; b = basilar papilla; cc = crus commune; cd = cochlear duct; lm = lagenar macula; lsd = lateral semicircular canal; mn = macula neglecta; od = otic duct; psd = posterior semicircular canal; sm = saccular macula; u = utriculus; um = utricular maculus; usd = utriculo-saccular duct. (a), (b), (c), (d), (f) and (g) from Romer, A.S. (1977) *The Vertebrate Body, 5th Edition*. Copyright © 1977 W. B. Saunders (e) from Baird, I. L. (1974) *Handbook of Sensory Physiology Vol. V/1* (H. Autrum et al., eds). Copyright © 1974, Springer-Verlag.

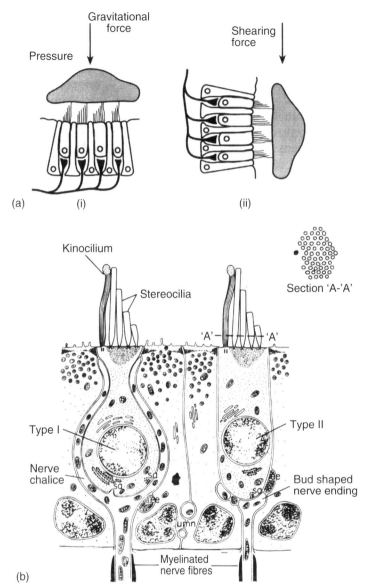

Figure 9.9 (a): Positions of the hair cells in (i) the utriculus and (ii) sacculus and lagena. (b): Two types of hair cell in the maculae and cristae of the membranous labyrinth: Type 1 amphora-shaped cells and Type II cylindrical cells. Type I cells are surrounded by a chalice-shaped nerve ending. At the top right of the figure a sectional view A–A′ is shown through the cilia of the Type II cell. The kinocilium is represented by the filled circle. ee = efferent nerve endings; sa = synaptic area; umn = unmyelinated nerve endings. Courtesy of A.J. Benson.

the head is moved forward/backward or up/down, the inertia of the otoliths ensures that the stereocilia of the hair cells will be bent in one direction or another. In the second case, when the head is stationary, the linear acceleration of the otoliths caused by gravity causes them to weigh down on the underlying hair cells. This gravitational force will act in different directions on the hairs when the head is placed at different angles. These various bending forces are

sensed by the stereocilia in the way discussed in the preceding section. The information is signalled to the brain along fibres of the vestibular nerve.

The three semicircular canals are disposed in the three dimensions of space. They spring from the utriculus (Figure 9.8) and each has a spherical enlargement, known as the **ampulla**, where it communicates with the aforesaid chamber. The canals, like the rest of the membranous vestibule, are filled with endolymph. Within the ampullae are elevated sensory areas, known as **cristae**, from which, once again, sensory hair cells spring. The tips of the hairs are embedded in a tall gelatinous cupule, which all but blocks the ampullary passage-way and swings to and fro like a swing door.

The semicircular canal system has evolved to detect angular accelerations of the head in space. When the head rotates in any of the three dimensions of space, the inertia of the endolymph in the semicircular canals will at first lag behind. Ultimately, viscous interaction with the walls of the tubes would impart movement to the fluid, which would then rotate in unison with its containing structure. However, the initial lag of the endolymph behind the movements of its containing ducts means that the 'swing-doors' of the ampullar cristae are forced open. In other words, the gelatinous cupule and the embedded stereocilia are distorted. Once again, impulses in fibres of the vestibular nerve are initiated. Note, however, that it is the angular acceleration that is detected, not the constant angular velocity which might be induced by spinning over a lengthy duration (say 20 s or more).

The sensory input from the utriculus, sacculus and semicircular canals is integrated with input from the eyes, from receptors in the muscles, joints and skin, to initiate reflexes which maintain the normal orientation of the animal with respect to gravity and which counteract externally applied accelerations in all planes. The majority of these reflexes is mediated by spinal and brain stem regions; there is very little involvement of the cortex.

9.3.2 Phonoreception

9.3.2.1 Fish

It is known that many fish are sensitive to sound. We noted above that the lateral line system may well be involved at low frequencies. There is, however, mainly from ablation studies, evidence that both the sacculus and the lagena are involved in detection of higher frequencies. Amongst the bony fish the swim bladder is sometimes pressed into service as a 'hydrophone'. In the squirrel fish (Holocentridae), for instance, the swim bladder is extended so that it abuts the auditory region of the skull. In the Ostariophysi (carp, goldfish, tench, minnow, catfish, etc.) a yet more complex adaptation is found. Four anterior vertebrae are modified to form the so-called

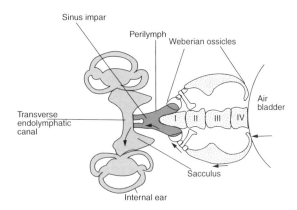

Figure 9.10 Weberian ossicles. The figure shows a horizontal section through the anterior region of the body of a carp (*Cyprinus carpio*). The arrows indicate the direction of vibrations from the swim bladder to the sacculus. I, II, III and IV indicate the four vertebrae from which the ossicles are derived. Modified from Romer, 1970.

Weberian ossicles. These connect the swim bladder to a backwardly directed, perilymph-filled, vesicle, the **sinus impar**. The sinus impar, in turn, connects with a transverse endolymphatic canal that communicates with the sacculus (Figure 9.10). The saccular otoliths possess wing-like extensions that can detect the movement of endolymph within the chamber. The vibrations picked up by the swim bladder are transmitted via the ossicles to the perilymph of the sinus impar and thence via the transverse canal to the winged otoliths of the sacculus. Conditioning experiments have shown that the catfish, *Ameiurus*, can detect frequencies up to 13 kHz and has good frequency discrimination (a minor third – 1.2:1). Removal of the malleus, one of the Weberian ossicles, reduces sensitivity by a factor of up to a hundred.

9.3.2.2 Amphibia

In the amphibia the ear has had to adapt to detect pressure changes in the atmosphere, a much more rarefied medium than water. In anurans (e.g. frogs) a middle ear has developed so that these pressure changes (sound) are transmitted from a slightly sunken tympanic membrane by a bony shaft, the columella auris, to the chambers of the membranous labyrinth. In the urodeles, such as the salamander, no columella or middle ear develops. Urodeles are, however, not deaf. They are responsive to sound by way of the labyrinth and skin mechanoreceptors. Figure 9.8

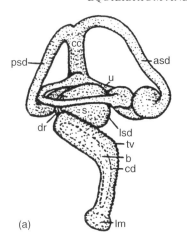

(a)

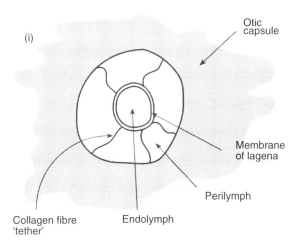

(i)

Otic capsule

Membrane of lagena

Perilymph

Collagen fibre 'tether'   Endolymph

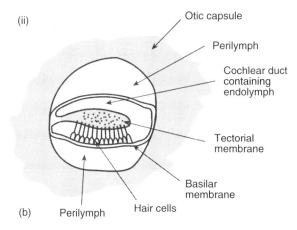

(ii)

Otic capsule

Perilymph

Cochlear duct containing endolymph

Tectorial membrane

Basilar membrane

(b)   Perilymph   Hair cells

shows that in the inner ear the lagena undergoes some extension and in the Anura (frogs and toads) there is also a comparatively well developed papilla basilaris. These two parts of the labyrinth are largely responsible for amphibian hearing. Frogs have been conditioned to sounds over a range from 50 to 10 000 Hz. The auditory sensitivity is particularly significant in the breeding season when croaking serves to attract both sexes to water.

Amphibia, as with all the other tetrapod land fauna, are responsive to the direction from which sound emanates. Unlike the mammals, but like the reptiles and birds, their tympanic membranes are not simple pressure detectors. In the case of amphibia the buccal cavity acts as a resonator and communicates pressure waves via the eustachian tubes to the interior surface of the ear drums. The ear drum is thus exposed to pressure variations on both its exterior and interior face. Thus, with amphibia (and also with reptiles and birds) the directionality of an impinging sound wave can be determined by signalling the response of the tympanic membrane to the intensities and phases of two opposing pressure waves.

9.3.2.3 Reptilia

It is in the reptiles, however, that we meet the true beginnings of the cochlea which assumes such importance in birds and mammals. In alligators, for example, the lagena, although not increasing greatly in length, becomes attached to the sides of the surrounding otic cavity so that three distinct canals are formed (Figure 9.11b). An associated development is the enlargement of the **basilar papilla** (Figure 9.11a). A rudiment of this can be found in the amphibia but

Figure 9.11 (Opposite) (a): Membranous labyrinth of crocodile. asd = anterior semicircular canal duct; b = basilar papilla; cc = crus commune; cd = cochlear duct; dr = reunient duct; lm = lagena macula; lsd = lateral semicircular canal duct; psd = posterior semicricular canal duct; s = sacculus; tv = tegmentum vasculosum. From *Handbook of Sensory Physiology* (ed Kerdel and Neff),1974, p. 188, fig 13A (Baird) with permission from Springer-Verlag. (b): Diagrammatic transverse sections to show to show the formation of a three-channel cochlear duct in the reptiles. (i) The lagena of fish and amphibia floats free (except for some collagen fibre 'tethers') in the perilymph filling the bony labyrinth. (ii) The lagena becomes attached to the sides of the bony labyrinth to form the cochlear duct. Hair cells based on the basilar membrane have their sensory hairs embedded in the tectorial membrane.

it is far better developed in the reptiles, especially the crocodiles and alligators, and is destined to play a highly significant rôle in birds and mammals. It consists of a strip of hair cells growing from the basilar membrane of the cochlear (lagena) covered by a continuous gelatinous membrane. This membrane, the **tectorial membrane**, assumes the major role in the detection of vibrations.

The tympanic membrane is often depressed beneath the body surface so that the beginnings of an external auditory meatus (L = opening) appear and, as in the anurans, a columella spans a middle ear chamber, conducting vibrations to the membranous labyrinth in the inner ear. Snakes are the exception to all this, having neither external auditory meatus nor middle ear chamber. They do, however, retain the columella, which becomes attached to the quadrate bone of the jaw articulation. Snakes are thus rather insensitive to air-borne vibrations but exquisitely sensitive to vibrations in the ground.

Although the anatomy shows some evolutionary advance over the amphibian, there is little evidence that the auditory sense is very different. Tortoises are very sensitive to sounds in the range 80–130 Hz; alligators respond up to and beyond 1000 Hz; lizards can detect frequencies up to 10 kHz. But there is little to suggest any ability to discriminate between different frequencies.

9.3.2.4 Birds

Penultimately we arrive at the birds. Here the anatomy has evolved in an interestingly similar way to that which we shall find in the mammals (Figure 9.12a). The lagena has become significantly elongated and retains the three-channel organization which, as we saw above, first appeared in the reptiles. The upper canal is termed the **scala vestibuli**, the middle the **scala media** and the lower canal, the **scala tympani**. A transverse section (Figure 9.12b) shows that the basilar papilla has once again grown in extent and can now be regarded as an **organ of Corti**. We shall discuss this in more detail when we come to the mammalian ear below. The width of the basilar membrane increases towards its distal end, which suggests that low frequency notes are detected at this end. Beyond the far end of the cochlea the original macula of the lagena persists. This, too, is believed to be particularly responsive to low frequencies. The ear has now three distinct chambers, an external auditory meatus leading to a tympanic membrane, a middle ear chamber crossed by a columella and three irregular shaped bones and an inner ear containing the membranous labyrinth.

Most birds are, of course, extremely sensitive to sound. It is of great importance in their social life. Bird calls are species-specific and in some song-birds there is good evidence that fledglings learn local dialects. It has been found that some cave dwelling birds use sound to provide echolocation (*Steatornis*, the Venezualan oil bird, *Collacalia*, an Asian swift) but there is no evidence for their having developed the ultrasonic sensitivity that is so characteristic of bats. Finally, directional sensitivity has evolved to a state of great precision in nocturnal hunters such as the owl (Section 10.3).

9.3.2.5 Mammalia

In mammals the auditory part of the ear, the cochlea, reaches its evolutionary peak. The faintest sound-wave humans can detect has a force of about 0.001 dyne/cm^2 or about 10^{-16} watt/cm^2. This corresponds to a pressure change of 20 μPa. at the tympanic membrane. The frequencies that humans can detect range from 20 Hz to 20 kHz although the top of the range diminishes with age. A trained ear can discriminate between frequencies of 1000 and 1002 Hz. These remarkable abilities are largely due to the greatly developed cochlea. As Figure 9.8g shows it is no longer straight, or slightly curved, as in the birds, but twisted into a spiral not unlike the shape of a snail's shell. A sectional view is shown in Figure 9.13a. It can be seen that the three canals, the scalae vestibuli, media and tympani, which we met first in the reptiles, persist and Figure 9.13b shows that the basilar papilla has developed into the complex organ of Corti.

Before we can discuss how this delicate and intricate structure works, we need to look briefly at the anatomy of the entire mammalian ear. Figure 9.14a shows that both the external and the middle ear have undergone considerable development. In many species the pinna is large and highly moveable. It plays a significant role in determining the source of sound. Humans still retain, in a largely vestigial form, the muscles which in other species move the pinna. The external auditory meatus is comparatively long and, to prevent invasion by unwanted strangers, is protected by hairs and wax secretions.

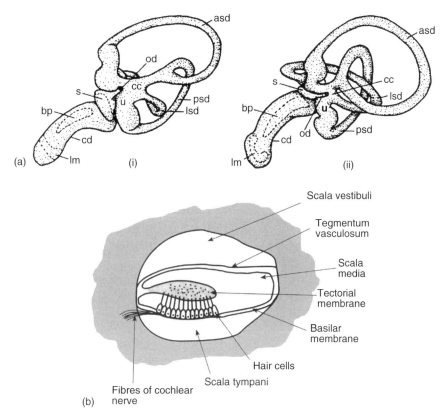

Figure 9.12 (a): Membranous labyrinth of (i) Anserine bird (goose, *Anser*) and (ii) Passerine bird (thrush, *Turdus*). Note differences in semicircular canals, saccule and cochlear duct. asd, psd, lsd = semicircular canals; bp = basillar papilla; cc = crus commune; cd = cochlear duct; lm = lagena macula; od = otic duct; s = sacculus; u = utriculus. From Baird, 1974: with permission from Springer-Verlag (b): Transverse section through the cochlear duct of a bird. From *Handbook of Sensory Physiology* (ed Kerdel and Neff),1974, p. 197, fig 17A and B (Baird) with permission from Springer-Verlag.

The tympanic membrane marks the division between the outer and middle ear. The middle ear chamber is kept at atmospheric pressure by the passageway provided by the **eustachian tube**, which opens into the pharynx. This, of course, is important. The tympanic membrane is delicate and any large disparity in the pressure on either side will lead to its rupture. The vibrations caused by sound on the tympanic membrane are transmitted across the middle ear chamber by the auditory ossicles: the **malleus**, **incus** and **stapes**. These, proverbially the smallest bones in the human body, are attached to the wall of the middle ear chamber by ligaments and muscles. The muscles, the tensor tympani (running to the malleus) and the stapedius (running to the stapes) contract in unison to high intensity sounds. They thus serve to protect the delicate inner ear from the damaging effects of excessive vibration. Finally, the 'footplate' of the stapes is attached to the membrane covering the **oval window (fenestra ovalis)** by an annular ligament. In a condition known as **otosclerosis** the footplate becomes fused with the bony surrounds of the oval window. It is one of the commonest forms of impaired hearing in Caucasian adults (prevalence 0.2–1%), the mean age of onset is the third decade of life and 90% of those affected are under the age of 50. Stapes microsurgery significantly improves hearing thresholds. But this is only a treatment of the symptom. The underling causes are many and various – some environmental, some genetic. Mutations in any of at least seven genes, scattered over the genome (*OTSC1, 2, 3, 4, 5, 6* and *7*), have been shown to cause the condition. Recently another gene, *TGBF1*, which encodes a growth factor involved in the embryology of

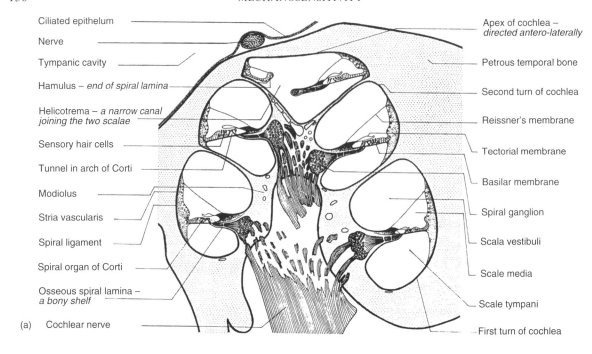

Ciliated epithelum

Nerve

Tympanic cavity

Hamulus – *end of spiral lamina*

Helicotrema – *a narrow canal joining the two scalae*

Sensory hair cells

Tunnel in arch of Corti

Modiolus

Stria vascularis

Spiral ligament

Spiral organ of Corti

Osseous spiral lamina – *a bony shelf*

(a)   Cochlear nerve

Apex of cochlea – *directed antero-laterally*

Petrous temporal bone

Second turn of cochlea

Reissner's membrane

Tectorial membrane

Basilar membrane

Spiral ganglion

Scala vestibuli

Scale media

Scale tympani

First turn of cochlea

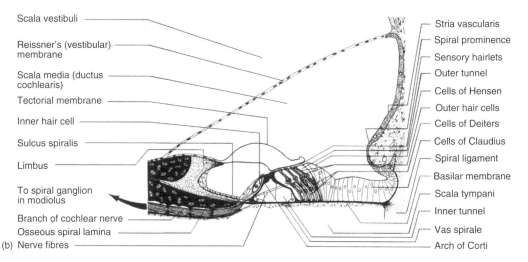

Scala vestibuli

Reissner's (vestibular) membrane

Scala media (ductus cochlearis)

Tectorial membrane

Inner hair cell

Sulcus spiralis

Limbus

To spiral ganglion in modiolus

Branch of cochlear nerve

Osseous spiral lamina

(b) Nerve fibres

Stria vascularis

Spiral prominence

Sensory hairlets

Outer tunnel

Cells of Hensen

Outer hair cells

Cells of Deiters

Cells of Claudius

Spiral ligament

Basilar membrane

Scala tympani

Inner tunnel

Vas spirale

Arch of Corti

Figure 9.13   (a): The cochlear duct is wound in the form of a snail's shell. The sectional view in the figure is taken vertically through this 'snail shell' conformation. (b): The scala media and organ of Corti are shown in more detail. From Freeman, W.H. and Bracegirdle, B. (1976) *An Atlas of Advanced Histology*, p. 113, with permission from Elsevier.

the ear, has also been shown, when defective, to be associated with the disorder.

Let us now return to our consideration of physiology of the cochlea. To simplify matters, Figure 9.14b shows the cochlea unwound from its spi-

ral into a straight tube. We have just seen that when atmospheric pressure waves, which we experience as sound, impinge on the tympanic membrane, the vibration is transmitted to the oval window. The membrane covering this window thus transmits

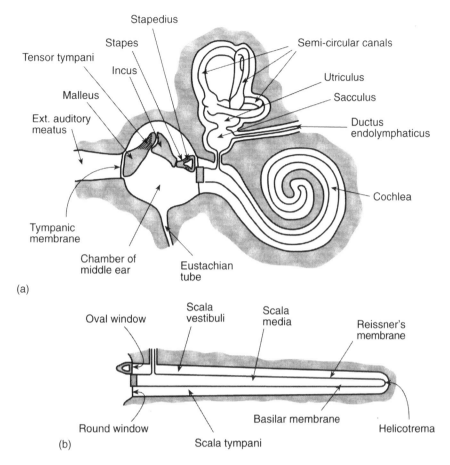

Stapedius

Stapes

Tensor tympani

Incus

Malleus

Ext. auditory meatus

Semi-circular canals

Utriculus

Sacculus

Ductus endolymphaticus

Cochlea

Tympanic membrane

Chamber of middle ear

Eustachian tube

(a)

Oval window

Scala vestibuli

Scala media

Reissner's membrane

Round window

Scala tympani

Basilar membrane

Helicotrema

(b)

Figure 9.14 (a): Anatomy of the mammalian ear. (b): Conceptual diagram of the cochlea unwound to form a straight tube. Further explanation in text. From Smith, C. U. M. (1970) *The Brain: Towards an Understanding*. Copyright © 1970, Faber & Faber.

the pressure changes to the perilymph of the inner ear. Now consider Figures 9.13b and 9.14b. As the membrane covering the oval window moves inward, the pressure in the scala vestibuli increases. Reissner's membrane is forced down and this increases pressure in the scala media until this, in turn, is released by a movement downwards of the basilar membrane. The consequent increase in pressure in the scala tympani is finally released by a bowing outwards of the membrane covering the **round window (fenestra rotunda)**. These movements are, of course, effectively instantaneous.

Now, as we can see from Figure 9.13b, there is another membrane in this system which has yet to be mentioned: the **tectorial membrane**. We noted the

origin of this membrane from the papilla basilaris in sections 9.3.2.2 & 9.3.2.3. This membrane, as membrane as the figure shows, rests upon two rows of hair cells. Indeed, the tips of the hairs are embedded in the membrane just as they were embedded in the gelatinous cupules we discussed earlier in this chapter. Unlike Reissner's membrane and the basilar membrane it floats comparatively freely in the endolymph and in consequence any changes in hydrostatic pressure will affect it equally on all sides. It follows that such pressure changes, especially rapid changes, will not cause it to move up and down in unison with the other two membranes.

Next let us consider the hair cells. Figure 9.13b shows that there is a single row of inner hair cells, separated by a small space from three or four rows of outer hair cells. These cells each develop from 50 to 100 stereocilia but differ from the hair cells we have considered so far in lacking kinocilia. They do, however, develop a prominent centriole where a kinocilium might have been expected. A surface view shows that the stereocilia take the form of a 'W' or 'U' with the base directed toward this centriole (Figure 9.15). The tips of the stereocilia are embedded in the tectorial membrane, whilst the bases of the hair cells are attached to the basilar membrane, making synaptic contact with dendritic endings of the cochlear nerve.

The synapses are interesting. Figure 9.16 shows a multitude of synaptic vesicles (probably containing glutamate) clustered around a dense body which, like the synaptic ribbons of vertebrate photoreceptors, probably serves to muster the vesicles prior to release. There are a number of other specializations in the presynaptic active zone that are designed to ensure prompt and efficient release of transmitter. The Ca^{2+}-channels are both highly concentrated and of a type which reacts very rapidly to small changes in membrane polarity. These two features ensure a near-instantaneous release of transmitter in response to membrane depolarization. There are also two mechanisms that ensure a rapid termination of transmitter release. There is an avid Ca^{2+} buffer in the hair cell cytoplasm and a rapid repolarization of the membrane is ensured by a local clustering of Ca^{2+}-activated K^+-channels. All these specializations help to prevent the rapid response to mechanical distortion of the hair bundle being lost in sluggish synaptic signalling at the hair cell's base.

There is a striking difference between the inner and outer hair cells. Whereas the inner hair cells make contact with up to ten afferent fibres, the outer hair cells are far less richly innervated. Some 90% of the afferent fibres in the cochlear nerve derive from synaptic endings on the row of inner hair cells. Figure 9.16 shows that the base of an inner hair cell contains many synaptic vesicles and also 'dense bodies' (synaptic ribbons) and other accessory structures. Efferent fibres of the cochlear nerve are also present. Figure 9.16 shows, further, that these fibres make synaptic contact with the dendritic endings of the afferent fibres. This suggests that the there is feedback control which can set the sensitivity of the system. In contrast the outer hair cells, though

sparsely innervated by afferent fibres, have a powerful efferent innervation. The efferent fibre endings are large and filled with transmitter vesicles. In Box 9.1 we see that the outer hair cells are able to contract. It seems, therefore, that this powerful efferent innervation also allows the brain to 'set' the sensitivity of the cochlea by altering the distance between the tectorial and basilar membranes (we shall return to this when we consider the physiology of cochlear fibres in Chapter 10).

As might be expected with so delicate and precise a mechanism, many things can go wrong and induce deafness. With the great increase in knowledge of the human genome in recent years several hundred 'deafness' genes have been discovered. These genes are distributed over all 22 autosomal chromosomes as well as on the X-chromosome. Many of them are linked to other (nonauditory) abnormalities but at least a dozen appear to stand alone; they are, in other words, nonsyndromic, although other conditions may ultimately be shown to be linked to them. Of course, not all of these hundred or so genes affect the ear or the hair cells. Many of them will influence more central parts of the auditory system. But those that do affect the hair cells allow the beginnings of a genetic dissection of these vital structures. A gene has, for instance, been shown to encode a potassium channel in the outer hair cells; connexin genes have also been shown to have a significant part to play in potassium homeostasis; and, quite recently, a gene, *OTOF*, which encodes a protein called otoferlin expressed in inner hair cells, has been tracked to chromosome 2. There is evidence to show that otoferlin is involved in the lining-up of vesicles alongside the 'dense body' or 'synaptic ribbon' which, as we saw above, is characteristic of hair cell synapses. More detail of these gene malfunctions is given in Box 9.2.

Next let us turn our attention to the crux of the matter. We have seen that the basilar membrane vibrates in response to incoming sound. But we have also seen that the tectorial membrane remains comparatively stationary. The stereocilia of the hair cells are thus subjected to mechanical distortion. We have also seen that their tips project into the K^+-rich endolymph. The resulting depolarizations can be detected by microelectrode recording. They mimic accurately the imposed sound frequencies. Such potentials are known as **microphonic potentials**. The microphonic depolarizations (receptor potentials) lead

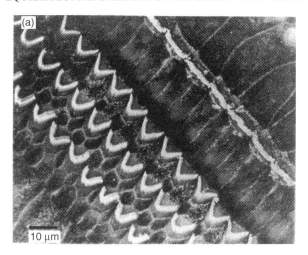

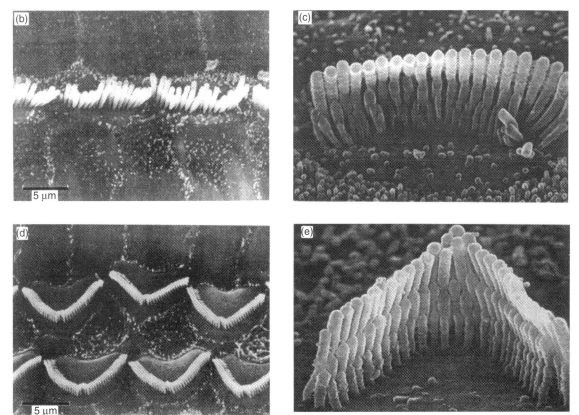

Figure 9.15 Scanning electron micrographs of hair cells in the organ of Corti. The tectorial membrane has been removed and the microscope looks down on the basilar membrane. (a) Three rows of outer hair cells (note U-disposition) and one row of inner hair cells. (b) Stereocilia on the inner hair cells form a nearly straight row. (c) Higher magnification of inner hair cell (75 000×). (d) Stereocilia on the outer hair cells are smaller and arranged in a U-pattern. (e) Higher magnification of stereocilia on outer hair cells (125 000×). (a), (b) and (d) from Pickles, J.O. (1988) *An Introduction to the Physiology of Hearing* by permission of Academic Press Ltd.

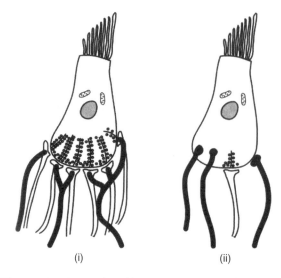

(i)   (ii)

Figure 9.16   Innervation of inner and outer hair cells in the organ of Corti. The schematic figure shows afferent fibres (white) and efferent fibres (black). (i) Inner hair cell. The efferent fibres make synaptic contact with the dendritic endings of the afferent fibres. (ii) Outer hair cell. The efferent fibres synapse directly on the hair cell which makes rather few synapses (only one shown) with sensory (afferent) fibres.

to the release of transmitter substances on to the dendritic endings of the cochlear afferent fibres.

Thus we see that at the very heart of the hugely complex mammalian ear are hair cells, somewhat modified, it is true, but essentially the same as those which we met first in the lateral line canals of our aquatic ancestors. We shall see that something of the same sort can be said of the other organs of special sense. The molecular mechanisms evolved early in evolutionary history have been retained but built over time into enormously intricate and sophisticated organs.

One of the evolutionary imperatives which forced the development of the mammalian cochlea was the necessity to discriminate different auditory frequencies. We saw that this ability was present to a small extent in fish, amphibia and reptiles. In birds and mammals it has undergone great development. We noted above that the frequency range of the human ear runs between 20 Hz and 20 kHz with some deterioration of the upper range with age. We also noted that humans and other mammals have extremely good frequency discrimination within their auditory

ranges. Our next question must, therefore, be: how is the frequency discrimination achieved?

It might be thought that the problem has an easy solution. Why shouldn't the cochlear nerves be phase-locked with the incoming pressure waves of the sound? Why, in other words, shouldn't a tonal frequency of 20 Hz be signalled by an impulse frequency of 20 Hz and a tonal frequency of 15 kHz be signalled by an impulse frequency or 15 kHz? There are two obvious difficulties with this simple solution. First, as we noted in Chapter 2, impulse frequency in sensory nerves normally signals intensity. The nervous system might find a way round this but the second difficulty is more intransigent. The biophysics of nerve fibres necessitates a refractory period of about 2 ms after each impulse. It follows (as we noted in Chapter 2) that single fibres cannot convey more than about 500 impulses per second. Above about 500 Hz some other means of frequency discrimination must be employed.

Two principal mechanisms seem to be at work. First there is evidence (Chapter 10, Figure 10.5) that cochlear fibres can phase-lock to sound frequencies above 500 Hz by not responding to every cycle. It is consequently believed that, at the lower end of the frequency spectrum (below some 5 kHz), groups of cochlear nerve fibres may combine to deliver an impulse frequency matching the tonal frequency to some cerebral centre. This is known, for obvious reasons, as the **volley theory**. A second, and considerably more important, mechanism is based upon the observation that the basilar membrane increases in width from the round window end to the helicotrema (or, in the case of birds, to the macula of the lagena). The human basilar membrane, for instance, increases in width from 100 to 500 μm over its 33 mm length (Figure 9.17). This suggested to Hermann von Helmholtz, back in the nineteenth century, that it might be compared to a sheet of tuned resonators. High frequency tones would cause maximum disturbance at the round window end and low frequency tones toward the helicotrema. Careful observation by von Bekesy and others has largely confirmed Helmholtz's hypothesis. It has been found that a complex waveform travels along the entire basilar membrane but the position where it displays maximum amplitude is, as Helmholtz supposed, related to its frequency. Helmholtz's conjecture is, again for obvious reasons, known as the **place theory** of

BOX 9.1 BIOPHYSICS OF OUTER HAIR CELLS

We have noted that cochlear hair cells are classified into two types: inner and outer (Figure 9.13). They vary in their dimensions in different parts of the cochlea. At the base of the guinea pig cochlea the *outer hair cells* are about 20 μm in length and have short stiff stereocilia, whilst at the apex they are 80 μm long with correspondingly lengthy and flexible stereocilia. This variation in length affects not only their mechanical but also their electrical properties. It can be shown that they exhibit spontaneous electrical oscillations across their boundary membranes. The period of these oscillations varies in different parts of the cochlea. Near the round window, at the base of the cochlea, the short, stiff, outer hair cells display rapid spontaneous oscillations; further up towards the helicotrema, the lengthier cells show slower oscillations. There is a coupling between the dimensions of the cell and the period of spontaneous electrical oscillation. Because the dimensions of the outer hair cells vary regularly from base to apex of the cochlea, the spontaneous oscillations match the auditory frequency to which the underlying basilar membrane is tuned. Thus, when an incoming auditory signal induces mechanical vibration in the basilar membrane, the resulting electrotonic flows caused by opening and closing ion channels in the stereocilia amplifies this pre-existing oscillation. This is known as '**electrical resonance**'. The hair cell acts as a tuned amplifier. This increases the ear's sensitivity by two orders of magnitude.

The variation in electrical resonance from base to apex of the cochlea implies that the population of ion channels in the hair cells must also vary in a regular manner from round window to helicotrema. This implication has been verified by the finding that the numbers of both Ca^{2+} and Ca^{2+}-activated K^+ (K_{Ca}) channels decrease as the characteristic frequency diminishes. Investigations of the chick cochlea have shown, furthermore, that each of the 10 000 or so hair cells presents a unique population of ion channels. Not only does each hair cell present a different number of channels but the channels themselves have different biophysical characteristics. A beginning has been made on the molecular biology of this fascinating system. It has been shown that the different K_{Ca}-channels are derived by alternative mRNA splicing at seven different sites on the primary transcript.

Electrical resonance is not the only mechanism the outer hair cells have for increasing the sharpness of the tuning. It can be shown that the electrical response is coupled to a mechanical response. Depolarizations lead to a shortening of the hair cell length; hyperpolarizations have the opposite effect, causing an elongation of the cell. This electromechanical coupling is due to a voltage sensitive protein, **prestin**, which changes its cross-sectional area in response to transmembrane voltage. At points of maximum sensitivity the response of the hair may be as large as 30 nm/mV. The means by which voltage changes across outer hair cell membranes are transduced into length changes are beginning to be understood. It appears that both active movements of the cell body and active movement of the sensory hairs are involved and the proteins responsible for these movements have recently been identified. Clearly both movements increase the specificity of the cell to particular frequencies. The greater the electrical resonance, the greater the mechanical movement and this, in turn, feeds back to increase the tensional forces between stereocilia and tectorial membrane. This, in its turn, leads to greater opening probabilities of the mechanosensitive channels on the stereocilia. It is also believed that the whole system can work in reverse. Spontaneous, or afferent-induced, motion of the hair cells may cause movements in the basilar membrane and pressure changes in the scala media and elsewhere which, ultimately, are relieved by movements of the tympanic membrane. This is responsible for the spontaneous **otoacoustic emissions** that have been detected in human and other mammalian ears. Whether these movements are also responsible for some instances of tinnitus is still a matter of controversy.

The mammalian cochlea is a truly remarkable molecular mecahanism. It is sensitive to pressure changes of less than a billionth of a standard atmosphere and the hairs on the hair cells are sensitive to

(*Continues*)

(Continued)

deflections of less than the diameter of an atom. Research on the precise ways in which this extraordinary sensitivity is achieved is continuing and we still have not arrived at final agreed answers. The interested student should consult the references given below.

REFERENCES

Fettiplace, R. and Hackney, C.M. (2006) The sensory and motor roles of auditory hair cells. *Nature Reviews Neuroscience*, **7**, 19–29.

Holton, T. and Hudspeth, A.J. (1983) A micromechanical contribution to cochlear tuning and tonotopic organisation. *Science*, **222**, 508–10.

Rosenblatt, K.P. *et al.* (1997) Distribution of Ca^{2+}-activated K^+-channels isoforms along the tonotopic gradient of the chicken's cochlea. *Neuron*, **19**, 1061–75.

LeMasurier, M. and Gillespie, P.G. (2005) Hair cell mechanotransduction and cochlear amplification. *Neuron*, **48**, 403–15.

frequency discrimination. To discriminate between different frequencies the brain has only to 'look' at where along the basilar membrane the maximum impulse frequency in the cochlear nerve originates.

In recent years Helmholtz's place theory has been extended and amplified by the finding that hair cells themselves are tuned to respond to some frequencies rather than others. This tuning is a function of the molecular anatomy and cytology of the cell. It is found that the hair cells and their stereocilia differ in size and flexibility in different parts of the basilar membrane. At the round window end they are small and comparatively stiff, at the helicotrema end they are large and flexible. This, combined with specific populations of ion channels, determines their electrical characteristics (Box 9.1). Each hair cell is tuned to react maximally to a particular stimulus frequency. Indeed, there is some evidence to suggest that this tuning is under feedback control in the cochlea. The basilar membrane and its hair cells are thus far more complex than the strings of a piano or the plates of a xylophone. Nevertheless, Helmholtz guessed the gist of it over a century ago. The intricate electromechanical tuning of hair cells, and their feedback modulation, is superimposed on the underlying mechanism of maximum disturbance at a particular part of the basilar membrane being related to frequency of incoming sound.

Many mammals are sensitive to far higher frequencies than the human ear can detect. By conditioning experiments involving vibrissae and/or pinnae it can be shown that many small mammals are sensitive to sound up to 100 kHz. The humanly audible squeaks of mice and shrews are mostly at the lower end of their frequency range. Much of the social communication between these mammals occurs beyond the range of the human ear. Dogs also have good high frequency hearing, their upper limit being in the region of 35 kHz. This feature has been made use of by manufacturers of ultrasonic dog whistles. The domestic cat, however, has a frequency range

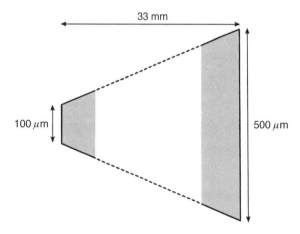

Figure 9.17 Schematic figure of basilar membrane. The membrane is uncoiled and straightened out. In humans it is about 33 mm long and ranges from about 100 μm at the round window end to about 500 μm at the helicotrema. Further explanation in text.

BOX 9.2 GENETICS AND DEAFNESS

Several hundred genes are now known to be involved in different forms of hearing loss (see reference to OMIM in bibliography, http://www.nslij-genetics.org/search_omim.html). Between 1/1000 and 1/2000 children are born with a profound hearing impairment. Inherited hearing disorders are conventionally divided into **syndromic** (associated with defects in the external ear or associated more generally with other organ systems) and **nonsyndromic** (no other visible abnormalities or medical problems).

Syndromic impairments include Waardenburg syndrome (WS), Branchio-otorenal syndrome, Stickler syndrome, Usher syndrome (of which there are three subtypes and several sub-sub-types), Pendred syndrome, Jervell and Lange-Nielsen syndrome (JLNS) and a number of others. All these conditions are due to autosomal mutations. Two X-linked syndromes are also known: Alport syndrome and Mohr-Tranebjaerg syndrome.

Nonsyndromic deafness is caused by mutations in a large number of genes, scattered throughout the genome. In addition, mutations in at least two **mitochondrial genes** lead to hearing loss and, as all mitochondria are inherited from the oocyte, these conditions are passed through the female line.

The very large number of gene mutations causing deafness indicates the extreme delicacy and complexity of the auditory apparatus. We noted in Section 9.3.2 that at least eight genes are associated (when defective) with one of the commonest forms of deafness – otosclerosis. Defects in many of the genes encoding components of the hair cells – cadherin 23, prestin and so on – also cause deafness. This multiplicity means that only a few of the better known conditions can be discussed in this Box. For fuller accounts the student should consult the references cited below. A good place to start is Smith and van Camp's, 2007 discussion.

Usher Syndromes. Usher syndromes are the most common forms of hereditary deaf–blindness. There is an incidence of 1/23 000.

The three clinical subtypes – USH1, USH2 and USH3 – all present varying degrees of hearing impairment and vestibular dysfunction coupled with progressive visual loss due to retinitis pigmentosa. USH2A is the most common of these subtypes.

It has been shown that USH2A is due to mutations in a gene located on chromosome 1 (1q41), *USH2A*, which encodes a 5213 amino acid protein called **usherin**. Usherin has four major domains. Several different transcripts of *USH2A* have been identified. Some of them are translated as transmembrane (TM) proteins. A TM transcript containing a 71 amino acid sequence has been located at the base of differentiating stereocilia, where it is involved in the filamentous linkages between bundles of actin microfilaments in adjacent stereocilia.

Mutations in *USHA2A* TM transcript accounts for the disorganized hair bundles characteristic of USH mouse models and, hence, could well be responsible for the hearing impairments of humans suffering Usher syndrome. This 'long' transcript is not found in the retina or other tissues. On the other hand, shorter transcripts, lacking the 71 amino acid domain, are present in abundance. These transcripts are located in basement membranes and it is concluded that the **retinal** symptom of Usher syndromes – retinitis pigmentosa – is due to mutations in these shorter transcripts.

We saw in Chapter 5 that homologues of *USHA* genes can be found in the sea urchin genome. We have just noted the extreme complexity of the molecular genetics of *USHA* in mammals. Not only are there several subtypes and sub-sub-types, all showing somewhat different symptoms, but as indicated above the gene responsible for even a single subtype is differentially expressed, by differential transcription, in different tissues. Presumably this 'downstream' complexity, as well as the multiplicity of genes (scattered through the human genome on chromosomes 1 q41, 11p15.1, 3q21-q25, 10q21-q22,

(Continues)

(*Continued*)

5q14, 3p24-23, 10q21-q22, 21q21, 17q2.3, 21q22.3), has evolved through the more than half billion years that have elapsed since the common ancestor of the echinoderms and chordates existed.

Connexin Deafness. About 20% of all hearing loss and 50–80% of all nonsyndromic loss is due to a mutation of agene located on chromosome 13 (13q11–q12) and known as *GBJ2*. This gene codes for a gap junction protein, Connexin 26 (Cx26). Although this gene is subject to many mutations the most common is a G → A transition at codon 70 (in the shorthand of molecular biology, G70A). This leads to a premature 'stop' codon and thus a truncated protein being synthesized. Cx26 is expressed in stria vascularis, basilar membrane, limbus and spiral prominence of the cochlea (Figure 9.13). It follows that gap junctions in these structures are defective. It is believed that this defect prevents the proper recycling of K^+ from synapses at the bases of the hair cells back into the K^+-rich endolymph via the stria vascularis. This disrupts the functioning of the organ of Corti which, in turn, causes deafness. It has been suggested that the unusually high prevalence of mutated *GBJ2* in the population is due to the attraction between, and then marriage of, similarly challenged men and women. Connexin 26 is not the only gap junction protein responsible for gap junction deafness. Mutations in other gap junction genes, *GJB1*(Cx32), *GJB3*(Cx31) and *GJB6*(Cx30) also lead to hearing impairment. Further detail may be found on the connexion deafness homepage (www.davinci.org.es/deafness).

Potassium Channel (KCNE1) Deafness. Jervell and Lange-Nielsen syndrome (JLNS1) is a congenital deafness associated with heart disease. It is due to mutations on the *KCNE1* gene located in chromosome 21 (21q22.1–q22.2). It can also result from mutations in the *KCNQ1* gene located in the same region of chromosome 21. It is very rare, having an incidence in England, Wales and Ireland of one child in 1.6–6 million. It is of interest in this section as mutations in the gene have somewhat the same outcome, though through a very different pathway, as the connexin defects of the previous section. The gene codes for a potassium channel (the MinK channel) that is expressed not only in cardiac tissue (hence the heart disease) but also in the stria vascularis of the cochlea. These channels are involved in the secretion of the K^+-rich endolymph which is essential for the function of the cochlear hair cells. Mutations in the *KCNE1* gene lead not only to defective cochlear hair cells but also, because of the reduced secretion of endolymph, collapse of Reissner's membrane and profound deafness.

Concluding Remarks. These three examples out of several hundred show the detailed complexity of the contemporary research into many causes of deafness. Will such work lead to improved therapy and perhaps cure? Time will tell. At the very least it will prevent clinicians prescribing the wrong remedies for seemingly similar hearing deficiencies.

REFERENCES

Adato, A. *et al.* (2005) Usherin, the defective protein in Usher syndrome type IIA, is likely to be a component of interstereocilia ankle links in the inner ear sensory cells. *Human Molecular Genetics*, **14**, 3921–32.

Connexin-deafness homepage at http://davinci.org.es/deafness/.

OMIM (Online Mendelian Inheritance in Man) at http://www.nslij-genetics.org/search_omim.html.

Smith, R.J.H. and van Camp, G. (2007) Deafness and hereditary hearing loss: overview. *GeneReviews*, http://www.genetests.org.

much the same as our own. Cetacea, on the other hand, emit and respond to sounds well up towards and including 100 kHz. They may use these sounds in social life and there is evidence that some species, for example Dolphins (*Delphinus*), also use them for echolocation. The intensity and continuity of their sound emissions increase as they approach obstacles or search for food.

9.3.3 Bat Sonar

The real aficionados of echolocation are, however, the bats. There are two suborders: the Microchiroptera and the Megachiroptera (flying foxes). There are some 680 species of microchiropteran bats. Most are insectivorous but a number of species are frugivorous and some have become carnivorous, feeding on frogs, lizards, fish, birds and small mammals. Three species, the vampires (family: Phyllostomatidae), feed entirely on blood. The most interesting, from the auditory point of view, are clearly the insectivorous species. They accomplish the extremely demanding task of catching and consuming insects on the wing. Some species hunt in the open sky above tree level, others have specialized in the more difficult but, if successful, more rewarding task of foraging the far richer population of insect life amongst the canopies of the trees. Still others find their prey in the yet more acoustically 'cluttered' terrestrial surface, amongst fallen leaves and twigs and so on. There is evidence that the echolocation systems of species hunting in different habitats have adapted to cope with the different problems presented.

In all cases they continuously emit sharp bursts of frequency-modulated sound. In *Myotis* the burst of sound, or 'click', commences at 80 or 90 kHz, modulating down to end a couple of milliseconds later at 30–35 kHz. These bursts of sound are emitted at the rate of some 30 per second whilst the bat is in flight and the rate rapidly increases when prey insect or an obstacle is approached. Other bats emit sounds at lower frequencies; indeed the bottom of the frequency range comes into the human auditory spectrum. We saw (Chapter 8) that moths and lace flies have evolved defence mechanisms to nullify bat echolocation systems. Bats have thus not only to adapt to hunting in different environments but also to counter insect defence techniques. We have still a great deal to learn about the measures and counter-measures which have emerged in this long predator–prey arms race. Further discussion of the bat echolocation system is given in Chapter 10.

Bat echolocation seems to have evolved independently in the two suborders of bat. Investigation of the megachiropteran fruit eating bats shows that, with the exception of one genus, *Rousettus,* none use echolocation. *Rousettus* emits 'clicks' at a much lower frequency than the microchiropteran bats

(modulating from 18–10 kHz) and the mechanism of emission is distinctively different. The Megachiroptera are far more visual animals than the largely crepuscular and nocturnal Microchiroptera and it has been suggested that they have evolved from a primate stem in contrast to the insectivore origins of the Microchiroptera.

It is with the Microchiroptera that the ear has reached its peak development. We shall see in Chapter 10 that large volumes of the brain are built around this sense, just as large volumes of the primate brain are built around the visual sense. The sensory world of the Microchiropterans is thus an auditory world. Indeed, the analogies between the visual system and the microchiropteran auditory system run deep. It can be shown, for instance, that a region of the bat basilar membrane plays an analogous rôle to that of the fovea in the mammalian retina (Chapter 17). Whether, as some have suggested, the qualia which the bat lives through as it navigates the world in the evening resembles the visual world of the peregrine falcon at midday, who can at present say. It must at present (and perhaps for ever) remain speculative just 'what it is like to be a bat'.

It is, however, pleasingly symmetric to end this chapter as we began it – with echolocation. The hair cell which we first met in the lateral line canals of the fish, remains remarkably unchanged but now housed in the extraordinarily intricate structure of the mammalian – in this case microchiropteran – inner ear. Instead of responding to the 'gentle touch of water', it now responds to the vastly gentler touch of the air.

9.4 CONCLUDING REMARKS

The vertebrate hair cell provides a prime example of how evolution, having once hit upon an effective mechanoreceptor, incorporates it into a vast variety of different structures, some of astonishing complexity. We shall meet with modified, immobile, cilia at the centre of other sense receptors as we proceed through this book: olfaction, vision. We have already noted that many insect neurosensory dendrite outersegments (though not, apparently, mechanoreceptors) are also modified, immobile cilia. This common design principle probably points towards some underlying feature in cell biology that we have, as yet, been unable to discern.

We have also seen, as we have made our way through this chapter, how the mechanosense, originally evolved to detect the abiotic environment, has, in its ultimate forms, become focused on fellow inhabitants of the living world. We saw the same progression in Chapter 8 where we considered not only insect acoustic systems, which allowed communication between conspecifics and detection of predator and/or prey, but also the sense of touch. This, too, we saw came to provide important channels of social communication. In the present chapter we have ended with bat attack sonar but we must not forget the hugely important role played by the auditory sense in communication between conspecific members of the birds and the mammals. We shall pick up this point with special reference to human auditory communication in the next chapter.

10

CEREBRAL ANALYSIS

Dual function of ear: equilibrium and phonoreception. **Vestibular pathway**: ipsilateral vestibular complex - co-ordination of movement and orientation - nystagmus - motion sickness - inebriation. **Auditory pathway**: cochlear fibres: characteristic frequencies - frequency threshold curve (FTC) - lateral inhibition; cochlear nucleus: principal subdivisions - stellate ('chopper') cells - bushy cells; superior olivary nucleus - EE and EI cells - direction of sound source; inferior colliculus; medial geniculus. **Mapping of auditory space in barn owls** - auditory pathways - interaural intensity and timing differences - spatial maps in inferior colliculus, and optic tectum. **Mammalian auditory cortex**: columnar histophysiology - trigger features - shifting patterns of excitation. **Bat auditory cortex**: sonic characteristics of chirps - comparison with human speech sounds - analysis in auditory cortex - single-cell recording - Q10dB tuning - detection of insect wing flutter - compensation for self-induced Doppler shifts - auditory fovea in cochlea - oto-acoustic emissions - texture detection (echo colours) - 'what is it like to be a bat?' **Human auditory cortex**: underpins human life-style - FM sounds - transitions - evolution - speech sounds (phonemes) - FM and CF components - VOT - categorical perception - recognition of speech sounds inborn - categorical perception in Japanese macaques - human linguistic environments shape inborn perceptions - co-articulation - challenges for computer scientists. **Linguistic cortices**: dominant hemisphere - planum temporale - Broca and Wernicke's areas - angular gyrus - arcuate fasciculus – the FoxP2 gene and neural basis of language. **Callosectomy**: lateralisation - left analytical, right holistic - hypothesis generator. **Concluding remarks**: unity in diversity; the distinctiveness of sensory qualia.

In Chapter 9 we followed the development of the ear in the vertebrates. We saw how it originated, in association with lateral line systems, mainly as an accelerometer. Anyone who has watched fish in an aquarium, or elsewhere, knows that they are active animals and may often have to orientate themselves without benefit of horizon or other visual clues. As evolution proceeded and a tetrapod land fauna emerged, this original function was retained and, in many forms, one thinks of the birds and the arboreal primates, became, if anything, yet more sophisticated. Added to this original function was, however, the increasingly important requirement to detect, in the aqueous or atmospheric medium, those gentle pressure waves that we subjectively experience as sound. In this chapter we follow inwards the

Biology of Sensory Systems, Second Edition   C.U.M. Smith
© 2008 John Wiley & Sons, Ltd

information picked up by ears and consider where it is sent and what is done with it. After brief accounts of the mammalian vestibular and auditory pathways, we shall turn to the mapping of auditory space in the brains of those highly evolved nocturnal predators, the owls. After outlining the mammalian auditory cortex we turn to a discussion of the cortices of those other extraordinary nocturnal predators, the insectivorous bats. Finally, we come to the human auditory system which, unlike that of the owls and bats, is not so much specialized for nocturnal navigation as for the human life style and its most characteristic feature, language.

10.1 THE MAMMALIAN VESTIBULAR PATHWAY AND REFLEXES

The anatomy of the vestibular pathway is highly intricate (Figure 10.1). Afferent fibres from the cristae of the semicircular canals and the maculae of the sacculus and utriculus run to Scarpa's (= vestibular) ganglion, close to the external auditory meatus, where they have their cell bodies. Then, after joining with cochlear fibres to form the vestibulocochlear nerve, they continue to the **ipsilateral vestibular complex** in the floor of the medulla, beneath the fourth ventricle. This complex consists of four significant nuclei: lateral (Deiter's), medial, superior and descending. There are also a number of minor nuclei and they are all interconnected by an intricate distribution of afferents and efferents.

The complex is also innervated by descending fibres from the cerebellum and reticular formation. In addition, each complex receives innervation from the contralateral complex. In some cases this contralateral innervation underlies a 'push–pull' mechanism. Cells driven by the cristae of one semicircular canal, for instance, also receive input from the cristae of the contralateral canal. As well as all this, the complex also receives input from the eyes and from proprioceptive fibres running up the spinal cord. The complex is thus an extremely important centre for the integration of information relating to movement and orientation. Figure 10.1 shows that, in addition to powerful interaction with the cerebellum and the oculomotor nuclei, the vestibular complex also sends fibres onwards to the cerebral cortex. These are believed to terminate in the postcentral gyrus close to the lower end of the interparietal sulcus. Epilepsies,

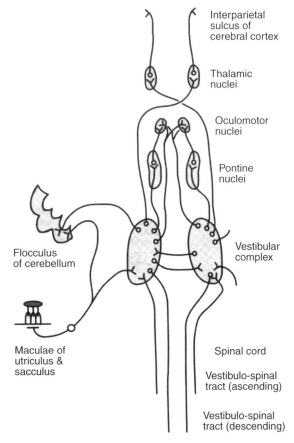

Figure 10.1 The major pathways of the vestibular system. For simplicity only ascending pathways in the brain stem and brain are shown. Further explanation in text.

which have their focus in this area, are usually preceded by an aura characterized by sensations of vertigo and disorientation.

The vestibular apparatus (as we saw in Chapter 9) detects both the stationary orientation of the head in space (otoliths) and its acceleration (cristae of the semicircular canals). It is supplemented by numerous somaesthetic receptors throughout the body (Chapter 7). To remove the rain of information from these sensors, it is necessary to suspend the body in water or confine it to an orbiting space craft. In these conditions the vestibular apparatus and the eyes are left to do the whole job. If, further, the subject is blindfolded, input from the membranous vestibule alone remains.

The role of input from the semicircular canals can be vividly demonstrated by sitting the subject in a rapidly rotating swivel chair. The eyes drift in the opposite direction to the rotation in an attempt to fix a stationary object and then (losing that object) jump rapidly in the direction of rotation to find another fixation point. Similarly, when the rotation is suddenly stopped the eyes move in the direction of the previous spin and then jerk rapidly in the opposite direction. This sudden change is due to the cristae of the semicircular canals suddenly being exposed to a wash of endolymph flowing in the opposite direction. These characteristic ocular movements are defined as **nystagmus**. They are caused by a three-neuron pathway from the semicircular canals to the vestibular nucleus, then to the oculomotor (or abducens) nuclei and, finally, to the extrinsic eye muscles (Figure 10.2).

The significance of this vestibulo-oculomotor reflex can be shown dramatically if vision when the ocular system is rotated is compared with vision when the head is kept still and the environment rotated around it. In the second case, detail of the spinning environment is very rapidly lost: at two rotations a second the target is merely a blur. In the first case, the subject sitting in a spinning chair suffers little loss of visual acuity below about 10 rotations a second.

Finally, it is worth saying a few words about **motion sickness**. This uncomfortable sensation is largely due to a mismatch of sensory input. In some cases this mismatch occurs in the vestibular apparatus itself. If the head is moved out of its normal orientation and rotated, the signals from the cristae are no longer correlated in the usual way with signals from the otoliths. Another source of motion sickness is a mismatch of cues from the eyes and the vestibular apparatus. Below decks in a rough sea, the eyes report no relative motion between the head and the rest of the cabin whilst the vestibuli are reporting violent

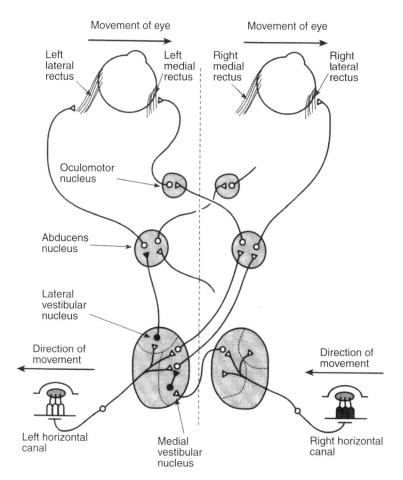

Figure 10.2 Some of the nerve pathways underlying the eye movements of nystagmus. Excitatory fibres white; inhibitory fibres black. When the head rotates to the left the hair cells in the ampulla of the left horizontal semicircular canal are stimulated. Impulses travel in the vestibular nerve to the vestibular nucleus. From there inhibitory fibres (black) transmit to the abducens nucleus. These synapse with excitatory fibres which terminate on the left lateral rectus (extrinsic eye muscle). This muscle is, consequently, inhibited. A second pathway, via the contralateral abducens and oculomotor nuclei excites the left medial muscle. The eye turns to the right. At the same time impulses from the right horizontal semicircular canal are inhibited (the hair cells are bent in the hyperpolarising direction). The inhibitory interneuron in the contralateral vestibular nucleus is switched off. Activity thus flows through the pathway from the left vestibular nucleus to the right abducens nucleus to the right rectus muscle. It consequently contracts and pulls the right eye to the right. The figure is necessarily simplified: only some of the many reciprocal connections are shown.

motion. The disabling symptoms of seasickness are induced. It is also worth noting that excessive intake of alcohol also leads to sometimes calamitous disorientations. This is due to ethanol altering the specific gravity of endolymph so that the cupulae of the semicircular canals no longer float, but feel the force of gravity and, consequently, cause the hair cells of the underlying cristae to send unusual signals along the vestibular nerves.

10.2 THE MAMMALIAN AUDITORY PATHWAY

We saw in Chapter 9 that about 90% of the afferent cochlear fibres originate at synapses with the inner hair cells. The cochlear fibres run through the spiral ganglion (Figure 10.2) where their cytons are located and then on to the cochlear nucleus. From there further fibres transmit the auditory information via nuclei in the brain stem, midbrain and thalamus to the auditory cortex in the temporal lobe of the brain (Figure 10.3).

As Figure 10.3 shows, the auditory 'pathway', unlike the somaesthetic and visual systems but like the vestibular pathway discussed above, passes through a large number of subcortical nuclei before it reaches the cerebral cortex. The number of such nuclei depends on whether one is inclined to 'lump' or 'split': some anatomists recognize only four, others up to fifty on each side of the system. These nuclei, moreover, should not be regarded as mere junction boxes on the way to the cortex. In many cases they integrate information directed at them from different sources

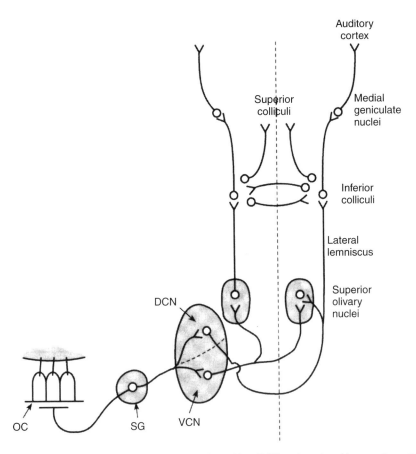

Figure 10.3   Auditory pathway. Major fibre pathways from the left cochlea. DCN = dorsal cochlear nucleus; OC = organ of Corti; SG = spiral ganglion; VCN = ventral cochlear nucleus. Further explanation in text.

and perform analyses and feature extractions. Indeed, it has long been known that the auditory cortex is not necessary to discriminate the physical dimensions of sound. This is done by the subcortical system. Instead, as we shall see in Section 10.4, the auditory cortex is concerned with very specific features of the auditory environment.

Let us examine the auditory pathway in a little more detail: first the cochlear fibres themselves, then the cochlear nucleus, the olivary nuclei, the inferior colliculus, the medial geniculate nucleus and, finally, the auditory cortex.

10.2.1 Cochlear Fibres

As with sensory fibres in most systems, there is a spontaneous background activity upon which is superimposed bursts of additional activity when the cochlea is stimulated. This evoked activity adapts over time. In Chapter 9 we discussed the 'place theory' of frequency discrimination and it follows that fibres originating from particular locations in the cochlear will be maximally sensitive to particular sound frequencies. The frequency to which the fibre is most sensitive is called the '**characteristic frequency**' (CF). Figure 10.4 shows that, as the intensity increases, the frequencies to which the fibre is responsive greatly increase. This again is to be expected from the physics of the basilar membrane. It will be remembered that a complex waveform travels along the membrane, peaking at the resonant frequency. The range of frequencies to which the fibre responds as the intensity increases is called its **frequency response area**. It can also be regarded as the fibre's receptive field. The boundary of this receptive field or frequency response area is called the frequency threshold curve (FTC) or, sometimes, **frequency tuning curve**.

The shape of the FTC shown in Figure 10.4 is characteristic of such curves. Its major feature is the sharp cut-off on the high frequency side. The sharpness of this cut-off is greater than the existing measurements of the waveform in the basilar membrane would suggest. In consequence it has been proposed that a 'second filter' mechanism exists in the cochlea. It may be that the active nature of the hair cells, especially the outer hair cells (Section 9.3.2; Box 9.1), is responsible for this sharpening of response.

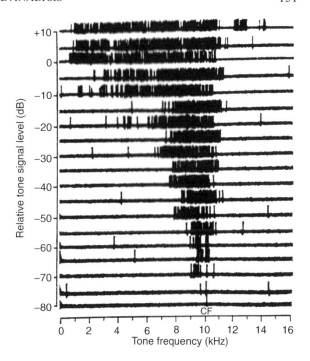

Figure 10.4 Frequency response area of a single cochlear fibre. A continous tone is swept through a range of frequencies at different dB levels. As the dB level is decreased the response becomes more and more focused until the frequency to which it is most sensitive is reached (CF = characteristic frequency). In this case it is 10 kHz. The boundary of the frequency response area is known as the frequency threshold curve (FTC). From Evans, E. F. (1972), *Journal of Physiology*, **226**, 263–87, with permission from Wiley-Blackwell.

Another feature of cochlear fibres that we meet in other sensory systems is a species of lateral inhibition. It can be shown that the response of a cochlear fibre to a tone of a given frequency can be inhibited by tones falling closely to one side or other along the frequency spectrum. We shall see, too, that lateral inhibition plays a role at 'higher' levels in the auditory system. It is also, as we shall see in Parts III and IV, of fundamental importance in other sensory systems.

It will be remembered from Chapter 9 that at low frequencies (below about 5 kHz) discrimination was accomplished by 'locking' the frequency of the incoming sound to the frequency of impulses in one or a group of cochlear nerve fibres. This proposition was called 'volley theory'. Electrophysiological recording from single cochlear fibres has provided support for this theory. Figure 10.5a shows a

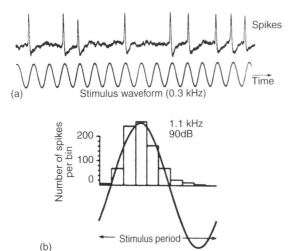

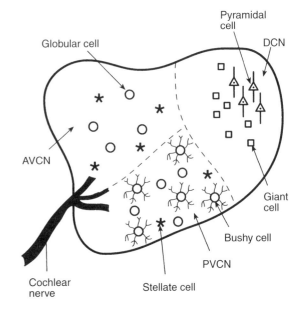

Figure 10.5 Phase locking of response in a single cochlear fibre to a 300 Hz tone. (a): It can be seen that the spike responses are aligned with the phase of the input signal. From Evans, E.F. (1972), *Journal of Physiology*, **226**, 263–87, with permission from Wiley-Blackwell. (b): Phase locking can be made more obvious if a histogram is constructed showing the number of spikes falling within a particular segment of the oscillating waveform. From Evans, 1982, Functional anatomy of the visual system, in *The Senses* (eds H.B. Barlow and J.D. Mollon). Copyright © 1982 Cambridge University Press.

Figure 10.6 Anatomy of cochlear nucleus. AVCN = anterior ventral cochlear nucleus; DCN = dorsal cochlear nucleus; PVCN = posterior ventral cochlear nucleus. Further explanation in text.

single coclear fibre firing in phase with a half-cycle of the sound frequency. This 'locking' can be visualized more vividly if a period histogram (Figure 10.5b) is constructed.

Finally, it is worth noting the response of cochlear fibres to 'clicks'. Here the stimulus is brief but covers a wide band of frequencies. In consequence, discharge is widespread and, if the intensity of the stimulus is sufficient, practically all the cochlear fibres will carry impulses.

10.2.2 Cochlear Nucleus

Figure 10.6 shows that the cochlear nucleus is divided into dorsal and ventral nuclei. The cochlear nerve fibres enter at the middle of the ventral nucleus, thus dividing it into an anteroventral and posteroventral nuclei. The nucleus thus has three principal subdivisions: **dorsal**, **anteroventral** and **posteroventral** nuclei. Cochlear fibres enter at the junction between the anteroventral and posteroventral nuclei and immediately branch to innervate all three nuclei.

The relationships of the cochlear fibres are carefully preserved in each of the three subdivisions of the cochlear nucleus. There is, in consequence, a map of the basilar membrane in each of the subdivisions. This map is said to have a tonotopic or cochleotopic (it amounts to the same thing) organization.

Microscopic examination of the cochlear nucleus reveals a number of distinct cell types: globular cells, pyramidal cells, giant cells, bushy cells, multipolar (=stellate) cells and so on. Microelectrode recording from these cells show that they have distinctively different responses to input from the cochlear nerve fibres. Most of the small globular cells respond rather similarly to the cochlear nerve fibres. The **stellate cells**, on the other hand, respond to steady input by a regular series of impulses. In consequence they are known as '**chopper cells**'. The frequency of the response varies from one chopper cell to another. It is likely, therefore, that these cells signal the different frequency components of a sound up to about 800 Hz. In contrast the **bushy cells**, whose dendritic arborizations spread widely across the posteroventral nucleus, respond only to the onset of a signal. This response, as we shall see, is probably important in **sound localization**. In the dorsal nucleus cells more complex responses are to be found. There is good evidence of lateral inhibition. A single tone can sometimes reduce or totally eliminate activity in a cell. It is likely that this mechanism sharpens discrimination between two similar tones and it may also increase sensitivity to frequency modulation in one direction rather than another. There are, as we shall see, strong analogies to these forms of information processing in the retina.

10.2.3 Superior Olivary Nuclei

This group of nuclei are to found in the ventral pons varolii. They are the first nuclei to receive input from both ears. They are of importance in correlating the input from the two ears and thus in locating the source of a sound. Three physiological types of cell are found; two are responsive to frequencies above 1 kHz and one responsive below 1 kHz. Let us consider them in order. The first type is known as *E–E cells*. They respond to similar variations in sound intensity at both ears. The second type, known as *E–I* cells, responds to differences in intensity at the two ears. These cells, in responding to head or pinna 'shadowing,' are clearly of significance in determining the source of a sound. The third type of cell, responsive to sound frequencies below 1 kHz, detects time delay between signals from the two ears. Some of the latter cells, the so-called '**critical delay**' cells fire only at a very specific interaural delay, perhaps 150 or 200 ms. Together, this array of cells is able to extract the horizontal direction of a sound source.

This ability to recognize the spatial location of a sound source is of great importance to all animals: it enables them to detect predators, prey and suitable conspecifics for mating and so on. Many mammals have large and highly mobile pinnae to their external ears that assist this direction finding. In addition, sound sources can be located, though far less effectively, monoaurally, using a single ear. This is accomplished by the ear's sensitivity to the way in which the frequency spectrum is altered by reflections from the torso, face and the various ridges and depressions of the pinna. Sound coming from different directions is reflected differently by these contours and a single ear is sensitive to these differences in spectral composition or auditory 'colour' and can thus determine the

direction of the source, especially whether it is above or below, in front or behind the head. But the most highly developed auditory direction finding system is not developed in the mammals at all. We shall see in the next section that those nocturnal hunters, the owls, have honed the ability to detect the sources of the tiny rustles and scurryings of their prey to an almost incredible degree of accuracy.

10.2.4 Inferior Colliculus

This region of the mid-brain evolves from the tectum of the lower vertebrates. In the anamniotes it is the final destination of the auditory fibres and hence of great importance. Its significance is much reduced in the mammals, where the final analysis of auditory information has shifted to the cerebral cortex. Nevertheless, it still forms a way-station in the mammalian auditory pathway and a cochleotopic map is present. Many of the cells show strong binaural drive. In addition, some cells do not respond to steady tones and only respond to frequency or amplitude modulated tones. This, as we shall see in Section 10.5, is particularly well shown in the Chiroptera.

10.2.5 Medial Geniculate Nucleus

This is the final junction before the auditory cortex is reached. It is innervated from the ipsilateral inferior colliculus and sends its output to the ipsilateral superior temporal gyrus, the primary auditory cortex. We shall return to the auditory cortex in Section 10.4. At this point we digress from our consideration of mammalian auditory systems to consider the somewhat different (though not radically different) system in the barn owl. As noted above, this system is of great interest as it contains perhaps the most highly evolved of all animal systems for detecting the source of minute sounds.

10.3 THE AVIAN AUDITORY PATHWAY AND THE MAPPING OF AUDITORY SPACE BY THE BARN OWL

The ability to detect the source of sound is of great importance to owls. They listen for the small noises made by their nocturnal prey. The barn owl (*Tyto alba*), like other owls, has many specializations for night-time hunting. Its wing feathers (as the ancients knew) have evolved to ensure silent flight, its eyes are proverbially large, ultrasensitive in low illuminations and positioned to provide excellent stereoscopic vision and last, but far from least, hearing is acute and acutely sensitive to location of a sound source. This can be demonstrated most easily by making use of the owl's habit of turning its head toward the source of an unexpected sound. The fitting of minute earphones, inactivation of one ear or the other by anaesthetics, and several other experimental techniques confirm the significance of the auditory system in this reflex orientation towards a sound source.

A bird's auditory pathway is, unsurprisingly, somewhat different from that of a mammal (Figure 10.7). To begin with, as we noted in Section 9.3.2, the tympanic membrane is exposed to sound pressure waves impinging on both sides. The signal transmitted across the middle ear chamber to the cochlea is thus more complex than in the mammalian ear. From the cochlea the cochlear nerve fibres run inwards to

the midbrain and each bifurcates, one branch running to the angular nucleus, the other to the magnocellular nucleus. From the angular nucleus a pathway leads up to the posterior lateral lemniscal nucleus on the contralateral side and from there to the auditory area in the inferior colliculus. This area consists of a core and a surrounding shell. Figure 10.7 shows that the projection from the posterior lateral lemniscal nucleus terminates in the shell. From the magnocellular nucleus, pathways project to the laminar nuclei on both the ipsilateral and contralateral sides. Following the circuitry upwards we can see that, after sending a branch to the anterior lateral lemniscal nucleus, the laminar nucleus projects to the core of the auditory area in the contralateral inferior colliculus. From the core a further pathway leads to the shell and from there the information is carried further to the external nucleus of the inferior colliculus and, ultimately, to the optic tectum and the archistriatal gaze fields of the forebrain.

The direction of sound is determined (as in mammals) by a combination of frequency specific

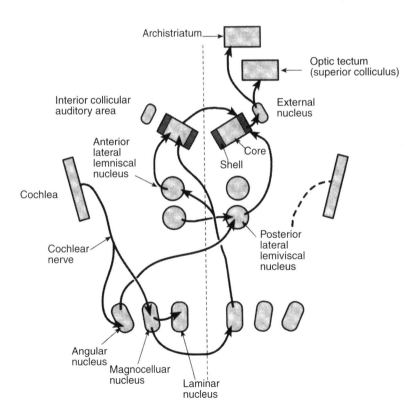

Figure 10.7 Auditory pathways in barn owl (simplified). For clarity the pathways from only one ear are shown. Explanation in text. After Konishi, M. (1993) and Cohen, Y.E. & Knudsen, E.I. (1999).

interaural intensity differences (IIDs) and frequency specific interaural timing differences (ITDs). To begin with, the owl's ears are slightly asymmetrical. The left ear is higher on the head, but points downward, whereas the right ear, situated lower on the head, points upward. The left ear is thus more sensitive to sounds coming from below the head and the right ear more sensitive to those coming from above. It can be shown that the owl is able to locate sound sources in the vertical dimension by comparing the intensity signal sent from each ear. If, for instance, the sound intensity at a given frequency (above about 3 kHz) delivered through earphones is greater in the left than the right ear, the owl bends its head downwards and vice versa. Interaural timing differences at a specific frequency (ITDs), however, cause the owl's head to swivel in the horizontal plane. In this case keeping the frequency and intensity constant but delaying the onset by 42 ms between left and right ears causes the owl to turn its head through 20°. Thus, by a combination of IIDs and ITDs, the barn owl is able to determine the direction from which a sound is coming in three-dimensional space.

The separation of ITDs and IIDs occurs early in the auditory pathway. Figure 10.7 shows that cochlear fibres deliver their signals to both the magnocellular and angular nuclei. It turns out that neurons sensitive to ITDs are concentrated in the magnocellular nucleus whilst those sensitive to IIDs are clustered in the angular nucleus. The cochlear fibres running to the magnocellular nucleus are locked to the phase of the incoming sound up to a frequency of about 10 kHz (Figure 10.8). They are insensitive to the intensity of the sound. The fibres running to the angular nucleus, on the other hand, are not phase locked but do respond to differences in sound intensity.

As Figure 10.7 shows, the magnocellular nucleus projects to the laminar nucleus. Here information from both ears is collated. Many of the cells of the laminar nucleus resemble the 'critical delay' cells of the mammal's superior olivary nucleus. The cells are coincidence detectors. They are activated only when signals from the two ears are delivered at approximately the same time. The owl's system is extraordinarily precise. The coincidence detectors can detect time differences as small as 10 ms. Given reliably constant transmission rates along the cochlear fibres and interneurons, coincidence detectors enable cells

in the laminar nuclei to determine time differences in the sound impinging on the two ears and thus the direction from which the sound comes (Figure 10.8).

Intensity differences at the two ears are compared in the posterior lateral lemniscal (PLL) nuclei (Figure 10.7). The processing depends on excitatory

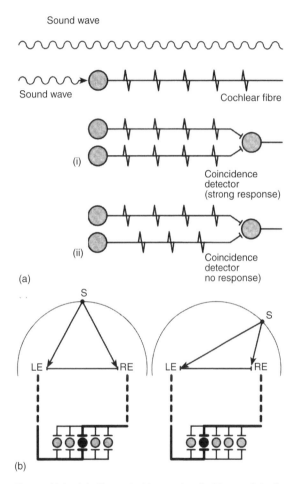

Figure 10.8 (a) Phase locking and coincidence detection. The cochlear fibre fires in response to every second peak in the sound wave. (i) If cochlear fibres from opposite ears converge on a coincidence detector the latter will fire if the two signals are delivered within a few tens of microseconds of each other; (ii) if the time differential is greater the detector will respond only weakly or not at all. (b) The principle of source location by way of interaural time differences (ITDs). A sound source (S) equidistant from the two ears will stimulate a certain coincidence detector (dark circle); a sound source further form one ear than the other will stimulate a different coincidence detector. LE = left ear; RE = right ear. Further explanation in text. Adapted from Konishi, M. (1993).

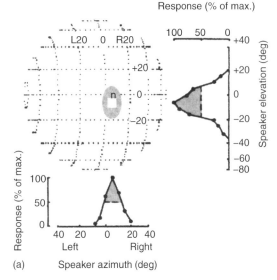

(a)

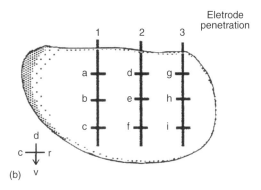

(b)

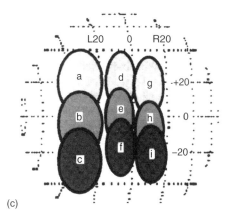

(c)

input arriving from the contralateral angular nucleus and inhibitory input arriving indirectly from the ipsilateral angular nucleus. In essence, the PLL cells compare the level of inhibition and excitation they receive at a given frequency and fire or not, as the case may be. In this way the intensity of the sound at the two ears is compared.

The signal from the coincidence detectors in the laminar nuclei is (as we noted above) projected upwards to the core of the inferior collicular auditory area. The intensity signal from the PLL nuclei is, in contrast, projected to the shell region of the same area. Both pathways finally combine in the external nucleus: it is here the information about IIDs and ITDs come together for the first time. Beyond the external nucleus of the inferior colliculus the auditory pathway branches once again. One branch runs to the optic tectum (corresponding to the mammalian superior colliculus) and the other branch runs on upwards to the forebrain and ultimately to the so-called 'gaze fields' in the archistriatum. These fields (corresponding to the mammal's frontal eye fields) project to motor nuclei which control the movement of head and eyes and the direction of gaze.

The cells responding to particular locations in auditory space are distributed regularly in both the external nucleus of the inferior colliculus and the optic tectum. In other words, these parts of the owl's midbrain contain maps of auditory space. The precision of the auditory maps in the barn owl far exceeds that found in mammals. The spatial tuning of cells in the owl's optic tectum turns out to be on the order of 40 ms (ITD) and 15 dB (IID) and these cells, as Figure 10.9 indicates, are positioned in such a way as to form a spatial map. It is believed that activity in this map is compared with activity in deeper layers of the tectum which represent gaze direction. The error signal between the two superimposed maps is

Figure 10.9 (*Opposite*) Map of auditory space in barn owl optic tectum. (a): Auditory spatial tuning of a neuron in the optic tectum. The response to noise bursts presented at various locations in the horizontal plain (azimuth) and in the vertical plane (elevation) are plotted below and to the right. The shaded area indicates the 'best area' for the neuron. (b): Schematic diagram of three electrode penetrations through the left optic tectum showing recording sites. (c): Auditory best areas recorded at the sites indicated in (b) projected on to spatial coordinates. From *Trends in Neurosciences, Vol. 22*, Cohen and Knudsen, p. 132, © 1999, with permission from Elsevier Science.

used to direct the gaze to the sound source. Further up the auditory system, in the archistriatal gaze fields, this spatial isomorphism is lost. Groups of cells representing similar positions in space are still grouped together to form clusters. There is, however, no topographic organization of the clusters. Cells in one cluster, tuned to a particular region of auditory space, abut cells in another cluster which are tuned to another, but unrelated, region of space. It is likely that this nonisomorphic organization of spatially tuned cells has to do with the fact that the forebrain is concerned with numerous more complex tasks: identification of sound source, selection of one auditory stimulus from a number of possible candidates for attention, recall of similar sound sources in the past and so on.

10.4 THE MAMMALIAN AUDITORY CORTEX

Let us return from our consideration of the mapping of auditory space in the alien brain of the barn owl to brains in our own branch of the evolutionary bush. In the primates, the auditory cortex is located in the inner surface of the superior temporal gyrus (Figure 10.10). In other mammals, for example the cat, it is spread over a large area of the lateral surface of the temporal lobe. It is divided into a core area (the primary auditory cortex, A1) surrounded by a belt of secondary and tertiary cortex. A1 receives input from the medial geniculate nucleus, whilst the surrounding belt areas receive input from other thalamic nuclei as well as from the medial geniculate. In consequence, they may be regarded as association and polysensory areas. Nevertheless, all of these areas contain a complete map of the cochlea, although the magnitude and orientation of the maps vary in the different areas.

The histological structure of the auditory cortex shows strong similarity to other sensory areas. There is, as customary, a six-layered stratification. Input fibres terminate in layer IV. Layer V projects back to the medial geniculate nucleus, layer VI to the inferior colliculus. Orthogonal to this six-layered stratification there is, as in other parts of the neocortex, a columnar structure. In some areas columns of cells show distinctive responses to binaural drive. These are areas where there is strong input from

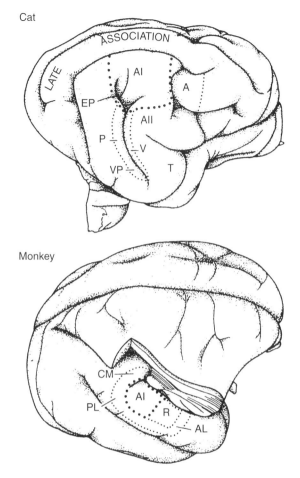

Figure 10.10 Locations and approximate boundaries of auditory cortices in the cat and monkey. Anterior to the right, posterior to the left. The cat's auditory cortex is located on the surface of the brain. AI = primary auditory cortex; AII = secondary auditory cortex. A = anterior; V = ventral; VP = ventroposterior; P = posterior; T = temporal fields. The monkey's (owl monkey) auditory cortex is shown on the upper surface of the temporal lobe. The parietal cortex has been dissected away so that it can be seen. AI = primary auditory cortex; AL = anterolateral cortical, CM = caudomedial cortical, PL = posterolateral cortical, R = rostral cortical fields. From Brugge, J.F. and Reale, R.A. (1985) Auditory cortex, in *Cerebral Cortex* (eds A. Peters and E.G. Jones), with kind permission of Kluwer Academic Publishers.

callosal fibres so that the cells are innervated from both ears. **Summation columns** contain cells whose responses summate simultaneous input from both ears. In contrast, **suppression columns** contain cells which respond most strongly to input from one ear.

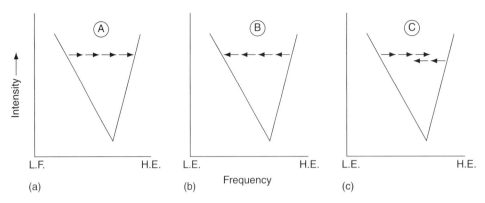

Figure 10.11 Responses of neurons in the auditory cortex of the cat to frequency modulated tones. The arrows in the figure indicate in which direction the frequency needs to change in order to trigger a response from the cell. In (a) the response was only obtained when the frequency was increasing throughout the range, whilst in (b) the response was only obtained when the frequency was decreasing. In (c) a response occurred when the frequency was increasing in the lower part of the range and decreasing in the upper part of the range.

If both ears are stimulated the response of the cells is diminished.

In addition to these binaural columns (comparable to the binocular columns of the primary visual cortex (Chapter 18)) the primary auditory cortex contains cells which respond to a number of special features of the auditory input. Instead of responding to pure tones or wide-band clicks and so on, as do neurons lower in the auditory pathways, many cortical cells are 'triggered' only by frequency modulated tones, either up or down, or in some cases both up and down (Figure 10.11). This specialization (again comparable to the visual cortex) has been carried further in mammals, where social vocalizations are important. It has, for example, been shown that the primary auditory cortex of macaques and squirrel monkeys contains cells triggered only by conspecific calls, indeed, in some cases, by the calls of specific individuals.

Thus we can see, as we reach the auditory cortex, that a close analysis of the auditory input is taking place. Specific cells in the cortex respond to 'on' and 'off', to 'clicks', to frequency modulations (up, down, up and down, rate of change), to location of the stimulus in space, to movement of the stimulus, to conspecific vocalizations and so on. The auditory cortex is, to borrow a Sherringtonian image, a moving pattern of excitation. It maps in a dynamic and as yet hardly understood fashion the auditory environment in which the mammal lives. Although the neurophysiologist is getting to know the units, he

has still hardly begun to understand how the whole shifting pattern is integrated, emphasized here, de-emphasized there, to form the unitary sound world which the animal experiences.

In the next section we shall consider how this supple system has been developed by the Microchiroptera to provide an astonishingly sensitive echolocation system: a system which takes the auditory system towards its physical limits. Then, in Sections 10.6 and 10.7, we shall see how the system has been developed in another way by the hominids to generate the all-important speech recognition cortices. It is not difficult to argue that the whole human phenomenon depends on the development of this cortex.

10.5 THE BAT AUDITORY SYSTEM AND ECHOLOCATION

Bats, like owls, are noctural hunters. Unlike owls they do not depend on sound emissions from prey animals. They take a much more active position. We saw in Chapter 8 that the insectivorous microchiroptera emit short bursts of high frequency sound. The sonic characteristics of these chirps vary in different species and there is evidence that the differences are related to different feeding strategies. Bats foraging in open skies and/or around the foliage of trees commonly emit chirps consisting of a constant frequency tone (CF) followed, when approaching a prey insect, by chirps of a rapidly descending frequency modulated tone (FM). In different species, the CF tone may be pitched at anything between 150 kHz to 30 kHz and may last only a few milliseconds or up to 60 ms. The FM tone is usually of very short duration, one or two milliseconds, and descends from over 100 kHz to below 30 kHz. This is of some interest for, as we shall see in the next section, human speech sounds also make use of CF and FM components, albeit at a much lower frequency. The bats, of course, use these sounds for echolocation. It is the reflections from obstacles or prey which interest the chiropteran auditory system.

Whereas the CF component is used for scanning the environment over a radius of up to 50m for likely prey insects, it is also valuable in detecting (by way of Doppler shifts) the movement of prey towards or away from the hunter. The FM component is used by most, if not all, bats to measure range as the creature moves in for the kill. The large number of frequencies in the FM sweep provides precise information about target movement, distance and other details. The echo-ranging is very precise. Behavioural experiments have shown that bats can pinpoint the source of an echo to within 0.3 cm at a distance of 30 cm. The neuronal mechanisms involved are located in the inferior colliculi and auditory cortices. Many neurons in these areas respond to pairs of stimuli separated by specific intervals and respond hardly at all to single stimuli. Two major classes are known. In one class the latency of response to a high intensity tone is longer than that to a weaker tone of the same frequency. As in the case of the owl's direction finding system, it is believed that the relevant cells make synaptic connection with a 'coincidence detector' neuron and the latter fires only when a very definite interval between emission and echo (i.e. target distance) occurs (Figure 10.12c). A second class of neurons is simply tuned to respond maximally to a definite interval between sound emission and echo return. Here we see, once again developed to an astonishing level of sophistication, the short-term memory characteristics which we have met elsewhere in the auditory system, especially in the mechanisms designed to detect sound source by comparison of time of arrival of binaural signals.

Microelectrode recording showed that over 50% of the cells in the auditory cortex of the little brown bat, *Myotis lucifugus,* responded best to pairs of FM pulses similar to those emitted by that species. The best responses were obtained to an intense first pulse followed by a fainter second pulse. Similar cells are found in the cortex of the American moustached bat, *Pteronotus parnelli*. In this species the biosonar pulses consist of an approximately 15 ms CF component followed by a brief FM component. Each pulse consists of four major harmonics which are conventionally labelled CF_{1-4} and FM_{1-4} (Figure 10.12a). Microelectrode investigation of cerebral cortex of *Pteronotus* shows that it has a complex organization well adapted to analysing these biosonar tones.

Figure 10.12b shows the large extent of the moustached bat's auditory cortex. It consists of a mosaic of subareas. Functional detail of these areas is shown in Figure 10.12d. The primary auditory cortex (A1) consists of a longitudinal strip of cortex where there is a systematic frequency map. At the posterior of the strip ((b) or A1b) the cells respond to comparatively low frequency tones (10–20 kHz) and at the anterior ((a) or A1a) they respond to high frequency tones, 100 kHz and above. Towards the anterior end of this strip is an area, (c), known as the Doppler shifted CF (DSCF) area, where cells are tuned to detect variations in the frequency of the second harmonic (CF_2) of the echo signal. This indicates the velocity of movement between target and bat. Just above A1a is a region (d) (CF/CF) where coincidence detector cells are tuned to respond to a CF tone and the second or third harmonic (CF_2, CF_3) of its echo. This area is also particularly sensitive to changes in the frequency of the echo signal caused by Doppler shifts. A similar organization is also found in a small area (e) known as the dorsal intrafossa (DIF) area. Above the CF/CF area are two cortical areas (f) and (g) where cells are triggered by FM tones. These cells, again, are coincidence detectors. Their maximal responses are elicited by the FM tone and the second, third or fourth harmonics (FM_2, FM_3, FM_4) of its echo. The timing between emission and echo is crucial. In (f), the FM–FM area, the delay ranges between 0.4 and 18 ms giving a range of 7–310 cm., whilst in (g), the dorsal fringe (DF) area, the optimal delay between tone and echo ranges between 0.8 and 9 ms, giving a range of 14–156 cm. Figure 10.12b shows that there are a number of other small areas in the bat's cortex which also have specialized functions in echolocation. Additionally, area (h), the ventral fringe (VF)

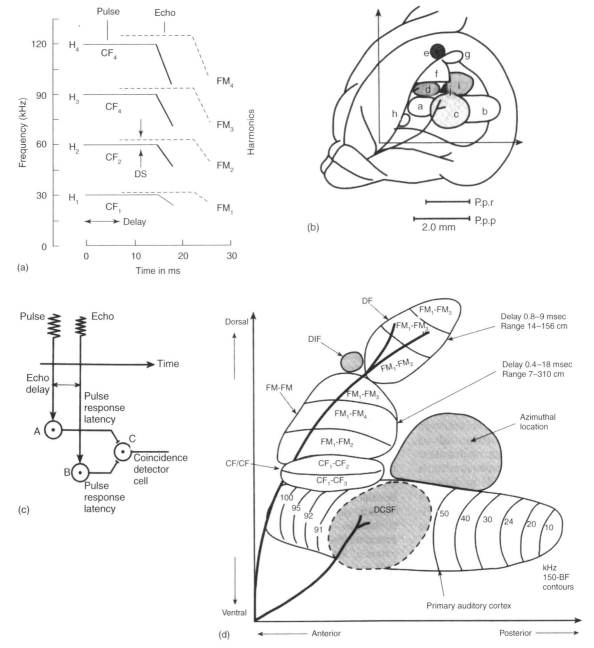

Figure 10.12 (a) Spectrogram of *Pteronotus* biosonar signal. The four harmonics ($H_{1,2,3,4}$) of the pulse are shown. The major harmonic, H_2, is emphasized. The Doppler-shifted echo is represented by the broken line. The echo delay is about 8 ms and the Doppler shift (DS) varied according to the frequency of the harmonic. From Suga, Yan and Zhang, 1997: with permission. (b) Dorsolateral aspect of *Pteronotus* auditory cortices. a = A1a; b = A1b; c = DSCF; d = CF/CF; e = DIF; f = FM-FM; g = DF; h = VF; i = DM. Scale bars are for P.p.r = Panamanian bat (*Petronotus parenelii rubiginosus*) and P.p.p (*Petronotus parnelii parnelii*). Adapted from Suga, 1995. (c) Coincidence detection hypothesis. The pulse triggers response in cell A with a long response latency. The echo triggers response in cell B with a shorter response latency. If impulses from A and B reach coincidence detector cell, C, at the same time they will summate and fire the cell. After Neuweiler, 1990. (d) Functional organization of *Pteronotus* auditory cortex. Expanded and schematized view of (b). The dark lines represent blood vessels. The major blood vessel runs on the Sylvian fossa. CF = continuous frequency tone; DCSF = Doppler shifted continuous frequency. DF = dorsal fringe; DIF = dorsal intrafossa; FM = frequency modulated tone. The primary auditory cortex (A1) is crossed by iso-best frequency (iso-BF) contours in kHz. Further explanation in text. Simplified from Suga, N., Yan, J. and Zhang, Y. (1997).

area, contains FM–FM cells and area (i) is believed to be concerned with azimuthal location.

The cells responding to the CF component in bat biosonar are usually extremely sharply tuned. A measure of tuning is to take the major harmonic (about 62 kHz in *Pteronotus*) and divide it by the width of the FTC 10 dB above threshold. This is known as $Q_{10\,dB}$. The larger the $Q_{10\,dB}$ value the sharper the tuning. It is found that auditory cells at the CF echo frequency have $Q_{10\,dB}$s of up to 600 compared with those outside the echo frequency range where the $Q_{10\,dB}$s may be only 20 to 30. It has been shown that these sharply tuned cells are particularly responsive to small changes in the CF echo frequency. These changes may be as small as 20 Hz, that is about 0.03% of the CF. This great sensitivity has an important biological significance. It is believed to provide the bat with information about fluttering insects. The movement of an insect's wings will cause amplitude modulations and Doppler shifts in the echo response (sometimes known as 'glints') sufficiently large to be detected by the bat's precisely tuned neurons. In *Pteronotus* these flutter detector cells are located in the DSCF area (Figure 10.12c). Indeed, moustached bats appear to be 'blind' to any insect which does not move its wings, even if it is only a few centimeters away. It is interesting to note that many moths have adopted the appropriate countermeasure of 'freezing' when they detect the chirp of an echolocating bat. It is also interesting to note the similarity with visual systems. As we shall see in Chapter 18 these, too, respond best to movement. Prey animals have once again learnt to 'freeze'.

Such extreme sensitivity to frequency has a drawback. The cells will be sensitive to Doppler effects not only from insect movements but also from the bat's own movements. When the bat moves towards its target the CF echo frequency rises. Horseshoe (*Rhinolophus*) and moustached bats compensate for this self-induced Doppler shift by automatically lowering the frequency of the emitted tone. It turns out that in each successive CF chirp the frequency is lowered by the amount by which the previous echo exceeded a set frequency. The return echo frequency is kept within 50 Hz of the characteristic or 'best' frequency.

All of this very precise echolocation demands an extraordinarily sensitive ear. It has been found that 50% of the length of the moustached bat's cochlear

is tuned to between CF + 9 kHz to CF −6 kHz and a similar great over-representation of the CF is found in the cochlea of the horseshoe bat (*Rhinolophus rouxi*). For obvious reasons this length of basilar membrane is called the **auditory fovea**. It seems that the extremely sharp tuning of CF cells in the auditory system is mainly due to the large expanse of basilar membrane devoted to that frequency. In other words, the accuracy of discrimination is related to the extent of the cerebral map devoted to tones at or near the CF (an analogy can be drawn with both the map of the retina in the primary visual cortex (Chapter 18) and the map of the body surface in the somaesthetic cortex (Chapter 8, especially Figure 8.20)). It is also believed that resonance of the basilar membrane in response to CF tones helps to sharpen the discrimination. This belief is strengthened by the observation that a strong '**otoacoustic**' emission comes from the ear in response to CF tones. In other words, when a loud tone just above the frequency of the CF tone is directed at the ear of *Pteronotus*, a loud response due to a strong resonance of the basilar membrane occurs. Otoacoustic emissions, albeit far weaker, have also been detected from other mammalian and, indeed, human ears. These echoic otoacoustic emissions should be distinguished from the spontaneous emissions (due to mechanical movements of the outer hair cells) which are discussed in Box 9.1.

Finally, as a yet further sophistication of the sonar system, both horseshoe and moustached bats (as well as some others) are able to detect the texture of the objects in their auditory environment. Sound waves will interfere with each other when they are reflected from the 'elevations' and 'declivities' of a rough surface. For instance, sound waves (like other waves) will destructively interfere if they differ by $\lambda/2$ (where λ the wavelength) and constructively interfere if they differ by λ. Hence if the elevations and declivities of a rough surface differ by $\lambda/4$, the echo beam from the declivity will travel $\lambda/4 + \lambda/4 = \lambda/2$ further than the beam reflected from the elevation. Hence we have the condition for destructive interference. If the frequency is high, say 155 kHz, as in *Hipposideros bicolour* and assuming velocity of sound in air as 344 m/s, then $\lambda/4$ is about 0.5 mm. Lower frequencies, of course, have longer wavelengths and hence will not allow the bat to detect such small variations in surface texture. Behavioural experiments have confirmed that many bats can indeed discriminate between different textured surfaces by this type of auditory analysis.

There is an analogy with colour vision. Just as white light is broken up into colours in the reflected beam by the surface properties of an object, so a broad band CF or downwardly directed FM echolocation emission from a bat is reflected back as a complicated wave front, full of destructive and constructive interferences. These are said to be **echo colours**. The ability to detect and analyse echo colours provides invaluable information about the environment. Any movement on the ground or amongst a litter of leaves and twigs, will change the echo colour of the returning signal. Experiment has confirmed that tiny movements of insects on the ground or in the foliage of trees cause detectable change in the echo colour. The echo colour of the returning acoustic wavefront also provides information concerning the nature of a rock face, whether for instance it is suitable for landing and roosting.

In a very influential paper the philosopher Thomas Nagel asked 'What is it like to be a bat?'. The preceding paragraphs have given some idea of the sophisticated information processing occurring within its auditory system. As Nagel says, their brains are evolved to 'make precise discriminations of distance, size, shape, motion and texture comparable to those we make by vision'. The neurophysiologist is beginning to be able to draw up schemes which catch the ongoing dynamics of the auditory system as the bat flits through the evening sky after its insect prey, avoiding the acoustic clutter of trees and bushes, detecting small movements of insect wings, homing in on a counter-manoeuvring moth. But, as Nagel insists, what it is like to be that bat, what experiences – qualia – it lives through remains conjectural. Many would say it can never be anything other than conjectural. This is the mind–body problem, a problem which we skirt in this book, touch on in Chapter 24, but mainly leave to philosophers for in-depth analysis.

10.6 THE HUMAN AUDITORY CORTEX AND LANGUAGE

Just as the barn owl's auditory system and the bat's auditory cortex have been developed to an astonishing level to serve their ways of life, so the hominid auditory cortex has been developed to a similar level of sophistication to underpin the human lifestyle. As was the case in the microchiropteran system, we find that, whilst nuclei lower in the brain contain cells responsive to continuous tones, most cells in the human auditory cortex only respond to frequency-modulated tones. There is good evidence from lesions, pathology and psychophysiology (microelectrode work is obviously unavailable) to show that it is particularly responsive to brief sounds varying with respect to each other and involving rapid frequency transitions. The auditory cortex of the dominant hemisphere is also particularly good at detecting the relationship between brief sounds and determining whether one follows the other or whether they both occur together. It will be seen below that all these abilities are basic to the recognition of human speech sounds. Over tens of millions of years the auditory system has played a vital role in predator–prey wars by quickly detecting slight rustles, tiny cracklings and snappings of twigs and detecting where such tiny alarm signals are originating. With the hominids it has built on these sensitivities to provide the crucial faculty upon which the human lifestyle depends.

Because speech comes so naturally to us, we seldom stop to consider how remarkable it is. In literate cultures we assume that it consists of a stream of words, such as those on this page. But this is far from being the case. Linguists have anatomized language into a small number of elemental sounds. These are called **phonemes**. In the word 'pit', for example, there are three phonemes: /p/, /i/ and /t/. Change any phoneme and a different meaning results: kit, pet, pie. Phonemes, however, are not themselves utterly constant. They vary according to where they are placed in a sentence. These variants are called allophones. Consider, for instance, the /t/ phoneme. If the tongue contacts the alveolar ridge above and behind the teeth, as in 'eight', the alveolar phoneme is produced. If the tongue is placed further forward, against the teeth, as in 'eighth', another allophone, the dental allophone, is generated. The /t/ phoneme lends itself to a number of such allophonal variants. Disregarding, for the moment, allophones, standard southern English is said to have 20 vowel phonemes and 24 consonant phonemes.

Phonemes can be analysed spectrographically. When this is done, they are shown to consist of a number of discrete bands of acoustic energy at different frequencies. These frequency bands are called

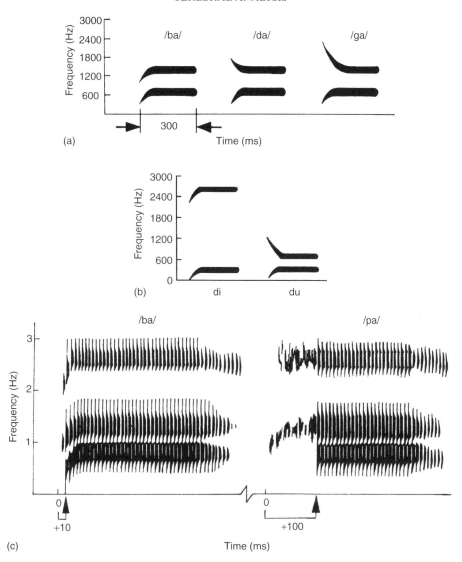

Figure 10.13 Spectrograms of human speech sounds. (a) Shows the importance of the initial short FM in distinguishing different phonemes. (b) Different spectrograms provide the same heard consonant. (c) The importance of voice onset time (VOT). Further explanation in text. After Gazzauiga (1979).

formants. The lowest formant of a phoneme is called the first formant (F1), the next highest the second formant (F2) and so on. Most of the energy is carried by the first two formants. Figure 10.13a shows that the spectrogram of consonant–vowel monosyllables, such as /ba/, /da/ and /ga/, consist of two parts: an initial very short FM phase succeeded by a more prolonged CF phase.

The figure shows that the consonants /b/, /d/ and /g/ are due to very rapid (tens of milliseconds)

FM segments either up or down going. The CF segments persist over a few hundred milliseconds and give the vowel sound. Different voices, higher or lower pitched, will deliver the formants at different positions on the frequency ordinate, but the relationship between the formants must remain constant if the same vowel is to be heard. Figure 10.13b shows an interesting instance where, although most of us hear the same consonant, the sound spectrograms are very different. When /d/ is placed before /i/ the

FM segment of each formant rises; whilst when /d/ is placed before /u/ it falls. This is a first instance of the difficulty of fitting the physical signal to the heard speech sound. Finally, figure 9.13c shows the importance of Voice Onset Time (*VOT*) in distinguishing consonants. Listeners perceive /p/ when VOT exceeds 30 ms, below that time a /b/ is perceived. It is clear then, as argued above, that effective operation of the speech cortex depends on the ability to detect rapid FM tones and sharp transitions.

The significance of this ability was dramatically supported by one of the seminal experiments in auditory physiology. In 1957, Liberman and his colleagues prepared a series of consonant–vowel (CV) monosyllables consisting of two formants each. They then varied the FM start of the second formant in a continuous manner and asked the subject to compare it with an unvarying standard and say when they heard a difference. For instance, F2 in Figure 10.13a might have been varied, gradually changing it from upgoing, through horizontal to downgoing. Liberman's results are shown in Figure 10.14. As the FM segment of F2 is changed the subject at first 'hears' /b/; then suddenly a transition occurs and he 'hears' /d/. There is a switch from one phonemic category to another. This **categorical perception** is not found when nonspeech sounds are synthesized and varied in a similar way. In this case, perception of the sound varied in a continuous fashion. There was no 'step' change. Similarly, categorical transitions are not demonstrable when the CF segments corresponding to vowel sounds are changed.

Categorical perception of speech sounds is inborn in human infants. Infants as young as one month old were presented with synthesized speech sounds and nonspeech sounds. Their attention was monitored by observing their teat sucking behaviour. When categorical transitions of speech sounds were played over the loud speaker, their teat sucking pattern changed; when similar transitions in nonspeech sounds were presented, no such behavioural change was observed. Several other features of the adult language-recognition system have also been shown to be present in very young infants. There is nowadays little doubt that humans are born 'prepared' to speak. The auditory system is not a *tabula rasa* which develops speech recognition simply by extensive exposure to speech after birth. In this, as we shall see, it is similar to the visual system.

It is interesting to note that humans are not alone in this preparedness. No other animals, of course, speak in the sense that humans do, but many other mammals and birds use vocal communications. Quite a large variety of species have been investigated for evidence of categorical perception of species-typical calls. These species include mice, macaques and marmosets. In all cases, good evidence for categorical discrimination has been found. In Japanese macaques (*M. fuscata*) the analysis has been taken further. These monkeys produce some 80–90 different vocalizations. Two of these vocalizations can be distinguished on the criterion of whether a FM element occurs early or late in the call. By using operant conditioning techniques, it was shown that these macaques could distinguish between these elements. Other types of macaque – pigtailed and bonet macaques – require extensive training to distinguish these segments of the calls. If, on the other hand, all the monkeys were required to distinguish the calls on the basis of some other feature of the vocalization, the Japanese monkeys fell far behind the others in mastering the task. The Japanese macaques thus

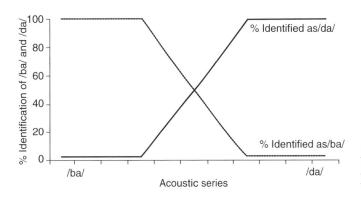

Figure 10.14   Categorical perception of /ba/ vs /da/. The acoustic properties of the phoneme are varied continuously. The switch from identifying /ba/ to identifying /da/ is (comparatively) discontinuous.

seem to have developed a specific dialect that is inaccessible to other macaques.

This, of course, is similar to human language. The underlying biological preparedness is shaped by the linguistic environment into which the child is born. Again, we shall note similarities in the visual system. Innumerable experiments have shown that visual neurology is laid down in plan form, leaving its finer details to be moulded by experience. In the case of speech, there is good evidence that the moulding begins before birth. The mother's voice is transmitted to the uterus by bone conduction. On birth, an infant will suck on a teat to hear a tape of its mother's voice over that of another woman and even when it is played a song or a poem heard prenatally. As infancy grades into childhood and then adulthood, the phonetic contrasts which can be detected become restricted to those of the native language. For instance, Werker and Tees showed, with respect to English and Hindi, that discrimination between certain contrasts in English were lost to Hindi speakers and, vice versa, certain contrasts in Hindi were lost to English speakers as early as twelve months old.

Not only has the auditory cortex to pick up and discriminate between the extremely rapid transients

underlying categorical perception but it also has to cope with an extraordinarily rapid input of information. It can deal with up to 60 phonemes per second, more than twelve times the number of nonspeech sounds it can distinctly perceive in the same time. Furthermore, if we look at the sound spectrogram of simple English sentence such as 'I see it' (Figure 10.15), we can see that it bears rather little relation to what we seem to hear.

The auditory system (again like the visual system) has, in a sense, to 'impose' meaning on this complex input. This, as we shall see in the next section, is largely the job of an area at the posterior of the primary auditory cortex known as Wernicke's area. Speech does not consist of a string of phonemes, each clearly separated from its neighbours, but a complex signal in which each phoneme is affected by both previous and subsequent phonemes. For instance it is well known (and a source of much patronising comment) that many English speakers find difficulty in pronouncing 'law and order' it often coming out as 'lore and order'. The speech signal is produced by the human vocal apparatus in '**coarticulated**' fashion, each part reflecting that which has gone before and that which is to come later. There is no invariable

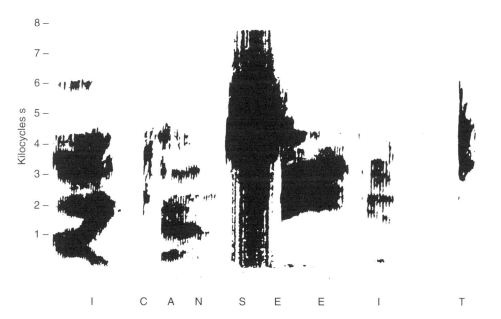

Figure 10.15   Sound spectrogram: 'I can see it'. The ordinate records the frequency of time in kHz and the abscissa records time. The sentence has been spoken very clearly. In the normal run of things the words are far less clearly separated. It is also found that the form of the consonants is strongly dependent on both the preceding and the following vowels. Note how the word 'it' is composed of two bursts of sound energy more widely separated than the bursts representing the different words.

BOX 10.1   BROCA AND WERNICKE

Aphasia, a disorder of symbolic thought and expression, has been noted since antiquity. J.W. Goethe, in *Whilhelm Meister's Appprenticeship* (1796), provides a good early description. 'Altogether unexpectedly my father had a shock of palsy; it lamed his right side and deprived him of the proper use of speech! We had to guess at everything he required; for he could never pronounce the word he intended. There were times when this was terribly afflicting to us... His impatience mounted to the highest pitch; his situation touched me to the inmost heart.' Only in the nineteenth century, however, was a beginning made on understanding its causation in cerebral pathology. Physicians including Gall and Pinel at the beginning of that century contributed accurate descriptions of aphasia after apoplexy (stroke). It became clear that these disabilities were invariably accompanied by paralysis of the right side of the body, suggesting pathology in the left hemisphere. These early contributions were followed by publications from Marcel Dax, Jean Baptiste Bouillard and Bouillard's son in law, Simon Aubertin. But it was not until Paul Broca, in the 1860s, demonstrated that lesions of the posterior part of the left third frontal convolution were the cause of aphasia (or aphémie, as he called it) that the true relation between pathology and speech impairment began to be understood.

Paul Broca (1824–1880) was born at Sainte-Foy-la-Grande between Bordeaux and Bergerac. His father was a country doctor and formerly a surgeon with the Napoleonic army. Paul Broca was a brilliant and precocious student and became the youngest prosector and secretary of the *Société Anatomique* ever appointed. He made significant contributions to many branches of medicine, publishing altogether over 500 papers and treatises in a not overlong lifetime. In addition to his fame in relating aphasia to lesion in a specific region of the cerebral cortex, Broca is also remembered for founding the science of Anthropology in France. He published on both Cro-Magnon man and trephination in the neolithic period and in 1859 founded the *Société d'Anthropolgie de Paris* and a School and Institute of Anthropology. In 1880 he was elected a lifetime member of the French Senate to represent 'France and Science' but although of strong physique and great energy he only held this position for six months, dying on 8 July 1880 at the comparatively early age of 56.

Carl Wernicke (1848–1905) was a less powerful character than Broca. Although he enjoyed almost the same lifespan as the Frenchman, he did not have an equally wide ranging impact on science and society. Unlike Broca, who possessed a charismatic, fiery personality and great talents as raconteur and bon viveur, Wernicke was taciturn and reserved. He was born the son of a civil servant in upper Silesia and after graduating in medicine at Breslau grasped the opportunity of working for six months with Theodor Meynert in Vienna. This short period seems to have inspired Wernicke and he ever afterwards looked back on Meynert as his master. Although Wernicke published in many branches of neurology, especially ophthalmology, the work for which he is remembered is a small treatise published in 1874 when he was 26: *Der aphasische Symptomenkomplex*. In this monograph he attempted to correlate the various different types of aphasia with lesions in different parts of the cerebral cortex and in the subcortical fibre tracts. His guiding concept and strongly held conviction was that mental disorders had their correlates in disorders of the brain. The distinction between psychiatry and neurology was, he felt, misplaced and artificial: 'Geisteskrankheiten sind Gehirnkrankheiten' (mental diseases are brain diseases). At the same age as Paul Broca, 56, in the full flow of his career, having just moved to a Chair in Psychiatry at Halle, he had a fatal accident whilst riding his bicycle in the Thuringian forest and died on 15 June 1905.

(Continues)

(*Continued*)

REFERENCES

Goethe, J.W. (1796) *Wilhelm Meisters Lehrjahre*, trs. 1842 T. Carlyle, *Wilhelm Meister's Apprenticeship*, Vol. 11, Chapman and Hall, London, p. 197.

Goldstein, K. (1970) Paul Broca (1824–1880), in *The Founders of Neurology*, 2nd edn (eds W. Haymaker and F. Schiller), Charles C. Thomas, Springfield.

Goldstein, K. (1970) Carl Wernicke (1848–1904), in *The Founders of Neurology*, 2nd edn. (eds W. Haymaker and F. Schiller), Charles C. Thomas, Springfield.

Riese, W. (1947) The early history of Aphasia. *Bulletin of the History of Medicine*, **21**, 322–34.

relation between acoustic property and phonetic category. Figure 10.15 emphasizes that it is impossible to map phonetic category onto acoustic signal.

The auditory system is exquisitely sensitive to the subtleties of coarticulation, to size and shape of the vocal tracts of different speakers and the rate at which vocalizations are emitted, to phonetic context, not only to consonants but also to vowels, the latter often providing information about emotional state. It would take us too far into the vast and well worked field of psycholinguistics to review the current state of knowledge. The interested student can make a start by examining some of the books and reviews listed in the bibliography. Suffice it to say, in ending this section, that it is small wonder that so little progress has been made in the computer understanding of speech. The auditory system is profoundly parallel in its processing, dependent on context and action-orientated.

10.7 LATERALIZATION AND THE NEUROANATOMY OF LANGUAGE

In the great majority of humans the anatomical areas most involved with speech are situated in the left hemisphere (Table 10.1). In these instances the left

Table 10.1 Cerebral lateralization and handedness

Handedness	Dominant Hemisphere (%)		
	Left	Right	Neither
Left or ambidextrous	70	15	15
Right	96	4	0

After Kandel *et al.* (1991).

hemisphere is consequently known as the **dominant hemisphere**. Anatomical examination of the hemispheres shows a distinct structural dissimilarity between them. The Sylvian fissure is longer and reaches further towards the top of the cerebrum in the left hemisphere than in the right hemisphere. If the upper surface of the temporal lobes are compared, it can be shown that in 65% of the cases the left **planum temporale** is far greater in extent than it is in the the right (Figure 10.16a). In 11% of the cases the right was greater than the left and in 24% of the cases there was no significant difference. The fact that an asymmetrical planum temporale can already be detected in the foetus suggests that the human brain is primed to develop asymmetrical cerebral hemispheres.

Although the major anatomical substrata of speech are located in the dominant hemisphere, many other areas of the brain are also involved. As might be expected of so important a function, many parts of both cerebral hemispheres play a part (Figure 10.16c). Furthermore, there is good evidence nowadays to implicate subcortical structures such as the thalamus and the caudate nucleus. Nevertheless, a useful and widely used 'first approximation' is still that proposed by Damasio and Geschwind and shown in Figure 10.16b. It is largely derived from observations of stroke and other lesion-induced speech loss with subsequent post mortem neurohistology. The names given to the crucial areas, **Broca's area**, **Wernicke's area**, are those of the investigators who first reported these correlations between linguistic loss and neural damage.

As Figure 10.16b indicates, the first area concerned with speech is Wernicke's area. This lies just posterior to the primary auditory cortex. In Brodmann's cytoarchitectonic numerology, the primary auditory cortex is area 41 and Wernicke's area is

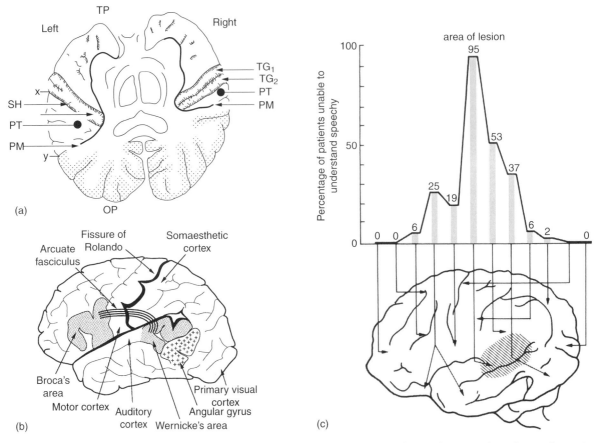

Figure 10.16 (a) Horizontal section through the human brain at the level of the Sylvian fisure to show the much greater extent of the planum temporale on the left than on the right. The posterior margin of the planum temporale (PM) slopes backwards more steeply in the left hemisphere than the right, and the right margin (formed by the sulcus of Hershl (SH)) slopes forward more steeply. The planum temporale on the left thus extends from the position marked by 'x' to that marked by 'y'. There is a single transverse gyrus of Hershl (TG) on the left but two on the right (TG$_1$, TG$_2$). OP = occipital pole; TP = temporal pole. After Geschwind *et al.*, 1968. (b) Language areas in the brain. The left cerebral hemisphere is shown from the side. Further explanation in text. (c) Although the major speech centres are as shown in (a) and (b) many parts of the cortex involve themselves in this definitively human function. From Young, J.Z. (1978), '*Programs of the Brain*', p. 184, Fig. 16.3, by permission of Oxford University Press.

area 22. It is to Wernicke's area that signals caused by speech are directed after arriving at the primary auditory cortex. Lesions to this area affect the ability to comprehend or interpret the speech sounds as linguistically meaningful. Similarly, visual stimuli from the written word also make their way to Wernicke's area. The pathway here is from the primary visual cortex (Brodmann 17) to the secondary visual cortex (Brodmann 18) and then via the **angular gyrus** (Brodmannn 39) to Wernicke's area. Damage to any

of these areas impedes both the ability to understand the written word and to name a visual object.

Wernicke's area is connected to Broca's area by a tract of fibres known as the **arcuate fasciculus**. If this is interrupted, it becomes impossible to repeat a heard or a written word. Broca's area itself is central to computing the complex of muscle activity required to articulate a word. It is, as can be seen from Figure 10.16b, closely adjacent to the region of the primary motor cortex which maps facial and laryngeal musculature. As mentioned above, the scheme outlined in the preceding paragraphs is necessarily a simplification of the full neuroanatomy. It does, however, provide the core of the system and many linguistic disabilities (aphasias) can be traced to lesions in its various elements.

It is interesting, finally, to note that recent work on rhesus macaques (*Maccaca mulatto*) has shown that these primates, which shared a common ancestor with humans no later than some 25–30 million years ago, possess a brain region dedicated to the analysis of species-specific calls. Experiments in which brain activity in response to nonbiological sounds was compared to that in response to monkey vocalizations showed that, whereas nonbiological sounds elicited activity in wide areas of the auditory cortex, species-specific calls elicited activity focused in the area immediately around the Sylvian fissure. These perisylvian areas are the monkey homologues of Broca's and Wernicke's areas in humans. There is, however, no evidence of lateralization. Nevertheless, it is possible to speculate that brain areas dedicated to language emerged very early in hominid evolution and developed slowly and incrementally during millions, perhaps tens of millions, of years. It may be that these areas along with other areas of the brain devoted to processing input of social relevance (see the face recognition systems discussed in Section 18.4 and the mirror neurons on Section 23.8) make up the neural substrate on which human language has developed.

10.8 LANGUAGE AND THE *FOXP2* GENE

Scans of the human genome have shown that mutations on genes located on at least four chromosomes (2, 13, 16 and 19) lead to speech impairments However, the most exciting development has been the discovery in 2001 that mutations of a gene, the *FOXP2* gene, located on chromosome 7 (7q31) lead to acute difficulties in both the comprehension of language and its production as speech.

FOXP2 is a member of a large family of similar genes. They all encode transcription factors which include a sequence of amino acids known as the forkhead box, hence Fox. This domain binds to specific nucleotide sequences in DNA which act as promoters for a number of genes. *FOXP2* thus controls the expression of a number of other genes. Unfortunately, at the time of writing these genes and their protein products remain unknown. *FoxP2* genes are found in a number of other vertebrates, as far down the phylogenetic tree as alligators. They are thus very ancient and, as we shall see, very stable.

The identification of *FOXP2* as a 'language gene' emerged from genetic analysis of a family discovered in 1990. This family (code named KE) was found to have exhibited an inherited inability to understand and produce grammatical speech through three generations. The trait was passed down as the effect of a single autosomal dominant gene. Isolation and molecular analysis of this gene showed that in members of the KE family an arginine (R) to histidine (H) transition had occurred in position 553 of the amino acid sequence of the FOXP2 protein (R553H). This position is right in the middle of the forkhead box. It is plausible to suppose that this alteration in the amino acid sequence interferes with protein's ability to bind onto the appropriate DNA sequences and this, in turn, will disable the promoters of a number of genes.

The outcome of this point mutation (substitution of an adenine (A) for a guanine (G)) on the relevant part of the *FOXP2* DNA multiplies up through the complexities of brain biology to engender the disastrous disability from which members of family KE suffer. Members of this family have little or no cognitive handicap but experience great difficulty in language comprehension and in carrying out the coordinated articulations necessary for speech. They have difficulty, in other words, in controlling the vocal apparatus responsible for speech sounds and difficulty in understanding sentences and applying grammatical conventions. Neuroimaging studies, especially fMRI, showed underactivity in Broca's area., but defects were also found in other parts of the brain including other parts of the cortex, the basal ganglia and the cerebellum – all areas involved in the control of motor activity. It is worth remembering that the fine control of the larynx, tongue and mouth is absent from the chimpanzees and other great apes, and it has often been suggested that this is a major reason for their failure to evolve rudimentary speech. These neuroimaging studies are consistent with laboratory investigations of the expression zones of *FoxP2* in mice. The gene was shown to be expressed not only in the cerebral cortex, but also in the thalamus, midbrain, cerebellum and medulla. The gene is also involved in programming the proper development of the lungs, also involved in the physiology of articulate speech.

As mentioned in Section 5.3, the *FOXP2* gene appears to have been under considerable selection pressure during the most recent phase of human evolution. The gene, as mentioned above, is very ancient and is, in general, highly conserved. The human FOXP2 protein differs from zebra finch FoxP2 by only seven amino acids (common ancestor some 300Ma ago) and from mouse FoxP2 (common ancestor 75Ma ago) by only three amino acids. Yet human FOXP2 differs from chimpanzee FoxP2 (common ancestor 5Ma ago) by two amino acids, a very considerable acceleration and sequence variation in human populations suggests that this change occurred no longer ago than 200 000 years (Section 5.3). It is interesting to note that the human version of *FOXP2* has also been found in DNA extracted from Neanderthal fossils.

Humans are, however, not the only organisms in which *FoxP2* has been implicated in the development of vocal communication. The vocalizations of mice, in which the gene has been 'knocked out', are subtly different and they lack their characteristic isolation calls. It has also been found that *FoxP2* is highly variable in echolocating compared with nonecholocating bats suggesting, once again, that it is involved in audiomotor coordination. Finally, it has been implicated in song learning in songbirds. It has been shown, for instance, that two *Fox* genes (*FoxP1* and *FoxP2*) are expressed in the brain nuclei that control their vocalizations. Zebra finches learn their songs by listening to an adult tutor bird. Once learnt the song hardly changes. In contrast, canaries modify their song throughout life. It can be shown that *FoxP2* expression is accentuated during the zebra finch learning periods and during the July and August singing seasons of wild canaries. The situation is, however, not straightforward in either zebra finches or canaries. Several other genes are in play, as are changing hormone levels. Nevertheless, it is interesting that *FoxP* genes appear to have a rôle to play in the vocal communications of forms as distantly related as humans and songbirds.

FoxP2, and other *FoxP* genes and their protein products, are the subject of intensive research. The original work on the KE family instanced the crucial importance of *FoxP2* in human language comprehension and speech. Subsequent work has broadened the focus to include audiomotor communication in other mammals and birds. The effect of this single gene in controlling the on/off switches of an unknown number of other genes is felt throughout the intricately interconnected motor areas of the brain. It is, moreover, as noted above, far from the only gene concerned with the development and maintenance of human language. The dramatic newspaper reports in 2001 of the finding of a 'gene for language' overstated the position. Nevertheless, the isolation of this gene and its study in a wide variety of communicating animals is likely to provide insights into the learning and mastery of language, one of mankind's defining and most precious possessions.

10.9 CALLOSECTOMY AND AFTER

Turning back to our discussion of the neural basis of language in the human cerebral cortex, it will be recalled, from Section 10.7, that recognition and production of language is confined to one cerebral hemisphere, the so-called dominant hemisphere, in most of us the left hemisphere. The major connection between the dominant and the subdominant hemisphere is a large tract of fibres, the corpus callosum. A less important tract, the anterior commissure, also runs between the two hemispheres. Although for many years the functional significance of the corpus callosum was deeply unclear, animal experiments in the mid-1950s showed that it plays a crucial role in coordinating the activity of the two hemispheres. If it and the **crossed visual fibres** of the optic chiasma (Section 18.1.2) are sectioned, it could be shown that conditioned reflexes taught an animal through one eye could not afterwards be elicited by displaying the conditioned stimulus to the other eye. The information was confined to just one hemisphere. Then, in the 1960s, Sperry and others carried out a series of careful studies on human patients who had had their corpus callosi sectioned to alleviate otherwise intractable epilepsy. At first these patients seemed perfectly normal on recovery. Their epilepsy, instead of spreading from a focus in one hemisphere to involve the other as well, was satisfactorily confined to a single hemisphere. Apart from a splitting headache (as the joke insists) the behaviour of these so-called 'split brain' patients seemed perfectly normal.

But, as is nowadays common knowledge, this was not in fact the case. The deficiency shown by these patients is one of the most interesting and thought-provoking of all neuropsychological dysfunctions. Sperry and his colleagues were, in essence, able to show that the same defects as had previously been demonstrated in experimental animals could also be demonstrated in humans. Split-brain patients, of course, possess unsectioned optic chiasmata. Saccadic eye movements normally ensure that information from each eye reaches both hemispheres. But if very brief stimuli were delivered (by means of a tachistoscope) the confounding action of the saccades could be countered and it could be arranged that information flashed to the left visual field was delivered to the right hemisphere and vice versa. When information was flashed in this way to the right hemisphere, the split-brainer would deny all knowledge of having seen it. In other words, the information confined in the right hemisphere had no way of gaining access to the linguistic centres in the left hemisphere.

Although in such circumstances the individual would vehemently deny being aware of the information flashed to the right hemisphere, it can nevertheless be shown that it had reached and been processed in the right hemisphere. The right hemisphere controls the left hand. If the individual is asked to indicate in some way with the left hand what has been flashed into the right hemisphere he can do so. This, of course, raises fascinating problems for philosophers of mind.

Further analysis of callosectomised patients shows that the two cerebral hemispheres are biased towards different abilities (Figure 10.17). It is often said that the left hemisphere, the linguistic hemisphere, is adapted to analytic tasks, whilst the right hemisphere is better at holistic activities. There is, undoubtedly, some truth in this conclusion but only a certain amount of truth. The right hemisphere is capable of simple language comprehension and the left of some holistic appreciation. In the normal individual they work together, complementing each other. This cooperation is, perhaps, more complete in women than men. There is, in other words, some

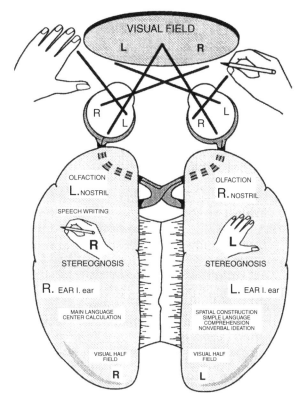

Figure 10.17 Lateralization of human cerebral hemispheres. The figure shows specializations of the two hemispheres. It also indicates that these specializations are more a matter of emphasis than sharp differentiation. The right hemisphere, for instance, possesses some ability to comprehend language; the left hemisphere considerable ability to appreciate holistic pattern.

evidence that hemispheric specialization (such as it is) is more marked in men an in women.

Finally, it must be re-emphasized that experimental analysis of the neuropsychology of split-brain individuals requires extreme care and technical sophistication. The brain, especially the sensory brain, is adept at drawing conclusions from almost imperceptible clues. It is a hypothesis generating engine. This, again, has been forced upon it during the long evolutionary war of predator and prey. If a snapping twig, an unusual stripe, a half-heard rustle, is not immediately completed into a pattern, if meaning isn't immediately extracted, the prey, the dinner, will escape, or, from the other perspective, the jump to safety will be delayed a split second too long and life will end. Hence any clue provided to the left hemisphere of a split-brainer will be used and a correct answer to the experimenter's question provided, even if the information is firmly locked in the subdominant hemisphere. It is only by controlling for all these factors that the remarkable features of split-brain responses have been elucidated.

10.10 CONCLUDING REMARKS

This is the final chapter of this section. We have travelled a long way from the simple mechanoreceptors of prokaryocytes and roundworms with which we started. We saw how they have been incorporated into ever more complex sensory systems. We reviewed the subtle systems of stretch and strain detectors which provide our sixth or kinaesthetic sense. We looked at the delicate and highly sensitive tactile hairs of the insects and saw how they were developed into vibration detectors and ultimately tympanal organs or 'ears'. We saw, also, how systems, originally evolved to detect changes in the abiotic environment, have become profoundly caught up in detecting and communicating with other living forms. The calls of cicadas sound all around the Mediterranean littoral and stirred the mythopoeic imagination of classical Greece. We marvelled at the sonic contest between bat and moth and touched on the shifting complexity of the bat's auditory brain. The extraordinary precision with which those silent nocturnal predators, the owls, can detect and swoop on their unsuspecting prey also shows the sophistication that can be achieved by the mechanosenses. Auditory communication is also highly significant in social intercourse and reaches peaks in songbirds and yet further peaks in humankind. We examined (all too briefly) some aspects of the human linguistic brain and of our beginning understanding of its genetic basis. The human world is full of talk. The ongoing revolution in communications is spreading human talk as a network over the planet's surface. But also we saw, as we went through these pages, how the subjective aspect of the mechanosenses varies. Although at the centre of the labyrinth of physiology there still remains the molecular biology and biophysics of membrane-embedded stretch sensitive channels yet, subjectively, how different is the sensation of touch from that of sound. Once again we find ourselves on the fringes of the great unsolved problem of the modern world: the problem of mind.

PART II: SELF ASSESSMENT

The following questions are designed both to help you assess your understanding of the topics covered in the text and to direct your attention to significant aspects of the subject matter. The sequence of questions follows the sequence in which the subject matter is presented in the text. It is thus easy to refer back to the appropriate page or pages. After reading each chapter and/or each section you should look through these questions and make sure you know the answers and the issues involved.

CHAPTER 6: MECHANOSENSENSITIVITY OF CELL MEMBRANES

6.1   Why is the molecular biology of stretch receptors less well known that that of other types of receptor?

6.2   With reference to Appendix A, discuss the technique of patch clamping as applied to *E.coli*. Why is the size of *E.coli* a problem and what can be done to side-step it?

6.3   What do the acronyms MscL and MscS stand for? How do we know that they are separate entities?

6.4   Provide a brief outline of the way in which the MscL channel was isolated and purified.

6.5   By means of a graph indicate the mechanosensitivity of this channel.

6.6   How many MscL subunits are believed to be grouped together to form a mechanosensitive channel?

6.7   How do MscL and MscS channels respond to membrane stretch?

6.8   Discuss two possible roles for stretch receptors in bacterial membranes.

6.9   Explain the difference between poikilo-osmotic and homeo-osmotic animals. Which are the most common?

6.10   Where are osmoreceptor cells located in the mammalian brain?

6.11   Where do the axons of the osmoreceptor cells terminate?

6.12   Which hormones do the osmoreceptor axons liberate?

6.13   What effect on the osmolarity of the ECF do the hormones have?

6.14   Draw a diagram showing the feedback neuroendocrine loop which controls the osmolarity of the internal environment

6.15   Describe the electrophysiological evidence which confirms the sensitivity of the MCNs to variations in osmolarity of the ECF.

6.16   Describe experiments which show that membrane stretch is related to the electrophysiology of the MCNs.

6.17   With reference to the patch clamp results explain why the channels in the MCNs are described as 'stretch inactivated (SI)' channels.

6.18   Explain how hypertonicity in the ECF leads, via the SI channels, to an increased frequency of impulses in the MCN axons and hence a countervailing decrease in hypertonicity.

6.19   Which congenital muscular disease might be due to mutations of SI-channel genes?

Biology of Sensory Systems, Second Edition   C.U.M. Smith
© 2008 John Wiley & Sons, Ltd

CHAPTER 7: KINAESTHESIA

7.1   What input other than from muscles, joints and tendons is processed to maintain body equilibrium in space?

7.2   What role do the abdominal muscles play in the life of long bodied decapod crustacea?

7.3   What form do the stretch receptors take in *Homarus vulgaris*?

7.4   What effect does stretch have on the neurosensory cell innervating (a) RM1 and (b) RM2?

7.5   Why is the RM2 neurosensory cell known as the 'fast adapting' cell and the RM2 neurosensory cell known as the 'slow adapting' cell?

7.6   What role do the accessory fibres play?

7.7   With reference to Section 6.2.1 compare the part played by the motor fibres to crustacean RMs with that played by gamma motoneurons on mammalian skeletal muscle.

7.8   What rôle do hair sensilla play in insect kinaesthesia?

7.9   How do campaniform sensilla differ from hair sensilla and where are they mostly found?

7.10 Draw a diagram of a scolopidium. What and where is the scolopale?

7.11 What is a chordotonal organ and where are they found?

7.12 What are the subgenual organs and where are they found? What stimuli are they adapted to detect?

7.13 Explain how insects such as dragonflies and houseflies maintain equilibrium during flight.

7.14 Define a 'motor unit'. Does this unit vary in size in different parts of the body?

7.15 How do mammalian intrafusal fibres resemble crustacean receptor muscles?

7.16 Name the three types of mammalian intrafusal fibre and indicate their different responses to stretch.

7.17 Distinguish between the fusimotor and skeletomotor systems of motoneurons.

7.18 Describe, with the aid of a diagram, the feedback loops involved in the coactivation control of skeletal muscle contraction in mammals.

7.19 Are the reflex mechanisms in the spinal cord restricted to the homonymous muscle? If not, which other muscles are involved?

7.20 What different categories of proprioceptive information do the group Ia and group II fibres carry to the CNS?

7.21 Distinguish between dynamic and static gamma motoneurons.

7.22 What is meant by 'fusimotor set'.

7.23 Compare and contrast the response characterisitics of spindle endings and Golgi tendon organs. Are these two types of proprioceptor often associated with each other?

7.24 How does the response of Golgi tendon organs depend on the frequency of the stimulating stretching force?

7.25 Sketch a figure to show the wiring diagram underlying muscular response to stimulation of a Golgi tendon organ.

7.26 Name the three types of receptor associated with most joints and indicate their adequate stimuli.

7.27 Review the many different sensory systems and feedback loops which constitute a mammal's 'sixth' or 'kinaesthetic' sense and consider how far the metallic artefacts of present-day robotics have to develop before they can begin to compete.

CHAPTER 8: TOUCH

8.1   Why are neurobiologists interested in the tiny soil nematode worm *C. elegans*?

8.2   How were *mec* genes discovered?

8.3   What do the acronyms ALML, ALMR, PLML, PLMR, AVM and PVM stand for?

8.4   What characteristic ultrastructural feature do the touch receptor neurons display? Look back to Chapter 6: is there any similarity between the ultrastructure of *C. elegans* touch receptors and insect mechanoreceptors?

8.5   Name two *degenerins*. What are the products of these two genes and what mammalian structure do these products resemble?

8.6   Name three nondegenerin *mec* genes. What are their protein products?

8.7   Draw a diagram representing a hypothetical construct of these MEC proteins to form a mechanosensitive organelle.

8.8   Where are TRP receptors found in *C. elegans*?

8.9 Name three types of arachnid mechanoreceptor.

8.10 What is 'stochastic resonance' and how is it significant in explaining the sensitivity of arachnid trichobothria?

8.11 How do lyriform organs detect mechanical stress in arachnid exoskeletons? What rôle do these organs play in a spider's life?

8.12 Sketch a diagram showing the general features of an insect hair sensillum.

8.13 Do insect hair sensilla respond to different sensory modalities?

8.14 Where is the tubular body found and what is its function?

8.15 Which TPR channels are found in the membrane of the tubular body? What does the acronym 'nompc' stand for?

8.16 How are modified cilia involved in gustatory and olfactory sensilla?

8.17 Describe the use made of tarsal vibration detectors by some aquatic insects. Can such insects detect the position of their prey? If so, how? Do you see a similarity with the detection of the source of sound by vertebrates (refer forward to Chapter 10)?

8.18 Describe the two types of acoustic detector developed by insects.

8.19 What is Johnston's organ and where is it found? What is its function in mosquitoes and midges?

8.20 Explain the difference in the stimuli which affect acoustic sensilla and tympanic organs.

8.21 Describe the structure of a typical insect tympanal organ.

8.22 Discuss some of the functions for which insect tympanal organs are used.

8.23 Referring forward to Chapter 9 (Section 9.3.2.5), explain why physiology does not permit moth ears to discriminate between the different frequencies of bat sonar calls.

8.24 Explain why *D. scalestes* is a more successful parasite than *D. phalenodectes.*

8.25 Discuss the possible significance of moth sound emissions as a defence against bat attack. What is Batesian mimicry?

8.26 Which are the fast adapting and which the slow adapting touch receptors in mammalian skin?

8.27 What type of stimulus affects Pacinian corpuscles? How is the histological structure of the corpuscle adapted to its function?

8.28 What is 'glabrous' skin?

8.29 Do all the mechanoreceptor afferent fibres enter the dorsal (posterior) horn of the spinal cord's grey matter?

8.30 Sketch a diagram to show where the primary and secondary somaesthetic areas are located.

8.31 In which of the three Brodmann areas of the somaesthetic cortex do the somaesthetic fibres terminate?

8.32 In which layer of the cortex do the somaesthetic fibres terminate?

8.33 Why is a column of cells in the somaesthetic cortex regarded as computational module?

8.34 What is meant by the term 'somaesthetic homunculus' and why is it so distinctively nonisomorphous?

8.35 Describe experiments on mouse vibrissae which demonstrate the lability of the somaesthetic cortex.

8.36 What similar work on human touch sensitivity complements the mouse vibrissae experiments?

8.37 Review some of the instances in which touch sensitivity is fundamental to social interaction between individuals.

CHAPTER 9: EQUILIBRIUM AND HEARING: THE USES OF HAIR CELLS

9.1 Draw a diagram of a typical mammalian hair cell.

9.2 What is Brownian motion? How does it limit the sensitivity of hair cells?

9.3 Distinguish between kinocilia and stereocilia.

9.4 What effect does movement of stereocilia towards the kinocilium have on membrane potential? Away from the kinocilium? Orthogonally to the kinocilium?

9.5 What molecular and biophysical mechanisms are responsible for the membrane potential changes of Q 9.4? How rapid are these changes?

9.6 Describe the 'tip links' model of hair cell stimulation.

9.7 Are TRP channels present in stereocilia? If so which?

9.8 What evidence suggests that the *C. elegans* mechanosensitive channel and the ion channels of hair cells are related?

9.9 Describe the molecular mechanisms which may be responsible for adaptation in hair cells. Does *C. elegans* show anything similar?

9.10 How is depolarization of the hair cell membrane linked to the release of neurotransmitter from its base?

9.11 How are hair cells organized and what role do they play in the lateral line systems of fish?

9.12 Are lateral line systems developed in aquatic reptiles (e.g. sea snakes, turtles, etc.) and/or mammals (e.g. porpoises, seals, etc.)?

9.13 Distinguish between the membranous vestibule and the membranous labyrinth.

9.14 How many semicircular canals are developed in the most primitive of living vertebrates?

9.15 Which chambers of the ear constitute the membranous vestibule?

9.16 Which part(s) of the membranous vestibule detect linear and which parts angular acceleration of the head?

9.17 How do perilymph and endolymph vary in their ionic constitution? Which resembles an extracellular fluid and which an intracellular fluid?

9.18 Where are the hair cells located in the untriculus and sacculus?

9.19 Where are otoliths found?

9.20 Which nerve carries information to the brain from the equilibrium sensors in the ear?

9.21 What are cristae and where are they found in the membranous vestibule?

9.22 Are the semicircular canals sensitive to constant angular velocity of the head?

9.23 Are the Weberian ossicles homologous or analogous to the auditory ossicles in the mammalian ear?

9.24 What significant anatomical change occurs to the lagena in the reptilia?

9.25 In what way does the width of the lagena's basilar membrane vary in birds?

9.26 What structure does the bird's basilar papilla develop into in the mammals?

9.27 What is otosclerosis and why does it cause deafness? Discuss possible treatments.

9.28 With the aid of a diagram explain the sequence of pressure changes which underlie sound detection in the mammalian cochlea.

9.29 What evidence is there that there is feedback control of cochlear sensitivity? (Refer also to Box 9.1)

9.30 What are microphonic potentials?

9.31 What neurophysiological problems are set by the task of discriminating between different frequencies at 500 Hz and above?

9.32 What is the 'volley theory' and what the 'place theory' of frequency discrimination? How has the 'place theory' been extended by recent investigations?

9.33 Who was Hermann von Helmholtz and what was his major contribution to our understanding of cochlear physiology? (Refer also to Box 3.1)

9.34 Discuss some of the genetic defects to which the ear is subject (refer also to Box 9.2).

9.35 Describe the main features of the echolocation sounds emitted by insectivorous bats.

9.36 Looking forward to Chapters 14 (olfaction) and 17 (retina), list the various sensory cells in which cilia have been modified to detect environmental happenings.

CHAPTER 10: CEREBRAL ANALYSIS

10.1 List the parts of, and inputs to, the medullary vestibular complex. What is meant by 'push–pull' innervation from the two sets of semicircular canals?

10.2 How may information pertinent to equilibrium from the membranous vestibule be isolated from other relevant input?

10.3 What is nystagmus and how may it be demonstrated?

10.4 Discuss the causes of some forms of motion sickness.

10.5 What is meant by the 'characteristic frequency (CF)' of a cochlear fibre. Can it be said to be an instance of the Muller–Helmholtz theory of specific nerve energies?

10.6 Explain how the frequency response area of a cochlear fibre may be regarded as its receptive field.

10.7 What is meant by 'lateral inhibition'? How does the response of cochlear nerve fibres show this type of inhibition?

10.8 Does electrophysiological recording from single cochlear fibres provide evidence for volley theory?

10.9 How is the basilar membrane represented in the cochlear nucleus?

10.10 Describe the response of stellate cells and bushy cells to input from the cochlea.

10.11 How are cells in the superior olivary nuclei involved in determining the direction of a sound source?

10.12 What behavioural response is used to show the owl's ability to detect the spatial position of a sound source?

10.13 Which features of sound does the owl's brain use to determine the direction of its source? Where are these features first extracted? Which feature is used to determine the direction of the source in the vertical plane and which in the horizontal plane?

10.14 Explain how coincidence detectors are used to compare the time at which sound impinges on owl's left and right ears.

10.15 Explain how excitatory and inhibitory synapses are involved in determining the azimuthal direction from which sound emanates.

10.16 What is meant by 'spatial tuning'?

10.17 Where are maps of auditory space located in the owl's brain? To what use are they put?

10.18 What is believed to be the significance of the nontopographic organization of spatially tuned cells in the owl's archistriatum? To which part of the mammal's brain is the archistriatum analogous?

10.19 Where is the auditory cortex located in (a) primates, (b) cat and bat?

10.20 In which layer of the auditory cortex do fibres from the medial geniculate nucleus terminate? How does this compare with the somaesthetic cortex (Section 8.6), the visual cortex (Section 18.2.1)?

10.21 What are the preferred trigger stimuli of many of the cells in the auditory cortex?

10.22 In macaque visual cortex there is evidence for the existence of face recognition cells (Section 18.4). Are analogous cells present in macaque auditory cortex?

10.23 Describe the type of sound emitted by foraging bats.

10.24 How are cells in the bat auditory cortex adapted to analyse the animal's sonar?

10.25 Define $Q_{10\,dB}$. Explain why the larger the value of $Q_{10\,dB}$, the more sharply the cortical cell is 'tuned'.

10.26 Are bats sensitive to moth wing movements? If so, explain how.

10.27 How do some bats compensate for self-induced Doppler shifts in the echo from the emitted tone?

10.28 What is the 'auditory fovea' and why has it been given that name?

10.29 What is an otoacoustic emission and how is it produced?

10.30 Can bat sonar systems detect surface textures and, if so, how?

10.31 There is said to be an analogy between the echo signal from a rough texture or jittery source and colour in the visual modality. Explain.

10.32 To what sound stimuli is the human auditory cortex particularly sensitive?

10.33 Define a 'phoneme' and a 'formant'.

10.34 Give an example to show the importance of 'voice onset time (VOT)'.

10.35 What is 'categorical perception'? Does it occur with nonspeech sounds? Is it inborn?

10.36 Is there evidence for categorical perception in nonhuman animals?

10.37 What evidence is there that the ability to perceive speech sounds is moulded by early experience? Does something similar happen in other primates?

10.38 Explain what is meant by 'coarticulation'.

10.39 In which cerebral hemisphere is the planum temporale usually best developed?

10.40 Sketch the positions of the major areas concerned with speech in the dominant hemisphere.

10.41 Explain the role of Wenicke's area and the angular gyrus.

10.42 How is Wernicke's area connected to Broca's area? What is the consequence of interrupting this connection?

10.43 What is the significance of the anatomical position of Broca's area?

10.44 Is there any evidence for speech area primordia in nonhuman primates?

10.45 Name the major tract of fibres connecting the two cerebral hemispheres.

10.46 Why is it necessary to cut the optic chiasma as well as the corpus callosum in animal split-brain experiments?

10.47 Why is a tachistoscope employed to project images in experiments on callosectomized humans?

10.48 How is it known that, in spite of a split-brain subject's denial, information directed at the right hemisphere arrived there and was processed?

10.49 In what way are the abilities of the two cerebral hemispheres biased in humans?

10.50 Is there any evidence that men's cerebral hemispheres are more specialized than women's?

PART II: NOTES, REFERENCES AND BIBLIOGRAPHY

CHAPTER 6: MECHANOSENSITIVITY OF CELL MEMBRANES

The molecular biology of the mechanosensitive channels in *E. coli* is discussed in Hamil and McBride (1994), Sukharev *et al.* (1994, 1997, 2005); Anishkin and Kung (2005) provide a recent review of the X-ray diffraction work and biophysical analysis, including excellent illustrations. An account of poikilo-osmotic animals, their physiology and behaviour, may be found in textbooks of comparative physiology, for example Prosser and Brown (1962) which, although dated, still provides a good survey of classical data. Up-to-date information on mammalian osmoreceptors is presented by Bourque and Oliet (1997) whilst information on the neuroendocrinological and neurophysiological feedback loops underlying mammalian homeo-osmosis is to be found in any modern textbook of those subjects.

Anishkin, A. and Kung, C. (2005) Microbial mechanosensation. *Current Opinion in Neurobiology*, **15**, 397–405.

Blount, P. *et al.* (1996) Structure and function of the bacterial mechanosensitive channel. *EMBO J.*, **18**, 4798–805.

Bourque, C.W. and Oliet, S.H.R. (1997) Osmoreceptors in the central nervous system. *Annual Review of Physiology*, **59**, 601–19.

Hamil, O.P. and McBride, D.W. (1994) The cloning of a mechano-gated membrane ion channel. *Trends in Neurosciences*, **17**, 439–43.

Prosser, C.L. and Brown, F.A. (1962) *Comparative Animal Physiology*, W.B. Saunders, Philadelphia.

Sukharev, S.I. *et al.* (1994) A large-conductance mechanosensitive channel in *E. coli* encoded by *MscL* alone. *Nature*, **368**, 265–8.

Sukharev, S.I. and Anishkin, A. (2005) Mechanosensitive channels: what we can learn from 'simple' model systems? *Trends in Neurosciences*, **27**, 345–51.

Sukharev, S.I., Blount, P., Martinac, B. and Kung, C. (1997) Mechanosensitive channels of *Escherichia coli*: the *MscL* gene, protein and activities. *Ann. Rev. Physiol.*, **59**, 633–57.

CHAPTER 7: KINAESTHESIA

The structure and functioning of insect sensilla are extensively described by McIver (1985). Further detail is given by Altner and Prillinger (1980) whilst Blum (1985) provides a more general account. The biophysics of mechanosensitive sensilla is described by French (1988), and both Gong *et al.* (2004) and Walker, Willingham and Zuker (2000) discuss channel biophysics. Field and Matheson (1998) provide an exhaustive review of chordotonal organs. One of the best accounts of general entomology (morphology, anatomy, systematics) is still that of Imms (1946). Kinaesthesia in mammals is discussed in texts of neurophysiology and neuroscience, for example Kandel, Schwartz and Jessel (1991) and a detailed review is given by McCloskey (1978). Other detail may be found in Hunt (1990), Jami (1992) and Matthews (1981).

Insects

Altner, H. and Prillinger, L. (1980) Ultrastructure of invertebrate chemo-, thermo- and hygroreceptors and its

Biology of Sensory Systems, Second Edition   C.U.M. Smith
© 2008 John Wiley & Sons, Ltd

functional significance. *International Review of Cytology*, **67**, 69–139.

Blum, M.S. (ed.) (1985) *Fundmentals of Insect Physiology*, John Wiley & Sons, Inc., New York.

Field, L.H. and Matheson, T. (1998) Chordotonal organs of insects. *Advances in Insect Physiology*, **27**, 1–228.

French, A.S. (1988) Transduction mechanisms of mechano sensilla. *Annual Review of Entomology*, **13**, 39–58.

Gong, Z. *et al.* (2004) Two interdependent TRPV channel subunits, inactive and Nanchung, mediate hearing in *Drosophila*. *Journal of Neuroscience*, **24**, 9059–66.

Imms, A.D. (1946) *A General Textbook of Entomology*, 6th edn, Methuen, London.

McIver, S.B. (1985) Mechanoreception, in *Comprehensive Insect Physiology, Biochemistry and Pharmacology*, Pergamon Press, Oxford.

Moulins, M. (1976) Ultrastructure of chordotonal organs, in (ed. P.J. Mill), *Structure and Function of Proprioceptors in the Invertebrates*, Chapman and Hall, London.

Pringle, J.W.S. (1938) Proprioception in insects lll: the function of hair sensilla at joints. *Journal of Experimental Biology*, **15**, 467–73.

Walker, R.G., Willingham, A.Y. and Zuker, C.S. (2000) A *Drosophila* mechanosensory transduction channel. *Science*, **287**, 2229–34.

Mammals

Hunt, C.C. (1990) Mammalian muscle spindle: peripheral mechanisms. *Physiol. Rev.*, **70**, 643–63.

Jami, L. (1992) Golgi tendon organs in mammalian skeletal muscle: functional properties and cnetral actions. *Physiological Reviews*, **72**, 623–66.

Kandel, E.R., Schwartz, J.H. and Jessel, T.M. (eds) (1991) *Principles of Neuroscience*, Elsevier, New York.

Matthews, P.B.C. (1981) Evolving views on the internal operation and functional role of the muscle spindle. *Journal of Physiology*, **320**, 1–30.

McCloskey, D.I. (1978) Kinaesthetic sensibility. *Physiological Reviews*, **58**, 763–820.

Wilkinson, R.S. and Fukami, Y. (1983) Responses of isolated Golgi tendon organs of cat to sinusoidal stretch. *Journal of Neurophysiology*, **49**, 976–88.

CHAPTER 8: TOUCH

Touch sensitivity in *C. elegans* is discussed by Huang and Chalfie (1994), Hong and Driscoll (1994) and Tavernarakis and Driscoll (1997), and both Christensen and Corey (2007) and Ronan and Gillespie (2007) describe the part played by TRP channels in the nose rays. The structure of the amiloride sensitive Na^+-channel is described by Canessa (1994). The commonality of molecular mechanisms across nematodes, insects and vertebrates is reviewed by Garcia-Anoveros and Corey (1997). An excellent introduction to the spiders is provided by Foelix (1982) and Barth's many publications, especially Barth (2002, 2004), provide detail. Insect mechanoreception is described by Frazier (1985), Michelsen and Larsen (1985) and Schwartzkopff (1974); tympanal ears are reviewed in Hoy and Robert (1996). K.D. Roeder was responsible for much of the pioneering work on the neurophysiology and behaviour of moths in response to bat attack sonar: Roeder (1975); more recent work on moth acoustic physiology and behaviour is discussed in Spangler (1988). The original work on the columnar structure of the mammalian somaesthetic cortex is reported in Mountcastle (1957). Investigations of the plasticity of the somaesthetic cortex are described in Woolsey and Van Der Loos (1970) Cowan (1979), Jenkins *et al.* (1990), Elbert *et al.* (1995), Hamilton and Pascuel-Leone (1997), Yaest and Simons (1997) and an overview is provided by Buonomano and Merzenich (1998). The physiology and endocrinology of the 'de-arousal' induced by self- or mutual grooming is reviewed by Spruijt, van Noof and Gispen (1992).

Caenorhabditis Elegans

Christensen, A.P. and Corey, D.P. (2007) TRP channels in mechanosensation: direct or indirect activation? *Nature Reviews Neuroscience*, **8**, 510–21.

Hong, K. and Driscoll, M. (1994) A transmembrane domain of the putative channel subunit MEC-4 influences mechanotransduction and neurodegeneration in *C. elegans*. *Nature*, **367**, 470–3.

Huang, M. and Chalfie, M. (1994) Gene interactions affecting mechanosensory transduction in *Caenorhabditis elegans*. *Nature*, **367**, 470–3.

Kerkut, G.A. and Gilbert, L.I. (1985) *Comprehensive Insect Physiology, Biochemistry and Pharmacology*, Pergamon Press, Oxford.

Ronan, D. and Gillespie, P. (2007) Metazoan mechanotransduction mystery finally solved. *Nature Neuroscience*, **8**, 7–8.

Tavernarakis, N. and Driscoll, M. (1997) Molecular modelling of mechanotransduction in the Nematode *Caenorhabditis elegans*. *Annual Review of Physiology*, **59**, 659–89.

Spiders

Barth, F.G. (2002) *A Spider's World: Senses and Behaviour*, Springer, Berlin.

Barth, F.G. (2004) Spider mechanoreceptors. *Current Opinion in Neurobiology*, **14**, 145–422.

Foelix, R.F. (1982) *Biology of Spiders*, Harvard University Press, Cambridge, Mass.

Harris, D.J.P. and Mill, P.J. (1977) Observations on the leg receptors of *Ciniflo* (Araneida: Dictynidae) 1 External mechanorecptors. *J. Comp. Physiol.*, **119**, 37.

Insects

Frazier, J.L. (1985) Nervous system: sensory system, in *Fundamentals of Insect Physiology* (ed. M.S. Blum), John Wiley & Sons, Inc., New York.

Hoy, R.R. and Robert, D. (1996) Tympanal hearing in insects. *Annual Review of Entomology*, **41**, 433–50.

Michelsen, A. (1974) Hearing in invertebrates, in *Handbook of Sensory Physiology*, Vol. **V/1** (eds H. Autrum, *et al.*), Springer-Verlag, Berlin.

Markl, H. and Tautz, J. (1975) Sensitivity of hair receptors in caterpillars of *Barathra brassica* L. (Lepidoptera, Noctuidae) to particle movement in a sound field. *Journal of Comparative Physiology*, **99**, 79–87.

Michelsen, A. and Larsen, O.N. (1985) Hearing and sound, in *Comprehensive Insect Physiology, Biochemistry and Pharmacology*, Vol. **6** (eds G.A. Kerkut and L.I. Gilbert), Pergamon Press, Oxford.

Roeder, K.D. (1975) Neural transactions during acoustic stimulation of noctuid moths, in *Sensory Physiology and Behaviour* (eds R. Galum, *et al.*), Plenum, New York.

Schwartzkopff, J. (1974) Mechanoreception, in *The Physiology of Insecta*, 2nd edn (ed. M. Rockstein), Academic Press, New York.

Spangler, H.G. (1988) Moth hearing, defense, and communication. *Annual Review of Entomology*, **33**, 59–81.

Mammals

Cowan, W.M. (1979), The development of the brain. *Scientific American*, **241** (3), 116–21.

Elbert, T. *et al.* (1995) Increased cortical representation of the fingers of the left hand in string players. *Science*, **270**, 305–7.

Buonomano, D.V. and Merzenich, M.M. (1998) Cortical plasticity: from synapses to maps. *Annual Review of Neuroscience*, **21**, 149–86.

Hamilton, R.H. and Pascuel-Leone, A. (1998) Cortical plasticity associated with Braille learning. *Trends in Cognitive Sciences*, **2**, 168–74.

Iggo, A. (1982) Cutaneous sensory mechanisms, in *The Senses* (eds H.B. Barlow and J.D. Mollon), Cambridge University Press, Cambridge.

Jenkins, W.M. *et al.* (1990) Functional re-organisation of primary somatosensory cortex in adult owl monkeys after behaviourally controlled tactile stimulation. *Journal of Neurophysiology*, **63**, 82–104.

Mountcastle, V.B. (1957) Modality and topographic properties of single neurons of cat's somatic sensory cortex. *Journal of Neurophysiology*, **20**, 408–34.

Woolsey, T.A. and Van Der Loos, H. (1970) The Structural organisation of layer IV in the somatosensory region (S1) of mouse cerebral cortex. The description of a cortical field composed of discrete cytoarchitectonic units. *Brain Research*, **17**, 205–42.

Yaest, R. and Simons, D. (1997) Barrels in the desert: the Sde Beku workshop on neocortical circuits. *Neuron*, **19**, 231–37.

General

Canessa, C.M. (1994) Amiloride sensitive epithelial Na^+-channel is made of three homologous subunits. *Nature*, **367**, 463–7.

Garcia-Anoveros, J. and Corey, D.P. (1997) The molecules of mechanosensation. *Annual Review of Neuroscience*, **20**, 567–95.

Spruijt, B.M., van Noof, J.A.R.A.M. and Gispen, W.M. (1992) Ethology and neurobiology of grooming behaviour. *Physiological Reviews*, **72**, 825–52.

White, J.G. (1985) Neuronal connectivity in *Caenorhabditis elegans*. *Trends in Neurosciences*, **8**, 277–83.

CHAPTER 9: EQUILIBRIUM AND HEARING: THE USES OF HAIR CELLS

Hudspeth has been prominent in developing an understanding of the biophysics and molecular biology of hair cells. The two papers listed below, Hudspeth (1989, 1992), provide an overview of his work and his 1997 paper gives a valuable summary of the whole field. Other investigators are pursuing the topic as indicated, Gillespie and Corey (1997), in particular, providing an intriguing account of the way in which sensory adaptation may occur. A brief review of the genetics of deafness is given by Griffith and Friedman, 1999) and Yasunaga *et al.* (1999) describe the isolation of a gene causing nonsyndromic deafness. Pickles (1988) provides an overview account of the physiology of hearing with particularly good scanning electronmicrographs of cochlear hair cells. Lateral line systems are reviewed by Flocke (1971), Prosser and Brown (1962) and Sand (1984). The evolution of the membranous labyrinth is discussed in Romer (1970) and in more detail by Baird (1974) and Wever (1974). Clack (1997) reviews the evolution of the ear in the tetrapod vertebrates.

Hair Cell Biophysics

Flocke, A. (1965) Transducing mechanisms in lateral line canal organ receptors, in (ed. L. Frisch), *Sensory Receptors, Cold Spring Harbor Symposia in Quantitative Biology, XXX*, Cold Spring Harbor, New York.

Gillespie, P.G. (1995) Molecular machinery of auditory and vestibular transduction. *Current Opinion in Neurobiology*, **5**, 449–55.

Gillespie, P.G. and Corey, D.P. (1997) Myosin and adaptation by hair cells. *Neuron*, **19**, 955–58.

Gillespie, P.G., Dumont, R.A. and Kachar, B. (2005) Have we found the tip link, transduction channel and gating spring of the hair cell? *Current Opinion in Neurobiology*, **15**, 389–96.

Griffith, A.J. and Friedman, T.B. (1999) Making sense of sound. *Nature Genetics*, **21**, 347–49.

Hackney, C.M. and Furness, D.N. (1995) Mechanotransduction in vertebrate hair cells: structure and function of the stereociliary bundle. *American Journal of Physiology*, **268**, C215–21.

Hudspeth, A.J. (1989) How the ear's works work. *Nature*, **341**, 398–404.

Hudspeth, A.J. (1992) Hair-bundle mechanics and a model for mechanoelectrical transduction by hair cells, in *Sensory Transduction* (eds D.P. Corey and S.D. Roper), Rockefeller Press, New York, pp. 357–70.

Hudspeth, A.J. (1997) How hearing happens. *Neuron*, **19**, 947–50.

Pickles, J.O. (1988) *An Introduction to the Physiology of Hearing*, Academic Press, New York.

Pickles, J.O. and Corey, D.P. (1992) Mechanoelectrical transduction by hair cells. *Trends in Neurosciences*, **15**, 254–58.

Yasunaga, S. *et al.* (1999) A mutation in OTOF, encoding otoferlin, a FER-1-like protein, causes DFNB9, a nonsyndromic form of deafness. *Nature Genetics*, **21**, 363–69.

Lateral Line Canal

Flocke, Å. (1971) The lateral line organ mechanoreceptors, in *Fish Physiology*, Vol. **V** (eds W.S. Hoar and D.J. Randall), Academic Press, New York, pp. 241–63.

Prosser, C.L. and Brown, F.A. (1962) *Comparative Animal Physiology*, W.B. Saunders, Philadelphia.

Sand, O. (1984) Lateral line systems, in *Comparative Physiology of Sensory Systems* (eds L. Bolis, R.D. Keynes and S.H.P. Maddrell), Cambridge University Press, Cambridge.

Evolution of the Ear

Art, J.J. (1984) Auditory function at the receptor level in reptiles, in *Comparative Physiology of Sensory Systems* (eds L. Bolis, R.D. Keynes and S.H.P. Maddrell), Cambridge University Press, Cambridge.

Baird, I.L. (1974) Anatomical features of the inner ear in submammalian vertebrates, in *Handbook of Sensory Physiology* Vol. **V/1** (eds H. Autrum, *et al.*), Springer-Verlag, Berlin.

Chung, S.-H., Pettigrew, A. and Anson, M. (1978) Dynamics of the amphibian middle ear. *Nature*, **272**, 142–47.

Clack, J.A. (1997) The evolution of tetrapod ears and the fossil record. *Brain, Behaviour and Evolution*, **50**, 198–212.

Feng, A.S. and Shofner, W.P. (1981) Peripheral basis of sound localisation in anurans, acoustic properties of the frog's ear. *Hearing Research*, **5**, 201–16.

Romer, A.S. (1970) *The Vertebrate Body*, 4th edn, W.B. Saunders, Philadelphia.

Wever, E.G. (1974) The evolution of vertebrate hearing, in *Handbook of Sensory Physiology* Vol. **V/1** (eds H. Autrum, *et al.*), Springer-Verlag, Berlin.

Vestibular System

Benson, A.J. (1982) The vestibular sensory system, in *The Senses* (eds H.B. Barlow and J.D. Mollon), Cambridge University Press, Cambridge.

Freeman, W.H. and Bracegirdle, B. (1976) *An Atlas of Advanced Histology*, Heinemann, London.

Smith, C.U.M. (1970) *The Brain: Towards an Understanding*, Faber and Faber, London.

CHAPTER 10: CEREBRAL ANALYSIS

The vestibular pathway is described in detail in Wilson and Jones (1979). It is worth noting that both nystagmus and motion sickness are open to adaptation. In the case of nystagmus, experiments with inverting spectacles have shown that after a week or so of adaptation, it will be reversed. Similarly motion sickness normally disappears after a few days or weeks. Animal experimentation has shown that this adaptation depends on the flocular lobe of the cerebellum and its projections to the vestibular system. Thus, for most of us, sea sickness is a temporary phase on a long voyage. The significance of the subcortical nuclei in the auditory pathway is discussed by Neff, Diamond and Casseday (1975) and Masterton (1992). Konishi (1992, 1993) and Cohen and Knudsen (1999) describe the results of neurophysiological investigation of the highly developed auditory brain of the barn owl. The owl's auditory brain is equalled by that of the bat and three valuable papers are listed which give information on the subtle neurophysiology underlying the microchiropteran echolatory way of life (Neuweiler, 1990; Suga, 1995; Sullivan, 1986). Suga, who has made the major contribution to this work, has also been interested in relating bat auditory mechanisms to those at work in the human speech cortices (Suga, 1995). Otoacoustic emissions from human and other mammalian ears are reviewed in Probst, Lonsbury-Martin and Martin (1981). The human auditory cortex is described by Brugge and Reale (1985) and its most sophisticated operation, human language is, as emphasized in the text, a vast subject and one which has been investigated for centuries. Stephen Pinker (1994) still gives one of the best modern surveys and the other references listed below report investigations of its neurobiological substrata. Harnad, Steklis and Lancaster (1976) edit a comprehensive overview of its evolutionary origins and development whilst Fisher, Lai and Monaco (2003) and Scharff and Haesler (2005) review the significance of the *FoxP2* gene. Although there has not been space in the text to consider birdsong, in many respects the only analogue of language in the nonmammalian world, the publications of Bottjer and Arnold (1997), Brenowitz, Margoliash and Nordeen (1997), Nottebohm (2005) and Breneowitz and Beecher (2005) can form starting points for those interested in contemporary analyses and Pepperberg (2000) reviews the work on parrots which suggests that these birds, at least, may have the rudiments of grammar. Finally, the philosopher, Thomas Nagel, asks the question which we must all have pondered and shows that it leads to the heart of the mind–brain problem (Nagel, 1974).

Subcortical Pathways

Brenowitz, E.A., Margoliash, D. and Nordeen, K.W. (1997) An introduction to birdsong and the Avian song system. *J. Neurobiol.*, **33**, 495–500.

Evans, E.F. (1972) The frequency response and other properties of single fibres in guinea pig cochlear nerve. *Journal of Physiology*, **226**, 263–87.

Evans, E.F. (1982) Functional anatomy of the visual system, in *The Senses* (eds H.B. Barlow and J.D. Mollon), Cambridge University Press, Cambridge.

Masterton, R.B. (1992) Role of the central auditory system in hearing: the new direction. *Trends in Neurosciences*, **15**, 280–4.

Neff, W.D., Diamond, I.T. and Casseday, J.H. (1975) Behavioural studies of auditory discrimination: central nervous system, in *Handbook of Sensory Physiology: Auditory System*, Vol. **V/2** (eds W.D. Keidel and W.D. Neff), Springer-Verlag, New York.

Wilson, V.J. and Melville Jones, G. (1979) *Mammalian Vestibular Physiology*, Plenum Press, New York.

Auditory Space in Barn Owls

Adolphs, R. (1993) Bilateral inhibition generates neuronal responses tuned to interaural level differences in the auditory brainstem of the barn owl. *Journal of Neuroscience*, **13**, 3647–68.

Cohen, Y.E. and Knudsen, E.I. (1999) Maps versus clusters: different representations of auditory space in the midbrain and forebrain. *Trends in Neuroscience*, **22**, 128–35.

Konishi, M. (1992) The neural algorithm for sound localisation in the owl. *Harvey Lectures*, **86**, 47–64.

Konishi, M. (1993) Listening with two ears. *Scientific American*, **268** (4), 34–41.

Koppl, C. (1997) Phase locking to high frequencies in the auditory nerve and cochlear nucleus magnocellularis of the barn owl, *Tyto alba. Journal of Neuroscience*, **17**, 3312–21.

Primate Auditory Cortex

Brugge, J.F. and Reale, R.A. (1985) Auditory cortex, in *Cerebral Cortex* (eds A. Peters and E.G. Jones), Plenum Publishing, New York.

Whitfield, I.C. and Evans, E.F. (1965) Responses of auditory neurons to stimuli of changing frequency. *Journal of Neurophysiology*, **28**, 655–72.

Gil-da-Costa, R., Martin, A., Lopes, M.A. *et al.* (2006) Species specific calls activate homologs of Broca's and Wernicke's areas in the macaque. *Nature Neuroscience*, **9**, 1064–70.

Bat Echolocation

Neuweiler, G. (1990) Auditory adaptations for prey capture in echolocating bats. *Physiological. Reviews*, **70**, 615–41.

Suga, N. (1995) Processing of auditory information carried by species-specific complex sounds, in *The Cognitive Neurosciences* (ed. M.S. Gazzaniga) MIT Press, Cambridge, Ma., pp. 295–313.

Suga, N., Yan, J. and Zhang, Y. (1997) Cortical maps for hearing and egocentric selection for self-organisation. *Trends in Cognitive Sciences*, **1**, 13–20.

Sullivan, W.E. (1986) Processing of acoustic temporal patterns in barn owls and echolocating bats, similar mechanisms for the generation of neural place representations in auditory space. *Brain Behav. Evol.* **28**, 109–21.

Human Auditory Cortex and Speech

Damasio, A.R. and Geschwind, N. (1984) The neural basis of language. *Ann. Rev. Neurosci.*, **7**, 127–47.

Eimas, P.D. *et al.* (1971) Speech perception in infants. *Science*, **171**, 103–4.

Fitch, R.H., Miller, S. and Tallal, P. (1997) Neurobiology of speech. *Annual Review of Neuroscience*, **20**, 331–53.

Geschwind, N. *et al.* (1968) Isolation of the speech area. *Neuropsychologia*, **6**, 327–40.

Harnad, S.R., Steklis, H.D. and Lancaster, J. (eds) (1976) Origins of language and speech. *Annals of the New York Academy of Science*, **280**, 1–914.

Liberman, A.M. *et al.* (1957) The discrimination of speech sounds within and across phoneme boundaries. *Journal of Experimental Psychology*, **54**, 358–68.

Miller, J.L. and Eimas, P.D. (1995) Speech perception: from signal to word. *Annual Review of Psychology*, **46**, 467–92.

Pinker, S. (1994) *The Language Instinct*, Penguin, Harmondsworth.

Springer, S.P. (1979) Speech perception and the biology of language, in *Handbook of Behavioural Neurobiology, Neuropsychology*, Vol. **2** (ed. M.S. Gazzaniga), Plenum Press, New York.

Suga, N. (1995) Processing of auditory information carried by species-specific complex sounds, in *The Cognitive Neurosciences* (ed. M.S. Gazzaniga), MIT Press, Cambridge, Ma, pp. 295–313.

Werker, J. and Tees, R.C. (1992) The Organisation and reorganisation of human speech perception. *Annual Review of Neuroscience*, **15**, 377–402.

Young, J.Z. (1978) *Programs of the Brain*, Oxford University Press, Oxford.

Language and the *FoxP2* Gene

Breneowitz, E.A. and Beecher, M.D. (2005) Song learning in birds: diversity and plasticity, opportunities and challenges. *Trends in Neurosciences*, **28**, 127–32.

Fisher, S.E., Lai, C.S. and Monaco, A.P. (2003) Deciphering the genetic basis of speech and language disorders. *Annual Review of Neuroscience*, **26**, 57–80.

Gang, L. *et al.* (2007) Accelerated FoxP2 evolution in echolocating bats. *PloS ONE*, **2** (9), e900. doi: 10.1371.

Lai, C.S. *et al.* (2001) A forkhead-domain gene is mutated in a severe speech and language disorder. *Nature*, **413**, 519–23.

Nottebohm, F. (2005) The neural basis of birdsong. *PloS Biology*, **3** (5), e164, doi: 10.1371/journal.pbio.oo 30164.

Pepperberg, I.M. (2000) *The Alex Studies: Cognitive and Communicative Abilities of Grey Parrots*, Harvard University Press, Boston, MA.

Scharff, C. and Haesler, S. (2005) An evolutionary perspective on FoxP2: strictly for the birds. *Current Opinion in Neurobiology*, **15**, 694–703.

Callosectomy

Sperry, R.W. (1964) The great cerebral commissure. *Scientific American*, **210** (1), 42–52.

General

Bottjer, S.W. and Arnold, A.P. (1997) Developmental plasticity in neural circuits for a learned behaviour. *Annual Review of Neuroscience*, **20**, 459–81.

Hudspeth, A.J. (1997) How hearing happens. *Neuron*, **19**, 947–50.

Nagel, T. (1974) What is it like to be a bat. *Philosophical Review*, **83**, 435–50.

Probst, R., Lonsbury-Martin, B.L. and Martin, G.K. (1991) A review of otoacoustic emissions. *Journal of the Acoustical Society of America*, **89**, 2027–67.

PART III: CHEMOSENSITIVITY

When from a long distant past nothing subsists, after the people are dead, after the things are broken and scattered, still, alone, more fragile, but with more vitality, more unsubstantial, more persistent, more faithful, the smell and taste of things remain poised a long time, like souls, ready to remind us, waiting and hoping for their moment, amid the ruins of all the rest; and bear unfaltering, in the tiny and almost impalpable drop of their essence, the vast structure of recollection.

Marcel Proust: *Remembrance of Things Past (Swann's Way)* trs. C.K. Scott Moncrieff

All animals are sensitive to their molecular environment. This is important not only in food discrimination, but also in mating, mother–infant relations, territoriality and other social behaviours. In the vertebrates the senses of smell and taste lead into evolutionarily ancient parts of the brain. This perhaps accounts for their emotional resonance: a resonance which was famously caught by Marcel Proust, when the taste of a tea-soaked madeleine (a variety of tea cake) brought back such vivid memories that he felt himself to have finally recaptured past time. This, too, emphasizes that the ancient 'smell brain' has developed connections into the neocortex. These connections have in fact been traced through the thalamus to the orbito-frontal cortex (smell) and the post central gyrus and insula (taste).

Unlike the mechanoreceptors of Part Two, all metazoan chemoreceptors (so far as is presently known) make use of 7TM receptors and G-protein membrane biochemistry to transduce the external stimulus into an intracellular signal (Chapter 1). Chemoreception is thus not nearly so instantaneous as mechanoreception. What chemoreceptor cells lack in rapidity of response is, however, more than made up for in sophistication. It has been estimated that up to 2% of the mammalian genome may be taken up with genes specifying about 1000 different olfactory receptor molecules. The mammalian vomeronasal organ takes up another 100–200 genes. Similarly, a large percentage of the *Drosophila* genome (and by implication that of other insects) is also devoted to olfactory receptor molecules. The chemoreceptors of the nematode, *Caenorhabditis elegans*, are grouped into four large unrelated families and, again, involve over 1000 genes. In spite of this large number of genes, the chemosensory behaviour of *C. elegans* is quite restricted: feeding, egg laying, mating. Unlike the case in mammals, each chemosensory cell of *C. elegans* expresses several 7TM receptors.

The 7TM proteins in all these different systems seem to have evolved independently. This serves to emphasize the suspicion that we know very little of the nature of the 'taste worlds' in which other animals live. Although trained humans can discriminate at least 10 000 different odors, many animals and perhaps most mammals can recognize many more. They live in far richer worlds of tastes and scents and smells.

The chemical senses are customarily classified into three: **general chemical sense, olfaction and gustation**.

Biology of Sensory Systems, Second Edition   C.U.M. Smith
© 2008 John Wiley & Sons, Ltd

All organisms display the general chemical sense. We have only to allow a drop of acid to contact our skin to recognize that this is the case in ourselves. This sense is mediated by free nerve endings in the skin. Some vertebrates have, in addition, a fourth chemosensory system consisting of **solitary chemoreceptor cells (SCCs)**. This system is most well developed in two species of teleost fish: the sea robins (*Prionotus spp.*) and rocklings (*Ciliata spp.*). The SCCs are scattered in epithelium covering the fins and are involved in food detection and sensing of predators. But the chemical senses that are of most interest to us in this book are the latter two: olfaction and gustation. For here the chemical sensitivity is greatly heightened and, most importantly, exquisite discrimination between different chemical stimulants has evolved.

We shall begin in Chapter 11 with a brief account of chemosensitivity in prokaryocytes. We shall see that the techniques of molecular biology have provided a nearly complete understanding of this simple but all-important process in *Escherichia coli*. We shall then go on, in Chapter 12, to look at the very important role chemoreceptors play in monitoring the constitution of the 'internal environment' in mammals. In Chapter 13 we shall take up the topic of gustation, the sense of taste and then, in Chapter 14, finish this part of the book with an account of olfaction, the sense of smell.

11

CHEMOSENSITIVITY IN PROKARYOCYTES

Primordial emergence of chemosensitivity - motile bacteria - structure and functioning of prokaryotic flagella - 'smooth' and 'tumbling' motion of *E. coli* - chemotaxis - binding and receptor-transducer (R–T) proteins - sensory adaptation - genetic analysis of R–T proteins - biochemistry of the intracellular signalling pathway between R–T and effector - sensory adaptation caused by methylation. **Concluding remarks**: running a sensory system into the molecular ground.

Chemosensitivity undoubtedly emerged very early in the history of life on earth. From the beginning, prokaryocytes were immersed in an aqueous medium. An ability to sense the chemical consitution of this medium could not have been anything but crucial to survival. We may speculate that, once having hit upon a satisfactory mechanism, there was little pressure to change it. As in the case of the mechanoreceptors we considered in Part Two, the evolutionary process cannot go back and start over. It elaborates and develops what it has hit upon. It 'tinkers' with what it has until it adjusts it to near perfection. Nevertheless, as we shall see, the molecular biology of chemosensitivity in bacteria such as *Escherichia coli* and *Salmonella typhimurium* is in some ways markedly different from that which lies at the basis of olfaction and gustation in the Metazoa.

There is no doubt that contemporary motile bacteria are sensitive to the chemical substances in their environment. It has long been known that they will swim up a concentration gradient of an attractant chemical. They can both sense the material in the environment and act on the sensation. How do they do it?

Motile bacteria are propelled by flagella. Prokaryotic flagella are far simpler than those of the eukaryotes. They consist of a single tubular array of flagellin subunits twisted into a helix. They also have a very different mechanism for producing motion. Instead of the sliding filament system believed to be at work in eukaryotic flagella, they have the distinction of being the only organic structures so far known to employ a rotary mechanism (Figure 11.1). The cellular end of the flagellum is rotated at about 100 revolutions per second by a mechanism energized by a transmembrane hydrogen ion gradient.

11.1 CHEMOSENTIVITY IN *E. COLI*

Most flagellated bacteria have more than one flagellum. *E. coli* has five to ten. When they all rotate

---

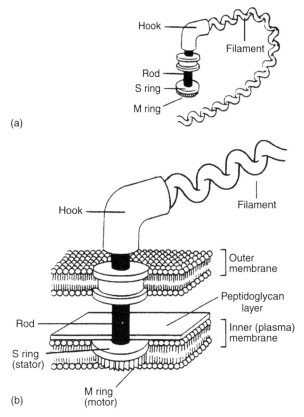

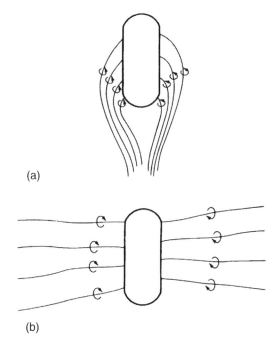

(a)

(b)

Figure 11.2 Anticlockwise and clockwise rotation of bacterial flagella. (a) anticlockwise rotation. The flagella stream together as a single bundle and propel the bacterium forward. (b) Clockwise rotation. The individual flagella pull away from the bacterium. According to the varying pull of the different flagella the bacterium veers from one side to the other and tumbles over itself hither and thither.

Figure 11.1 Rotary mechanism of a bacterial flagellum. The motile machinery penetrates both the outer and inner membrane boundary membranes of the bacterium. Energy derived from a proton gradient across the membrane causes the M-ring to rotate relative to the S-ring (or stator) at about 100 revolutions per second. The stator is held steady by embedment in the peptidoglycan layer of the inner membrane. A rod links the M-ring to a 'hook' and thence to the helical flagellar filament. A bearing in the outer membrane acts as a seal. From Adler, J. (1983) Cold Spring Harbor Symposia in Quantitative Biology, XLVIII, 2, 803–4. Copyright © 1983, Cold Spring Harbor Laboratory Press.

in the anticlockwise direction, the bacterium swims forward smoothly. Things, however, are very different if they rotate in the clockwise sense. In this case, because of the helical structure of the flagellum, the flagella all pull outwards resulting in an irregular 'tumbling' motion (Figure 11.2).

If the swimming of a bacterial cell is followed under a microscope it is seen to consist of a series of smooth 'runs' (several seconds) interspersed with episodes (about 0.1 s) of chaotic tumbling. When the cell comes out of its tumble, it will set off smoothly again but in a completely random direction. If, however, the cell is placed in a gradient of chemical attractant it is found that when the swimming is in the direction of the source, fewer tumbles occur than when it is moving in any other direction. The net result is that the bacterium migrates up the concentration gradient towards the source of the attractant (Figure 11.3).

Clearly this phenomenon provides a valuable system for the investigation of the general problem of chemoreception. The flagella of a bacterium may be attached to a glass slide and the rotation of the cell observed in response to various chemicals. The genetics of *E. coli* are, of course, very well known, so the sensory system may also be examined by genetic techniques.

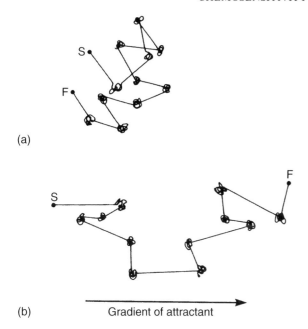

(a)

(b) Gradient of attractant

Figure 11.3 Bacterial migration along a concentration gradient of chemical attractant. (a) Path in the absence of an attractant gradient. The swim alternates between periods when the flagella rotate in an anticlockwise sense giving a smooth straight 'run' and periods when they rotate in a clockwise sense when the bacterium 'tumbles'. The direction the bacterium is facing when the tumbling ends is completely random, hence the next run will be in a random direction. The bacterium thus makes no consistent progress but swims in an erratic circular course. (b) Path in the presence of an attractant. The duration (and hence length) of the run between tumbles is increased when the bacterium is moving up the attractant gradient and decreased when it is moving in the opposite direction. Hence, although periodic tumbles still occur and randomize the direction of the run, the overall movement of the bacterium is nevertheless up the gradient towards the attractant's source. S = start; F = finish.

It has been shown that detection of attractant (or repellant) molecules is by way of transmembrane proteins. There are two mechanisms. In the first, an attractant molecule interacts with a **binding protein (BP)** in the bacterium's periplasmic space, causing a conformational change so that it 'fits' one or other of the transmembrane proteins. This has been shown to be the case with sugars and peptides. Several such BPs have been isolated: for example galactose binding protein (GBP), ribose binding protein (RBP), maltose binding protein (MBP) and dipeptide binding protein (DBP). In the second mechanism, the

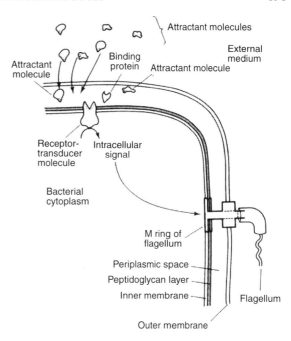

Figure 11.4 Interaction of attractant molecules with binding and receptor–transducer molecules. Attractants are of two types. Either they fit the active site of the receptor–transducer molecule directly, or they are 'adapted' to do so by attaching to a binding protein in the periplasmic space. In either case, the activated receptor–transducer molecule generates a signal (Figure 11.6) which affects the direction of rotation of the flagellar motor and, hence, the frequency of tumbling.

attractant interacts with the transmembrane protein directly. Amino acids are examples of this second category. The transmembrane proteins have the ability to affect the rotation of the flagella. In other words, they are able to transduce the signal represented by the attractant molecule as well as detect it. To distinguish them from the binding proteins in the periplasmic space they are known as **receptor–transducer (R–T) proteins** (Figure 11.4).

This system has one other very important feature. It shows sensory adaptation. This, as we have seen, is a feature of all sensory systems. In the case of *E. coli*, it is found that a sudden immersion in attractant suppresses tumbling. But after a time it begins to be seen again and, in a few minutes, returns to its normal frequency. This adaptation, moreover, is restricted to the specific attractant molecule. Addition of a different attractant inhibits the tumbling in the usual way. The biological significance of adaptation or desensitization is obvious.

11.1.1 Molecular Genetics

Because its molecular biology is so well known, *E.coli* provides a valuable system for examining all these processes.

11.1.1.1 Binding Proteins (BPs)

The detailed molecular structure of a number of binding proteins has been determined. The GBP has, for instance, been successfully subjected to high resolution X-ray diffraction studies and its overall architecture and binding site configuration solved. It has been shown to consist of two 'wings' separated by a crevice which contains the binding site. When the site is occupied by the substrate – galactose or glucose – the wings 'close' by moving towards each other through an angle of $18°$. This alteration in three-dimensional conformation enables the binding protein to interact with the appropriate transmembrane R–T molecule. There is evidence that other binding proteins have a similar three-dimensional conformation. It is interesting to note that both insect olfactory sensilla (Chapter 14, Section 14.1.2) and mammalian olfactory cilia (Chapter 14, Section 14.2.2) also make use of binding proteins to capture oderant molecules and carry them to membrane olfactory receptor molecules.

11.1.1.2 Receptor–Transducer (R–T) Proteins

The genes for a number of the R–T proteins in *E. coli* have been isolated by the techniques of molecular genetics and their nucleotide sequences determined. The best known of these genes are the *tsr*, *tar*, *trg* and *tap* genes. They encode four R–T proteins: Tsr, sensitive to serine (attractant) and leucine (repellant); Tar, sensitive to aspartate and maltose (attractants) and Co^{2+} and Ni^{2+} (repellants); Trg, sensitive to galactose and ribose attached to binding proteins (attractants); and Tap, sensitive to dipeptides attached to binding proteins.

From the nucleotide sequences the amino acid structure of these R–T proteins can be deter-

mined and hydropathic analysis performed to predict membrane-spanning segments. All four of the proteins consist of over five hundred amino acids and appear to have two transmembrane sequences. In this respect they are radically different from the 7TM receptor proteins of vertebrate gustatory and olfactory cells. On the other hand, there is strong homology between the four bacterial R–T proteins, especially in the cytoplasmic domain where the processes of signalling to the flagellar apparatus and sensory adaptation occur.

Figure 11.5 indicates that the R–T molecule is held in the membrane so that an amino acid sequence of about 150 residues projects into the periplasmic space. This forms the attractant and/or repellant binding site. The major part of the molecule from about residue 215 to the carboxy terminal end lies in the bacterial cytoplasm. This part of the molecule is

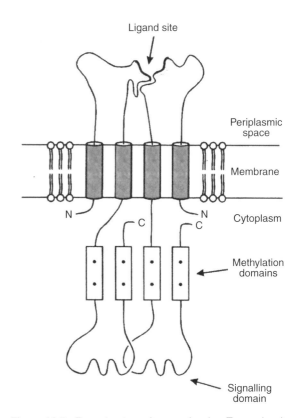

Figure 11.5   Receptor–transducer molecules. Two molecules are shown. As the figure shows they associate closely together to form a dimer. Each contributes to the ligand site. The cytoplasmic methylation and signalling domains are shown.

highly conserved across the four R–T proteins studied, generates the signal to the flagellar apparatus and is involved in the adaptation mechanism. The fully formed R–T protein is a dimer built of two of these 50 kDa polypeptides. There is evidence that they are randomly distributed in the plasmalemma.

11.1.1.3 Signal Transduction

Chemotactic signalling is initiated by the binding of the attractant molecule or of the attractant binding molecule complex to the periplasmic domain of the R–T molecule. There is evidence that this causes a conformational change which is transmitted through the membrane to alter the configuration of the cytoplasmic domain. This altered cytoplasmic domain then initiates a biochemical signalling cascade which ultimately affects the activity of the flagellum.

Genetic analysis has allowed the elements of this signalling pathway to be isolated and analysed. It consists of four significant proteins: **CheA**, **CheW**, **CheY** and **CheZ** (Che for 'chemotactic'). CheA and CheY transmit the 'tumble' signal from the receptor–transducer to the flagellum (Figure 11.6). When CheY attaches to the flagellar motor, it causes the flagellum to rotate in a clockwise direction, thus inducing tumbling. This pathway is inhibited when an attractant molecule binds externally to the binding protein and the complex so formed attaches to an appropriate R–T molecule. When, however, a repellant binds to the binding protein the opposite effect occurs, the receptor–transducer is activated, the pathway to the motor is, in its turn, activated and the flagellum turns in clockwise sense. Hence in the presence of an attractant, the bacterium will move up the concentration gradient and, in the presence of a repellent, will continue random tumbling. When neither attractant nor repellant are present, a balance of activation and deactivation ensures that smooth runs are interspersed with tumbles.

The biochemistry responsible for activation and deactivation is shown in Figure 11.6. When a repellant attaches to an R–T protein, the cytoplasmic domain of the latter binds CheW and induces the self-phosphorylation of CheA. CheA's phosphate group is rapidly passed on to CheY. It is only the phosphorylated form of CheY which can induce clockwise motion in the flagellum. The final protein in the

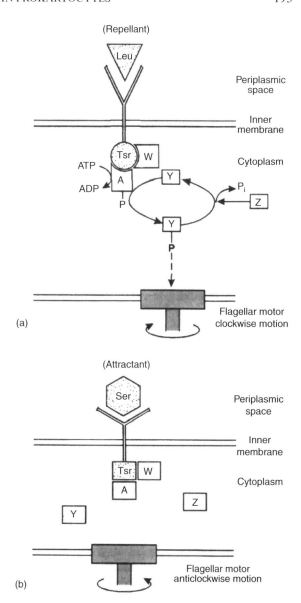

(a)

(b)

Figure 11.6 Molecular signalling in the *E. coli* chemosensory system. (a) The Tsr receptor–transducer protein accepts a repellant molecule (Leu). CheW and CheA are activated. CheA accepts phosphate from ATP and passes it on CheY. CheY diffuses to the flagellar motor and induces a clockwise rotation and hence tumbling. CheY is eventually dephosphorylated by CheZ. (b) The Tsr receptor–transducer accepts an attractant molecule (Ser). The consequent conformational change inactivates CheA and CheW so that CheY remains unphosphorylated and consequently inactive. The flagellum resumes its anticlockwise motion and the bacterium swims smoothly forward. A = CheA; W = CheW; Y = CheY; Z = CheZ. Data from Bourrett, Borkovich and Simon, 1991.

system, CheZ, eventually dephosphorylates CheY and thus terminates its influence.

Sensory adaptation occurs when the bacterium finds itself in an unvarying concentration of attractant. This is due to methylation of the R–T protein. For this reason these proteins are sometimes referred to as methyl-adapting chemotaxis proteins (MCPs). That adaptation is due to methylation was shown by the isolation of mutants in which methylation domains of the R–T proteins (Figure 11.5) were inactivated. Such mutants did not adapt; in the presence of an attractant they would cease tumbling for hours, even days, instead of for only a minute or so. It appears, therefore, that when a R–T protein is deactivated by binding an attractor, it exposes extra methylation sites. An enzyme, methyl transferase, attaches up to eight methyl groups. This increases the activity of the R–T protein again and, by the signalling system described above, causes tumbling to commence once more.

The great virtue of this system lies in the fact that the genetics of E. coli are so well known and so easily manipulated. The same system is at work in Salmonella typhimurium. The fact that these two bacteria (one a parasite within the gut of mammals, the other in the eggs of birds) have evolved separately for at least 150 million years suggests that similar chemosensitive mechanisms are probably widespread in the bacteria. There are good prospects for following up the successful genetic analysis of the R–T proteins and the cytoplasmic signalling system to provide a complete understanding of bacterial chemotaxis. This would provide the first instance in which a complete sensory motor system has been run into its molecular ground.

11.2 CONCLUDING REMARKS

The chemosensitivity of E. coli, perhaps even more than the mechanosensitivity we considered in Chapter 5, provides tempting opportunities for analysis by the extremely powerful methods of modern molecular biology. Over the last twenty or thirty years the application of these techniques has, as we saw above, disclosed the molecular mechanisms at work in great detail. We are approaching a complete understanding of how the bacterium not only senses chemicals in its aqueous environment but also reacts to them, either by moving towards or away from their source. The integrated activity of all the R–T proteins determines the swimming of the prokaryocyte in a complex chemical environment. The molecular mechanisms mimic in small the hugely more complex olfactory and gustatory physiology of members of the animal kingdom. Although the intracellular chemotactic signalling pathway probably has no counterpart in the world of the Metazoa, the role of the binding and R–T proteins foreshadows the molecular biology of animal gustatory and olfactory receptor cells. Indeed, it does more than merely foreshadow it. Molecular biologists have been able to stitch together elements of S. typhimurium, tar protein and mammalian insulin receptor to produce a functional R–T protein and there is also evidence that CheY and the Ras proteins of mammalian intercellular signalling have some evolutionary relationship. Although the eukaryocytes and later the animals broke away from the bacterial kingdoms inconceivably long ago (Figures 4.2 and 4.3), we can nevertheless still discern faint traces of their common ancestry.

12

MAMMALIAN CHEMO-ENTERORECEPTORS

Claude Bernard and the milieu intérieur: chemoreceptors monitor crucial parameters of the milieu intérieur - partial pressure (Pa) of respiratory gases is one such parameter. **Location of PaO$_2$ and PaCO$_2$ receptors**: carotid bodies, aortic bodies, medullary cells - evolutionary origin of carotid bodies - carotid labyrinth. **Histology**: type 1 and type 2 (sustentacular) cells - type 1 cells associated with large capillaries and afferent nerve endings - contain dense-cored catecholamine vesicles - form synaptic appositions with afferent nerve endings. **Physiology**: high blood flow rate - effect of varying PaO$_2$ and PaCO$_2$ - increased PaCO$_2$ stimulates - carotid bodies more sensitive than aortic bodies - reflex effect on respiratory rate - similar effect caused by fall in PaO$_2$ - medullary cells more sensitive than either carotid or aortic bodies - hypercapnia - reflexes other than respiratory to changes in PaCO$_2$ and PaO$_2$. **Biochemistry**: PaO$_2$ below normal closes specific K$^+$-channels - depolarisation - opening of voltage-dependent Ca^{2+}-channels - release of catecholamines on to afferent nerve endings - maybe membrane-bound haem protein senses PaO$_2$; PaCO$_2$ above normal - increased internal H$^+$ - H$^+$/Na$^+$ exchange - Na$^+$/Ca^{2+} exchange increases internal Ca^{2+} - release of catecholamines on to afferent nerve endings. **Concluding remarks**: crucial role of enteroreceptors - only when something is amiss are we conscious of their importance.

Every student beginning physiology is presented with Claude Bernard's famous dictum: 'La constance du milieu intérieur est la condition de la vie libre'. Bernard was a nineteenth-century experimental physiologist who was born near Villefranche in 1813. His major contribution was, as he says, 'to urge the belief that animals have really two environments: a *milieu extérieur* in which the organism is situated, and a *milieu intérieur* in which the tissue elements live'. This concept has proved enormously productive. We nowadays know that all the major parameters of a mammal's internal environment – pH, O$_2$, CO$_2$, temperature, osmotic pressure, hydrostatic pressure, glucose concentration and so on – are kept remarkably constant. It has been argued that this ability to stabilize the internal environment has been largely responsible for the great evolutionary 'success' of the mammals and birds. These so-called 'higher vertebrates' have been able to make a living throughout the globe, from the Arctic to the Antarctic, from, in the words of the hymn, 'Greenland's icy mountains to India's coral strand'. It can

Biology of Sensory Systems, Second Edition   C.U.M. Smith
© 2008 John Wiley & Sons, Ltd

also be argued that the great evolutionary advantage that maintaining a constant internal environment has conferred on these animals has forced the development of their extraordinarily complex anatomy and physiology. For much of this complexity is, precisely, to ensure that the internal environment, the medium which bathes the body's cells, is maintained at its optimal condition.

We saw, in Chapter 6, that mechanoreceptors located in the plasma membranes of the magnocellular neurons of the mammalian hypothalamus monitored variations in the osmolarity of the extracellular fluid (ECF). Similarly, in Chapter 7, we saw how other mechanoreceptors played crucial roles in monitoring the body's posture and the ongoing state of its muscles and joints. In this chapter we shall see how chemoreceptors are indispensable in monitoring the chemical parameters of the internal environment. They form an array of detectors feeding information about the partial pressures (Pa) of oxygen (O_2) and carbon dioxide (CO_2) and the hydrogen ion content (pH) of the blood, its glucose content and so on into the central computer of the CNS. Mechano- and thermoreceptors play similar roles for blood pressure and temperature. It would lead us too far into the thickets of cardiovascular physiology to attempt any complete account of these sensors and the reflexes they induce. That is more properly the province of textbooks of physiology and endocrinology. However, it would not be proper to give an account of chemoreceptors without some reference to one of these vital enteroreceptors. In this chapter we shall look at the monitoring and control of the partial pressures of the **respiratory gases, O_2 and CO_2**, in the ECF. The partial pressure of carbon dioxide is also related to the pH of the ECF, for carbon dioxide combines with water (H_2O) to give carbonic acid (H_2CO_3), which dissociates to give H^+ and HCO_3^-. Although blood plasma has powerful buffering systems that tend to mop up excess H^+ ions, this is not always the case in other compartments of the ECF.

12.1 LOCATION OF MAMMALIAN CHEMORECEPTORS FOR PaO₂ AND PaCO₂

The *carotid bodies*, located on the internal carotid artery just past the point at which the common carotids bifurcate, are the most important peripheral

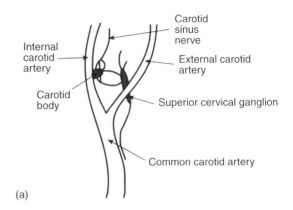

(a)

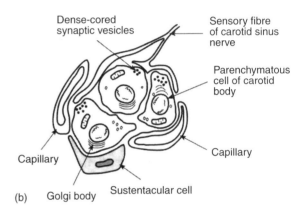

(b)

Figure 12.1 (a) Position of a carotid body at the bifurcation of the common carotid artery. Innervation is via the carotid sinus nerve and the superior cervical ganglion. (b) Cellular structure of a fragment of carotid body. Two types of cell are shown: parenchymatous, or type 1, and sustentacular or type 2. The proportion of parenchymatous chemoreceptor cells to sustentacular cells is about 3–5 to 1. Further explanation in text. After Gonzalez, C. et al. (1992).

chemo-enteroreceptors for respiratory gases in the mammalian body (Figure 12.1). They also contain important stretch receptors sensitive to arterial blood pressure. Other significant respiratory gas chemoreceptors take the form of **aortic bodies** on the arch of the aorta and its major branches. The latter are not found in all mammals. They are, for instance, present in dogs and cats, but not in rabbit, mouse or rat. On the other hand, abdominal chemoreceptors are well developed in mouse and the rat. They are located on the stomach wall, adjacent to the vagus nerve as it leaves the oesophagus and in the coeliac and hepatic plexuses. In addition to these peripheral receptors, '**central' chemoreceptors**, highly sensitive to the partial pressures of oxygen (PaO_2) and the partial pressures of carbon dioxide ($PaCO_2$), are located bilaterally in the **medulla**.

The evolutionary origin of mammalian carotid bodies provides an interesting study in comparative anatomy and physiology. The sequence of diagrams in Figure 12.2 shows that they evolved from the third aortic arch of our Piscean ancestors. In the amphibia we see that the gill capillaries have been transformed into the so-called **carotid labyrinth**, which ensures that only the most oxygenated blood reaches the brain. By the time we reach the reptiles and the other amniota, a further transformation has occurred and the structure is well on the way to becoming the chemoreceptor which monitors PaO_2 and $PaCO_2$ in our own blood.

12.2 STRUCTURE

All the peripheral chemoreceptor tissue has much the same histological constitution. The **carotid bodies** consist of two types of cell (type 1 or parenchymatous and type 2 or sustentacular) associated with a dense network of large capillaries (Figure 12.1). **Type 1** *cells* are the commonest. They have the ultrastructure of secretory cells with well formed Golgi bodies, endoplasmic reticulum and (unlike other secretory cells) contain a large population of **dense-cored synaptic vesicles** containing **catecholamines**. Associated with these cells are not only large capillaries but also numerous nerve fibres. Many of the dense-cored synaptic vesicles of the type 1 cells gather near synaptic appositions between these cells and nerve fibres. Although most of the nerve fibres are sensory there are also some parasympathetic efferents. The sensory fibres leaving the carotid bodies belong partly to the pharyngeal branch of the glossopharyngeal nerve (cranial IX) and partly to a branch of the vagus nerve (cranial X). The sensory fibres innervating the **aortic bodies** belong to the vagus nerve. Enveloping type 1 cells are a smaller number of sustentacular type 2 cells.

12.3 PHYSIOLOGY

The rate of blood flow through the carotid body is very high: about 21/min per 100 g of tissue. It is thought that this is due to direct passage through vessels connecting the entry and exit points. If this turns out to be the case, it is consistent with the evolutionary origin of the tissue discussed above. It has been known for many years that both the carotid and aortic bodies monitor the quantity of oxygen and carbon dioxide in the blood. More recently this has been subjected to detailed investigation. It has been shown that, when PaO_2 is held constant, the carotid bodies are sensitive to increases in $PaCO_2$ (Figure 12.3a), whilst the aortic bodies are largely unaffected. When $PaCO_2$ is held constant, both carotid and aortic bodies respond to falls in PaO_2 by increased impulse frequency in their afferent fibres, although the carotid bodies are more responsive than the aortic bodies (Figure 12.3b). On the other hand, the aortic bodies, but not the carotid bodies, are sensitive to carboxyhaemoglobinaemia (HbCO) when PaO_2 and $PaCO_2$ are held constant (Figure 12.3c). This implies that when the oxygen content of the blood is reduced due to anaemia or some other reason, it is the aortic rather than the carotid bodies which signal the defect.

It has been known for many years that stimulation of the carotid and/or aortic chemoreceptors leads to increases in respiration. The effect is much stronger from carotid than from aortic stimulation. The significance of the reflex is clear. An increase in $PaCO_2$ in the blood, beyond the normal level of about 40 mm Hg, causes an increase in ventilation which acts in a negative feedback fashion to bring the $PaCO_2$ back to normality. Similarly, though to a lesser extent, decreases in PaO_2 lead to increases in respiratory activity.

The peripheral chemoreceptors are, of course, only part of the story. As mentioned in Section 12.1, central chemoreceptors in the medulla also sensitively monitor $PaCO_2$. Carbon dioxide diffuses very easily from the cerebral circulation into the cerebrospinal fluid (CSF). Here it is hydrated to form carbonic acid (H_2CO_3). This quickly dissociates to give H^+ and HCO_3^-. Unlike blood plasma, CSF contains virtually no proteins which can buffer the hydrogen ions. Thus any rise in $PaCO_2$ in the CSF, a condition known as **hypercapnia**, leads to a decrease in pH, which excites the central chemoreceptors. These receptors are richly connected to the medullary respiratory centres. Excitation by increased H^+ concentration leads to increased respiratory activity. Both depth, and to a lesser extent rate of breathing, is increased. The peripheral and central chemoreceptors

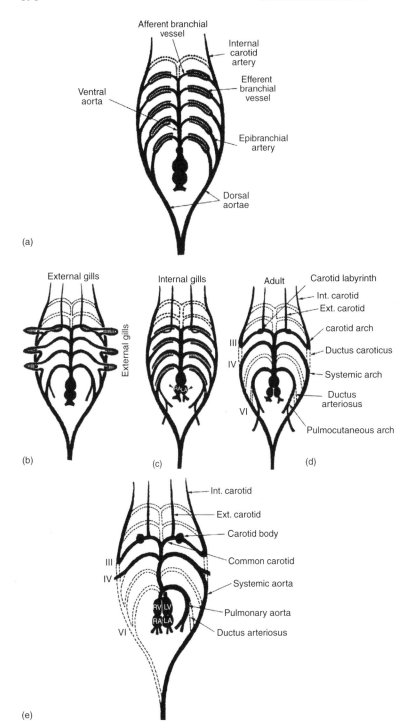

(a)

(b)   (c)   (d)

(e)

Figure 12.2 Evolution of the carotid bodies. (a): Aortic arches of a fish. The ventral aorta runs beneath the oesophagus and branchial vessels carry the blood up via the gills to the dorsal aorta above the gut. (b)–(d): Aortic arches in frog tadpole to frog adult. (b) = tadpole with external gills; (c) = transitional stage; (d) = adult frog. Note the origin of the carotid body. (e) = Aortic arches and carotid body in mammal. After Grove, A.J. and Newell, G.E. (1945).

thus work in cooperation with each other. The central chemoreceptors in fact play the dominant role: they are responsible for about 70% of the reaction to increased $PaCO_2$.

Although the most obvious reflex response to stimulation of the carotid and aortic chemoreceptors is increased respiratory activity leading to enhanced alveolar ventilation, careful investigation has shown a number of other consequences. These investigations have mostly involved the carotid bodies, as the aortic bodies are difficult to stimulate in isolation. Even investigation of the carotid bodies requires the use of sophisticated physiological techniques to prevent output from the medullary chemoreceptors, and from stretch receptors in the lungs, over-riding and confounding the response. When this is done, a number of of reflex responses to carotid body output can be shown. These include bradycardia (slowing of the heart rate) and sympathetic-induced decreases in coronary, splanchnic, renal and skeletal muscle circulations. There are also complex effects on the cerebral circulation. The circulation in the superficial cerebral cortex seems to be increased whilst that to deeper areas of the brain is decreased. In general, all of these outcomes emphasize what Walter Cannon called 'the wisdom of the body': they all tend to reduce the quantity of carbon dioxide diffusing into the blood. In addition, it has been shown that if afferent fibres from the carotid bodies are sectioned, an animal's behavioural response to hypoxia is abolished. The behavioural response to hypoxia varies according to the degree that oxygen is lacking. In dogs it increases from mild arousal to frantic search for escape.

In summary, we can see that the carotid and central chemoreceptors play crucial roles in maintaining the

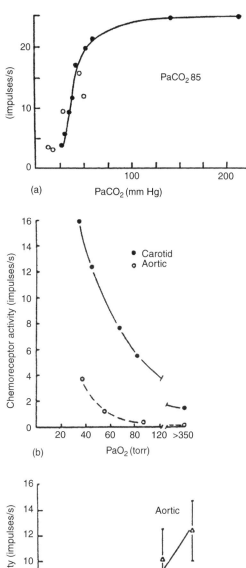

Figure 12.3 Response of carotid and aortic bodies to changes in partial pressures (Pa) of CO_2 and O_2. (a): Discharge (impulses/s) in a single afferent fibre from carotid body when PaO_2 is held constant and $PaCO_2$ varied. (a) From Biscoe, T.J., Purves, M.J. and Sampson, S.R. (1970), *Journal of Physiology*, **208**, 121–31. Copyright © 1970, The Physiological Society and Blackwell Publishing. (b) Discharge (impulses/s) from carotid and aortic bodies when $PaCO_2$ is held constant and PaO_2 varied. (c) Discharge (impulses/s) from carotid and aortic bodies when PaO_2 is at physiological levels and HbCO is varied. Note differences in aortic and carotid body responses. (b) and (c) From Marshall, J.M. (1994) Peripheral chemoreceptors and cardiovascular regulation. *Physiological Reviews* **74**, 543–94. Reproduced by permission of the American Physiological Society.

Figure 12.3

levels of respiratory gases and pH in the body's ECF. The maintenance of PaO_2 is particularly important for animals that move through significant differences in altitude; the maintenance of $PaCO_2$ is vital to compensate for the changing quantities of carbon dioxide in the ECF as the body's musculature (and other organs) undertake varying amounts of work.

12.4 BIOCHEMISTRY

Can we follow this intricate homeostatic physiology down to the molecular level and find (as we found in Chapter 6 when discussing mechanoreceptors) the molecular sensors at the core of the system? Recent work begins to suggest that we can, indeed, do just this. Let us take the oxygen sensor first. It is this that ultimately triggers the panic response to hypoxia mentioned at the end of the preceding section. The molecular situation is, as usual, very complex and it is difficult to isolate single crucial mechanisms. Oxygen is so important for mammalian cells that it would be surprising if there were not a great deal of failsafe redundancy built in. It can, however, be shown that, when PaO_2 in the immediate environment of the carotid body falls below resting values of 80 to 100 mm Hg, the type 1 cells are activated. As PaO_2 continues to fall, specific K^+-channels are closed. Reduction in K^+ permeability leads to depolarization. This, in turn, opens voltage-dependent Ca^{2+}-channels. The influx of Ca^{2+} triggers (as is usual) the release of the catecholamines, especially dopamine and norepinephrine, which (as we saw above) are highly concentrated in type 1 cells. These, in turn, initiate activity in fibres of the carotid sinus nerve (a branch of the glossopharyngeal nerve) which are in close proximity to the cells. The glossopharyngeal nerve (cranial nerve IX) runs to respiratory centres in the medulla oblongata which regulate breathing and blood pressure.

How does decreased PaO_2 cause the K^+-channel to close? This is a question to which the answer is still much in dispute. It may be that low partial pressures of oxygen in the surroundings affect the internal energy metabolism of type 1 cells leading to a decrease in levels of ATP. This in itself might cause ATP-dependent K^+-channels to close; or it might lead to release of Ca^{2+} from mitochondria and thus trigger catecholamine release. However, the most pop-

ular theory at the time of writing is that an oxygen sensitive haem protein is closely associated with the K^+-channels in the cell membrane. The hypothesis suggests that, just as haemoglobin and myoglobin alter their three-dimensional conformation in response to oxygenation, so this putative membrane-bound haem protein alters its conformation. This alteration in structure affects an adposed K^+-channel protein, changing its open/shut probability. This hypothesis is shown diagrammatically in Figure 12.4.

The carotid bodies and the medullar chemoreceptors are also, as we noted, highly sensitive to $PaCO_2$. The molecular mechanism at work here, as we have again already noted, appears to depend on the formation of carbonic acid from carbon dioxide and water and its dissociation into H^+ and HCO_3^-. H^+ diffuses into the chemoreceptor cell leading to a drop in cytosolic pH. When cytosolic pH falls, it activates a mechanism which exports protons in exchange for

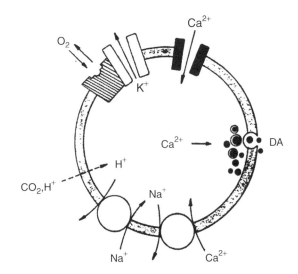

Figure 12.4 Cellular mechanisms which transduce low PaO_2 and increased $PaCO_2$ into neurotransmitter release by carotid chemoreceptor cells. Reduction in PaO_2 is sensed by a membrane receptor (shown at top of figure) which causes an adposed K^+-channel to close. The consequent depolarization opens Ca^{2+}-channels and the influx of Ca^{2+} initiates the release of neurotransmitter. Increased $PaCO_2$ causes increased influx of H^+, which drives a pump bringing Na^+ into the cell. This, in turn, activates an antiport mechanism which brings Ca^{2+} into the cell and this, again, causes the release of neurotransmitter. Further explanation in text. From Gonzalez, C. *et al.* (1994) Carotid body chemoreceptors: from natural stimuli to sensory discharges. *Physiological Reviews* **74**, 829–98. Reproduced by permission of the American Physiological Society.

Na^+ (Figure 12.4). It can be shown that type 1 cells (and central chemoreceptors) also possess a powerful Na^+–Ca^{2+} antiporter in their membranes. This means that internal Na^+ is exchanged for external Ca^{2+} (Figure 12.4). This antiport mechanism is stimulated by increases in internal Na^+ levels. Hence the upshot of raised plasma $PaCO_2$ is an increase in levels of Ca^{2+} within the type 1 cells. Again this leads to the release of catecholamine neurotransmitter onto the surrounding nerve fibres and an increase in impulse frequency in the sensory nerves.

12.5 CONCLUDING REMARKS

This short chapter has concentrated on just one of the many chemo-enteroreceptors present in the mammalian body. There is a multitude of others and the topic of sensory physiology tends to merge into that of endocrinology and biochemistry as the subject is pursued. But, just as the intricate bodies of the higher animals could not survive without the great system of entero-mechanoreceptors we described in Chapter 6, so they would equally quickly succumb without the multitude of entero-chemoreceptors touched on in this chapter. Enteroreceptors ensure that the essential parameters of the environment in which the body's cells live are continuously optimized. Their work goes largely unrecognized by the conscious brain; it is only when something goes awry that we become aware of their importance. Then, as the unfortunate dog deprived of its oxygen supply knew only too well, their messages fill consciousness.

13

GUSTATION

Gustation and olfaction not always distinguishable - universal in animal kingdom - platyhelminthes - annelida - mollusca. **Insects**: **Tabinids** - chemosensory sensilla - gustation and olfaction distinguished - proboscis extension in flies and butterflies - tarsal and labellar sensilla - electrophysiological recording - form of gustatory sensilla - distribution - fine structure of labellar sensilla - biophysics - comparison with vertebrate myelination; **Drosophila** – Gr genes - molecular biology of gustatory receptors – maps in sub-oesophageal ganglion. **Mammals**: biological significance - complex neurology - comparison with other senses - subjectively multifarious - analysable into combinations of sweetness, saltiness, sourness, bitterness plus umami and water - qualia related to biological objectivity; **taste buds** - location - fungiform, foliate and circumvalate papillae - innervation - cellular constitution - rapid cellular turnover; **taste receptor cells (TRCs)** - true receptor cells - stimulus transduction - generalist or specialist? - electrophysiology – T1R and T2R 7TM receptors - molecular biology of sweet, umami, salt, sour, bitter and water transduction; **central projections** - gustatory information is relayed via the medulla and thalamus to two gustatory areas in the cerebral cortex. **Concluding reamrks**: much remains to be learnt from future research - commercial interests

In the last chapter we looked at the crucial role which chemoreceptors facing inwards – chemo-entoreceptors – play in maintaining a constant internal environment. In this chapter and the next we shall consider two groups of chemoreceptors that face outwards and are designed to monitor the chemical constitution of the external environment. We customarily distinguish these exteroreceptors into those that are specialized to detect taste and those that are specialized to detect odours. This distinction is reasonably clear in tetrapod vertebrates such as ourselves. Taste, **gustation**, is generally regarded as a contact sense. The stimulating molecules have to be in solution and in contact with the receptor. In contrast,

olfaction is a distance sense. The chemical molecule is wafted to the sense receptor on atmospheric currents. There are obvious difficulties with this classification. At the cellular level, and even more so at the molecular level, the receptor mechanisms can be much the same. Furthermore, the distinction is difficult to apply to aquatic animals where the stimulating chemicals are, of necessity, in solution. Nevertheless, with all these provisos, we shall, for convenience, divide our consideration of the specialized chemical exteroreceptors into two chapters, considering gustation in this chapter and olfaction in Chapter 14.

Gustation is, of course, universal in the animal kingdom. *Caenorhabditis elegans* is known to show extreme sensitivity to environmental chemicals such as acetone. Planariae have chemoreceptors in their heads which function during feeding and hence may be regarded as gustatory receptors. Charles Darwin in his great study on earthworms (*Lumbricus*) showed that they could discriminate between red and green cabbage and between carrot and celery leaves. Terrestrial snails use chemoreceptors to locate edible material. Perhaps the most interesting, because the most thoroughly researched, invertebrate gustatory systems are, however, to be found amongst the members of the great class Insecta.

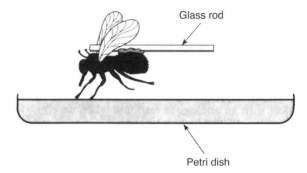

Figure 13.1   Testing a blowfly for tarsal chemosensitivity.

13.1 GUSTATION IN INSECTS

13.1.1 Tachinid Flies

Something has already been said of insect sensory sensilla in Chapters 7 and 8. It will be remembered from those chapters that sensilla are frequently multimodal. Hence chemosensitive sensilla often contain mechanosensitive neurosensory cells. It is also difficult to make the conventional distinction into gustatory and olfactory sensilla. Should water receptors, for example, be distinguished from hygroreceptors? Generally speaking, we can define gustatory receptors as those which detect substances in the liquid phase, dissolved, perhaps, on the surfaces of leaves, whilst olfactory receptors detect molecules in the gas phase, often with extraordinary sensitivity. We shall consider insect olfaction in Chapter 14.

The study of insect gustation received great impulse first from the work of Minnich and then from that of Dethier on the **reflex proboscis extension** of butterflies and blowflies to stimulation of the tarsi with nutrient solutions. The experimental set-up is quite simple. The fly is attached to a glass rod and its tarsi dipped into a petri dish of solutions of different constituents at different concentrations (Figure 13.1). The experimenter watches to see if the proboscis is extended, or if the extension is inhibited.

Subsequently, similar chemosensitivity has been demonstrated in the large chemosensory hairs extending from the **labellum of tachinid flies**, such as the blowflies *Calliphora* and *Phormia*. When the tarsal chemoreceptors are stimulated, the labellum extends so that these hairs come in contact with and test the solution. It has proved possible to make electro-physiological recordings from both the tarsal and the labellar chemosensory hairs. The impulse frequency, as would be expected, increases with concentration of the test solution. A single labellar sugar receptor will respond differently to different sugars, although the impulse frequency always increases with concentration (Figure 13.2). Nevertheless, there is some specialization. Four groups of chemosensitive hairs have been distinguished on the labellum of the blowfly; they are optimally sensitive to, respectively, sugars. cations, anions and water. The sugar sensitive sensilla are also responsive to some amino and fatty acids, whilst the water receptor is inhibited by salts. In other insects, although water, sugar and salt sensitive sensilla are usually found, other receptors are specialized to fit the animal's feeding habits. Hence, phytophagous insects and caterpillars usually have receptors sensitive to the chemicals of the food plant.

The chemosensitive sensilla themselves are normally either uniporous or multiporous (Figure 13.3a). Contact (gustatory) sensilla are usually uniporous, whilst distance (olfactory) sensilla, to increase their sensitivity, are usually multiporous. Gustatory sensilla take the form of hairs or pegs of various shapes and sizes and are usually multimodal. The hairs on the labellum of muscid and tachinid flies are, for example, uniporous and lengthy (several hundred microns) whilst those on the tarsi are mostly much shorter (a few tens of microns). The latter have been classified into four morphological types: type A (short, about 30 µm, numerous, contain sugar or salt receptors); type B2 (about 70 µm, only on ventral side of tarsus, sugar sensitive); type B3 (project laterally from the distal end of each of the last four tarsomeres and a group on the fifth tarsomere, about

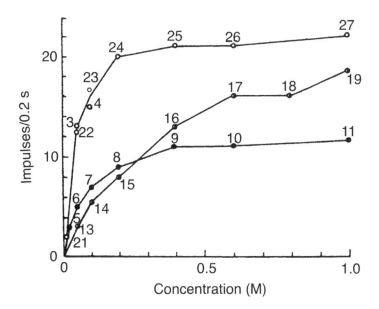

Figure 13.2 Response curves to sucrose, glucose and fructose in the fleshfly *Boettcherisca peregrina*. 0.2 M sucrose (×) was given as control. Number attached to each symbol indicates the order of stimulation. O = sucrose; ◑ = glucose and ● = fructose. (NB: Half filled ◑ for glucose; filled ● for fructose). From Morita, H. and Shiraishi, A. (1968), *J. Gen. Physiol.*, **52**, 559–583. Copyright © 1968, Rockefeller Press.

70 µm in length, sugar and salt sensitive); type D (the longest of all, about 200 µm, a pair on each tarsomere and two pairs on the first and fifth tarsomeres, sugar and salt sensitive). The distribution of these hairs on the tarsus of the prothoracic leg of the blow fly is shown in Figure 13.3b.

If the structure of a single gustatory sensillum from the labellum of *Phormia* is examined in more detail, we find that it contains four chemosensory and one mechanosensory cell. The chemosensory cells send their dendritic outersegments along the length of the sensillum to terminate just beneath the pore. Their axons run to the suboesophageal ganglion. The mechanosensory cell possesses a tubular body and is similar to the mechanosensory cells described in Chapter 8. Its axon also runs to the suboesophageal ganglion.

A diagrammatic representation of the relationship of the chemosensory cell with its surroundings is given in Figure 13.4a. It can be seen that it is sheathed in the customary three supporting cells. The chemosensory cell itself is surrounded by a glial cell; outside this is an inner sheath cell (thecogen cell). The thecogen sheath cell forms the ciliary sinus (Chapter 8) which surrounds the junction between the inner and outersegment of the dendrite and secretes a cuticular sheath surrounding the out-

ersegment. The ciliary sinus is thus continuous with the space between the outersegment and its cuticular sheath. This space is filled with the fluid secreted into the ciliary sinus by the inner sheath cell. The intermediate sheath cell (trichogen cell) and outer sheath cell (tormogen cell) form the sensillar sinus. This sinus, as the figure shows, is continuous with the outer space of the sensillar shaft.

It can be shown that, when the gustatory sensillum is in contact with its adequate stimulus, the tip of the outersegment is depolarized (I_m: Figure 13.4). We shall meet with an analogous response when we come to consider the rather better understood hair cells of the vertebrates. This depolarization spreads electrotonically (I_{o1} and I_{o2}) down the outersegment until it reaches the inner segment. The circuit is completed by a flow of current (I_o) via the ciliary sinus and sensillar sinus, through the outer space of the sensillar shaft, back to the tip (Figure 13.4(b)). Depolarization of the base of the outersegment spreads to the initial segment of the gustatory axon, where impulses are initiated.

The organization of the insect chemosensory sensillum is in many ways analogous to the myelination of vertebrate axons. In the latter case, the electrotonic spread is greatly enhanced by the presence of a high resistance myelin sheath. In the insect

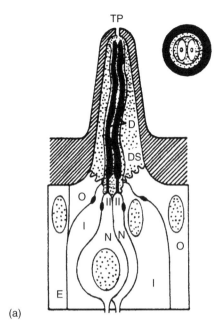

(a)

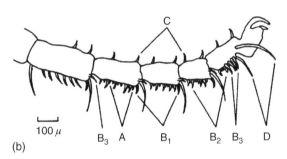

(b)

Figure 13.3 (a) Uniporous gustatory sensillum. D = dendritic outersegments; DS = dendritic sheath; E = epidermal cell; I = inner sheath cell; N = neurosensory cell; O = outer sheath cell; TP = terminal pore. Transverse section of the sensillum at top right of the figure. From Blum, 1985: with permission. (b) Tarsus of the prothoracic leg of blowfly from the side to show chemosensory sensilla. Tactile sensilla omitted. The different types of hair are labelled A, B1, B2, B3, C, D. Explanation in text. From Kerkut, G.A. and Gilbert, L.I. (eds) (1985) *Comprehensive Insect Physiology*, Nervous System: Sensory, Vol. 6. Copyright © 1985, Oxford University Press.

sensilla, the place of myelin is taken by the cuticular sheath surrounding the outersegment. This enables efficient electrotonic or cable conduction to occur down the quite lengthy (several hundred microns) sensilla which many insects develop.

Turning, finally, to the chemosensory molecules themselves we find that the most incisive work has been done on the fruit fly, *Drosophila*, which forms the subject of the next section. It is likely that the molecular biology discussed there applies not only to fruit flies but also to the Tabinid flies discussed in this section and to other insects as well.

13.1.2 *Drosophila*

Because its genome is so well known (Chapter 5), *Drosophila* has proved an excellent model in which to study the molecular biology of the insect gustatory system – and not only insect gustatory systems. For *Drosophila* responds to many of the same gustatory stimuli as mammals: sugars, salts, alchohols and so on. Taste receptor cells (TRCs) are found in many parts of the insect's body: proboscis, mouth parts, legs, wings, ovipositor and so on. Chemosensory hairs or bristles, as in the Tachinids, usually contain two to four gustatory cells and a single mechanosensory cell. The dendrites of the gustatory cells extend into the bristle and the sensory neuron projects to the brain. Gustatory neurons from the proboscis, mouth parts and some from the leg project to the suboesophageal ganglion, whilst those from the legs mostly project to segmental ganglia.

Searches of the genome database have revealed 60 *gr* genes encoding 68 gustatory receptors. All code for 7TM proteins of about 480 amino acids. Although the sequences of these putative gustatory receptors are extremely diverse, they nevertheless all have a significantly similar 33 amino acid sequence towards the C-terminal end. *Drosophila* gustatory receptors show no sequence similarity to the mammalian T1R and T2R gustatory receptors (Section 13.2).

The identification of gustatory receptors has allowed experimentalists to determine which sensory hairs are responsive to which gustatory stimuli. The Gr5a receptor is, for instance, expressed in 25–50% of all proboscis chemosensory neurons. It has been further possible to show that mutations in the gene encoding this receptor leave the insect unable to detect sugars. This finding, along with other supporting evidence, indicates that these receptors are sugar detectors. Similarly, mutation of another gustatory receptor gene, coding for the Gr66a receptor, which is found in about 25% of proboscis chemosensory cells, leads to flies unable to detect 'bitterness', for example caffeine. This sharp discrimination of 'sweetness' from 'bitterness' is, as we shall see below, also characteristic of the mammalian gustatory system.

Because of the comparative simplicity of the *Drosophila* nervous system (some 100 000 neurons) and the fact that gustatory neurons project directly to the suboesophageal ganglion, it is possible to begin the task of following the taste information inwards to its final destination. Is the gustatory surface **mapped** in the brain (as the mammalian somaesthetic, auditory and visual surfaces are mapped)? Or, is information about different tastes segregated so that there are patches where 'bitterness', patches where 'sweetness', patches where 'saltiness' and so on are analysed? These questions have been answered by tracing the projections of gustatory neurons into the suboesophageal ganglion. It was shown that gustatory neurons originating in the mouth parts terminated in front of those originating in the proboscis and those, in turn, terminated in front of those originating in the legs. This suggests that the gustatory sensory surface is indeed topographically mapped in the fly's brain. But, it has also been shown that within this topographic map taste quality is also localized. Thus 'sweetness' neurons from the proboscis terminate together in a patch entirely separate from the patch where 'bitterness' neurons from the same area of the proboscis terminate. Thus the answer to the question, as is so often the case in biology, is not a clear cut yes or no, but a bit of both.

Finally, it is possible to see the biological advantage of the fly's gustatory organization. The brain is informed of where the gustatory information is coming from and is thus able to adjust its behaviour

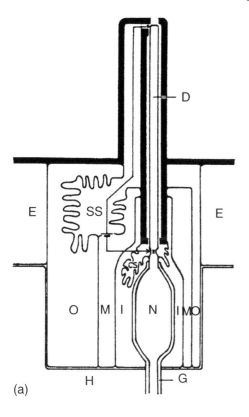

(a)

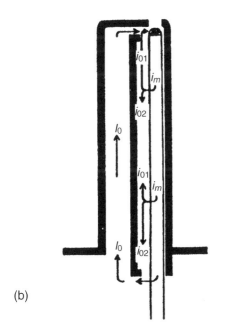

(b)

Figure 13.4 (*Opposite*) (a) Diagrammatic representation of blowfly gustatory sensillum. Only one outersegment is shown. Note the thick cuticle with which it is surrounded. cs = ciliary sinus; D = dendritic outersegment; E = epidermal cell; G = glial cell; H = haemocoele; I = inner sheath cell; M = intermediate sheath cell; N = neurosensory cell; O = outer sheath cell; ss = sensilla sinus. From Kerkut and Gilbert, 1985: with permission. (b) Biophysics of the gustatory sensillum. i_m = membrane current; i_{o1} and i_{o2} = longitudinal current within outersegment sheath toward the tip and base respectively; I_o = longitudinal current in the outer lumen. Explanation in text. (a) Adapted from Kerkut, G. A. and Gilbert, L. I. (eds) (1985).

accordingly. In addition, the brain is also informed of what taste is being detected at each bodily location and this also is significant in governing the fly's behavioural response.

Let us now move from insect gestation to the much more complex systems developed in the vertebrates and, in particular, the mammals. Although these systems are many orders of complexity removed from those of the insect, they nevertheless show some overall similarity. It is not absurd to believe that investigations of the much more amenable, yet highly sensitive, systems developed over the vast stretches of evolutionary time by the insects will help direct some of the questions asked by investigators of mammalian gustatory systems.

13.2 GUSTATION IN MAMMALS

The sense of taste is well developed in all vertebrates. In this section, however, we shall confine ourselves to the mammals and, in particular, humans. Taste provides vital information about food material already in the mouth, the last moment before conscious control is lost. Is it nutritive or poisonous? Is it customary or novel? Did it have beneficial or noxious effects on previous occasions? Not surprisingly, taste has a complex neurological basis. It is compounded of input from the gustatory receptors principally in the tongue but also in the epiglottis, the upper third of the oesophagus and the soft palate. Input relating to roughness, texture, temperature and smell is also significant. Memory and cultural upbringing also play a part. What is tasty in one culture is disgusting in another.

Tastes, like smells, are multifarious. In this they differ from the mechanosenses such as touch. Touch seems always to have the same quality, merely varying in intensity. Smells vary along both qualitative and quantitative axes. In this they resemble that other, and far more sophisticated, mechanosense, hearing, as well as vision. But how should we describe our taste sensations? We have all heard (and some of us have smiled) at wine aficionados' descriptions. They try to bring up all sorts of associations, some visual, some social, some geographic, some climatic to describe their experience. Are taste sensations simply unanalysable, a potentially infinite continuum, or can they be shown to be due (like colours) to the

permutations and combinations of a much smaller number of elements? Historically there has been much debate on this subject but ultimately the latter view seems to have won through. Our contemporary understanding stems from the proposal by Hans Henning in 1922 that human taste could be analysed into four basic qualities: **sweetness, saltiness, sourness** and **bitterness**. In addition, investigators nowadays recognize the pleasant taste of monosodium glutamate called (from the Japanese) **umami**, which is distinctively different from the four classical tastes, and, finally, **water**.

This subjective classification relates to objective biology. The pleasant hedonic tone of sweetness and umami relate to high calorie, easily digestible food. Fruits and berries often advertise this fact by displaying vivid colours to the visual system. Saltiness, sourness and water are all related to the ionic and pH regulation of the 'internal environment'. Bitterness is regarded as a warning sign: the ingested material is dangerous. This objective analysis suggests that the gustatory systems of nonhuman animals would have a similar (though far from identical) organization. This has been shown to be the case in many vertebrate species. Whether their subjectivity is similarly similar is, of course, another question altogether.

13.2.1 Taste Buds

From fifty to a hundred gustatory receptor cells are grouped into **taste buds**, which are located on projections known as papillae. The human tongue has four types of papillae: **filiform, fungiform, foliate** and **circumvallate**. The filiform papillae do not possess any taste buds. Their function is entirely mechanical, giving the tongue its rough abrasive character – more strongly developed in many mammals, for example the domestic cat, than in humans. The other three types of papillae all carry taste buds. **Fungiform papillae**, named after their resemblance to button mushrooms, are grouped mainly on the front and the front edges of the tongue (Figure 13.5). Taste buds, mostly (but not all) sensitive to sweetness and saltiness, are buried in the surface epithelium of these papillae. Because of their rich blood supply, they are visible as small red spots on the front of the tongue. **Foliate papillae** are found in a set of three to eight parallel folds (hence their name) towards the rear edge of the

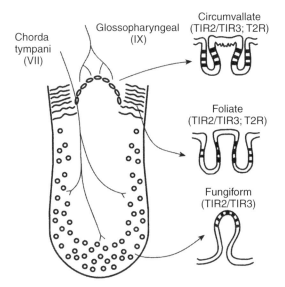

Chorda
tympani
(VII)

Glossopharyngeal
(IX)

Circumvallate
(TIR2/TIR3; T2R)

Foliate
(TIR2/TIR3; T2R)

Fungiform
(TIR2/TIR3)

Figure 13.5 Tongue and taste buds. The tongue is shown from its superior aspect. Sectional views of the three types of taste-bud-bearing papillae are shown in the right hand column. The dark patches indicate the position of the taste buds. The location of the T1R and T2R taste receptor molecules is indicated. Further explanation in text.

tongue. The majority of receptor cells in these taste buds are sensitive to sourness or acidity. **Circumvallate papillae** are, as their name indicates, somewhat sunken papillae surrounded by a deep moat that separates them from the rest of the tongue's surface. Eight or nine of these papillae form a V-shape on the rear of the tongue. About 250 taste buds develop in their wall and in the wall of the surrounding trench of each papilla. They are most sensitive to sourness and bitterness. The walls of these papillae also possess secretory glands which help, with the motion of the tongue, to rinse out the moat. As mentioned above, other taste buds are located in the epiglottis, the upper third of the oesophagus and the soft palate. Although there are some small differences in taste sensitivity across the tongue, the old idea of a strong segregation with sweetness detectors towards the front and bitterness detectors towards the back has not been confirmed by modern investigations.

The innervation of the taste buds is far more complex than that of the olfactory receptors, which will be considered in Chapter 14. Those in the anterior part of the tongue are innervated by the **chorda tympani** branch of the **facial nerve** (cranial nerve VII), whilst the rear of the tongue is served by the **glossopharyngeal nerve** (cranial nerve IX). The non-tongue taste buds are innervated by a branch of the **vagus nerve** (cranial nerve X).

The anterior two thirds of the tongue is also innervated by the mandibular branch of the trigeminal nerve (cranial nerve V). This nerve carries information relating to temperature, texture, pain and so on. These sensations add to those derived from the taste buds and olfactory system to provide the total experience of the ingested material. Indeed, most cuisines make use of these additional sensory inputs to characterize their foods. It is also the case that cultural factors, rather than nutritional factors, determine the palatability, ensuring, for instance, that those which are normally served hot are acceptable whilst the same foods served cold are not, and vice versa.

13.2.1.1 Cellular Structure of Taste Buds

A taste bud is a group of 50 to 100 cells arranged together rather like the segments of an orange and surrounded by the epithelial cells of the papilla (Figure 13.6c). There are two classes of cell: principal (or chief) cells and basal cells. There are three types of principal cell: type 1 (or dark) cells, type 2 (or light) cells and type 3 cells. Type 1 and type 3 cells are generally **taste receptor cells** (**TRCs**) whilst type 2 cells are usually supportive. This tentative assignment of function is due to the fact that their roles vary across species and, indeed, from one part of the tongue to another. The apices of all three types of principal cell are joined by tight junctions. They cluster together and project into the taste or gustatory pore. This pore is filled with secretions and opens on to the surface of the papilla.

Type 1 cells form up to 65% of the cell population of rabbit taste buds. Their apices develop a rich brush-like set of 30–40 microvilli. The apex also contains numerous dense granules that contain secretions which are voided into the gustatory pore. The walls of type 1 cells are thrown into many sheet-like wings, which sheath unmyelinated fibres and neighbouring type 2 cells. Synapses are made between type 1 cells and neurons in the mouse but not in the rabbit.

Type 2 cells constitute about 20% of the taste bud cells. Their apices are filled with electron-dense material and are produced into a number of blunt microvilli that protrude into the taste pore. Synapses

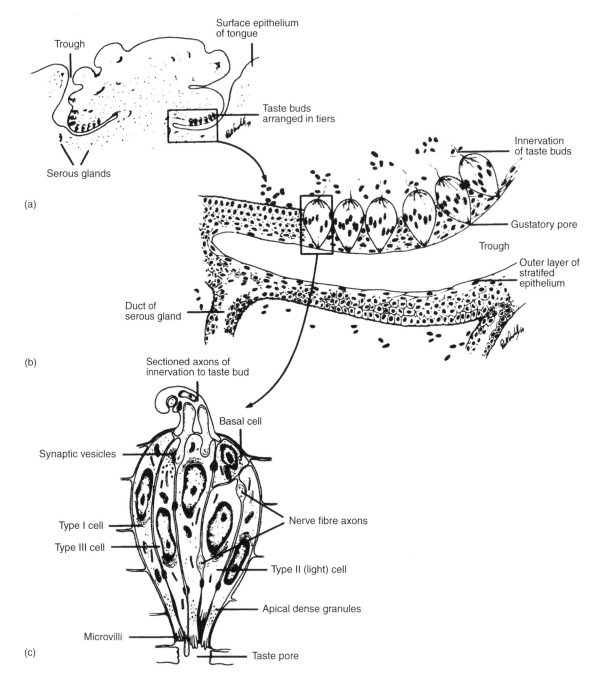

Figure 13.6   Taste buds. (a) Position of taste buds in a circumvallate papilla; (b) enlargement of (a); (c) single taste bud. From Keverne, '*The Senses*', 1982, p. 40, Fig. 19.1 by permission of Cambridge University Press.

are formed with neurons in the mouse but (again) not in the rabbit.

Type 3 cells, which form less than 10% of the taste bud cells in the rabbit, develop a single large microvillus that protrudes well into the taste pore. Unlike the other two types, which sometimes do and sometimes do not develop synapses, these cells seem always to make synapses with adjacent neurons and, consequently, can always be regarded as gustatory receptor cells.

All the taste bud cells have a very short life span and are continuously replaced. Radioactive labelling of epithelial cells surrounding rat taste buds showed that daughter cells moved into the taste bud at the rate of one very ten hours. Once in the taste bud their life expectancy was no more than about ten days. During this time the cell moves from the periphery of the bud to the centre. At the end of their short life the taste bud cells are either phagocytosed or undergo apoptosis. This rapid turnover of taste bud cells perhaps accounts for the difficulty of assigning precise functions to each type.

Taste receptor cells (TRCs), unlike olfactory cells, are true receptor cells. Sensory nerve fibres enter through the basal lamina of the bud (where they lose their myelin sheaths) and run up between the cells. They are sheathed by the membranous extensions of the type 1 (dark) cells. One fibre normally innervates more than one TRC and, vice versa, one receptor cell is usually served by more than one fibre. As taste bud cells are in constant turnover, nerve fibres are continuously searching out new synaptic contacts.

13.2.1.2 Molecular Biology

As in the case of olfactory cilia (Chapter 14), there has been continuing argument over whether TRCs are generalists or specialist. Does an individual cell respond to just one or more than one of the six primary tastes? It turns out that the gustatory and olfactory systems differ in this regard. In contrast to the olfactory system, it appears that many gustatory cells are 'generalist'. This conclusion has emerged from studies of the receptor molecules involved. The situation is not, however, quite straightforward. It appears that, while TRCs dedicated to 'sweetness' detect a large number of different 'sweet' substances by possessing one low-affinity sweetness receptor, TRCs

cells dedicated to 'bitterness' possess a large number of different high-affinity bitterness receptors.

These findings are consistent with recordings from single nerve fibres from the front of the rat and hamster tongue. These recordings identify some fibres (N-fibres) with maximum responses to sodium chloride (saltiness) with lesser responses to hydrochloric acid (sourness). Other single fibres (H-fibres) respond best to hydrochloric acid, with lesser responses to sodium chloride and quinine (bitterness). But, once again, there are many species differences and the fact that the branches of one sensory nerve fibre may innervate several TRCs has to be borne in mind. Investigation of the molecular biology and biophysics of single TRCs is technically difficult and the research to date often reveals a complicated situation.

Molecular biologists have identified two families of taste receptor genes: *T1R* and *T2R*. The *T1R* family consists of three genes, *T1R1, T1R2* and *T1R3*. These genes all encode GPCRs with large extracellular domains which are believed to be involved in binding tastant molecules (Figures 13.7a and 13.7b). The second family of taste receptor genes, the *T2R* family, consists of about thirty members, which again code for GPCRs (Figure 13.7c). These genes are distantly related to those which code for opsin.

Sweetness. Members of the T1R family function together as heterodimers to detect sugars and amino acids. T1R2 and T1R3 act together to detect all natural sugars and artificial sweeteners and T1R1 and T1R3 together detect amino acids. T1R2/T1R3 heterodimers are mostly found in the foliate and circumvallate papillae. Members of the T2R family of receptor molecules are also found in taste receptor dendrites of these papillae. T1R1/T1R3 heterodimers are mostly located in the fungiform papillae at the front of the tongue.

When T1R2/T1R3 are activated by an appropriate tastant molecule, a G-protein signalling system is activated. Evidence suggests that the G-protein α-subunit is very similar to the transducin of photoreceptor outersegments (Chapter 17) and it has consequently been named **gustducin**. It is expressed preferentially in the tongue. The gustducin activates a PLC system (Figure 13.8, see also Figure 1.10), which in turn leads to the activation of TRPM5 cationic channels and thus depolarization of the cell. Finally, the depolarized membrane initiates the opening of Ca^{2+} gates and this, together with IP_3 triggered

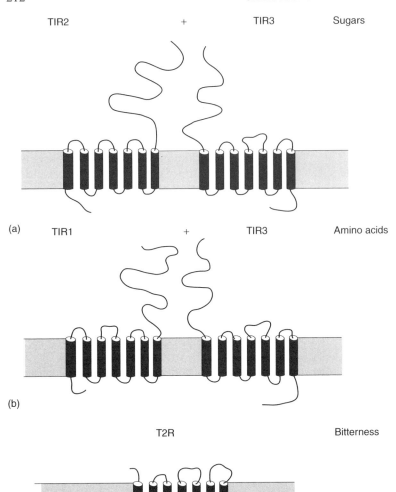

TIR2   +   TIR3   Sugars

(a)

TIR1   +   TIR3   Amino acids

(b)

T2R   Bitterness

(c)

Figure 13.7 Taste receptor molecules. Plan views of the T1R and T2R families of taste receptor molecules. (a) Heterodimers of T1R2 and T1R3 recognize sugars and other sweet tastants; (b) heterodimers of T1R1 and T1R3 recognize amino acids; (c) T2Rs of which there are thirty different members recognize bitterness (after Scott, 2005).

release of Ca^{2+} from the ER, causes the exocytosis of transmitter into the synaptic gap. The biochemistry is outlined in Figure 13.8.

It is interesting to note that the *T1R2* genes of different mammals express proteins with slightly different amino acid sequences. It can be shown, for instance, that human T1R2 is activated by aspartame (Nutrasweet), whilst mouse T1R2 is not. If mouse *T1r2* gene is replaced by the human gene, the animal is immediately able to detect and respond to aspartame. Vice versa, it appears that both domestic and wild cats lack a functional T1R2 receptor due to a deletion in the relevant gene, which leads to a premature stop codon. Cats do not appreciate what seem to us sweet tastes. Could blockers of T1R2 have the same effect in humans?

Umami. This is the name given to the taste of certain Japanese food – dried katsuwo fish (*Katsuwonus pelamis*), the kombu seaweed (*Laminaria japonica*) and so on. It is also characteristic of chicken broth and cheeses such as Roquefort and Parmesan. It is distinctively different from sweetness, although it

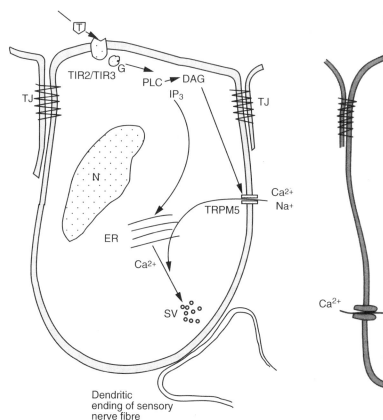

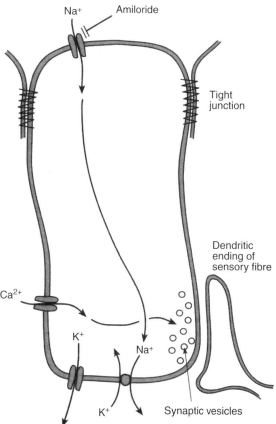

Figure 13.8 Transduction routes for sugar and nonsugar sweet tastants. Explanation in text. DAG = Diacylgycerol; ER = endoplasmic reticulum; G = gustducin; N = nucleus; PLC = phospholipase C; SV = synaptic vesicles; T = tastant molecule; TJ = tight junction.

Figure 13.9 Transduction route for salty tastants. Na^+ enters an amiloride-sensitive channel and is ultimately pumped out of the cell by a $Na^+ + K^+$ pump at its base. The current leaves by cation (possibly K^+) channels at the base of the cell. The depolarization opens Ca^{2+}-channels and the inflowing Ca^{2+} initiates release of transmitter on to the dendrite of a sensory fibre. Further explanation in text. After Lindemann, B. (1996).

also has a pleasant hedonic quality. Its most significant active ingredient is l-glutamate although some other amino acids, small peptides and nucleotides are also effective. A series of experiments indicates that the umami receptor is a T1R1/T1R3 multimer. This receptor, as we noted above, is most strongly affected by glutamate, although other amino acids activate it to a lesser extent. The 'downstream' biochemistry is believed to be the same as for the sweetness detector: gustducin → PLC → DAG → TRPM5 → membrane depolarization → Ca^{2+} inflow → transmitter exocytosis.

Finally, it should be noted that taste preference studies in mice where the T1R1/T1R3 genes have been 'knocked-out' shows that some ability to recog-

nize 'umami' tastes persists. Thus it is likely that some less prominent means of recognizing amino acids in food exists in these cells.

Saltiness. The detection of salt is of great importance to the animals; it is crucial for the ionic homeostasis of the internal environment. It has been shown that Na^+ affects salt sensitive TRCs by entering a Na^+-specific ion channel (Figure 13.9) rather than involving the membrane biochemistry of a G-protein system. This has been demonstrated by making use of the Na^+-channel blocker, **amiloride**. This guanidinium compound is a well established external blocker of epithelial Na^+-channels (ENaCs).

Note that these channels are in no way related to the voltage-gated Na^+-channels of excitable membranes. In the presence of submicromolar concentrations of amiloride on the mucosal surface of a fungiform papilla, impulse frequency in gustatory nerve fibres in response to sodium chloride was found to be significantly diminished. Patch clamping of single TRCs also showed that Na^+ influx was abolished in response to amiloride. It is concluded that the influx of Na^+ depolarizes the TRC leading to the release of transmitter on to the adjacent nerve terminal.

Deeper molecular insights into the nature of the amiloride sensitive Na^+-channel have been obtained by the cloning of a homologous channel from rat distal colon. ENaCs are now known to consist of three 75 kDa subunits. Each of the different subunits (α, β and γ) makes two passes through the membrane. ENaCs are members of the degenerin family of channels, which are widely expressed in epithelial cells throughout the body. The use of antibodies raised against this ENaC has enabled the amiloride-sensitive channels of TRCs to be located. They are not only present in TRCs but also in the epithelial cells surrounding the taste buds. It is believed that the Na^+ pathways in these surrounding cells modulate the activity of the TRCs themselves.

The fact that saltiness is not detected through a G-protein membrane coupling system but directly through an ion channel underlies the finding that response to sodium chloride is very rapid. In rats and hamsters the latency of response to sodium chloride is <50 ms compared to >300 ms for saccharine. The response also adapts very quickly, often in less than one minute. The molecular mechanism of adaptation is still unknown.

Salt sensitivity is under hormonal control. Addition of aldosterone to the vascular perfusate of frog tongue increases the response of the glossopharyngeal nerve to sodium chloride application. This effect is seen some 3–6 h after the perfusion. In other tissues it has been shown that, in periods of less than about 10 h, aldosterone increases the 'open' probability of pre-existing Na^+-channels, thus increasing sensitivity. Whether this mechanism also obtains in TRCs is not yet known. The other hormone which affects salt sensitivity is antidiuretic hormone (ADH). Application of this hormone also causes a slow increase in glossopharyngeal nerve response to salt application to the tongue. ADH is released from the pituitary when the osmolarity of the plasma increases. If at the same time it makes the TRCs more sensitive to sodium chloride an animal is likely to cut down its intake of salty food and thus compensate for this increased osmolarity. These exteroreceptive controls on the osmolarity of the plasma evidently complement the enteroreceptive controls discussed in Chapter 6.

Sourness. The detection of acidity is also of great importance in maintaining the homeostasis of the internal environment. In this case it is the pH balance that is affected. The detection of acidity is also important in helping animals to avoid unripe, and hence nutritionally suboptimal, fruit and avoiding spoilt food. The sour taste is believed to be due to dissociated H^+. H^+, like Na^+, seems to affect TRC membrane channels directly. A number of different mechanisms have been found in different vertebrates. In amphibians such as the mud puppy, *Necturus*, H^+ blocks K^+ leak channels (Figure 13.10a). As K^+ leak channels play a significant role in maintaining the resting potential across biomembranes (Chapter 2) blockage will lead to depolarization. This, in turn, leads in the customary way to exocytosis of transmitter substance from synaptic vesicles. In the hamster and, possibly the rat, a different mechanism exists. In this case (Figure 13.10b) H^+ passes through amiloride-blockable Na^+-channels. This flow of cations into the TRC will also cause depolarization and consequent release of transmitter.

Bitterness. Like sourness, bitterness causes aversive reactions. Foodstuffs which taste bitter (for instance plant alkaloids such as quinine, strychnine, etc., the cyanide of 'bitter almonds', as well as metabolic waste products such as urea) are rejected. A large number of other substances also taste bitter and it may be that some plants and invertebrates have evolved to have a bitter taste to prevent being eaten. In some cases this may be an example of Batesian mimicry: the organism is not itself harmful but mimics those which are and thus survives by deception.

Once again there seem to be a multiplicity of transduction mechanisms. The most important are the blockage of K^+-channels (although this seems to be a rather indiscriminate mechanism) and, more specifically, mechanisms working through a *T2R* G-protein system. This second mechanism (Figure 13.11) is very similar to that already described for detecting sweetness. The *T2R* receptors are 7TM proteins that

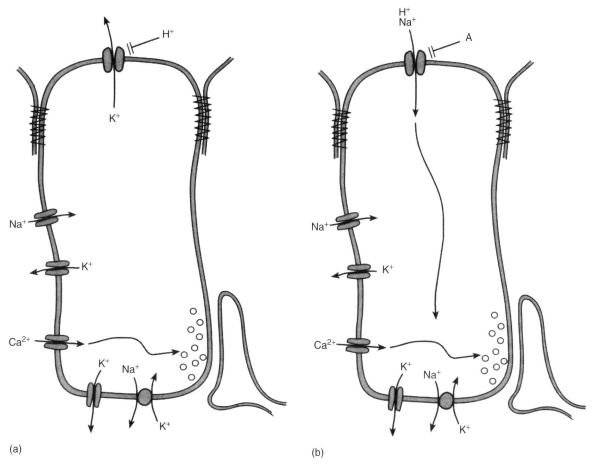

Figure 13.10 Transduction routes for sour tastants. (a) *Necturus*. H^+ blocks a K^+-channel, hence inducing depolarization, the opening of Ca^{2+}-channels and the release of transmitter. (b) Hamster and (probably) rat. H^+ passes through Na^+-channels that can be blocked by amiloride (A). The consequent depolarization again causes inflow of Ca^{2+} and release of transmitter. Further explanation in text. After Lindemann, B. (1996).

have an approximately 40% sequence homology with the T1R sweetness receptors although they lack a lengthy carboxyterminal chain (Figure 13.7). They are located preferentially in **circumvallate** and to a lesser extent in **foliate papillae**. Humans have some 25 *T2R* genes and 35 *T2r* genes have been identified in the mouse. Different T2R receptors recognize different bitter chemicals. mT2R5, for instance, recognizes cyclohexamide and hT2R14 detects picrotoxin (the prefix 'h' means 'human', prefix 'm' means 'mouse'). Unlike the T1R sweetness detectors the T2Rs are highly specific. Mice lacking mT2R5 cannot detect cyclohexamide, although they care-

fully avoid other bitter compounds. When a T2R receptor receives an appropriate ligand, a gustducin collision–coupling biochemistry leads to the activation of a PLC/TRPM5 cascade (as described above for sweetness detectors) and release of transmitter substance from the taste receptor cell onto the dendrites of a sensory fibre.

Both sweetness and bitterness receptor mechanisms show a strong resemblance to those which we will find at work in olfactory cilia and photoreceptor outersegments. There is, however, a significant difference. Instead of cyclic nucleotides (cGMP) holding channels **open**, thus maintaining the cells in a

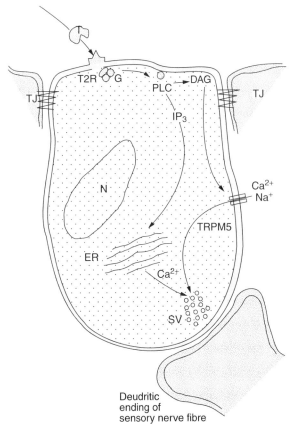

Figure 13.11 Bitter tastant interacts with a T2R receptor molecule and, via gustducin, activates PLC. DAG opens TRPM5 channels in the TRC membrane leading to depolarization. This opens Ca^{2+}-gates in the membrane; IP_3 also releases Ca^{2+} from intracellular stores in the ER The increased internal Ca^{2+} triggers release of transmitter. DAG = Diacylglycerol; ER = endoplasmic reticulum; G = gustducin; N = nucleus; PLC = phospholipase C; SV = synaptic vesicles; T = tastant molecule; TJ = tight junction Further explanation in text.

depolarized state until it is removed by the transducin collision–coupling mechanism and so allowing **hyperpolarization** (Chapter 17), the DAG second messenger in TRCs **opens** previously closed TRPM5 channels leading to **depolarization**.

Water. Ingestion of adequate quantities of water is essential to maintain appropriate osmolarity of the body fluids. Saltiness detectors, as described above, play an important role in maintaining this balance but there is also good evidence for the existence

of water detectors. The glossopharyngeal nerves of frogs and the chorda tympani nerves of mammals, for instance, contain nerve fibres that respond to the application of water to the tongue. Other fibres respond to the application of sodium chloride.

It can be shown that whereas aqueous solutions of sodium acetate do not inhibit the response of water detectors, solutions of sodium chloride and choline chloride do. In consequence, it has been proposed that activation of water detectors depends on chloride channels in the TRC apical membranes. Decreasing external concentrations of chloride activate these channels, leading to an increased secretion of Cl^- and this in turn leads to a depolarization of the TRC.

It has also been found that, subjectively, the 'taste' of water is affected by what precedes it on the tongue. If the preceding substance is quinine or citric acid, water tastes sweet, whereas if it is sodium chloride or sucrose it appears bitter. This suggests that there is significant interaction between water receptors and those of the other tastes.

As with the other taste mechanisms discussed in this section, there are probably other biochemical routes and research is still very active.

13.2.2 Central Projections

As noted above, TRCs are true receptor cells. On depolarization they release transmitter onto the dendritic endings of sensory fibres belonging to the VIIth, IXth and Xth cranial nerves. Figure 13.12 shows that the fibres in all three gustatory pathways terminate in the **solitary nucleus** of the medulla. The solitary nucleus is a complex formation and also receives input from many parts of the viscera. The gustatory fibres terminate within this complex in a thin strip known as the gustatory nucleus. From the gustatory nucleus connections are made upwards to small cells (parvocellular) of the **ventral posterior nucleus** of the thalamus. The gustatory information is then projected onwards to terminate in two gustatory areas in the cortex. The first gustatory area lies in the postcentral gyrus (Brodman's area 3b), and the second lies deep in the Sylvian fissure on the outer surface of the insula. Both these gustatory areas are close to the somatosensory area of the tongue (Figure 8.20).

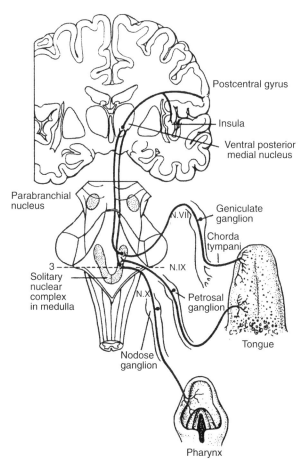

Figure 13.12 Gustatory pathways into the brain. Explanation in text. From Kandel, Schwartz and Jessel (1991) *Principles of Neurosciences*, 3e, Copyright © 1991, Simon and Schuster.

13.2.3 Labelled Lines or Population Profile?

Does the brain recognize different tastes by noting which gustatory fibres are active or by noting the pattern of activity in the whole population of fibres? There is evidence for both mechanisms but the consensus at the time of writing is moving towards the latter theory. This consensus is helped by the preponderating view that taste cells are 'generalists' rather than 'specialists' (see above). The 'across-fibre' pattern theory is also supported by recordings from the chorda tympani nerve of hamster when the taste buds are exposed to different concentrations of the same tastant or different tastant molecules which cause the same (or very similar) taste sensation. It can be shown that, when the concentration of a tastant, such as sodium chloride, is varied, the pattern of impulses in 40 chorda tympani fibres remains the same, although the frequency in each fibre increases or diminishes with the intensity of the stimulus. The whole pattern of activity, in other words, increases or decreases in intensity whilst the overall profile remains unchanged. Similarly, stimuli inducing the same (or closely similar) taste sensations – sweeteners, such as saccharine, sucrose, fructose, sodium salts such as sodium chloride and sodium nitrate ($NaNO_3$), or acids such hydrochloric, citric and acetic acids – generate similar patterns of activity across the forty fibres. This neurophysiological evidence is backed up by behavioural experiments which show that hamsters do not discriminate between the sweeteners or between the salts.

13.3 CONCLUDING REMARKS

Contact chemoreceptors (gustatory receptors) are clearly of great importance in the life of all members of the animal kingdom. Being heterotrophic organisms, animals depend on finding and ingesting appropriate food. The central pathways of gustatory fibres in the mammal show how close the final destination of gustatory input is to sensory fibres carrying other information about the tongue. But it is not only the reflex responses of the tongue which are triggered by gustatory input, it is also the larger scale feeding behaviour of the whole animal. In many cases just one unfortunate response to ingested material, one occasion which might lead hours later to vomiting, is sufficient to ensure that that particular taste reflexly prevents ingestion on future occasions. We are just beginning to understand the biophysical and biochemical mechanisms that are at work in TRCs and in the gustatory receptors of other animals which allow this acute taste discrimination. We are also at the beginning of understanding how the TRCs are integrated into the overall physiology and nutritional behaviour of an animal. Finally, turning to a more applied aspect, it is clear that multibillion pound interests centre on gustatory physiology. Not only the food and drink industries but also pesticide and herbicide manufacturers will benefit from a deeper understanding of gustation in the animal kingdom.

14

OLFACTION

Insects: hygroreceptors - humidity important for small animals - mechanical distortion of sensillum - sensillum often shared with thermoreceptor; **olfactory sensilla** - oderant binding proteins (OBPs) - pheromones - many types - pheromone binding proteins (PBPs) - molecular biology - Drosophila olfactory system - Bombyx antennae - extreme sensitivity; **central processing**: Drosophila antennal lobes – protocerebrum and mushroom bodies. **Mammals: olfactory epithelium** - extent varies according to lifestyle - turbinals - histology - sensory neurons - regenerate throughout life - spatial organisation; **olfactory neurosensory cells (ORNs)** - structure - olfactory binding proteins (OBPs) - olfactory cilia - generalist or specialist? - sensitivity - olfactory receptor proteins (Ors); **molecular biology of ORNs** – Olfactory genes - CNG channels - isolation - functionality - patch clamping of ORNs – biophysics - sensory adaptation - graded response - anosmias; **central processing** - cribriform plate - olfactory bulb - mitral, tufted, periglomerular cells - glomeruli - bulb compared with retina - neurochemistry - olfactory tract - pyriform lobe (uncus) - thalamus - orbito-frontal cortex. **Vomeronasal organ**: location - epithelium - ORNs - different molecular biology - separate evolutionary history - pheromones - projection to accessory olfactory bulb - amygdala and hypothalamus - emotion. **Concluding remarks**: sigificance of chemosenses in inter-individual communication.

We noted in Chapter 13 that the distinction between taste and smell, between gustation and olfaction, so obvious in our human world, is often far from being so obvious in other members of the animal kingdom. This is especially the case in many invertebrate forms. Amongst the vertebrates the two senses are reasonably distinct, even in aquatic forms, with separate sense organs and neurology. Many fish, especially the cartilaginous fish, such as sharks and dogfish, have excellent olfactory senses being able, in the case of sharks to detect blood and other body fluids in the water from considerable distances. Many bony fish also have excellent olfactory abilities. Migratory fish, such as salmon, are able to detect their home streams after their period in the ocean by way of their olfactory sense. If the olfactory sacs are plugged, salmon are at a loss in determining which stream to ascend. In air breathing terrestrial forms, however, the division between the two chemosenses becomes far sharper. Consequently, in this chapter we shall restrict ourselves to a discussion of two fully terrestrial animal groups, the insects and the tetrapod chordates. We shall start with a consideration of insect olfaction and then go on to an account of the rather better known (because more intensively researched) olfactory systems of vertebrates.

14.1 INSECT OLFACTORY SYSTEMS

In Chapters 7 and 8 we looked at the structure and physiology of insect sensory sensilla. Then, in Chapter 13, we examined in some detail the structure and functioning of insect contact chemoreceptors, or gustatory receptors. Much of what was said in those chapters also applies here. With the exception of hygroreceptors, insect olfactory receptors are normally housed within multiporous sensilla.

14.1.1 Hygroreceptors

We saw in Chapter 13 that one of the types of neurosensory cell found within contact uniporous sensilla was a water receptor. Hygroreceptors, which detect humidity, are obviously closely allied to water receptors. But, as they typically have no opening to the exterior, they are best classed alongside olfactory receptors as distance receptors. Atmospheric moisture has no way of accessing the neurosensory cells within the sensillum. Instead, mechanical distortion of the sensillum in response to different humidity is believed to be the adequate stimulus. The sensilla are normally short pegs with an inflexible socket into the cuticle. Sensilla of this type have been found on the antennae of all insects which have been carefully examined. In spite of the importance of hygroreception, it appears that hygroreceptors are not very well represented amongst the sensory hairs on insect antennae; in the cockroach *Periplaneta americana*, for instance, only about 100 of the 54 000 sensilla on each antenna is a hygroreceptor.

The distortion induced by changes in humidity may be either a bending of the sensillum or perhaps a swelling of the sensillar cuticle which puts pressure on the dendritic outersegment. The neurosensory cell is thus considered to be essentially a mechanoreceptor, although the tubular bodies so characteristic of mechanosensitive dendrites (Chapter 8) have yet to be identified with certainty. If bending is, indeed, the adequate stimulus, it is obviously important that the sensillum is protected from the normal collisions of everyday insect life. It is thus not surprising that these

scarce hygroreceptive sensilla are set well down under cover of thickets of lengthy mechanosensitive hairs and are often surrounded by a cuticular collar or set into a declivity.

Hygroreceptive sensilla normally contain more than one neurosensory cell (Figure 14.1). Quite generally there are three and sometimes four such cells. In the triadic organization shown in Figure 14.1 two

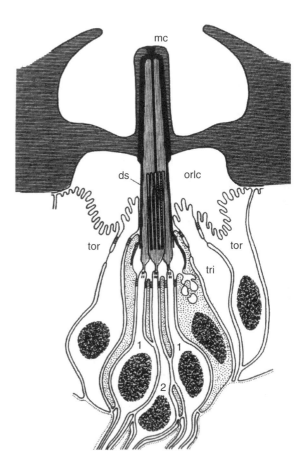

Figure 14.1 Hygro–thermal sensillum. This figure shows a typical 'peg' sensillum containing a triad of sensory neurons. Two type 1 cells (hygroreceptors) share the sensillum with a single type 2 cell (thermoreceptor). Whereas the type 1 cells have lengthy wide diameter dendrites which completely fill the peg, the type 2 cell has a short deeply invaginated dendrite which does not extend as far as the peg. ds = dendritic sheath; mc = moulting channel; oric = outer receptor lymph cavity; tor = tormogen cell; tri = trichogen cell; thecogen cells are stippled. With permission, from the Annual Review of Entomology, Volume 30, © 1985, by Annual Reviews http://www.annualreviess.org.

hygroreceptor cells share the sensillum with a thermoreceptor. This bimodality seems a common design principle throughout many orders of insect. It is clearly of crucial importance for a small animal, such as an insect, to have precise information about the temperature and humidity of environments in which it finds itself. More will be said of insect thermoreceptors in Chapter 20.

14.1.2 Olfactory Sensilla

Insect olfactory neurosensory cells are usually confined within multiporous basiconic or trichoid sensilla (Figure 14.2) located on the antennae and maxillary palps. Odorant molecules striking the sensilla are first adsorbed on the waxy cuticle and then diffuse through the pores into the lymph-filled interior. The odorant molecules first interact with **odorant binding proteins (OBPs)**, which not only solubilise hydrophobic odorants in the lymph but also adapt them to fit the active sites of receptor molecules in the olfactory receptor cell membranes. The similarity with the bacterial receptor-transducer proteins discussed in Chapter 11 is striking. There may also be analogous molecules in the olfactory mucus of vertebrates.

Insects live in a world saturated with 'semiochemicals', that is chemicals which carry specific meanings. They may signal reproductive opportunity (sex pheromones), danger (alarm pheromones), trails (trail pheromones), gathering together or on to a host (aggregation pheromones), dispersal (spacing or epideictic phermones) and so on. As is appropriate, considering their huge importance for survival of the species, the sex pheromones are the most effective of all. It has been calculated that the male silkworm moth, *Bombyx mori*, is sensitive to a single molecule of the female pheromone, **bombykol**.

Moth sex pheromone receptors have provided valuable preparations for olfactory scientists. They are arguably the most sensitive of all olfactory systems. Perhaps the most well known odorant binding proteins (OBPs) are those which bind these pheromones. The antennal sensilla of the giant silk moth, *Antherae polyphemus*, have been shown to contain a 15 kDa protein which very specifically binds the sex pheromone released by the female of the species. The sensilla lymph also contains

a pheromone-specific esterase which breaks down the pheromone, thus preventing too long-lasting an action. Similar highly specific OBPs have been found in other moths. They are nowadays known as **pheromone binding proteins (PBPs)**. In addition to PBPs, numerous other OBPs (sometimes referred to as general-odorant binding proteins (GOBPs)) have been identified in insect olfactory sensilla. In *Drosophila melanogaster* different forms of the highly abundant 14 kDa GOBPs are found in sensilla springing from different subregions of the antenna. It seems likely that this regionalization of GOBPs in the fruit fly plays a role in odour discrimination.

Figure 14.2 shows that the sensillum houses the dendritic outsegments of olfactory neurosensory cells, or olfactory receptor neurons (*ORNs*). Olfactory receptor molecules are inserted in the membranes of these outsegments. In all likelihood they resemble those which have been isolated

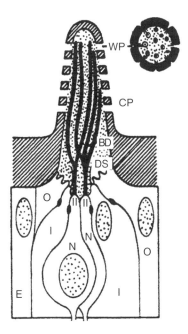

Figure 14.2 Multiporous basiconic olfactory sensillum. The sensillum may contain up to 40 neurosensory cells and the outsegments (as shown) are frequently branched. BD = branched dendritic outsegments; CP = cuticular process; DS = dendritic sheath; E = epidermal cell; I = inner sheath cell; N = neurosensory cell; O = outer sheath cell; WP = wall pore. From Frazier (1985), with permission from John Wiley & Sons, Inc.

in *Drosophila* (see below). There is increasing evidence that, as with the gustatory systems discussed in the last chapter, the PLC, IP_3, DAG system is involved. This implies that a G-protein membrane signalling system is at work. This brings insect olfactory cells into line with the vertebrate systems, which we shall discuss below. The biochemistry leads, as in the vertebrates, to a generator potential in the dendrite: usually a depolarization, but sometimes a hyperpolarization. In the first case an action potential is initiated in the olfactory axon, in the second case any potential action potential is inhibited.

The detailed understanding of the genetics and genetic technology of *Drosophila* has allowed considerable progress to be made in understanding the molecular basis of its olfactory system. In addition to the ease of genetic manipulation, another great advantage of the fruit fly system is its simplicity compared with that of the vertebrates. It consists of no more than about 3000 neurons. Numerous olfactory mutants have been identified. Molecular analysis shows that many of these may be traced to defects in the PLC, IP_3, DAG cascade.

Drosophila olfactory sensilla are located primarily on the third antennal segment (funiculus) and on the maxillary palps. About 200 basiconic, 150 trichoid and 60 coeloconic sensilla are located on the funiculus and a further 60 basiconic sensilla are found on each palp. Each sensillum normally contains three chemosensory and one mechanosensory neurons.

Genetic techniques have revealed a family of about 60 *Or* genes encoding some 62 7TM olfactory receptor molecules. It has been shown that the *Or* genes are quite distinct from the *Gr* genes that were discussed in Section 13.1.2 and few (if any) of the latter encode receptors which have an olfactory function. They also show no sequence similarity to vertebrate *Or* genes. As already mentioned, the olfactory receptor molecules (*Ors*) are located in the dendritic outersegments of the ORNs. Each ORN expresses only one type of Or.

Drosophila antennae develop, as noted above, four types of sensilla: large and small basiconic, trichoid and coeloconic. The maxillary palps only develop basiconic sensilla. A basiconic sensillum may contain three or four ORNs, each expressing a different Or. It appears, furthermore, that sensilla of a particular type house sets of ORNs with a similar odour response profile. Thus, large basiconics

(class ab1) house ORNs sensitive to isoamyl acetate (banana), 2,3-butanedione (butter or sweat), carbon dioxide and methyl salicylate (wintergreen mint) and so on; trichoids (smaller cone-shaped sensilla) house a different set of ORNs, whilst the thin basiconics of the maxillary palp house a different set again (Figure 14.3a). Moreover each of these sensillum types forms a spatially restricted subpopulation on either the third antennal segment (1200 neurons) or the maxillary palp (120 neurons) (Figure 14.3b). In this respect, as we shall see later in this chapter, insect chemosensory surfaces differ from those of vertebrates. Vertebrate olfactory surfaces show no (strong) spatial patterning: differentially sensitive olfactory cells are distributed comparatively randomly in the mucosa.

The sensilla fields on the antennae of the silk moth, *Bombyx mori*, are, as would be expected, far more luxuriant than those in *Drosophila*. In the male moth there are about 17 000 long (100 μm) and thin (2 μm diameter) sensilla forming a lattice on the branches of the antennae (Figure 14.4). This lattice work of sensilla is able to concentrate odorants, especially the sex pheromones of the female, by a factor of 1.5×10^5 when an air current at 60 cm/s is directed through them for 1s. The neurons from the sensilla terminate, like those of *Drosophila*, in a number of glomeruli in the antennal lobes of the deuterocerebrum. These will be discussed further in the next section. In moths they are very distinct and in some, in particular, the sphinx moth, *Manduca sexta*, it has been possible to create detailed maps of 'odour space'.

The intensely active life of many insects is lived in a world full of the bugle calls of chemicals. Can insects be said to experience emotions? It seems unlikely. How can we ever know? But if they did, we can imagine that their marked trails, the molecules wafting against their searching antennae, the odorants rising from surfaces of leaves and the interiors of blossoms, provide powerful surges of nostalgia, hope, excitement and despair. We cannot hope to answer the 'hard question' of what it feels like to be an insect (if anything at all!) but we can make some progress in understanding the workings of their brains. Although much work has been done on the representation of odours in moth antennal lobes and deuterocerebrum, the simpler organization found in the fruit fly, *Drosophila,* has proved, once again, to provide the best experimental preparation.

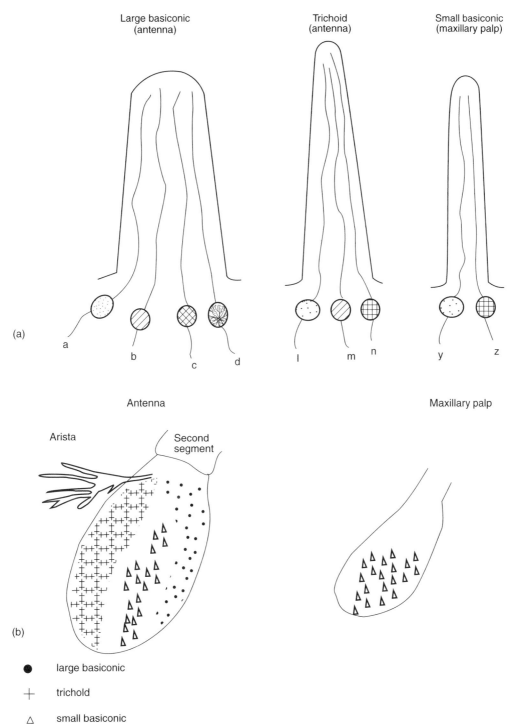

Figure 14.3 ORNs in *Drosophila* antennal and maxillary palp sensilla. (a): the three major types of sensilla are shown. Each contains the dendrites of ORNs which express a particular Or, symbolized by a, b, c and so on; (b): distribution of sensilla types on the antenna and maxillary palp. After Couto, A., Alenius, M. and Dickson, B.J. (2005).

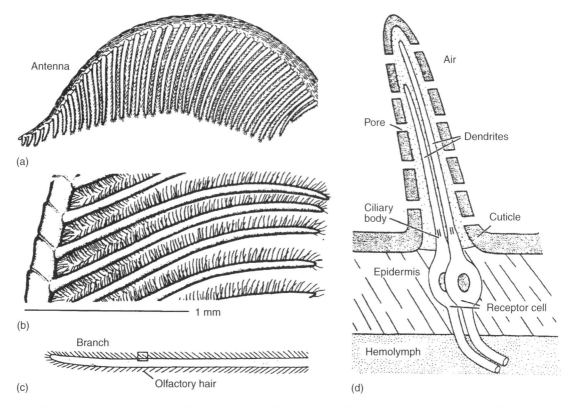

Figure 14.4 Antenna of male silk moth, *Bombyx mori*. (a): Single antenna; (b): Enlargement of antenna; (c): Single branch; (d): Single olfactory hair. From Schneider, 1977, '*Readings from Scientific American: The insects*' with permission from Lorelle Raboni.

14.1.3 Central Processing In *Drosophila* Antennal Lobes

Neurons from *Drosophila* sensilla project to the ipsilateral antennal lobe of the deuterocerebrum where they terminate in about 50 spherical aggregations of cells known as **glomeruli**. This is a low number compared with that found in many other insects: 53 in *Manduca sexta* (sphinx moth), 125 in *Periplaneta americana* (cockroach) and over 1000 in *Locusta migratoria*. It is also, as we shall see in Section 14.2.4, much smaller than in the 1800–2000 in a typical mammal.

The comparative simplicity of the *Drosophila* olfactory system has allowed it to be analysed in great detail. Indeed, almost the entire set of neural connections between the antennae and the antennal lobe has now been mapped. An important general principal has emerged – some indeed have called it the central

dogma of olfactory biology: **one neuron, one type of Or; one glomerulus, one type of ORN** (Figure 14.5). There are, however, many exceptions to this olfactory central dogma. It has been found that in a small number of ORNs two different Ors are expressed and (more rarely) two different types of ORN terminate in the same glomerulus.

Finally, it has been found that there is a correlation between sensory surface, type of sensillum and glomerular position. Thus it has been found that whereas ORNs from trichoid sensilla project to the dorsolateral region of the antennal lobe, ORNs from basiconic and coeloconic sensilla terminate medially and posteriorly and those from the maxilla and palp are directed to the central anterior region. This spatial distribution is somewhat reminiscent of the spatial distribution of gustatory neurons, which we noted in Chapter 13. It is thus not absurd to imagine that the pattern of activity in the antennal lobe

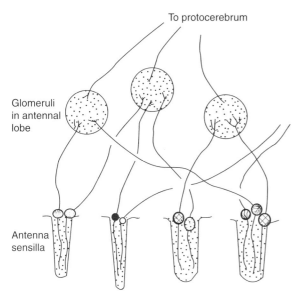

To protocerebrum

Glomeruli
in antennal
lobe

Antenna
sensilla

Figure 14.5 Schematic diagram to show the organization of *Drosophila* olfactory system. ORNs from the antennal sensilla send their fibres to glomeruli in the antennal lobe of the deuterocerebrum. The system is organized so that each glomerulus receives input from only one type of ORN. A further set of fibres carries the olfactory information to the mushroom bodies in the protocerebrum. See text.

reflects the various dimensions, both qualitative and quantitative, of the chemical environment surrounding the fly. We see below that a somewhat similar spatial representation of odour quality (chemical structure of the odorant molecule) is found in the olfactory bulb of mammals although, in mammals, there is no representation of the topography of the sensory surface.

However, the antennal lobes are not, of course, the final destination of olfactory information in the *Drosophila* brain. Projection neurons carry the information on from the antennal lobe glomeruli to the fly's mushroom bodies and protocerebrum. It has been found that projection neurons from single glomeruli terminate in the protocerebrum in a very determinate fashion. In other words, the pattern of axonal arborization developed in the protocerebrum by projection fibres from a given glomerulus is always very much the same. At the same time, the axonal arborization of fibres from different glomeruli interdigitate so that olfactory information of different types and from different areas is distributed

throughout the entire brain. This suggests that third order neurons have the opportunity to integrate this sensory information so that appropriate behavioural responses can be computed.

14.2 MAMMALIAN OLFACTORY SYSTEMS

Let us now turn from the scented world of insects to the almost equally aromatic world of the mammals. The nasal cavity of most air-breathing vertebrates contains at least two distinct olfactory organs: first, and most important, the main olfactory epithelium covering the nasal turbinals and, second, the vomeronasal organ. We shall discuss each in turn.

14.2.1 Olfactory Epithelium of the Nasal Cavity

In the higher primates, including humans, the olfactory epithelium is comparatively small. This is consistent with the fact that odors hang less readily in the forest canopies. The higher primates are, moreover, diurnal creatures specializing in the visual sense for exact judgment of distance and size. Nocturnal forms, where the visual sense is less important, generally develop their other two distance senses, auditory and olfactory, to a much greater degree. The magnitude of the olfactory epithelium in mammals varies from 2 to $4\,cm^2$ (humans), to $9.3\,cm^2$ (rabbits), to $18\,cm^2$ (dog) to $21\,cm^2$ in the domestic cat. It should be noted, however, that these figures do not give a true estimate of the 'acuity' of the olfactory surface, for they do not take into account the numbers of olfactory receptor neurons per unit area.

In mammals the olfactory epithelium is developed over a number of delicate plate-like bones, the **turbinal bones**, in the nasal cavity. The turbinals have the dual function of not only presenting the olfactory epithelium to the incoming air, which swirls around and is impeded by them, but also of warming that air before it proceeds to the lungs. Indeed, the presence or absence of turbinals in fossil skulls has been used to assess whether their long-dead owners were or were not warm blooded. The epithelium itself consists of three types of cell: supporting (glia-like) cells

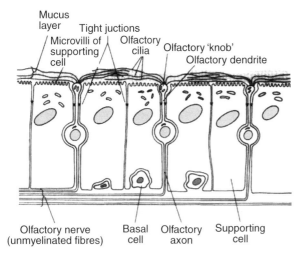

Figure 14.6 Olfactory epithelium. The lengthy olfactory cilia lie over the surface of the epithelium embedded in mucus. Tight junctions between the epithelial cells and between them and the olfactory neurosensory cells prevent any penetration of the intercellular space.

which secrete mucus; neurosensory cells or sensory neurons; and basal cells, which appear to be stem cells capable of dividing and forming new functional neurons throughout life (Figure 14.6) Olfactory cells are the only neurons in the mammalian body which renew themselves throughout life.

We shall see (or have already seen) that in the visual, auditory, somatosensory and, to a lesser extent, gustatory systems the sensory epithelium records spatial information. This mapping function is not well developed in the olfactory epithelium. To a first approximation, cells specialized in detecting specific odors are randomly distributed. However, closer examination does suggest that there are the beginnings of a spatial organization. 2-Deoxyglucose mapping (which enables the neurohistologist to detect active cells) reveals clusters of cells concerned with specific odorants. It appears, for instance, that butanol excites cells in anterior regions whilst limonene activates cells in the posterior parts of the mucosa. Recent work also suggests that the receptor cells are organized into anterior–posterior strips, called '**expression zones**'. There appear, although this remains a matter of dispute, to be three major nonoverlapping expression zones which overlap with a fourth smaller zone. The intricate shape of the nasal cavity

with its palisades of delicate turbinal bones makes it difficult to map these expression zones.

14.2.2 Olfactory Neurosensory Cells

Figure 14.6 shows that olfactory receptor neurons (ORNs) are bipolar with a single unbranched dendrite that squeezes up between the supporting cells to end in a small swelling – the olfactory knob. Up to twenty lengthy cilia project from the olfactory knob. The membranes of these cilia form the sensory membrane of the olfactory neuron. Normally the cilia lie embedded in the mucus, which covers the epithelium, forming a dense mat. Although the olfactory cell has the dual function of detecting the stimulus and transmitting the nerve impulse into the brain and is, consequently, a neurosensory cell, it is customary to call it a sensory neuron.

The mucus in which the olfactory cilia lie contains numerous small (20 kDa) proteins which are in many ways analogous to the odorant binding proteins (OBPs) of insect sensilla. They are secreted by glands in the nasal mucosa and are, in fact, found not only in the mucus covering the olfactory epithelium but also in that covering the purely respiratory epithelium. This fact, and their comparatively small size, suggest that they do not play the significant role of insect (or bacterial) OBPs. If anything, they have very broad-band affinities for odorant molecules and may simply capture them and present them to the ORNs.

The ultrastructure of olfactory cilia is not greatly different from that of other cilia. They contain the usual internal axoneme but are, in mammals at least, nonmotile. They are also unusually long and thin – ranging from 5 to 250 μm in length but often only 100–250 nm in diameter. We have already met this adaptation of an originally motile organelle, the cilium, to serve a sensory function in insect sensilla and vertebrate mechanoreceptors (kinocilia of hair cells) and we shall meet it again in vertebrate photoreceptors (rod and cone outersegments).

The bunch (between five and forty) of long thin cilia springing from the bulb of an olfactory cell undoubtedly increases the sensory surface area dramatically. Freeze–fracture electron microscopy shows, furthermore, that the membrane of each cilium contains a high density of globular particles. It is believed that these are the olfactory receptor molecules. We shall see in Chapter 17 that this is another point of analogy with rod and cone cell outersegments, for they are also densely populated with receptor molecules – rhodopsins or iodopsins.

The olfactory system is able to detect and discriminate between a large variety of odorants. As was the case with gustatory cells, it was long a matter of controversy whether an individual cilium is a generalist or a specialist; whether, in other words, each cilium responds to a number of different types of odorant molecule or to just one. In recent years evidence has accumulated to show that cilia in fact specialize. Vertebrate olfactory neurons adhere to the same central olfactory dogma that we noted for insect sensilla: one neuron, one receptor molecule. All the cilia springing from the bulb of an olfactory neuron express the same olfactory receptor molecule (Or) and hence all respond to the same odorant. The sensitivity is remarkable – humans can detect airborne odorants within the range 10^{-4} to 10^{-13} M. One of the signs of a bad head cold is a marked falling away of this delicate sensitivity. This is because the olfactory cilia become engulfed in the extra amount of mucus produced by the supporting cells.

14.2.3 Molecular Biology

14.2.3.1 Olfactory Receptor Proteins

A large family of genes encode olfactory receptor (Or) proteins. The completion of the human genome revealed some 360 olfactory receptor (Or) genes (plus 363 pseudogenes) whilst some 910 Or genes (plus 299 pseudogenes) have been identified in the mouse genome. Thus, if the mouse genome consists of approximately 24 000 genes (Chapter 5) then about 4% is devoted to olfaction. This gives some indication of the importance of the sense of smell in mice and its lesser importance in humans. This great family of Or genes all encode 7TM GPCRs. We shall see in Chapter 17 that rod and cone opsins also belong to this superfamily, as did the Grs we discussed in Chapter 13. The molecular biology of chemosensory cells thus once again finds parallels in rod and cone photoreceptors.

The 7TM olfactory receptor molecules differ from other members of the 7TM superfamily in show-ing great amino acid diversity in transmembrane domains 3, 4 and, especially, 5, and in the second and third extracellular loops. Looking back to Chapter 1, we can see that these domains form significant parts of the 'barrel of staves' embedded in the membrane. As it is likely that the extracellular loops and the interior of the 'barrel of staves' form the recognition site for odorant molecules, we can begin to see how different receptor molecules are adapted to recognize different odorants. It should be borne in mind, however, that whereas most G-coupled 7TM receptor proteins have rather precise affinities for their ligands, olfactory receptor proteins are believed to accept, with varying affinity, a range of stereochemically similar odorant molecules.

As indicated above, all the evidence shows that ORNs are 'specialists': in other words each expresses only one type of olfactory receptor molecule. However, the 'dogma' is not totally inflexible for, as noted above, a given receptor is stimulated by a small number of chemically related molecules. Vice versa, a single odorant molecule is recognized by a small number of different receptors. It follows that a given odorant is recognized by a specific group of Ors. This pattern of receptors provides its signature (Figure 14.7). The situation in the olfactory mucosa is, however, subtle and dynamic. Slight changes in the chemical structure of an odorant molecule change the group of receptors stimulated. Elimination of the carboxylic oxygen from octanoic acid, for instance, thus transforming it into octanol, a seemingly slight change, induces a large change in the perceived 'smell': from 'rancid and sour' to 'orange and rose-like' (Figure 14.7). Changes in concentration of an odorant molecule may also change the number of receptors stimulated and hence change the code signalled to the olfactory bulb. This matches well with our subjectivity. Several odorants change their 'smell' between dilute and concentrated. Indole, for instance, has a pleasant floral smell when dilute but is unpleasantly putrid when concentrated.

Finally, once the molecular structure of the olfactory receptor proteins became known, it became possible to study their distribution in the nasal mucosa. These studies confirmed that the olfactory epithelium was organized into distinct longitudinal zones (expression zones) that express different sets of OR genes. In the mouse each of the Or genes in a set is expressed in about 0.1% of the olfactory neurons and

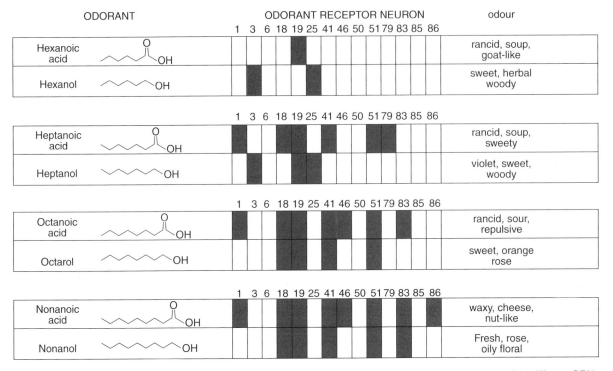

Figure 14.7 Recognition of closely related odorants by different combinations of receptors. The responses of 14 different ORNs to a series of fatty acids and alcohols. Different sets of ORNs are stimulated by the slightly different odorants and the perceived odour is often strikingly different. Note also that in some cases the ORN is only minimally activated. For further detail see text. Modified from Buck, 2004.

these neurons are distributed at random throughout the zone.

14.2.3.2 Membrane Biochemistry

The 7TM receptor in the olfactory cilium is (as usual) linked via a G-protein system to a membrane-bound effector. In most cases the effector is adenylyl cyclase (AC). In some cases, however, a PLC-β, IP$_3$, DAG system has been identified. The transduction mechanism of these latter Ors thus resembles that of the insect olfactory sensilla discussed in the previous section where there is increasing evidence that a PLC-β system operates. When cAMP is the second messenger it is found that it controls a narrow ion channel (Figure 14.8). Because the channel is controlled by a cyclic nucleotide it is called a cyclic nucleotide gated channel (CNG-channel). Although the olfactory CNG-channel was not the first to be isolated (that honour goes to rod cell channels) it is nowadays probably the best characterized.

14.2.3.3 CNG-Channels

Isolation of CNG-channels was first achieved by what has come to be traditional methodology. Firstly, a 63 kDa protein was purified from bovine rod and cone outersegments. When the protein was inserted into an artificial lipid bilayer, single channel currents could be detected in response to cGMP. Next, a bovine retinal cDNA library was probed by oligonucleotides representing sections of this protein. A clone coding for a 690 residue protein was isolated. When this was expressed in *Xenopus* oocyte it formed a functioning cGMP-gated channel. Using sequences derived from this protein, numerous other CNG-channels have been isolated from vertebrate photoreceptors, olfactory epithelia and, most recently, retinal ganglion cells.

To determine which regions of the amino acid chain are located in the membrane, a technique known as hydropathic analysis is employed. In essence, this merely means looking to see if certain stretches of the chain consist of predominantly

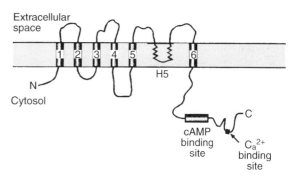

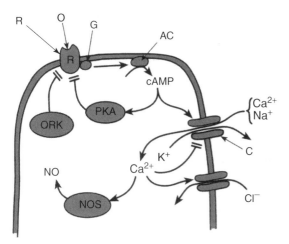

Figure 14.9 Subunit of CNG-channel. Four such subunits surrounding a central channel in the complete complex. Explanation in text.

Figure 14.8 Molecular biology of olfactory receptor cilia. On receipt of an appropriate odorant molecule (O), the odorant receptor initiates a G-protein collision–coupling process, which activates adenylyl cyclase (AC). The resultant cAMP opens a CNG-gated channel (C) in the membrane. Ca^{2+} and Na^+ flow inwards through this channel and K^+ outwards. Ca^{2+} has a number of effects (as shown in the figure). Further explanation in text. AC = adenylyl cyclase; C = CNG-gated channel; G = G-protein; NOS = nitric oxide synthase; O = odorant molecule; ORK = olfactory receptor kinase; PKA = phosphokinase A; R = odorant receptor.

14.2.3.4 Biophysics

The exceedingly delicate task of patch clamping an olfactory cilium has been accomplished and conductance channels which open in response to cAMP have been demonstrated. Because there are about 2400 channels/μm^2 on cilia compared with only about six channels/μm^2 on the olfactory knob and dendrite, studies of single channels have usually used the latter regions of the olfactory cell. Channels in these regions have been shown to have very similar biophysical characteristics to those on the cilia. In the absence of Ca^{2+} these channels respond to cAMP with a conductance of about 45 pS. Ca^{2+} and other divalent cations reduce this conductance to about 1.5 pS. These conductances can also be obtained by the application of cGMP, which is, perhaps, surprising as there is at present no evidence for cGMP in olfactory cells. It may be, however, that cGMP is the outcome of Ca^{2+} induced formation of nitric oxide (NO) from NO-synthase (Figure 14.8). It is known that the major target of nitric oxide is soluble guanylyl cyclase, which it activates. There are likely to be adequate supplies of GTP in the olfactory cell from which guanyl cyclase and form cGMP.

In the absence of Ca^{2+} blockade the CNG-gated channel is highly permeable to all monovalent cations: $Na^+ > K^+ > Li^+ > Rb^+ > Cs^+$. In the physiological situation Na^+, K^+ and Ca^{2+} flow down their electrochemical gradients, thus depolarising the cell. The depolarization of olfactory cells in response to odors can be observed by microelectrode recording techniques. Its magnitude varies with the concentration of odorant. This is an example of a generator potential. It initiates an action potential in

hydrophobic amino acids. When this is done with the CNG-channel protein, six hydrophobic segments are revealed. This implies that the channels have six transmembrane segments (Figure 14.9). This molecular structure resembles that of many well known voltage-gated channels: K^+, Na^+, Ca^{2+}, Cl^- and so on. Indeed, more detailed analysis shows that the fourth transmembrane segment, S4, is strongly homologous to the S4 voltage sensor of the voltage-gated channels. There is also a so-called β-'hair-pin' between S5 and S6. It will be recalled (Chapter 1) that a similar, so-called H5 domain, exists in voltage-gated channels, where it is believed to control the type of ion allowed through the channel. Unlike the voltage-gated channels, however, CNG-channels have a large C-terminal cytoplasmic domain that binds the cyclic nucleotide second messenger. It is believed, largely on the analogy of the well researched K^+-channel, that four of the CNG-channel proteins shown in Figure 14.9 form subunits of the complete channel. The tetramer has been shown to consist of two or three different types of CNG subunits. It is, in other words, a heterotetrameric complex.

the olfactory nerve fibre. The action potential propagates without decrement to the olfactory bulb in the forebrain.

14.2.3.5 Sensory Adaptation and Graded Response

One of the interesting features of isolated CNG-channels in olfactory cilia is that they do not become desensitized. This means that they do not become insensitive to renewed bursts of odorant. Sensory adaptation does, however, occur in the olfactory receptor cell. This seems to be largely due to the influx of Ca^{2+} ions, either directly acting back and suppressing the CNG-channel (Figure 14.8) or through their influence on calmodulin. The influx of Ca^{2+} ions through the CNG-channel also leads to desensitization of the 7TM receptor molecule.

The graded response to odorant concentration is due to the cAMP second messenger system increasing (or decreasing) the number of CNG-channels that are in the open state. In order to discriminate between different odours in real (biological) time the response has to be rapid. Experiment has shown that cAMP production peaks within 40–75 ms of odour application and falls back to zero within 100–500 ms. The amplification provided by the G-protein cascade ensures that numerous channels are activated by one burst of odorant. It has, however, been shown that the channel kinetics are rather slow. Their 'open' status may outlast brief pulses of cAMP by several hundred milliseconds. Continued activation of 7TM receptors by steady concentrations of odorant will thus ensure that the CNG-channel is kept steadily open by burst after burst of cAMP.

14.2.3.6 Anosmias

Genetic analysis of the human olfactory system has revealed several dozen specific anosmias. For instance, one person in ten is unable to detect cyanide and one in a thousand is insensitive to butyl mercaptan, the active agent in the stench emitted by skunks. These anosmias are probably due to deficiency in specific olfactory receptor molecules. Many are inherited in a Mendelian fashion. There is a clear analogy here with human colour blindnesses, which are also due to defective receptor proteins – in this case

iodopsins. In contrast to the genetics of the anosmias, the genetics of human colour blindness are comparatively well understood.

14.2.4 Central Processing

Olfactory cells, as we saw above, are neurosensory cells. Once the generator potential has reached a threshold magnitude, action potentials are initiated at the initial segment of the axon. Figure 14.10a shows that these axons pass through perforations in the cribriform plate to enter the olfactory bulb, which lies just above.

We have already made a number of comparisons between the olfactory and visual systems. Here we have another, for it has been remarked that the olfactory bulb shows some anatomical resemblances to the neural retina. The axons of olfactory receptor cells terminate by making complex synaptic contacts with the dendrites of **mitral cells** (so-called because their shape reminded early microscopists of a bishop's mitre), **tufted cells** and **periglomerular cells**. There is a convergence of about 1000 to 1, that is about 1000 olfactory axons converge on a single mitral arborization. About 25 mitral arborizations gather together to form a small spherical region known as a **glomerulus**. It follows that some 25 000 olfactory axons converge on a single glomerulus. There are some 2000 glomeruli in the rabbit olfactory bulb. Interspersed amongst the glomeruli are short axon periglomerular cells. These cells send an axon into one glomerulus and their dendritic arborization into a neighbouring glomerulus. There is good evidence to show that the periglomerular cells are inhibitory.

The perikarya of the mitral cells form a layer deeper in the olfactory bulb (Figure 14.10b). Interspersed amongst them are the cell bodies of **granule cells**. These cells, like the periglomerular cells, are inhibitory. It will be seen (Chapter 17) that this layered cellular organization of the olfactory bulb shows some resemblance to that of the retina. The main vertical transmission, carried by the axons of the mitral and, to a lesser extent, the tufted cells, is filtered (as it is in the retina) through two layers of horizontal modulation. Although there is certainly a resemblance, we shall see, when we come to Chapter 17, that the retina is considerably more complex.

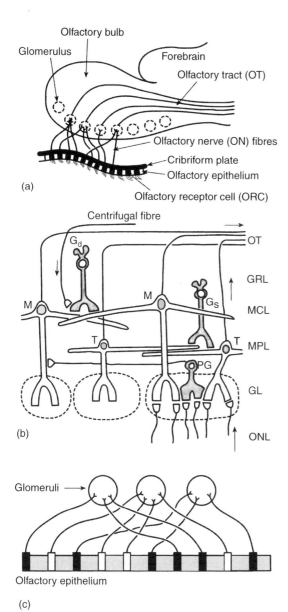

(a)

(b)

(c)

Figure 14.10 Olfactory bulb. (a) The figure shows olfactory axons passing through the cribriform plate to end in glomeruli in the olfactory bulb. (b) Basic circuit of the mammalian olfactory bulb. Layers: EPL = external plexiform layer; GL = glomerular layer; GRL = granule cell layer; OT = olfactory tract; MCL = mitral cell layer. Cells: G_d = deep granule cell; G_s = superficial granule cell; M = mitral cell; PG = periglomerular cell; T = tufted cell. Inhibitory cells stippled. Simplified from Shepherd, 1990. (c) Olfactory receptor cells (ORCs) specialized in detecting one or a few similar odorant molecules send their axons to the same glomerulus. Explanation in text.

Careful electron microscopy of the olfactory bulb has revealed some of the intricacy of the synaptic contacts. The neurochemistry is similarly intricate. About a dozen different neurotransmitters have been identified, including acetylcholine, nor-adrenaline, dopamine, GABA and several neuroactive peptides.

Is there any evidence to show that ORNs specialized in detecting the same odours project to the same glomeruli? In other words, does the second part of the olfactory central dogma apply: one glomerulus, one ORN? The answer to this question is largely in the affirmative. In recent years the sophisticated techniques of biochemical and molecular biological histology have been applied to the olfactory system. Horseradish peroxidase (HRP) injected into specific glomeruli can be shown to be retrogradely transported to a specific population of ORNs in the olfactory epithelium. Vice versa, the mRNA coding for specific receptor molecules in ORNs is detectable in their axons and their terminals within the glomeruli. It can be shown that this mRNA is only detectable in a small number or even a single glomerulus. It is concluded that the axons from ORNs expressing this odorant receptor all converge on one or a small subset of glomeruli. Thus, although ORNs responding to a small class of similar odorant molecules, or to single odorant molecule, may be distributed comparatively randomly in the expression zones of the olfactory epithelium, it appears that their axons converge on a small number of glomeruli, or even a single glomerulus (Figure 14.10c).

Moreover, the anatomical positions of these glomeruli are identical in different animals of the same species. A given odour thus elicits a similar pattern of activity in the glomerular population of the olfactory bulb of all members of the species (Figure 14.11). As the different odours activate different populations of ORNs (Figure 14.7) this pattern is complex and unique. If there are some 2000 glomeruli the number of different patterns is virtually unlimited. These patterns of activity can be visualized by 2-deoxyglucose histochemistry. It is fascinating to find that odours, like the inputs from other distance senses, are analysed by way of spatial maps in the central nervous system. It is also significant that, as noted in Section 14.1.2, the antennal lobes of insects, which share a common ancestor with vertebrates far back in the Precambrian, have evolved an almost identical system.

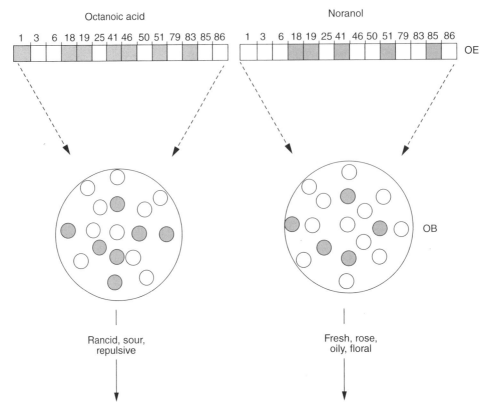

Figure 14.11 Spatial patterns of glomerular activity in the olfactory bulb represent different odors. Different odorants (octanoic acid, nonanol) activate different ORNs in the olfactory epithelium (OE). Each activated ORN runs to a specific glomerulus in the olfactory bulb (OB). The schematic shows that the two different odorants cause different patterns of glomerular activation in the bulb. These patterns are transmitted onward and ultimately perceived as two distinctively different odours. Compare figure with Figure 14.7. Modified from Buck, 2004.

From the bulb the olfactory information is transmitted to the brain by axons of the mitral (and tufted) cells that make up the olfactory tract. As Figure 14.12 shows, the tract courses beneath the frontal lobe to

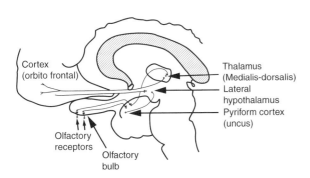

Figure 14.12 Central projections of the olfactory tract. Explanation in text.

terminate in one of the evolutionarily most ancient parts of the cortex: the pyriform lobe (or uncus). A further neuron carries olfactory information to the thalamus and a final fibre projects to the orbitofrontal neocortex. It may be that it is this pathway that triggers the emotional reaction which familiar odours and scents evoke.

14.3 THE VERTEBRATE VOMERONASAL ORGAN (VNO) AND PHEROMONES

The position of the vomeronasal organ in the mouse is shown in Figure 14.13. It is a blind-ending cul de sac beneath the main nasal cavity. It develops in the air-breathing tetrapod land fauna, although it appears to be comparatively inactive in humans and

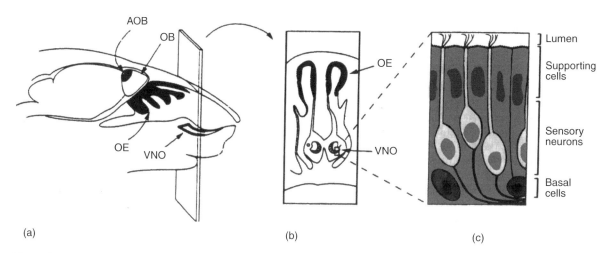

Figure 14.13 Mouse vomeronasal system. (a) Parasagittal section through nasal and vomeronasal organ. (b) Coronal section at position shown in (a). (c) Histology of the vomeronasal epithelium. AOB = accessory olfactory bulb; OB = olfactory bulb; OE = olfactory epithelium on turbinal bones; VNO = vomeronasal organ. From Liman, E. R. (1996) Pheromone transduction in the vomeronasal organ, *Current Opinion in Neurobiology*, **6**, 487, with permission of Elsevier Science.

old world primates. It possesses an olfactory epithelium which, at the cellular level, is indistinguishable from that covering the turbinals in the main nasal cavity. In other words, it consists of olfactory receptor cells (ORNs) (neurosensory cells) amongst supporting epithelial and basal cells. The ORNs, like those of the turbinal epithelium, regenerate throughout life. Instead of cilia, however, the ORNs develop thin microvilli.

The molecular biology of ORNs in the vomeronasal organ is also distinctively different from that of the turbinal ORNs. Although, like other ORNs, they possess a full complement of 7TM receptor molecules, these molecules bear no sequence resemblance to the 7TM receptor molecules in the other ORNs. They seem to have had a lengthy independent evolutionary history. Indeed, it has recently been demonstrated that two distinct 7TM receptor families exist in the vomeronasal mucosa, each thought to involve between 100 and 200 genes. These two families have been named V1R and V2R. Whilst the V1R family seems to be independently evolved, the other, the V2R family, with a lengthy extracellular N-terminal domain, appears to be related to the metabotropic glutamate receptor (mGluR). Referring back to Section 13.2.1.2, it is interesting to note that the TR1 'sweetness' receptor is also believed to be related to mGluR molecule. The

G-protein signalling system which is present in turbinal ORNs (Section 14.2.3.2 above) is not expressed in vomeronasal cells. At the time of writing, the transduction biochemistry is not certain: but it is probable that, instead of the preponderantly cAMP system of the nasal cavity, the vomeronasal ORNs use an IP_3 system (Figure 14.14). This difference, added to the dissimilarity of the 7TM receptor proteins, lends weight to the view that the vomeronasal and turbinal systems are derived by independent evolution. This view is further strengthened by the observation that CNG-channels are absent from VNO ORNs. Instead of CNG-channels, the VNO ORNs express channels belonging to the TRPC2 family of cation channels.

As the vomeronasal organ is not found in fish, it may be that the two olfactory epithelia were originally intercalated, only to be separated out during the evolution of terrestrial vertebrates. As it has recently been shown that both the nasal and vomeronasal systems detect hormones it would seem that this separation was never entirely complete.

That the vomeronasal organ is involved in detecting vertebrate pheromones has long been suspected. Snakes use the vomeronasal organ to track prey. However, the best authenticated examples of pheromones in mammals come from studies on the mating behaviour of the golden hamster. Male

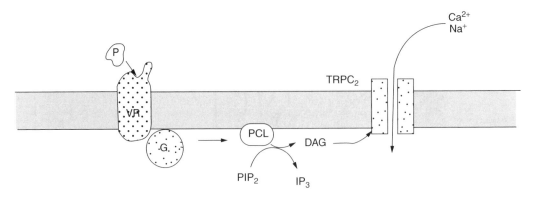

Figure 14.14   VNO transduction. A pheromone (P) activates V1R and/or V2R (VR) in the ORNs dendritic membrane. A G-protein system transmits this activation to PLC which, in turn, catalyses the hydrolysis of PIP_2 to IP_3 and DAG. DAG acts directly on TRPC2, opening the channel so that Ca^{2+} and Na^+ flow inwards. This leads to a generator potential in the ORNs dendrite. Modified from Liman and Zufall, 2004.

mounting behaviour is triggered by pheromones in the female vaginal secretions. Furthermore, the on-set of puberty in female mice is accelerated by male urine and delayed by female urine. These and other pheromone-induced behaviours are believed to be mediated through the vomeronasal organ. This research has been sharpened by the identification of TRPC2 channels in the VNO receptors in mice. It has subsequently been shown that when the gene for TRPC2 is eliminated ($Tprc2-/-$), mice lose both neurophysiological and behavioural responses to pheromones. There is a complete lack of electrophysiological response to dilute urine and male mice no longer react aggressively to other males and lose interest in females. Research is, at present, continuing and specific pheromone receptor molecules have yet to be characterized.

Afferent fibres from the vomeronasal epithelium project to the accessory olfactory bulb, posterior to the olfactory bulb (Figure 14.13). It is interesting to note that, like the turbinal olfactory epithelium, the vomeronasal epithelium is subdivided into zones. This subdivision is marked by the expression of different G-proteins in the apical compared with the basal region. These zones are preserved in the projection to the accessory olfactory bulb. The apical ORNs project to the anterior and the basal ORNs project to the posterior part of the bulb. The projection neurons terminate in glomeruli but, compared with the main bulb, these are comparatively poorly defined. Furthermore, there seems to be a distinct

difference in the mode of representation. Instead of a spatial map, which is so characteristic of the main bulb, the projection to the accessory bulb seems to be complex and many faceted. It is still the subject of research, using all the techniques of modern molecular neurobiology. It has been suggested that the complex nature of the representation may be related to the biological function of the system. It may be that the accessory bulb is primed to respond to the particular species-specific cocktail of chemicals in the appropriate pheromone and simply discard all others. The projection from the accessory bulb is, again, unlike that from the main bulb. Instead of projecting onwards to the cortex, the accessory bulb projects exclusively to parts of the limbic system: the amygdala and hypothalamic nuclei. These nuclei are known to be crucially involved in sexual and reproductive behaviour. Once again, the neuroanatomy is consistent with emotive response to 'something in the air', to the message in environmental chemicals.

Finally, as noted above, it appears that humans lack a functional vomeronasal system. Practically all the several hundred VNO receptor genes in humans, including the *TPRC2* receptor gene, are pseudogenes. It has been argued that the evolutionary loss of the VNO in hominids and old world monkeys is associated with the development of effective trichromatic colour vision. This, as suggested in Section 17.2.1.7, allowed sexual signals to be transmitted by the vivid coloration of skin and fur instead of by scents and odours. It is likely, however, that sexual signalling by chemical signals is only relatively reduced, for humans and other primates are by no means unaffected by pheromones; quite the contrary. Indeed it has been shown recently that it is a mistake to make too sharp a division between mammalian nasal and vomeronasal systems. There is now good evidence to show that both systems detect pheromones and that this information is not restricted to the limbic system but distributed to wide areas of the brain, including those which are regarded as cognitive.

14.4 CONCLUDING REMARKS

With this chapter we come to the end of Part Three. Although the chemosenses do not figure as largely in the human world as the mechanosenses (especially phonoreception) or the photosenses (vision) they play major roles in other forms of animal life. We have noted their deep significance in the life of insects. Their world, as we noted, is awash with chemical signals. It only takes a single pheromone molecule to tell the silk moth that a sexual partner is somewhere near. The lives of social insects are held together by trails and patches of semiochemicals. Once again, as we noted at the end of Part Two, detectors originally evolved to pick up signals relating to the abiotic world have developed into means of communication between living forms. This interindividual communication is not, of course, restricted to the insects. It is widespread through the animal kingdom. Who is not aware of the way the domestic dog marks out his territory? Nor is it restricted to infrahuman animals. Although our own chemosenses are nowhere near as acute as those of many other animals, bad smells and attractive perfumes play significant roles in our lives. Once again large commercial interests are concerned with the olfactory sense, as they were with gustation. The recent interest in the vomeronasal organ suggests that it is not only silk moths that are energized by pheromones emitted by the opposite sex.

PART III: SELF ASSESSMENT

The following questions are designed both to help you assess your understanding of the topics covered in the text and to direct your attention to significant aspects of the subject matter. The sequence of questions follows the sequence in which the subject matter is presented in the text. It is thus easy to refer back to the appropriate page or pages. After reading each chapter and/or each section you should look through these questions and make sure you know the answers and the issues involved.

CHAPTER 11: CHEMOSENSITIVITY IN PROKARYOCYTES

11.1   Describe the movement of prokaryotic flagellae. How does it differ from that of eukayrotic flagellae?

11.2   How does the direction of rotation of its flagellae affect the movement of *E. coli*? Which direction, clockwise or counterclockwise, induces 'tumbling'?

11.3   How does altering the number of 'tumbles' per unit time cause the bacterium to move towards the source of a chemical attractant?

11.4   Describe the biochemical mechanisms by which *E. coli* detects an attractant (or repellant) molecule.

11.5   How can sensory adaptation be demonstrated?

11.6   What rôle do binding proteins play? Refer forward to Chapter 14 and discuss their analogy with similar molecules in insect sensilla and mammalian olfactory cilia.

11.7   What effect does the phosphorylation of CheY have on the rotation of the flagellum?

11.8   How is the effect of CheY on the flagellar motor terminated?

11.9   Why are R–T proteins sometimes called MCPs?

11.10 How does the blockage of methylation domains on the R–T proteins affect bacterial motion? Explain how this accounts for sensory adaptation.

11.11 Is there any evidence that bacterial and mammalian chemosensory systems share a common ancestry?

CHAPTER 12: MAMMALIAN CHEMO-ENTERORECEPTORS

12.1   What evolutionary advantage is conferred on animals by the ability to maintain a stable 'internal environment'?

12.2   Explain how $PaCO_2$ is related to the pH of the ECF.

12.3   Where are chemoreceptors sensitive to $PaCO_2$ and PaO_2 located?

12.4   Discuss the evolutionary origin of the carotid labyrinth.

12.5   Which cells in the carotid body contain transmitter vesicles? Which neurotransmitter do the vesicles contain?

12.6   Which of the peripheral chemoreceptors is sensitive to oxygen deficiency due to anaemia?

12.7   How does respiratory rate change in response to a decrease in PaO_2 and/or an increase in $PaCO_2$?

Biology of Sensory Systems, Second Edition   C.U.M. Smith
© 2008 John Wiley & Sons, Ltd

12.8   Why is it difficult to determine the reflex responses initiated by the carotid bodies?

12.9   Explain the biochemical consequences of a fall in PaO_2 in type 1 cells of the carotid body.

12.10   Describe the biochemical consequences of a rise in $PaCO_2$ in the type 1 cells.

CHAPTER 13: GUSTATION

13.1   What is the difference between gustation and olfaction?

13.2   Describe how the proboscis extension reflex has been used to investigate insect gustation.

13.3   Where are chemosensitive hairs concentrated in dipteran insects?

13.4   Outline the biophysics of chemosensitivity in insect sensilla. How does the mechanism of electrotonic spread resemble that found in vertebrate myelinated axons?

13.5   Where are chemosensory hairs found in *Drosophila*?

13.6   To which part of the CNS do gustatory receptors on *Drosophila* proboscis project?

13.7   Is there any evidence that tastes are topographically mapped in *Drosophila's* CNS?

13.8   Explain how the organization of gustatory information in the fruit fly's brain relates to its behavioural response.

13.9   List the basic sensory qualia of human taste. How do they relate to the necessities of the biological world?

13.10   How are the taste buds distributed over the tongue and how are they innervated?

13.11   Draw a diagram to explain the cellular structure of a typical human taste bud.

13.12   Are taste receptors neurosensory cells or receptor cells?

13.13   Name the two families of taste–receptor genes and explain what type of protein they encode.

13.14   What is gustducin and where is it found?

13.15   Describe the molecular biology of one type of taste–receptor cell.

13.16   How does molecular biological investigation of rat colon cells promise to help our understanding of the saltiness receptor cell?

13.17   Describe how saltiness receptor cells are under hormonal control.

13.18   How does the molecular biology of bitterness-receptor cells both resemble and differ from that of rod and cone photoreceptors (refer also to Section 17.2.1.3).

13.19   What is the 'solitary nucleus', where is it located and what is its significance in gustation?

13.20   Where are the cortical gustatory areas located?

13.21   Comment on the commercial significance of research into the biology of gustation.

CHAPTER 14: OLFACTION

14.1   How and why are hygroreceptors distinguished from water receptors?

14.2   How are variations in humidity detected by insect hygrometric sensilla? Does this mechanism have any implications for the position and morphology of the sensillum?

14.3   Do hygroreceptive sensilla normally contain more than one neurosensory cell? If so, which other sensory modality is commonly represented?

14.4   How is the first step in the insect olfactory receptor mechanism similar to that found in bacterial chemoreception?

14.5   What is meant by the term 'semiochemical'? Gives some examples.

14.6   Describe the moth olfactory system.

14.7   In which part of an olfactory receptor neuron (ORN) are olfactory receptor molecules (Ors) embedded?

14.8   Describe the transduction biochemistry in ORNs. Do ORNs express more than one type of Or?

14.9   Where are *Drosophila* chemoreceptor sensilla located?

14.10   How do the *Drosophila* olfactory surfaces differ from those of mammals?

14.11   To which part of the insect brain do olfactory fibres project, and in what structures do they terminate?

14.12   What has been called the 'central dogma' of olfactory biology? Are there exceptions?

14.13 Where do projection fibres from the antennal glomeruli terminate?

14.14 What are the turbinal bones and what function do they serve in olfaction?

14.15 Does the olfactory epithelium have a topographical organization and, if so, what form does it take?

14.16 Describe two ways in which olfactory receptor cells differ from gustatory receptor cells.

14.17 Describe the conformation of an olfactory receptor protein. How is it believed to recognize an odorant molecule?

14.18 How does a pattern of activated Ors signal a specific odorant molecule?

14.19 Are ORNs distributed completely at random in the nasal mucosa?

14.20 Draw a diagram to illustrate the molecular biology responsible for the transduction of an odorant stimulus into a depolarization of the olfactory receptor cell.

14.21 Explain the molecular biology responsible for sensory adaptation and graded responses in olfactory cells.

14.22 Does the olfactory system show any analogies with inherited colour defects in the retina?

14.23 With reference to Chapter 17, explain the resemblance between the 'wiring' of the olfactory bulb and that of the retina.

14.24 What evidence is there that olfactory glomeruli are specialized to deal with particular odours?

14.25 Explain how the pattern of glomerular excitation in the olfactory bulb encodes the taste presented to the olfactory mucosa.

14.26 To which parts of the brain is the olfactory information delivered from the olfactory bulb?

14.27 In what ways is the vomeronasal epithelium similar and in what ways different from the nasal mucusa?

14.28 Describe the Or molecules expressed in the vomeronasal mucosa.

14.29 Which types of odorant molecules are the vomeronasal organ specialized to detect?

14.30 Describe the afferent pathway from the vomeronasal organ into the brain. Why is the destination of these afferent fibres particularly significant?

PART III: NOTES, REFERENCES AND BIBLIOGRAPHY

INTRODUCTION

Eisthen (1997) provides an account of the evolution of vertebrate olfactory systems, with particular reference to the origin of the tetrapod vomeronasal organs, the morphology of the receptor cells and the evolution of central projections; Whitear (1992) and Finger (1997) review the structure, function and central connections of vertebrate solitary chemosensory cells, whilst Prasad and Reed (1999) discuss the advances in understanding achieved by using the techniques of modern genetics to dissect the chemosensory system of *C. elegans*.

Eisthen, H.L. (1997) The evolution of vertebrate olfactory systems. *Brain, Behaviour and Evolution*, **50**, 222–33.

Finger, T.E. (1997) Evolution of taste and solitary chemoreceptor cell systems. *Brain, Evolution and Behaviour*, **50**, 234–43.

Prasad, B.C. and Reed, R.R. (1999) Chemosensation: molecular mechanisms in worms and mammals. *Trends in Genetics*, **15**, 150–3.

Whitear, M. (1992) Solitary chemoreceptor cells, in *Fish Chemoreception*, 2nd edn (ed. T.J. Hara), Elsevier, Dordrecht.

CHAPTER 11: CHEMOSENSITIVITY IN PROKARYOCYTES

Detailed accounts of bacterial chemosensitivity are to be found in the following publications.

Adler, J. (1983) Bacterial chemotaxis and molecular neurobiology. *Cold Spring Harbor Symposia in Quantitative Biology, XLVlll*, **2**, 803–4.

Bourrett, R.B., Borkovich, K.A. and Simon, M.I. (1991) Signal transduction pathways involving protein phosphorylation in prokaryotes. *Annual Review of Biochemistry*, **60**, 401–41.

Koshland, D.E. Jr (1981) Biochemistry and adaptation in a simple bacterial system. *Annual Review of Biochemistry*, **50**, 765–82.

Manson, M.D. (1992) Bacterial motility and chemotaxis. *Advances in Microbial Physiology*, **33**, 277–346.

Schuster, S.C. and Khan, S. (1994) The bacterial flagellar motor. *Annual Review of Biophysics and Biomolecular Structure*, **23**, 509–39.

Simon, M.I., Krikos, A., Mutoh, N. and Boyd, A. (1985) Sensory transduction in bacteria. *Current Topics in Membranes and Transport*, **23**, 3–15.

CHAPTER 12: MAMMALIAN CHEMO-ENTERORECEPTORS

Extracts from Claude Bernard's foundational *Leçons* are given in Fulton (1966) and Cannon (1932) is still a valuable resource. Accounts of the complex neurophysiology responsible for maintaining the level of respiratory gases in the ECF are given in textbooks of physiology. Detail of the peripheral chemoreceptors in the carotid bodies is provided by the publications listed below.

Bernard, C. (1878) *Leçons sur les Phenomènes de la Vie commune aux Animaux et aux Vegetaux*, Vol. **1** (ed. A. Dastre), Paris, p. 112.

Biscoe, T.J., Purves, M.J. and Sampson, S.R. (1970) The frequency of nerve impulses in single carotid body chemoreceptor afferent fibres recorded *in vivo* with intact circulation. *Journal of Physiology*, **208**, 121–31.

Cannon, W. (1932) *The Wisdom of the Body*, Kegan Paul, Trench, Trubner & Co. Ltd, London.

Fulton, J. (1966) *Selected Readings in the History of Physiology*, C.C. Thomas, Illinois.

Gonzalez, C. *et al.* (1992) Oxygen and acid chemoreception in the carotid body chemoreceptors. *Trends in Neurosciences*, **15**, 146–53.

Gonzalez, C. *et al.* (1994) Carotid body chemoreceptors: from natural stimuli to sensory discharges. *Physiological Reviews*, **74**, 829–98.

Grove, A.J. and Newell, G.E. (1945) *Animal Biology*, University Tutorial Press, London.

Haddad, G. and Jiang, C. (1997) O_2-sensing mechanisms in excitable cells: role of plasma membrane K^+ channels. *Annual Review of Neurosciences*, **59**, 23–43.

Marshall, J.M. (1994) Peripheral chemoreceptors and cardiovascular regulation. *Physiological Reviews*, **74**, 543–94.

McDonald, D.M. and Mitchell, R.W. (1975) The innervation of ganglion cells, glomus cells and blood vessels in the rat carotid body. *Journal of Neurocytology*, **4**, 177.

CHAPTER 13: GUSTATION

Taste is a huge and commercially important topic. The publications of the CCFRA, one of the largest food and drink research centres in the world, give some idea of the scope (http://www.campden.co.uk). Dethier's small book on the fly (1963) is a classic and gives detail of the proboscis extension experiments; Kerkut and Gilbert (1985) provide a comprehensive account of insect gestation and Dahanukar, Hallem and Carlson (2005) contribute a modern review. Keverne (1982) and Lindemann (1996) review mammalian gestation, and Scott (2005) provides an up-to-date review. Adler *et al.* (2000) and Nelson *et al.* (2001) describe the discovery of mammalian receptors for bitter and sweet tastes. The old idea, initially due to Hänig (1901) and developed by a process of 'graphical evolution' in textbooks over the years, that there is a strong segregation of sweet, bitter, sour and salty receptors across the tongue, is no longer accepted (Bartoshuk, 1993). Pfaffman first introduced the concept of a cross-fibre code for gustatory sensitivity (a summarizing review

is Paffmann, 1959); Erickson (1982) has sought to generalize this concept to apply to several other sensory modalities; Frank, Bieber, Smith (1988) describe the experiments on forty hamster chorda tympani fibres mentioned in the text.

Adler, E. *et al.* (2000) A novel family of mammalian taste receptors. *Cell*, **100**, 693–702.

Bartoshuk, L.M. (1978) Gustatory system, in *Handbook of Behavioural Neurobiology, Sensory Integration*, Vol. **1** (ed. R.B. Masterton), Plenum, New York.

Bartoshuk, L.M. (1993) The biological basis of food perception and acceptance. *Food Quality and Preference*, **4**, 21–32.

Blum, M.S. (ed.) (1985) *Fundamentals of Insect Physiology*, John Wiley & Sons, Inc., New York.

Dahanukar, A., Hallem, E.A. and Carlson, J.R. (2005) Insect chemoreception. *Current Opinion in Neurobiology*, **15**, 423–30.

Dethier, V.G. (1963) *To Know a Fly*, Holden-Day Inc, San Francisco, CA.

Erickson, R.P. (1982) The "across-fibre pattern" theory: An organising principle for molar neural function. *Contributions to Sensory Physiology*, **6**, 79–110.

Frank, M.E., Bieber, S.L. and Smith, D.V. (1988) The organisation of taste sensibilities in hamster chorda tympani nerve fibers. *Journal of General Physiology*, **91**, 861–96.

Hänig, D.P. (1901) Zur psychophysik des geshmacksinnes. *Philosophische Studien*, **17**, 576–623.

Henning, H. (1922) Psychologische studien am geschmacksinn. *Handbuch Biol. Arbeitsmeth*, **6A**, 627–40.

Kandel, E.R, Schwartz, J.H. and Jessel, T.M. (1991) *Principles of Neuroscience*, McGraw Hill, New York.

Kerkut, G.A. and Gilbert, L.I. (eds) (1985) *Comprehensive Insect Physiology, Nervous System: Sensory*, Vol. 6, Clarendon Press, Oxford.

Keverne, E.B. (1982) Chemical senses: taste, in *The Senses* (eds H.B. Barlow and J.D. Mollon), Cambridge University Press, Cambridge.

Lindemann, B. (1996) Taste reception. *Physiological Reviews*, **76**, 719–66.

Morita, H. and Shiraishi, A. (1968) Stimulation of the labellar sugar receptor in the fleshfly by mono- and disaccharides. *J. Gen. Physiol.*, **52**, 559–583.

Nelson, G. *et al.* (2001) Mammalian sweet taste receptors. *Cell*, **106**, 381–90.

Pfaffman, C. (1959) The afferent code for sensory quality. *American Psychologist*, **14**, 226–32.

Scott, K. (2005) Taste recognition: food for thought. *Neuron*, **48**, 455–64.

CHAPTER 14: OLFACTION

Detail of the structure and function of insect olfactory systems is given in Altner and Prillinger (1980), Altner and Loftus (1985) and Frazier (1985); Schneider (1977) and Mayer and Mankin (1985) discuss insect pheromones and Rospars and Hildebrand (1992) provide detail of the glomerular structure in the antennal lobes of a moth. Stocker (1994). Carlson (1996), Jefferis (2005) and Couto, Alenius and Dickson (2005) describe the olfactory system of that most well known of insects, *Drosophila,* whilst Vosshall and Stocker (2007) provide an up-to-date review. A comprehensive review of the well developed olfactory system in fish is given by Laberge and Hara (2001) and reviews of mammalian olfactory cells are provided by Schild and Restrepo (1998) and Schoenfeld and Cleland (2005), whilst Axel (2004) and Buck (2004) provide accessible accounts, with excellent colour slides, of the olfactory systems of *Drosophila* and mammals in their Nobel orations. Linda Buck also gives a valuable account of the cortical representation of the olfactory world. Shepherd (2003) provides authoritative discussions of the entire vertebrate olfactory system whilst Malnic *et al.* (1999) describe some of the subtleties of the olfactory sense. Buck (2004), Tirindelli, Mucignat-Caretta and Pryba (1998), Bargmann (1999) and Leon and Johnson (2003) discuss recent work on sensory representation in the accessory olfactory bulb. A useful overview of olfactory systems across the phyla can be found in Hildebrand and Shepherd (1997); Fernandez and Morris (2007) analyse the evolutionary relationship between colour vision and the VNO and Shepherd (2006) reviews evidence that pheromones affect not only the limbic system but large areas of the mammalian brain.

Insects

Altner, H. and Prillinger, L. (1980) Ultrastructure of invertebrate chemo-, thermo- and hygroreceptors and its functional significance. *International Review of Cytology*, **67**, 69–139.

Altner, H. and Loftus, R. (1985) Ultrastructure and function of insect thermo- and hygroreceptors. *Annual Review of Entomology*, **30**, 273–95.

Couto, A., Alenius, M. and Dickson, B.J. (2005) Molecular, anatomical, and functional organisation of the *Drosophila* olfactory system. *Current Biology*, **15**, 1535–47.

Carlson, J.R. (1996) Olfaction in *Drosophila*: from odor to behavior. *Trends in Genetics*, **12**, 175–80.

Frazier, J.L. (1985) Nervous system: sensory system, in *Fundamentals of Insect Physiology* (ed. M.S. Blum), John Wiley & Sons, Inc., New York.

Hallem, E.A., Ho, M.G. and Carlson, J.G. (2004) The molecular basis of odor coding in *Drosophila* antenna. *Cell*, **117**, 965–79.

Hallem, E.A., Dahanukar, A. and Carlson, J.R. (2006) Insect odor and taste receptors. *Annual Review of Entomology*, **51**, 113–35.

Jefferis, G.S.X.E. (2005) Insect olfaction: a map of smell in the brain. *Current Biology*, **15**, R668–70.

Gilbert, L.I. (ed.) (1985) *Comprehensive Insect Physiology, Biochemistry and Pharmacology*, Pergamon Press, Oxford.

Rospars, J.P. and Hildebrand, J.G. (1992) Anatomical identification of glomeruli in the antennal lobes of the male sphinx moth, *Manduca sexta. Cell Tissue Research*, **270**, 205–27.

Schneider, D. (1977) The sex-attractant receptor of moths, in *The Insects* (eds T. Eisner and E.O. Wilson), W.H. Freeman, San Francisco.

Schild, D. and Restrepo, D. (1998) Transduction mechanisms in vertebrate olfactory receptor cells. *Physiological Reviews*, **78**, 429–466.

Shepherd, G.M. (1990) *The Synaptic Organisation of the Brain*, Oxford University Press, New York.

Stocker, R.F. (1994) The organisation of the chemosensory system in *Drosophila melanogaster*: A review. *Cell Tissue Research*, **275**, 3–26.

Vosshall, L.B. and Stocker, R.F. (2007) Molecular architecture of smell and taste in *Drosophila. Annual Review of Neuroscience*, **30**, 505–33.

Vertebrates

Axel, R. (2004) Scents and sensibility: a molecular logic of olfactory perception, at http://nobelprize.org/nobel_prizes/medicine/laureates/2004/axellecture .html.

Bargmann, C.I. (1999) A complex map for pheromones. *Neuron*, **22**, 640–42.

Buck, L.A. (2004) Unravelling the sense of smell, at http://nobelprize.org/nobel_prizes/medicine/laureates/2004/buck-lecture.html.

Hildebrand, J.G. and Shepherd, G.M. (1997) Mechanisms of olfactory discrimination: converging evidence for common principles across phyla. *Annual Review of Neuroscience*, **20**, 595–631.

Liman, E.R. (1996) Pheromone transduction in the vomeronasal organ. *Current Opinion in Neurobiology*, **6**, 487–93.

Liman, E.R. and Zufall, F. (2004) Transduction channels in the vomeronasal organ, in *Transduction Channels in Sensory Cells* (eds S. Frings and J. Bradley), Wiley-VCH Verlag GmbH, Weiheim.

Fernandez, A.A. and Morris, M.R. (2007) Sexual selection and trichromatic colour vision in primates: statistical support for the pre-existing bias hypothesis. *The American Naturalist*, **170**, 10–20 and at doi. 10.1086/518566:2007.

Laberge, F. and Hara, T.J. (2001) Neurobiology of fish olfaction: a review. *Brain Research Reviews*, **36**, 46–59.

Leon, M. and Johnson, B.A. (2003) Olfactory coding in the mammalian olfactory bulb. *Brain Research Reviews*, **42**, 23–32.

Malnic, B. *et al.* (1999) Combinatorial receptor codes for odors. *Cell*, **96**, 713–23.

Matsunami, H. and Buck, L.B. (1997) Multigene family encoding a diverse array of putative pheromone receptors in mammals. *Cell*, **90**, 775–84.

Mayer, M.S. and Mankin, H.W. (1985) Neurobiology of pheromone perception, in (eds G.A. Kerkut, D. Schild and D. Restrepo), Transduction mechanisms in vertebrate olfactory receptor cells. *Physiological Reviews*, **78**, 429–66.

Schoenfeld, T.A. and Cleland, T.A. (2005) The anatomical logic of smell. *Trends in Neurosciences*, **28**, 620–27.

Shepherd, G.M. (2003) *The Synaptic Organisation of the Brain*, 4th edn, Oxford University Press, Oxford.

Shepherd, G.M. (2006) Smell brains and hormones. *Nature*, **439**, 149–151.

Tirindelli, R., Mucignat-Caretta, C. and Pryba, N.J. (1998) Molecular aspects of pheromononal communication via the vomeronasal organ of mammals. *Trends in Neurosciences*, **21**, 482–86.

PART IV: PHOTOSENSITIVITY

Consider, anatomise the eye; survey its structure and contrivance; and tell me from your own feeling, if the idea of a contriver does not immediately flow in upon you with a force like that of a sensation'.

David Hume, 1751/1779, *Dialogues concerning Natural Religion*, London

Charles Darwin recalled the time when, he said, the thought of the eye 'made him grow cold all over'. The eye has always been the type example of fitness for purpose in the argument from design. How could it have evolved? For how could anything less complete and unified, how could any intermediate stage, any half eye, be of use? This has always seemed to Natural Theologians the final unanswerable proof of their position. But we should not be so hasty. The human eye, the vertebrate eye, is far from being the only eye in the animal kingdom. We shall see in this Part that many other designs have evolved. All over the living world devices to detect the electromagnetic radiation streaming in from the Earth's star have developed.

The Universe is filled with electromagnetic radiation. Its wavelength (and hence the energy of its photons) varies widely (Figure I4.1a). Only a small segment of the electromagnetic spectrum has a significant impact on the surface of our planet (Figure I4.1b). The maximum energy of the solar radiation reaching the surface of the Earth is located at a wavelength of about 500 nm (57 kcal/mole photons). Higher energy ultraviolet photons (<300 nm) are absorbed by atmospheric ozone (O_3). This is just as well, as they are also absorbed – lethally – by proteins. We are well advised to be mindful of our ozone blanket.

The response of a molecule to light depends on its atomic structure – that is on its pattern of electrons. The most important molecular structures that the living world has hit upon for this purpose are pyrrole rings and carotenoids (Figure I4.2). Four pyrrole rings are incorporated into beautiful planar molecules, the porphryins, which form the photon-trapping centres of the chlorophylls. The carotenoids are yellow, orange and red fat-soluble pigments found throughout the living world and related to Vitamin A (or retinol) and, through Vitamin A, to the hugely important chromophore, *retinal*. Retinal, as Figure I4.2 shows, is merely the aldehyde of Vitamin A. Although most invertebrates can synthesize Vitamin A, vertebrate animals have lost this capacity. In consequence, it is a necessary constituent of the diet in these animals. There are, as Figure I4.2 shows, two forms of vitamin A – Vitamin A_1 and Vitamin A_2 – differing only by a double covalent bond between atoms 3 and 4 in the hexagonal ring. It follows that there are also two forms of retinal, $retinal_1$ and $retinal_2$. In addition, a third form of retinal, 3-hydroxyretinal, is found in some insects (especially Diptera and Lepidoptera) and in some squids.

Throughout the animal world photopigments consist of the chromophore, retinal, loosely bound, via a Schiff's base linkage, to an apoprotein, *opsin*. Opsin is a 7TM 'serpentine' protein with a molecular weight of about 40 kDa (Figure I4.3). These proteins are collectively known as **retinylidines**. Retinylidines have been isolated and analysed from a large number of vertebrate and invertebrate animals and, although they vary somewhat in magnitude, their opsin moieties all show the same 7TM structure. They all belong to a great superfamily of evolutionarily related proteins which includes not only the olfactory receptor proteins (Chapter 13) but also large

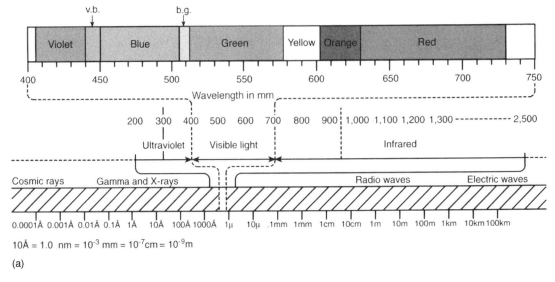

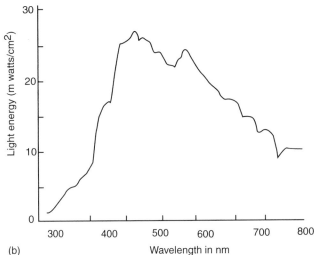

Figure I4.1   (a) Electromagnetic spectrum; upper part of figure in nanometers (nm). (b) Solar spectrum striking the surface of the Earth between 1 and 2 pm in central France.

number of synaptic receptor molecules. In recent years, it has been shown not only that the pigment of melanophores, **melanopsin**, shares this molecular design but that, in the form of **bacteriorhodopsin**, it is also to be found in the bacteria (Box I4.1). Once again it seems that once an effective solution to a problem has been hit upon, in this case detection of light, it is used over and again for one purpose or another. An outline of opsin evolution is given in Chapter 15, Box 15.1.

Detection of light is, of course, only the first event in photoreception. The detection must make a difference. It has to be signalled, first to the cell and then, in more complex systems, to the central nervous system. The 7TM structure of opsin gives the clue. As we noted in Chapter 1 and again when discussing chemoreception in Part Three such membrane-bound proteins are normally part of G-protein signalling systems. Opsin is no exception. In some ways photoreception might be regarded as

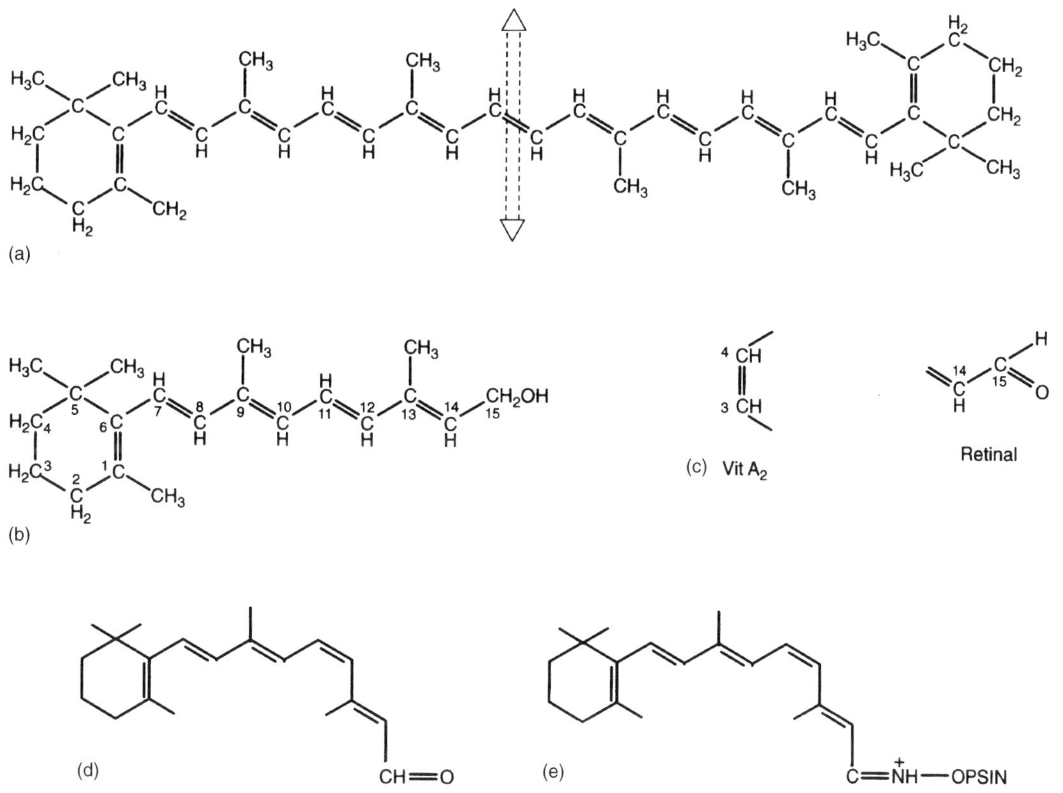

Figure I4.2 Molecular structures of carotene and its photoactive derivatives. (a) All-*trans* β-carotene. (b) Vitamin A₁. Note that it is the hydrolysis product of β-carotene. (c) Double bond between C_3 and C_4 creates vitamin A₂. Retinal is the aldheyde of Vitamin A (retinol). (d) 11-*cis* retinal₁ (note formalism). (e) Schiff base attachment of retinal₁ to lysine residue in opsin.

a specialized form of chemoreception. We saw in Part Three that odorant or tastant molecules caused a change in the conformation of the membrane-bound 7TM receptor, so that the alpha subunits of G-proteins were released to activate membrane-bound enzymes. and so it is with opsin. In this case, however, the odorant/tastant molecule is, in a sense, already attached to the 7TM receptor. It is the chromophore, retinal. The photon merely changes retinal's conformation so that it no longer fits its position in the opsin molecule. This causes the opsin to change its conformation and release neighbouring G-protein alpha subunits. These then activate, as before, specific enzymes in the photoreceptor cell's membrane. We shall look at this in more detail when we come, in Chapter 17, to the molecular biology and biophysics of vertebrate rod and cone outersegments.

So far in this Introduction we have been considering the molecular mechanisms which living organisms have evolved to detect light. But organisms do far more than merely detect the presence or absence of light. They make use of its physical characteristics to extract information about the environment, both biotic and abiotic, in which they struggle to survive. Let us look at some of these significant features.

Firstly, the fact that the wavelength of light in the visible spectrum is so small ensures that it travels in straight lines so that the edges of objects and the shadows they project are sharply defined (compare this with the less well defined shadows and edges of the acoustic world). Another consequence of the rectilinear propagation of light is the inverted image formed behind a pinhole. This phenomenon can, as Figure I4.4 shows, be regarded as the inverse of shadow formation.

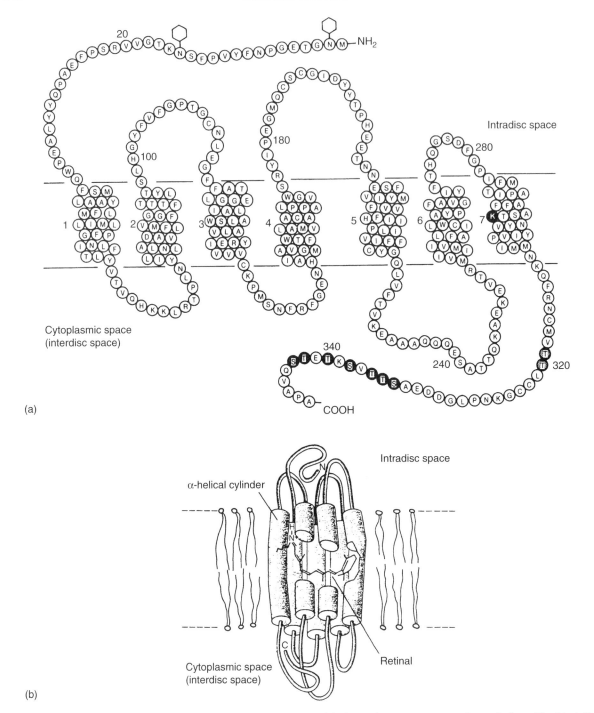

Figure I4.3 Molecular structure of bovine rhodopsin. The plan view (a) shows the seven transmembrane helices. The black K (lysine) residue is that to which retinal is attached. The N-terminal bears two oligosaccharide groups (represented by hexagons) and the stippled residues in the C-terminal are those which are phosphorylated by rhodospin kinase (Chapter 17). (b) Three-dimensional conformation of rhodopsin in a cell membrane. Note the orientation of opsin with respect to intradisc (extracellular) and interdisc (intracellular) compartments.

BOX I4.1   BACTERIORHODOPSIN

The membrane of *Halobacterium halobium*, a salt-loving bacterium belonging to the Archaebacteria, can be separated into three fractions: yellow, red and purple. The purple fraction can be formed into crystalline sheets which can be examined in the electron microscope. In addition to lipids it contains a 26 kDa protein. Because the fraction forms crystalline sheets, the structure of the protein can be examined in atomic detail. Because of its light sensitivity and 7TM 'serpentine' structure it is known as *bacteriorhodopsin*. It is the best characterized of all the rhodopsins. Like all the other rhodopsins, it consists of seven closely packed alpha helices extending through the membrane and, as with other rhodopsins, the protein is loosely bound to a *retinal* chromophore.

In halobacteria, such as *H. halobium*, ATP is generated by oxidative phosphorylation. In high oxygen tensions there is a switch to photosynthesis. The protons required for this process are translocated across the membrane by bacteriorhodopsin, which acts as a light-driven proton pump. It can be shown that two protons are moved from the inside to the outside for each photon absorbed.

The mechanism of this pumping action has been the subject of much research. It is known that the retinal is bound by a Schiff's base linkage (as in animal photopigments) to Lysine 216 (K216) of the opsin and makes contact with six out of the seven transmembrane helices. The retinal is in the all-trans conformation and lies across the tunnel between the helices, thus blocking the flow of protons. In proton pumping there is a light-induced switch from the all-trans to a 13-cis conformation. The retinal twists within the opsin 'tunnel' and transfers a proton from the cytoplasmic side to the extracellular side. In contrast to the rhodopsins of vertebrate retinae, the retinal does not detach and migrate away from its opsin apoprotein.

The amino acid sequence of bacteriorhodopsin is very different from that of animal opsins and this suggests that it may have had an independent evolutionary origin. This tentative conclusion finds support from the fact that retinal is in the 13-cis configuration rather than the 11-cis configuration of animal opsins. Nevertheless, the conformation of bacteriorhodopsin itself indicates that it belongs to the ubiquitous superfamily of 7TM 'serpentine' proteins, which have been pressed into service in so many different ways and places in the animal kingdom.

REFERENCES

Henderson, R. *et al.* (1989) Model for the structure of bacteriorhodopsin based on high resolution electron cryo-microscopy. *J. Mol. Biol.*, **213**, 899–929.
The internet provides a very useful summary of structural and functional detail at htt://monera.ncl.ac.uk/energy/brd.html

Secondly, white light is, of course, a mixture of all wavelengths between the short and the long end of the visible spectrum. When white light falls on a reflecting surface, some of these wavelengths may be absorbed and others reflected. In many of the more advanced photoreceptors, means of detecting different wavelengths have been evolved. Such animals are able to sense the colours of surfaces in their environment. This can be of great advantage in detecting ripe food, in sexual selection and in camouflage and predation.

Thirdly, not all surfaces reflect light. In many cases light is able to penetrate and pass through a material body. Such bodies are said to be transparent. But it is usually the case that, when light passes from one transparent medium to another, its velocity is altered. This has the consequence that, when the ray enters a denser medium, it is bent towards the normal (Figure I4.5a). This is known as refraction. The laws of refraction are dealt with in all texts of elementary physics. Refraction is of great importance in the design of image forming eyes. It is the refractive power

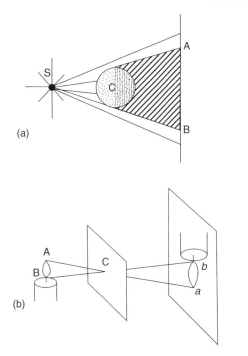

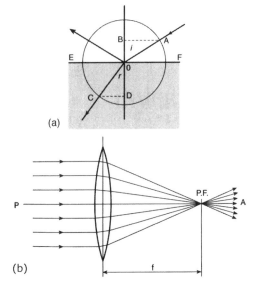

Figure I4.4 (a) Shadow cast by a point source of light. (b) Pinhole image.

Figure I4.5 (a) The second law of refraction: sin i/sin r = μ, the index of refraction. (b) Refraction by a convex lens. PA, the line passing through the centre of curvature of the two faces is known as the principal axis. If the incident beam is parallel to the principal axis the rays are brought to a focus at PF, the principal focus. The distance from the mid point of the lens to the principal focus is defined as the focal length, f, of the lens.

of lenses and corneas that focus images of objects on to retinae. The **focal length (f)** of the refractive system is the distance behind the mid point of the system to the point at which the rays converge (Figure I4.5b). The 'power' of a lens or other refracting system is defined as $1/f$ and measured in **Dioptres** (D). A lens of focal length one metre is defined as having a power of one Dioptre. A lens of focal length 25 cm has a power $1/0.25 = 4$ D. Converging lenses are regarded as positive and diverging lenses as negative (Figure I4.5).

Fourthly, and finally, most natural light is to some extent polarized. Ideally the electromagnetic oscillations constituting light occur in infinitely many planes evenly distributed throughout the 360° circle orthogonal to the direction of the ray. But in nature the oscillations in some of planes are absorbed. This may occur by atmospheric particles (Tyndall–Rayleigh effect) or during reflection and refraction at interfaces (Fresnel effect). Many animal photoreceptors can detect this slight polarization and use this information in orientation and direction finding (Chapter 21) (Figure I4.6).

Next let us look at some of the ways animal eyes have evolved to make use of these physical characteristics to form images. We have already noted (Figure I4.4) that light entering a **pinhole** creates an inverted image in the space behind. Numerous animal eyes make use of this fact. Perhaps the best known instance is that provided by the ancient sea-going mollusc, *Nautilus* (Figure 15.9). Some animal eyes make use of **reflection**. The most spectacular instance is provided by the scallop, *Pecten* (Section 15.2.3), but reflection is also pressed into service by some

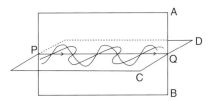

Figure I4.6 Plane polarized light. Instead of the oscillations occurring in all directions orthogonal to the direction of the beam (PQ) the figure shows only two planes being occupied: AB and CD.

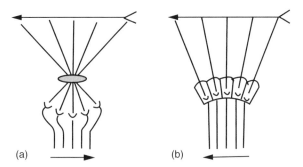

(a)

(b)

Figure I4.7 Concave and convex retinae. (a) Concave retina as in the vesicular eyes of vertebrates and cephalopod molluscs. (b) Convex retina as in the arthropod compound eyes. From Goldsmith, 1990: with permission.

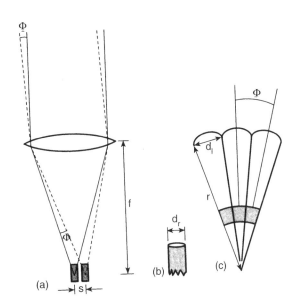

Figure I4.8 Acuity of eyes. (a) Vesicular. (b) Single receptor. (c) Compound. Explanation in text. d_i = diameter of lenslet; d_r = diameter of receptor; f = focal length; ϕ = angular separation of receptors; r = radius of curvature; s = spacing of receptors. From Goldsmith, 1990: with permission.

crustacea (Section 15.1.2) and, indeed, by a number of vertebrates (e.g. many fish (Section 19.3), mammals (Section 17.2.1.3, etc.)). Most image-forming animal eyes, however, depend on **refraction**. This may occur at a lens, which is often adjustable, or at an unadjustable cornea. The image is thrown upon a two-dimensional sheet of photoreceptors, very much as the lens of a camera throws an image on a strip of film. But there is an important difference. Whereas the strip of film in a camera is flat and orthogonal to the incoming light, the retinae of animal eyes are always curved (Figure I4.7). The curvature may be either concave or convex. In the first case, as found in vertebrate and cephalopod eyes, a single lens placed in front can focus an inverted image onto the retina. In the second case, as is found in the compound eyes of arthropods, an image can only be formed if a large number of tiny lenses, each responsive to a narrow cone of light, focus a mosaic image onto the retina. Note that the image in this latter case is not inverted.

One other feature of image-forming eyes is worth noting before we finish this introduction. This is their ability to resolve detail in the visual image. An important factor determining **resolving power** (or **acuity**) is the angular separation (ϕ) of the retinal receptor cells. Resolving power is proportional to $1/\phi$. In the case of a single lens eye, $1/\phi = f/d$, where 'f' is the focal length and 'd' is the distance between the receptors. Hence, resolving power in these eyes can be increased by increasing 'f' or decreasing 'd' or both. For an apposition type compound eye (Section 15.1), $1/\phi = r/d$ (once again) though in this case 'd' is the diameter of the ommatidial lens. These relationships are shown in Figure I4.8.

We noted above that resolving power can be increased by increasing 'f' or decreasing 'd'. There are, however, constraints on both these parameters. The magnitude of 'f' depends on the size of the eye and hence of the animal. When we look at the compound eye of a dragonfly, or the vesicular eye of a songbird, we recognize that this limit is being pressed to an extreme. Both eyes are about as large as the animal's head could support. Similarly, there are physical limits to the degree to which 'd' can be decreased. Taking the case of the vesicular eye, it is easy to see that the diameter of the photoreceptor cell outersegments cannot be decreased without limit. Furthermore, the outersegments must be sufficiently sensitive to discriminate between different luminant intensities in the image. To put it another way, resolving power is also limited by the **contrast sensitivity** of the photoreceptor cells. To discriminate one part of an image from another it is necessary that adjacent outersegments are subjected to differences in luminant intensity above their contrast sensitivity thresholds. If they are set too close together, the contrast will be too small to be detected. Physical considerations of this sort limit outersegments to a minimum diameter of about 1 μm and a separation of about 2 μm. Similar considerations apply to the compound eye. In this case, contrast sensitivity considerations place a lower limit of about 10 μm on facet diameter.

It will have become obvious from the foregoing discussion that the study of animal eyes involves a fascinating mixture of physics, biochemistry, molecular biology, physiology and zoology. In the first chapter of this Part (Chapter 15) we shall look at the design of some invertebrate eyes. Next, in the central three Chapters (16, 17 and 18), we shall consider in some detail the vertebrate eye and visual system as exemplified in humans. Then, in Chapter 19, we shall go on to consider some of the variations on this vertebrate theme.

15

INVERTEBRATE VISION

Ubiquity and antiquity of photoreceptors: homologies in early development - common ancestor? **Two major photoreceptor cell designs**: rhabdomeric and ciliary - differing biophysics. **Two major eye designs**: vesicular and compound. **Evolution of vesicular eye**: eyespots - flat eyes - pinhole eyes -vesicular eyes. **Evolution of compound eye**: simple ocelli - aggregate eye - compound eye. **Ommatidia**: structure - optics - retinula cells - rhabdom - apposition and superposition designs - differing sensitivities and acuities - diurnal and nocturnal insects - Dipteran neural superposition - reflection eyes in decapods. **Scanning eyes**: sea snails - jumping spiders - mantis shrimps - Colpilia (crustacean). **Examples**: **protistan**: eyespots - light antennae - eyespot of Chlamydomonas - biophysics - ocelli of Dinoflagellates; **Nautilus pinhole eye** - structure - optics - retina; **Pecten mirror eye** - structure - double retina - one ciliary, one rhabdomeric - unusual biophysics; **Octopus vesicular eye** - convergent evolution - large size - structure - focusing - 'verted' retina - rhabdomeric retinula cells - molecular biology - optic pathway - 'deep retina'; **Limulus primitive compound eye** - structure - electrophysiology - retinula cells - eccentric cell - lateral inhibition - biological significance; **Ocellar eyes of jumping spiders**: structure and functioning. **Dipteran advanced compound eye** - apposition - physiology - colour vision - neural superposition in optic lamina - chiasma to the medulla - lobula. **Concluding remarks**: in what sense can it be said that invertebrates 'see'?

The physical characteristics of electromagnetic radiation, discussed in the introduction to Part Four, ensure that practically all animals have developed photoreceptors. Human eyes are restricted to wavelengths between about 400 to 750 nm and we self-regardingly refer to this part of the spectrum as being the visible part of the spectrum. Many animals can, however, detect shorter wavelengths (down to about 200 nm), in what we know as the ultraviolet, and other animals can detect wavelengths in the infrared up to about 1000 nm. We shall start this chapter by reviewing the design principles of invertebrate eyes. We shall then go on to examine in a little more detail some representative examples: protistan eyes (*Chlamydomonas*), molluscan eyes (*Nautilus*, *Pecten* and *Octopus*), arthropod eyes (*Drosophila*, *Limulus* and spider). We shall leave discussion of the vertebrate eye to Chapters 16, 17 and 19.

15.1 DESIGNS OF INVERTEBRATE EYES

Although, as Duke-Elder points out, photoreception is one of the last senses to be evolved, lagging behind

BOX 15.1   THE EVOLUTION OF OPSINS

When did opsins first begin? We saw in the Introduction to Part Four that they are ubiquitous proteins. They are found in the purple membrane of halobacteria, in the photoreceptor cells of both invertebrates and vertebrates, and in the light-sensitive pigment of the melanophores of frog skin, frog iris and several other places. In melanophores they mediate light induced melanosome movements and in the frog's iris they are thought to control constriction and dilation. We have also noted that opsins share the 7TM conformation with a large number of other proteins to which they are, consequently, related. These proteins include not only olfactory receptor proteins, some gustatory receptor proteins and possibly some thermoreceptor proteins but also many synaptic receptor proteins, for instance the muscarinic acetylcholine receptor (mAChR), the α and β adrenergic receptors (α and β ARs), the 5HT receptors and, indeed, most other metabotrobic synaptic receptors. Opsins are thus part of a great superfamily of similarly structured proteins which all share a similar G-protein membrane-signalling biochemistry.

The fact that the 7TM conformation is found in the Archaebacteria in the form of bacteriorhodopsin indicates that it is a very ancient structure. There is some evidence, as we note in other parts of this book, that it has been independently 'discovered' several times by the evolutionary process. But, since it is the crucial element of animal photoreceptors, it is probably monophyletic. A recent phylogeny is shown in Figure A.

One of the significant distinctions between vertebrate and invertebrate opsins lies in the response of the chromophore – retinal – to light. In the vertebrates, retinal (as we shall see) detaches from opsin and diffuses into other cells (retinal pigment epithelium, Müller cells) for regeneration. This is not the case with the invertebrate pigment. Here the chromophore remains in place and is available for repeated transformation from the *cis* to the *trans* form and back again without leaving its apoprotein, opsin. Very interestingly the melanopsin recently analysed from the South African frog, *Xenopus laevis*, resembles invertebrate opsin in this regard. It is possible that this 'foreign' characteristic is due to the fact that melancocytes are not necessarily associated with a regenerative tissue like retinal photoreceptors. In this regard it is noteworthy that melanopsin has also been found in a new class of retinal ganglion cells, the intrinsically photosensitive ganglion cells (ipRGCs) (Section 17.2.7.4). This has led some authorities to suggest that ganglion cells originated as rhabdomeric photoreceptors that have retained their axon and in most cases have lost their photoreceptor function.

The similarities of melanopsin to invertebrate rather then vertebrate opsins goes deep into its molecular structure. Its ability to retain retinal after photoactivation depends on its possession of an aromatic residue (tyrosine$_{103}$) in the third transmembrane helix, rather than the acidic residues which occupy that position in vertebrate opsins. Furthermore, it resembles invertebrate but differs from vertebrate opsins in possessing a lengthy C-terminal cytoplasmic 'tail'.

So how should we answer the question with which we started? We can assume with a fair degree of certainty that 7TM proteins and their associated G-protein membrane biochemistry were very early developments in evolutionary history. From this population of candidate molecules photosensitive variants arose. Did pigment cells precede photoreceptor cells, or vice versa? It has been argued that there was little point in pigment cells if there were no eyes to respond, aggressively or otherwise, to changes of colour or shading. Hence eyes came before pigment cells. On the other hand, pigmentation may have arisen for purposes other than camouflage or advertisement. It may, for instance, have arisen in association with thermoregulation, or for screening delicate structures from too intense an illumination. We do not, as yet, have enough evidence to decide. In either case, we can suppose that early cells which 'discovered' the photosensitive possibilities inherent in combinations of retinaldehyde and opsin lie at the root of both melanophore and photoreceptor evolution.

(Continues)

(*Continued*)

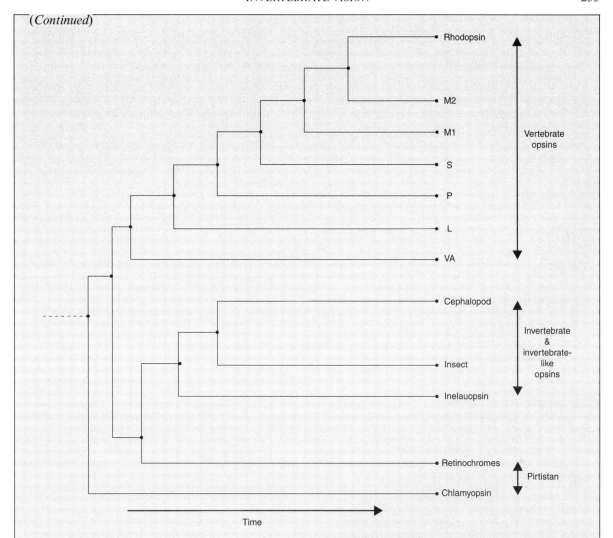

Figure A Phylogeny of opsins. The evolutionary relationship of some of the major opsins as deduced from their amino acid sequences is shown. The branch points represent gene duplications. The timing of these duplications is not represented in this dendrogram. It is interesting to note that the melanopsin of amphibian melanophores is, according to this analysis, grouped with the invertebrate opsins although, as shown, it is also related to the retinochromes which are found in both invertebrate and vertebrate eyes. L: long-wave (red) sensitive opsin; M1: blue-sensitive opsin; M2: green-sensitive opsin; P: pineal opsin; S: short-wave-sensitive opsin (all from chicken); VA: vertebrate 'ancient' opsin (from Atlantic salmon); cephalopod opsin from *Octopus*; insect opsin is *Drosophila* Rh1 opsin; chlamyopsin from *Chlamydomonas*. After Provencio, I. *et al.* (1998).

   The combination of opsin and retinaldehyde (retinal) is very versatile. We noted above that the detachment (or not) of retinal from its position deep in the opsin molecule depends on the presence of an acidic or aromatic amino acid side chain at an appropriate position in the third transmembrane helix. The wavelength of light to which retinal is most sensitive also depends on its amino acid environment within opsin. Looking back to Chapter 14 (Section 14.2.3), it is interesting to note that variations in the amino acid constitution of the 'barrel of staves' is also thought to be at least partly responsible for

(*Continues*)

(*Continued*)
the differential sensitivity of olfactory receptor proteins. In the case of opsin we shall see in Chapter 17 that at least three different amino acid substitutions can transform a green-sensitive into a red-sensitive pigment. Something further will be said about the evolutionary relationships of the human cone pigments in that chapter. But it must not be forgotten that, over geological time scales, opsins have evolved to fit the life needs of a great variety of animals. Variations in the amino acid sequences of the opsin molecule have generated pigments responding maximally (λ_{max}) to wavelengths from the ultraviolet into the far red end of the spectrum. The familiar red, green and blue iodopsins of the human retina are very far from being the only variants found in the innumerable retinae of the animal kingdom.

REFERENCES

Arendt, D. (2003) Evolution of eyes and photoreceptor cell types. *International Journal of Developmental Biology*, **47**, 563–71.

Arnhelter, H. (1998) Eyes viewed from the skin. *Nature*, **391**, 632–33.

Fryxell, K.J. and Meyerowitz, E.M. (1991) The evolution of rhodopsins and neurotransmitter receptors. *Journal of Molecular Evolution*, **33**, 367–78.

Provincio, I. *et al.* (1998) Melanopsin: an opsin in melanophore, brain, and eye. *Proceedings of the National Academy of Science*, **95**, 340–45.

Yokoyama, S. (1995) Amino acid replacements and wavelength absorption of visual pigments in vertebrates. *Molecular Biology and Evolution*, **12**, 53–61.

Yokoyama, S. (1996) Molecular evolution of retinal and nonretinal opsins. *Genes to Cells*, **1**, 787–94.

mechanoreception and chemoreception, it is of such importance to animal life that a vast array of different types of eye now exist. Many of these designs already existed in the Cambrian period, more than five hundred million years ago. For instance, fossils of the ubiquitous Trilobites of that period (now extinct) show well developed compound eyes. Contemporary eyes range from eyespots (or **stigmata**) through simple eyes, often known as **ocelli**, to the complex and highly evolved eyes of the arthropods, molluscs and vertebrates. It is fascinating to note (Box 15.2) that there is good evidence that the earliest steps in the development of all the more complex eyes, including the image-forming eyes, are controlled by the same genetic mechanisms. This provides a strong hint that in spite of the huge difference between, say, the compound eye of the house fly and our own large vesicular eye they, nevertheless, both had a common ancestor, probably back in the Precambrian period, before the Burgess shale, mentioned in Chapter 4, was laid down.

The simplest eyes – the simplest eyespots and ocelli – are not capable of forming an image. They can detect presence or absence of light and light in-tensity. Several are also capable of detecting the direction of a light source, either through their own structure or by being arranged at different parts of an organism's body. More complex eyes are able to detect patterns of light – images – and these, again, have evolved numerous times. Well known and independently evolved image-forming eyes are found in the Mollusca (especially the Cephalopoda), in the arthropods (compound eyes) and in the vertebrates. Several other phyla (the Annelida, perhaps some Cnidarians) have also evolved rudimentary image-forming eyes.

How are we to classify this huge diversity of photoreceptors? First, we can make a division between 'eyes' of unicellular and those of multicellular forms. Although a wide variety of photosensitive organelles have developed in the unicellular protista, they are all, necessarily, far simpler than the eyes of the metazoa. In Section 15.2.1 we shall look at the simple eyespot of the unicellular green alga *Chlamydomonas* as an example of a photoreceptor in a unicellular form. The eyes of multicellular forms are, as noted above, highly various. There are numerous classification schemes. At the

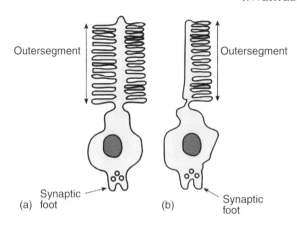

Figure 15.1 Two types of photoreceptor cell. (a) Rhabdomeric (b) Ciliary.

level of photoreceptor cells Eakin proposed a popular scheme in the early 1960s. He noted that there seemed to be two major types of photoreceptor cell in the Metazoa. In the first, developed by the **protostomes** (annelid–mollusc–arthropod), the photopigment was laid out in microvilli projecting from the walls of the cell. In the second, developed by the **deuterostomes** (echinoderm–chordate), the photopigment was incorporated into discs formed by invagination of the membrane of the cilium (Figure 15.1). These two distinctive designs are said to constitute the **rhabdomeric** and the **ciliary** types of photoreceptor.

Unfortunately this clear cut evolutionary distinction was not sustained by further research. Many exceptions were found. Some protostomes develop ciliary photoreceptors and some deuterostomes possess rhabdomeres. Furthermore, in the complicated eye of *Pecten*, the scallop, both rhabdomeric and ciliary receptors are found. It is interesting, however, to note that the two different photoreceptor designs are accompanied by a significant physiological difference. Whereas rhabdomeric receptors **depolarize** in response to illumination, ciliary receptors **hyperpolarize**. It is satisfying to find that this physiological difference holds even in the case of *Pecten*: its ciliary photoreceptors hyperpolarize whilst its rhabdomeric receptors depolarize. Unfortunately, there are exceptions even to this clear cut distinction. The Tunicate, *Salpa*, for instance, possesses rhabdomeric receptors (which as a deuterostome it shouldn't!) and

these hyperpolarize. Finally, *Amphioxus*, at the root of chordate evolution, has four photoreceptor systems, two of which are rhabdomeric (the microvillar organs of Hesse distributed along the nerve cord, and the Joseph cells) and two ciliary (the frontal eye and the lamellar body). Biology, as usual, refuses to obey the neat classificatory instincts of biologists.

If we turn from the structure of the photoreceptor cells to the multicellular eye itself, we find that metazoan animals have evolved a great variety of different designs. Again there are two main lines of development. One leads to the **vesicular eye**, which reaches its highest development in the chordates and molluscs, the other leads to the **compound eye**, which reaches its peak in the crustacea and insects.

15.1.1 Evolution of the Vesicular Eye

It is not difficult to understand how the vesicular eye evolved (Figure 15.2). In the beginning we may imagine that single photoreceptor cells developed in the epidermis. Such an organization is found in the epidermis of the earthworm, *Lumbricus terrestris*. From this it is no great step for them to aggregate together either just beneath the epidermis, as in some planaria (for example *Planaria gonocephala*), or in the epidermis itself to form so-called 'flat eyes'. Such 'eyes' are found in the epidermis of the some marine annelid worms. From this situation we can imagine that invagination leads first to a cupulate eye and then to a pinhole eye. A good example of a pinhole eye is provided by the primitive cephalopod mollusc, *Nautilus*. From the pinhole it is no great distance to the fully enclosed vesicular eye. In these eyes an image is formed on the retina either by a refractile lens or by refraction at the cornea or, often, both. In a few instances the image is also formed by reflection. We shall discuss examples of such eyes in Section 15.2.3. Vesicular eyes are best known in the vertebrates although, as we shall see in Section 15.2.4, highly evolved examples of these eyes are also found in cephalopod molluscs. We shall accordingly postpone detailed consideration of vertebrate vesicular eyes to later chapters. In Chapters 16 and 17 we shall look at one such eye, the human eye, in detail and consider other vertebrate vesicular eyes in Chapter 19.

15.1.2 Evolution of the Compound Eye

The evolution of compound eyes took a somewhat different route from that outlined in Figure 15.2. We start, again, with single photoreceptors but this time we have to imagine that the photosensitive cell lies at the bottom of a pigmented tube (Figure 15.3a). This has the advantage of directionality. Only light emanating from a certain point can stimulate the receptor at the bottom of its tube. The shadow of a passing object can be more precisely located. Again, as in the vesicular eye, it only requires a group of these simple ocelli to come together to form first an 'aggregate' eye, where the individual ocelli remain separate from each other, and then a true compound eye, in which

the sensory elements, the '**retinula cells**', are first grouped together to form **ommatidia** and then these ommatidia themselves are grouped to form the familiar multifaceted compound eye. Aggregate eyes are only developed in a few annelids (Figure 15.3d), arthropods and molluscs. The compound eye, on the other hand, is one of Nature's great inventions and is found throughout the Crustacea and Insecta. The spiders (Araneida), although using the same ommatidial elements as the other arthropods, dispense with separate lenses for each ommatidium and cover the whole system with a single cuticular lens.

Beneath each facet of a compound eye is a complex light-detecting structure. As Figure 15.3e shows, this consists of a **corneal lens**, **crystalline cone** and a group of seven or eight **retinula** cells forming a cylinder. This complex device is termed an **ommatidium**. Unlike many vesicular eyes there is no possibility of varying the focus. The lens and crystalline cone of the compound eye are not adjustable. They are made up of concentric lamellae of differing refractive index, the more central having greater RIs than the more peripheral. If the length of the lens and crystalline cone is equal to its focal length then an incident beam of parallel light is focused at the far end and emerges as a beam of divergent rays (Figure 15.3f(i)). If, however, the lens and crystalline cone is twice the focal length, then the beam emerges as a beam of parallel rays (Figure 15.3f(ii)).

The retinula cells are the photosensitive cells. In many arthropods all of them also send a nerve fibre to the optic laminae in the central nervous system. In other arthropods there is specialization: in the Dipteran insects, for instance, two retinula cells (R7 and R8) send fibres deep into the second optic lamina, while the others (R1 to R6) send only short fibres to the first lamina (Figure 15.18). In all cases, however, the retinula cells develop large number of microvilli. These constitute the **rhabdomere**. The rhabdomeres of the cylinder of retinula cells often interdigitate with each other to form the **rhabdom**. Incident light is focused on to the rhabdom by the corneal lens and crystalline cone. The visual pigments are concentrated in the rhabdomeres and in some insects each retinula cell expresses a rhodopsin sensitive to a different luminant frequency. In *Drosophila*, for instance, retinula cell 7 expresses a rhodopsin sensitive to ultraviolet (UV) light. Each ommatidium is shielded from its neighbours by pigment cells.

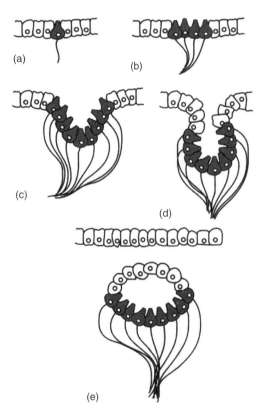

Figure 15.2 Evolution of the vesicular eye. (a) Simple photosensitive cell in epithelium; (b) Group of simple photosensitive cells forming a 'flat eye'; (c) Invagination of 'flat eye' to form a cupulate eye; (d) Further invagination leads to a pinhole eye; (e) Yet further invagination leads to a vesicular eye. The epithelium above the vesicular eye evolves into lens, cornea and so on.

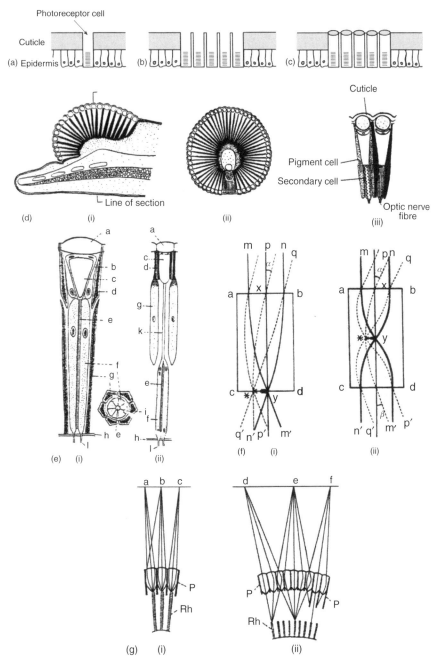

Figure 15.3 The evolution of aggregate and compound eyes. (a) Origin as a pigmented tube (in some cases recessed in the cuticle). (b) A number of tubes aggregate together. (c) Each tube acquires a cuticular lens to form an aggregate eye. (d) Aggregate eye in the polychaete worm *Branchioma vesiculoseum*. (i) Longitudinal section; (ii) Transverse section; (iii) Two photoreceptor units in more detail (From Milne and Milne, 1959). (e) Insect ommatidia. (i) Apposition type ommatidium; (ii) Superposition type ommatidium. Longitudinal and transverse sections are shown. a = cuticular lens; b = supporting cells; c = crystalline cone; d = iris pigment cell; e = rhabdom; f = retinula cell; g = retinula pigment cell; h = basement membrane; i = eccentric cell; k = translucent filament; l = nerve fibre. (f) Light path through crystalline cones. (i) Light path through the crystalline cone of an apposition eye; (ii) Light path through the crystalline cone of a superposition eye. (g) Image formation in compound eyes (i) Image formation in apposition eye; (ii) Image formation in a superposition eye. a–f = luminous points; P = pigment; Rh = rhabdom. At the right hand of the superposition eye the pigment is shown in the light adapted position. From Wigglesworth 1972. With permission from Kluwer Academic publishers.

Compound eyes, like vesicular eyes, are image-forming devices. There are a number of different designs and use is made of both refraction and reflection. In all cases only a partial image is formed in any given ommatidium. The full image is derived only from the integrated activity of the aggregate. There are three major ways in which this is done and, consequently, there are three different compound eye designs: **apposition**, **superposition** and **neural superposition** (Figure 15.4). In the apposition type, the lens and crystalline cone focus the incident beam on to the tip of the rhabdom (Figure 15.3g(i), Figure 15.4a). In the superposition type, the length of lens and crystalline cone is twice the focal length and the emergent beam is directed to the ommatidial cylinder of retinula cells some distance below (Figure 15.3g(ii), Figure 15.4b).

Apposition eyes are found in diurnal insects. They form relatively precise images of the environment. Superposition eyes tend to be developed by noctural and crepuscular insects. Sensitivity is increased because light from a number of lenses is focused on to a single retinula cluster. What they gain in sensitivity, though, they lose in accuracy. In most cases the superposition of the rays from the lens and cone is not precise enough to rival the resolving power of the apposition eye. This, however, has not proved to be the case in some nocturnal moths. Here the superposition is so precise as to give acuity as good as that of an apposition eye of the same dimensions. These moths gain an increase in sensitivity of between 100 and 1000 fold. Furthermore, even in superposition eyes, without so precise an optical build, the pigment in the pigment cells shielding one ommatidium from its neighbours is often able to migrate, so that a superposition eye can be transformed into a high resolution apposition type for daytime use.

In addition to the classical superposition type eye, some insects (for instance, Dipteran flies) have developed a yet more intricate system (Figure 15.4c). Here the rhabdomeres of the retinula cells are not fused to form a rhabdom but remain independent of each other. Each is thus an independent receptor cell. Its output is sent directly to the first lamina in the fly's optic lobe. A very precise neural wiring ensures that the output from retinula cells in adjacent ommatidia having the same field of view are sent to the same location in the first lamina (Figure 15.4c). This organization ensures that the sensitivity is equivalent to a superposition eye of the same dimensions. But it escapes the poor visual acuity of the superposition eye. The Diptera thus have the best of both worlds: a highly sensitive and a highly accurate eye.

A fourth type of compound eye has been developed by the long-bodied decapod crustacea (shrimps, prawns, crayfish and lobsters). These forms have superposition eyes but, instead of a lens and crystalline cone refracting the light on to deep clusters of retinula cells, another optical principle is used: reflection. In place of lenses and conical crystalline

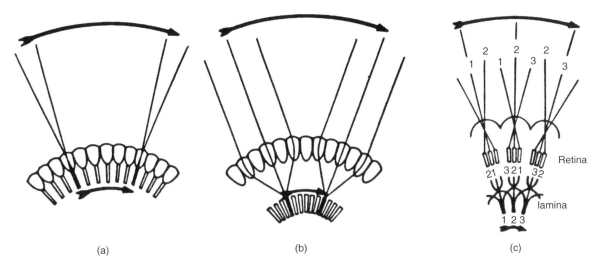

(a)   (b)   (c)

Figure 15.4   Three types of compound eye. (a) apposition; (b) superposition; (c) neural superposition.

cones these animals have box-like structures with 'mirror' walls. Light is reflected from these mirror walls on to the retinula cells where it forms, once again, an upright image. It is interesting that it is only the long-bodied decapods that have developed this type of compound eye, with its square facets; their near relatives, the brachyuran crabs, retain conventional apposition eyes and larval shrimps also show apposition eyes which only change into mirror-type superposition eyes at metamorphosis. It is not clear whether the ecology of the prawns and lobsters is sufficiently different from that of the crabs to merit this considerable anatomical reorganization. Finally, a fifth type of compound eye has been discovered quite recently in the swimming crab, *Portunus* (= *Macropipus*) and the hermit crab, *Eupagurus*. The eyes of these crabs are of the superposition type but combine both refraction and reflection. Their optics are complex and still being analysed. It may be that the compound eye which, after all, has had 500 million years in which to evolve and test out different optics, has still more surprises in store for the zoologist and sensory physiologist.

15.1.3 Scanning Eyes

All the eyes considered so far form a two-dimensional image on a sheet-like retina. The third dimension is added by central processing. But there are a few eyes where an alternative technique is used. In these eyes, developed in a few molluscs and arthropods, a narrow strip of photoreceptors is scanned over the visual scene. The free-swimming heteropod sea snails, which flap through the oceans by undulating the lobes of their feet as if they were fins, have eyes of this type. An example is provided by *Oxygyrus*, which has a retina three to six photoreceptors wide and over four hundred photoreceptors long. The eye scans the surroundings by tilting back and forth through a ninety degree arc at right angles to the photoreceptor strip. The downward movement is rapid (250°/s) followed by a slower upward scan (80°/s). Another example is provided by the anterior median (principal) eyes of jumping spiders (Salticidae). We shall discuss these in Section 15.2.6. The retina of these eyes consists of a strip of photoreceptors five to seven wide and about fifty long. The spiders move these eyes from side to side, orthogonal to the long dimension of the photoreceptor strip

and also rotate them when examining an interesting object. The lateral eyes of these spiders have, on the other hand, conventional two-dimensional retinae which detect movement. If and when this is detected the high resolution principal eyes are directed to scan that part of the surroundings. It is easy to draw an analogy with 'foveation', which plays a similar role in many mammalian eyes (Chapter 17). A final interesting example of a scanning eye is found in the mantis shrimps (Stomatopoda). In these crustaceans six rows of enlarged ommatidia form a strip in the centre of an otherwise standard two-dimensional compound eye. These enlarged ommatidia contain the colour visual pigments. To determine the colour of a visual stimulus the shrimp scans the colour strip back and forth across the scene.

We should not finish this section without mentioning the remarkable eyes of the small copepod, *Copilia* (Figure 15.5). These eyes have taken scanning to an extreme. Instead of a 'one-dimensional' strip of photoreceptors, they have reduced the system to 'zero dimension', a 'point'. A posterior lens scans back and forth through about 14° in the horizontal dimension and at a frequency of about 0.5–5 scans per second focusing light on to a single receptor. A single nerve fibre carries the output from the receptor to the brain.

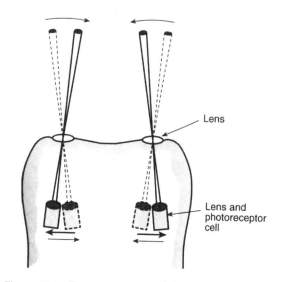

Figure 15.5 The scanning eye of the copepod crustacean *Copilia quadrata*. Each lens subtends an angle of about 3° and scans back and forth through 14° focusing light on a 'retina' consisting of a single photoreceptor cell. After Land, M.F and Fernald, R.D. (1992).

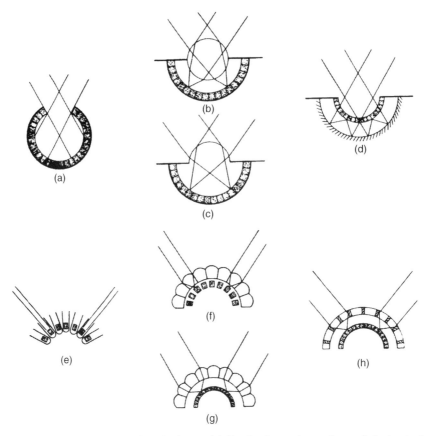

Figure 15.6 Major methods of image formation in animal eyes. (a) Simple pit eye of many lower phyla developing into the pinhole eyes of, for example, *Haliotis* (abalone) or *Nautilus*. (b) Eye with lens. (c) Corneal refraction. (d) Mirror eye. (e) Aggregate eye. (f) Apposition compound eye. (g) Superposition compound eye. (h) Reflecting superposition compound eye. Modified from Land, 1984; Land and Fernald, 1992.

From what has been said in this section, it is clear that over evolutionary time animal organisms have explored most of the possibilities for detecting light and forming images (Figure 15.6). It is extremely doubtful if contemporary engineers, given opaque, nonrigid, raw materials such as proteins and lipids, could come anywhere near the optical perfection of Nature's devices. Indeed, we might suspect that they wouldn't know where to start. We shall see, as we go on in this chapter and the other chapters in this Part, that animal photoreceptors (like the audioreceptors of Chapter 9) have evolved to the limits of what is physically possible. It is small wonder that (as we noted in the introduction) the structure and functioning of the eye made Charles Darwin experience more than one 'cold shudder'.

15.2 EXAMPLES OF INVERTEBRATE EYES

In this section we shall look in more detail at some examples of the many fascinating eyes developed in the invertebrates. We shall start by looking at eyespots or stigmata developed in unicellular organisms. The anatomical simplicity of these photoreceptors allows detailed biochemical analysis. We shall then turn our attention to some of the many eyes developed in the phylum Mollusca. After describing the primitive 'pinhole' eyes of *Nautilus* and the 'mirror' eyes of *Pecten*, the scallop, we reach the climax of the molluscan vesicular eye in the belemnoid cephalopoda, the octopi, squids and cuttlefish. These eyes, although evolved quite independently,

BOX 15.2 EARLY GENETICS OF EYES

We have already noted in several places the extreme antiquity of the visual pigment, rhodopsin. It is well represented in both the bacteria and the protista. Chemical analysis shows that the amino acid sequence of metazoan rhodopsins, although differing from one organism to another, is sufficiently similar to suggest a common ancestor in the remote past. Similarly, its 7TM disposition in cell membranes also indicates a common origin. Eyes, themselves, are, however, far more diverse. Although in most animal phyla they are restricted to simple eyespots, more elaborate systems can be found in six distinct phyla. These, moreover, are the most significant phyla: they contain 96% of contemporary animal species. We have seen something of their anatomical heterogeneity in this chapter.

The question arises: did this great variety of eyes arise independently or did they, too, have a common ancestry? Looking at the variety of structures and designs outlined in this chapter suggests a separate, or polyphyletic, origin. It may be the case that in some instances, for example the belemnite and vertebrate vesicle eyes, there are striking similarities, but these are, with very good reason, taken to be instances of convergent evolution rather than common ancestry. Whilst modern developmental genetics gives us no reason to doubt the latter conclusion, it is nevertheless beginning to gives us fascinating hints of common ancestry sometime before the proterostome/deuterostome divergence some 670 million years ago.

The evidence comes from the study of one of the genes, *Pax-6*, which is involved in the early development of eyes. As its suffix number indicates, *Pax-6* is a member of a large family of genes which regulates the transcription of other genes. The family plays an important rôle early in development, when its members control the transcription of cascades of other developmental genes. The nomenclature, *Pax*, refers to the fact that these genes all possess a 384 base pair (bp) sequence that encodes a 128 amino acid sequence which binds to DNA. This 384 bp sequence is known as the '*pa*ired bo*x*' (hence *Pax*) since it was first found in the pair rule genes which determine the early paired segmentation of *Drosophila* embryos. In addition to the paired domain all members of the *Pax* family share a highly conserved homeodomain.

Pax-6 has been found in many different species of animal from humans through insects and molluscs to round worms (nematodes) and ribbon worms (nemertines). In the early vertebrate embryo, *Pax-6* expression is at first widely distributed in the central nervous system and it can still be detected in the adult brain, especially in some of the nuclei of the forebrain, the substantia nigra of the midbrain and the granule cell layer of the cerebellum. So far as the forebrain is concerned, its expression becomes largely confined to the regions destined to develop into olfactory (olfactory epithelium and olfactory bulb) and optic (lens, cornea and optic vesicle) structures.

Mutations of *Pax-6* have disastrous effects. In the mouse they cause a condition known as small eye (Sey). In the heterozygous condition, *Sey* mice eyes have significantly smaller lenses and optic cups. Homozygous *Sey* is lethal. Early mice embryos (9.5 days) show no lens placode and the neural layers of the retina are highly abnormal. The olfactory placode, similarly, fails to develop, and the embryo shows no sign of nasal pits nor of an olfactory bulb. Clearly *Pax-6* plays a crucial role in the early development of eye and nose. Humans heterozygous for Se*y* suffer from a condition known as **aniridia**. In this condition there is a complete or partial failure of the iris to develop along with other defects including cataract, corneal opacity, glaucoma and so on. The incidence lies between 1/64 000 and 1/96 000. In addition, mutations of *PAX-6* can also lead to defects in the anterior chamber of the eye, including opacity of the central cornea, known as Peter's anomaly. In fact, differences in the degree of inactivation of *PAX-6* lead to a large number of ocular defects affecting numerous parts of the eye, especially the anterior chamber.

As indicated above, *Pax-6* is found throughout the animal kingdom. In all cases it plays a rôle in the early development of eyes. Furthermore, *Drosophila* geneticists have shown that it is possible to

(*Continues*)

(Continued)

transplant the gene into other parts of the embryo insect's anatomy, where it will induce 'ectopic' eyes. Eyes can be induced in legs, antennae, wings and so on. The insect can be covered with eyes! Further still, the mouse *Pax-6* will also induce ectopic eyes (not mouse eyes!) in *Drosophila*. Finally, it has been found that *Pax-6* from squid, normally essential in the early development of cephalopod's highly evolved eye, can also induce ectopic eyes in *Drosophila*.

All of these findings appear to point in one direction. They suggest that very early in development, perhaps at the stage represented by the platyhelminthes (Chapter 4), a genetic system evolved to programme the early stages of photoreceptor development. This system has remained, essentially unchanged, at the basis of all the huge variety of different animal eyes. Instead of a polyphyletic origin it may be that all eyes have a unitary origin. At the time of writing, the jury is still out. It has been found, for instance, that the first stages of eye development in *Drosophila* and vertebrates are not prevented by *Pax* null mutants and, furthermore, that planaria eye development proceeds to completion even when *Pax-6* is inactivated. But, taken together with the other evidences of unity at the molecular level that we have noted in this book, the story of the *Pax-6* gene reinforces the gathering vision of a remarkable unity in diversity throughout the animal kingdom. We look down through more than half a billion years and recognize ourselves.

REFERENCES

Callaerts, P., Halder, G. and Gehring, W.J. (1997) *Pax-6* in development and evolution. *Annual Review of Neuroscience*, **20**, 483–532.

Harris, W.A. (1997) *Pax-6*: Where to be conserved is not conservative. *Proceedings of the National Academy of Science*, **94**, 2098–2100.

Nilsson, D.-E. (2004) Eye evolution: a question of genetic promiscuity. *Current Opinion in Neurobiology*, **14**, 407–14.

Tomarev, S.I., Callaerts, P., Kos, L. *et al.* (1997) Squid *Pax-6* and eye development. *Proceedings of the National Academy of Science*, **94**, 2421–6.

are fully comparable in complexity and visual ability with the vesicular eyes of vertebrates. They form one of the most interesting cases of convergent evolution known in the animal kingdom. Finally, we shall turn to the phylum Arthropoda. Here we start by examining the structure and functioning of the primitive compound eye of *Limulus*, the King Crab (an Arachnid), then move to the highly evolved 'ocellar' eyes of the Salticid jumping spiders and end with that climax of the compound eye found in Dipteran insects.

15.2.1 Eyespots of the Protista

The term 'eyespot' is rather loosely applied. It may denote a photosensitive organelle in a unicellular organism, or it may refer to a single cell, or group of cells sensitive to light. In general, there are few if any optic nerve fibres and seldom any accessory structures such as lenses. Eyespots are found in flagellate protista, in the platyhelminthes and in the annelida. They are also occasionally found elsewhere. For instance they occur, as we noted in Section 15.1, in the *Amphioxus* nerve cord. Here they consist of small cluster of cells known as Hesse cells. In this section only protistan eyespots are considered.

Many different eyespots are developed by the flagellate protista. There are many types, ranging from simple coloured spots (known as **stigmata**) located in one or other part of the cell to the much more complex and certainly far larger **ocelli** of some marine dinoflagellates. It was long assumed that the coloured eyespot was the photoreceptor but this is no longer thought always to be the case. Indeed some phototactic protistans, such as the dinoflagellate *Gyrodinium*, show no trace of an eyespot. It seems that a visible eyespot is often no more than a part of the organism's photoreceptor apparatus. This apparatus is sometimes called a '**light antenna**'. Where eyespots exist, ultrastructural studies have shown that they all have some features in common. These include the possession of pigmented lipid droplets held together by one or more membranes. The pigment normally consists of one or more carotenoids (see Introduction) or rhodopsin and the membranes are often derived from chloroplast membranes.

One of the most intensively investigated stigma-type eyespots is that found in the free-swimming unicellular alga, *Chlamydomonas rheinhardtii* (Figure 15.7). It is situated at the edge of the chloroplast

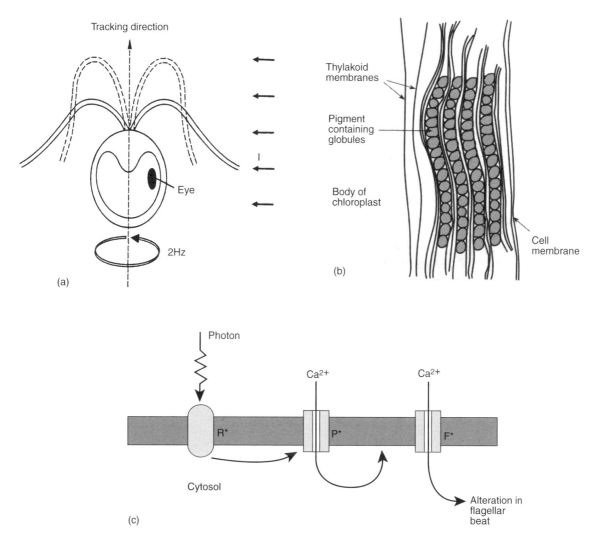

Figure 15.7 *Chlamydomonas* eyespot. (a): *Chlamydomonas* swims in the direction of the arrow rotating (counterclockwise) at 2 Hz. The beam of incident light (I) is consequently interrupted twice a second. The alga alters the movement of its flagellum until it moves directly toward the light source or (at high light intensities) directly away. (b): Drawing of a section through eyespot as seen in the electron microscope. Each layer of pigment globules is covered on its inner face by a thylakoid (i.e. chloroplast) double membrane. (c): Schematic to show the biophysical cascade induced by receipt of a photon by the *Chlamydomonas* rhodopsin. R* = activated rhodopsin; P* = activated photoreceptor channel; F* = activated flagellar channel. Explanation in text. After Foster and Smyth, 1980 and Harz, Nonnegasser and Hewgemann, 1992.

towards one side of the cell and consists of two to
four layers of closely packed globules sandwiched between chloroplast membranes. Careful electron microscopy has shown that, in front of the photosensitive spot, a lamellated structure develops which,
by constructive interference, ensures that the eyespot is sensitive to the direction of the incident light.
It has also been shown that the photosensitive spot
contains a rhodopsin somewhat similar to bacteriorhodopsin. This similarity is increased by the finding that retinal is in the 13-cis form. Although there
have been some recent reports which suggest the presence of a G-protein signalling system analogous to
that present in the complex eyes of vertebrates and
others, there is also evidence for a direct action on
a membrane Ca^{2+}-channel. In this latter schematic
(Figure 15.7b) incident light absorbed by rhodopsin
very rapidly ($<500\,\mu s$) opens a Ca^{2+}-channel (the
photoreceptor or P-channel) in the membrane. This
causes a membrane depolarization, which in turn
opens another set of Ca^{2+}-channels (the flagellar or
F-channels) in the vicinity of the flagellum.

The regular beat of the *Chlamydomonas* flagellum
pulls the alga forward in a spiral motion (rotation at
about 2 Hz), so that the eyespot intercepts light incident from the side every half second (Figure 15.7a).
The influx of Ca^{2+} through the F-channels (Figure 15.7c) alters the movement of the flagellum so
that the swimming direction is altered until the incidence of light is minimized. *Chlamydomonas* consequently swims towards the source of light so that its
photosynthetic apparatus can operate at optimal levels. At high light intensities the organism swims directly away from the light source.

Let us turn from the simple stigmata of *Chlamydomonas, Euglena* and so on to the far larger and
more complex ocelli of the dinoflagellates. Here again
we find many different types. It is believed that all
are modified chloroplasts. One of the most complex
is found in *Erythropsidinium*, a member of the order Warnowiales. The intricate structure of this organelle is shown in Figure 15.8. Very conspicuous
is a large refractile structure (called the crystalline
body or hyalosome) that is able to focus light on to
the retinoid. The retinoid consists of highly regular
(almost crystalline) layers of membrane above which
are large numbers of droplets containing carotenoids.
The biological significance of this magnificent photoreceptor is still in doubt. Like other dinoflagellates,

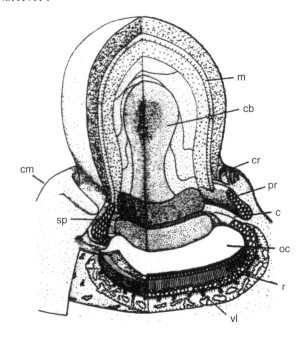

Figure 15.8 Ocellus of *Erythropsidinium* in longitudinal section. c = canal; cb = crystalline body; cm = cell membrane;
cr = constriction ring; m = mitochondria; oc = ocelloid chamber; pr = pigmented ring; r = retinoid; sp = scalariform plate;
vl = vesicular layer. From Dodge, J.D. (1991), reproduced by
permission of the author.

Erythropsidinium is not photosynthetic. Perhaps the
ocellus has evolved to detect prey or avoid predators.

15.2.2 The Pinhole Eye of *Nautilus Pompilius*

Nautilus pompilius, the pearly nautilus, belongs to
the most ancient subclass of the cephalopod molluscs. Fossil forms can be found as far back as 400
million years into the past. Nowadays it is to be
found swimming in moderately shallow waters of the
South Pacific. Its body is confined within a calcare-
ous, spirally-coiled shell into which it withdraws in
an emergency. Like other cephalopods it possesses
two large lateral eyes. But unlike other cephalopods
these eyes have no lenses and no vitreous humour
but pinholes which open directly into the surrounding seawater. The seawater directly bathes the well-
developed retinae. As mentioned above, they are perhaps the best known examples of pinhole eyes in the
animal kingdom.

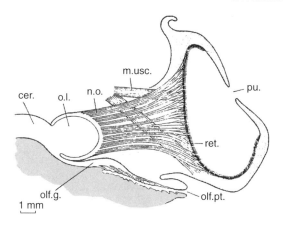

Figure 15.9 Pinhole eye of *Nautilus pompilius* in transverse section. cer = cerebral (supraoesophageal) cord; m = muscle; n.o. = optic nerves; o.l. = optic lobe; olf.g = olfactory ganglion; olf.pt = olfactory pit; pu = pinhole pupil; ret = retina. From Young (1965), *Phil Trans Roy Soc Lond B* **249**, p. 20, fig 8, with permission from the Royal Society.

A sectional view of the *Nautilus'* eye is shown in Figure 15.9. The orbit measures some $10 \times 15\,mm$ and the variable pinhole measures from 0.4 to 2.8 mm. The diameter of the pinhole is under muscular control but the action is slow (50 s to fully open; 90 s to constrict). The retina consists of some 4×10^6 close-set rhabdomeric photoreceptors. As these photoreceptors are only some $5–10\,\mu m$ in diameter the retina should be capable of good resolution (Part Four: Introduction). However, it has been calculated that the pinhole only provides a 2.3° minimal resolvable angle, which translates (using the formulae given in the Introduction and the dimensions of the *Nautilus'* orbit) to a lateral distance across the retina of no less than about 0.4 mm. *Nautilus* seems to have developed a retina far better than its optics can use! Indeed, investigation of the animal's lifestyle shows that it spends much of its time in light of low intensity, descending to a depth of some 300m during the day and ascending to about 150m at night. Why have such an excellent retina if it is never used? The *Nautilus* eye remains a mystery.

15.2.3 The Mirror Eye of *Pecten* (the Scallop)

Pecten belongs to the bivalve or Lamellibranch molluscs. It is closely related to the oysters. But unlike the other bivalve molluscs it is an active swimmer. It shoots through the water by clapping its shells together. Although some other bivalves develop eyes, they are little more than eyespots. The cockle, *Cardium edulis*, for instance, develops about 60 tiny photosensitive spots, no more than $50\,\mu m$ in diameter, and containing 12–20 ciliary-type photoreceptor cells. *Pecten*, however, develops as many as a hundred remarkable eyes on the perimeter of its mantle (Figure 15.10).

Pecten's eye has attracted scientific scrutiny for over a century. A sectional view is shown in Figure 15.11. It possesses a definite cornea, a cellular lens, a vitreous humour and, most intriguingly, no less than two retina. Each retina contains about 500 000 photoreceptor cells. Equally intriguingly there is a reflecting tapetum (or argentea) behind the proximal retina. Interestingly, a reflector is also found in the minute eye of *Cardium*. This mirror layer is composed of alternating layers of cytoplasm and guanine crystals. It forms an image on the distal retina. The function of the proximal retina is not clear, for the lens is not sufficiently powerful to form an image upon it. It may be that it merely responds to variations in the luminant intensity. If so, like the retina of *Nautilus* discussed above, it seems to be remarkably overspecified for the job. One final fascinating point should be remarked upon. As we noted in Section 15.1 above, the distal retina contains ciliary-type photoreceptors that hyperpolarize on illumination, whilst the proximal retina contains rhabdomeric photoreceptors which depolarize on illumination. There is one final twist to this extraordinary story. Although the ciliary photoreceptors of the proximal retina hyperpolarize in response to illumination, the biophysical mechanism is quite different from that found in vertebrate photoreceptors. Instead of closing CNG $Ca^{2+} + Na^+$-channels (Section 17.2.1.3) the scallop's ciliary photoreceptors open K^+-channels. *Pecten* seems to have independently evolved hyperpolarization. Why? Is it necessary that ciliary-type photoreceptors hyperpolarize? Is there a deep reason? As yet we have not the glimmerings of an understanding.

15.2.4 The Vesicular Eye of *Octopus*

The cephalopoda are classified into three subclasses: Belemnoidea (Dibranchiata), Nautiloidea (Tetrabranchiata) and Ammonoidea (Chapter 4). The

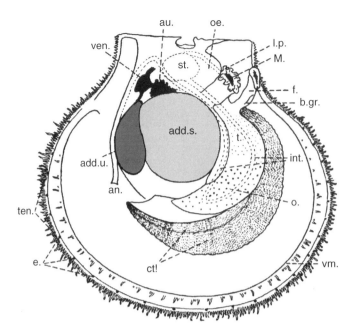

Figure 15.10 Anatomy of *Pecten*. The bivalve has been opened to show its internal anatomy. In life, when the animal is relaxed, the mantle and its tentacles project a small distance from the edge of the shell. e = eye; ten = tentacles. From Borradaile *et al.*, 1951.

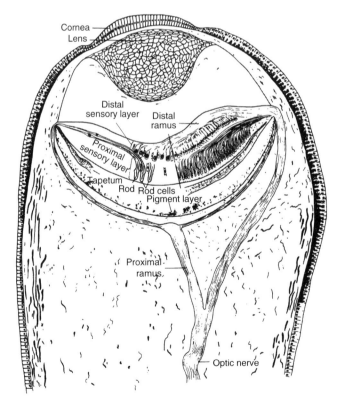

Figure 15.11 Eye of *Pecten* in section. The distal and proximal retinae (= sensory layers) are shown. Beneath the proximal retina is the reflecting tapetum (not fully drawn for the sake of clarity). Beneath the tapetum is a pigment layer. From Dakin, 1928.

members of the latter subclass are all extinct. We discussed the 'primitive' pinhole eyes of Nautiloids in Section 15.2.2 above; here we turn our attention to the remarkable vesicular eyes of the Belemnoidea. The belemnoids are classified into two orders: the decapod (ten armed) squids (*Loligo*) and cuttle fish (*Sepia*), and the octopod (eight armed) octopi (*Octopus*). The eye is very similar in both orders. It is celebrated amongst zoologists as an outstanding example of convergent evolution. It is not only almost identical in both belemnoid orders but its structure and functioning show striking similarities and equally striking dissimilarities to the eyes of fish. Yet the common ancestor of fish and cephalopods is way back half a billion years ago in the Precambrian period. It seems that over some five hundred million years, free-swimming vertebrates and cephalopods have felt their way to analogous solutions to the problem of visual distance detection. Students interested in the more philosophical aspects of biology may wish to ponder whether such striking convergences suggest, as we argued in Chapter 4, that evolutionary winnowing ultimately homes in on similar designs in very different lineages.

The two belemnoid lateral eyes are set on pedicles on either side of the head and protected by connective tissue and cartilaginous sheaths. They are always large and prominent. In a small octopus they may have a diameter of 10–15 mm but in the giant squid, *Architeuthis*, they have been reported to measure nearly half a metre (40 cm) in diameter! Extrinsic eye muscles ensure that the orbit is able to move in its socket and there is evidence for optokinetic reflexes somewhat similar (though less rapid) to those found in vertebrates. The iris is also well supplied with muscles so that the aperture of the rectangular pupil can be varied in response to varying light intensity. In front of the lens there is a cavity filled with an aqueous humour bounded anteriorly by a transparent cornea. In some forms the anterior chamber is open to the surroundings and hence filled with sea water. Behind the lens the orbit is filled with a vitreous humour which, as in the vertebrates, helps to hold the retina in place. The lens itself is held in position by a ciliary body but the method of focusing is radically different from that found in the vertebrates. Instead of altering the lens's curvature the ciliary muscles squeeze the orbit itself and thus, by putting pressure on the vitreous, force the lens

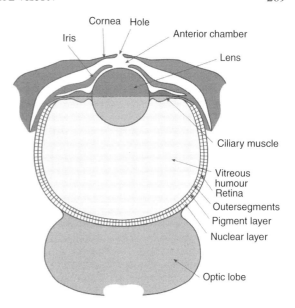

Figure 15.12 Belemnoid eye in section. The eye is formed by invagination of the surface epithelium (cp. *Nautilus*). It is lined by the retina and this lining continues anteriorly to form the posterior part of the ciliary muscle and the posterior part of the lens. In some forms the cornea is complete, in others a hole is left so that the anterior chamber is open to the surrounding sea water. Further explanation in text.

forward. In other words, the cephalopod eye focuses light on to its retina much as a camera focuses light on to photographic film. A silvery pavement epithelium – the argentea – covers the iris and extends some distance posteriorly. A cross-sectional view of a typical cephalopod eye is shown in Figure 15.12.

Perhaps the most interesting feature of the cephalopod eye is the retina. In both the decapoda and octopoda the photoreceptors are rhabdomeric and known as **retinula cells** (Figure 15.13a). The belemnoid retina does not suffer the embryologically-induced awkwardness of the vertebrate retina: the retinula cells are **not** covered by a neural retina and directed away from the incoming light but abut the vitreous humour and face outward. On the other hand, retinula cells resemble vertebrate rod cells (which are, of course, of the ciliary type) in being subdivided into an outer and inner segment. The outersegment is very long and thin ($200–300 \times 3\,\mu m$), and produces two sets of microvilli diametrically opposite each other and orthogonal to its long axis (Figure 15.13b). These

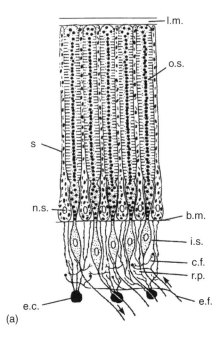

(a)

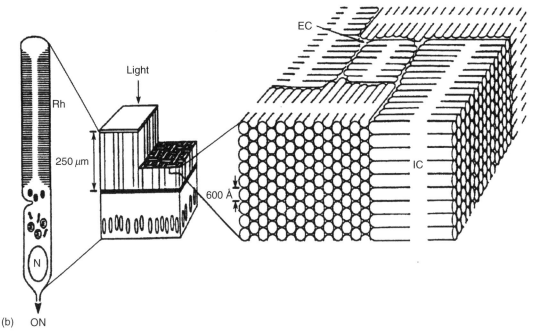

(b) ON

Figure 15.13 (a) Octopus retina in vertical section. The lengthy outersegments of the retinula cells are sandwiched between pigment cells. The inner segments of the retinula cells are located beneath a basement membrane and continue as fibres of the optic nerve into optic lobe. c.f. = collateral fibre of retinula cell; b.m = basement membrane; e.c. = epithelial cell; e.f = efferent fibre; i.s. = inner segment; l.m. = limiting membrane; n.s. = nucleus of supporting cell; o.s. = outer segment; r.p = collateral fibre; s = supporting cell (pigment filled). From Young, 1962a. (b) Detailed structure of the retina. The microvilli of the outersegments form a very precise mosaic. EC = extracellular compartment; IC = intracellular compartment; N = nucleus of retinula cell; ON = optic nerve fibre; Rh = outersegment. From Saibil and Hewat, 1987.

microvilli are also very long and thin ($1 \times 0.06\,\mu m$ (that is 60 nm)). They are also present in very large numbers: 200 000–700 000 in each row. There is good evidence that the photopigment, **rhodopsin**, is concentrated in the microvillar membranes. The centre of the outersegment is filled with pigment granules, which migrate towards the inner segment in the dark. There is also evidence that the outersegments themselves can contract. This happens during intense illumination. The inner segment contains a rich collection of mitochondria, pigment granules, membranes known as somal or myeloid bodies and the nucleus. From its inner end extends an axon which forms one of the fibres of the optic nerve leading into the optic lobe. The retinula cell is thus, unlike the vertebrate rod and cone cells, a neurosensory cell.

There are about 2×10^7 retinula cells in each *Octopus* retina and, as Figure 15.13a, shows their outersegments are packed closely together separated only by the thin pigment-filled processes of supporting cells. Their perikarya are located beneath a basal membrane and the nerve fibres leading away from their bases give off lateral branches which form a **plexiform layer**. This plexiform layer also contains glial cells and efferent fibres from the optic lobes. There is also evidence that gap junctions are made between the inner segments of the retinula cells, and between efferent and optic nerve fibre membranes. Although the plexiform layer cannot compare in intricacy with the plexiform layers of vertebrate retinae (Section 17.2), it nevertheless provides a basis for some initial processing of the visual information. The major business of processing the visual information occurs in the closely adposed optic lobe (Figure 15.14), which is sometimes called (after Cajal) the 'deep retina'.

Figure 15.13b shows that the outersegments of the retinula cells form a very precise mosaic. The microvilli of adjacent retinula cells are orientated at right angles to each other. This means that when the eye is held in its natural position the microvilli are orientated alternately in the vertical and horizontal direction. This is believed to be responsible for the cephalopod's well established sensitivity to the plane of polarized light (Chapter 21).

The molecular biology of belemnoid vision is in some ways similar to that of vertebrates, in others dissimilar. The major visual pigment is rhodopsin. Like vertebrate rhodopsin it consists of a 7TM protein,

opsin, and a chromophore, 11-cis retinal. In addition, another visual pigment, **retinochrome**, is found in the myeloid bodies of the retinula cell inner segments. This pigment is involved in the regeneration of rhodopsin. In the majority of cases there is only one type of rhodopsin in the retina, though in different belemnoid species its λ_{max} varies from 470–500 nm. In one bioluminescent deep sea squid (*Watasenia scintillans*), however, three different rhodopsins exist with λ_{max} at 470, 484 and 500 nm. Whether the colour vision implied by the presence of these three different photopigments is significant in the lifestyles of these bioluminescent squids is as yet unknown.

When light is absorbed by 11-cis retinal it is converted into the all-trans form (details in Section 17.2.1 (c)) and detaches from the opsin. The activated opsin then activates a G-protein system which in turn activates membrane-bound phospholipase C (Chapter 1, Section 4.2). This leads (as we saw in Section 1.4.2) to the synthesis of IP$_3$ and DAG and release of Ca^{2+} from intracellular stores at the proximal ends the retinula cell. The increased Ca^{2+} leads to a **depolarization** of the retinula cell membrane and this in turn initiates action potentials in the retinula axon. This, of course, is a major difference from the biophysics of vertebrate photoreceptor cells. We have already noted more than once that the latter hyperpolarize in response to illumination rather than depolarize.

The retinula cell axons form the optic nerve. Figure 15.14 shows that these fibres run out of the retina and cross over before entering the cortex of the optic lobe (the so-called 'deep retina'). Here they enter another plexiform layer and, the topological relations of the input fibres being preserved, an inverted representation of the image on the retina is presented. It has, however, proved very difficult to use microelectrode recording techniques on the belemnoid central nervous system. The detailed physiology of the optic lobes and the brain thus remains, at the time of writing, an enigma wrapped in a mystery.

15.2.5 Lateral Eyes of *Limulus*, the King or Horseshoe 'Crab'

Although *Limulus* (Figure 15.15a) is commonly referred to as a crab, it is in fact not a crustacean at all but a member of the subphylum Chelicerata,

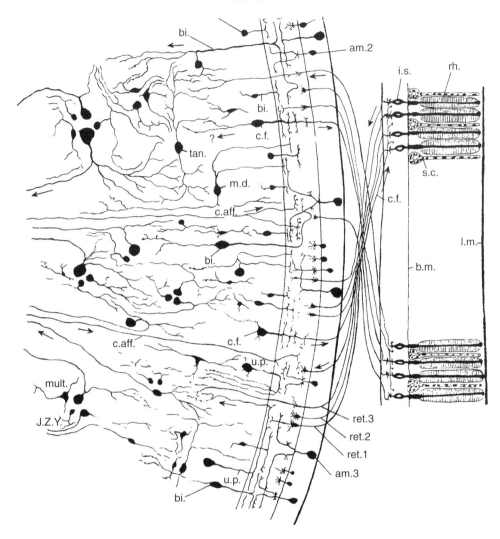

Figure 15.14   Octopus retina and 'deep retina'. The optic nerve fibres springing from the retinula cells cross over before entering the cortex of the optic lobe where they form the 'deep retina'. am 2,3 = amacrine cells of outer granule layer; bi. = bipolar cell; b.m. = basal membrane; c.aff. = afferent fibre from deeper regions; c.f. = centrifugal cell to superficial from deep retina; i.s = inner segment of retinula cell; l.m. = limiting membrane; m.d. = multidendritic cell; mult. = small multipolar cell; ret. 1,2,3 = retinal fibres of three diffferent types; rh = rhabdome of retinula cell; s.c. = supporting cell; tan = tangential cell; u.p.= unipolar cell. From Young (1962), *Phil Trans Roy Soc Lond B* **245**, p. 23, figs 1 & 4, with permission from the Royal Society.

more closely related to the spiders, scorpions and mites than to the crabs (Chapter 4). It is a primitive form, and fossil remains, not greatly different from living specimens, can be found preserved in Silurian strata dating back some 400 million years. Consistent with its ancient lineage is the primitive form of its compound eye. As Figure 15.15b shows, the ommatidia (about 850) are widely separate (not closely packed as in insect and crustacean eyes) and from

each springs a single optic nerve fibre. The simplicity of the anatomy soon attracted the attention of electrophysiologists, and Hartline and coworkers established that, in spite of the wide separation of the ommatidia, the eye nevertheless worked as a unit. In other words, the output from each ommatidium is affected by activity in its neighbours. Before considering this important physiology let us look at the anatomy in a little more detail.

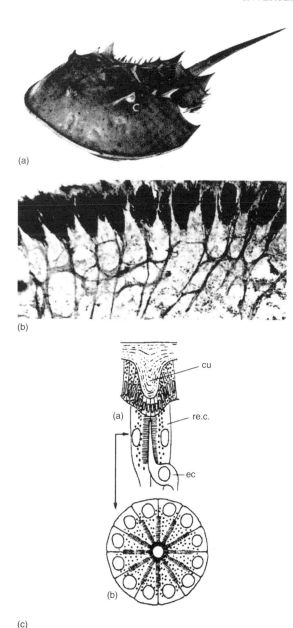

There is an as yet unconcluded debate concerning the relation of the *Limulus* ommatidium to those found in other arthropods. There is no corneal lens. There are a variable number of retinula cells (4–20) and, importantly, one or, more usually, two, '**eccentric cells**'. In contrast to those found in crustacea and insects, the retinula cells are purely sensory. Only the eccentric cells develop nerve fibres. These fibres constitute the optic nerve. However, the retinula cells resemble those in other arthropods in developing a column of microvilli, constituting a rhabdomere, in which the visual pigment, rhodopsin ($\lambda_{max} = 520$ nm), is located. The structure of the ommatidum is shown in LS and TS in Figure B15.15c.

When light of appropriate wavelength falls on the ommatidium, opsin is activated in the usual manner, leading to a sequence of biochemical events ending in depolarization of the retinula cell. This depolarization leads, in turn, to depolarization of the dendritic ending of the eccentric cell(s) and thus to generation of an action potential in the eccentric cell axon. The eccentric cell acts to integrate the responses of its surround of retinula cells. The action potential in the eccentric cell axon propagates towards the brain. However, as shown in Figure 15.16a, the axons send out collateral branches very soon after they leave the ommatidia. These fibres form the lateral plexus. It is here that what almost forms the type example of **lateral inhibition** occurs.

The effect of stimulating ommatidia in the vicinity of the ommatidium being studied is shown in Figure 15.16. If a pencil beam of light is shone on to an ommatidium, a steady tattoo of impulses (the frequency is dependent on intensity of stimulus) is propagated along the optic nerve fibre emanating from its eccentric cell(s). If, however, and without altering the intensity of the light on the ommatidium, another beam is switched on a short distance (1 or 2 mm) away, the frequency of impulses is at first completely interrupted and then markedly reduced. In other words, activity in the nerve fibre from the neighbouring ommatidia is transmitted via the lateral plexus to inhibit activity in the original fibre. The further away the neighbouring ommatidia are, the smaller is the effect.

Lateral inhibition is, as we have already seen and shall see again when we come to consider vertebrate visual systems, a very general feature of sensory systems. It is particularly easy to demonstrate in *Limulus* compound eye. It shows, as mentioned

Figure 15.15 (a) *Limulus polyphemus*, the king crab. The two lateral eyes (C) are situated on the external surfaces of the first lateral spines. From Duke-Elder, 1958: , (b) Lateral eye of *Limulus* in vertical section. The row of darkly stained objects is the ommatidia; the lateral plexus and optic nerve fibres are also easily visible. From Hartline, 1959. (c) Single ommatidium of lateral eye in (a) vertical section and (b) transverse section. cu = cuticle; re.c = retinula cell; ec = eccentric cell. From I.A. Meinertzhagen (1991), in J.R. Cronly-Dillon & R.L. Gregory, *Vision & Visual Dysfuntion, Vol 2*, p. 345, fig. 16.3 (a) and (b) reproduced by permission of the author

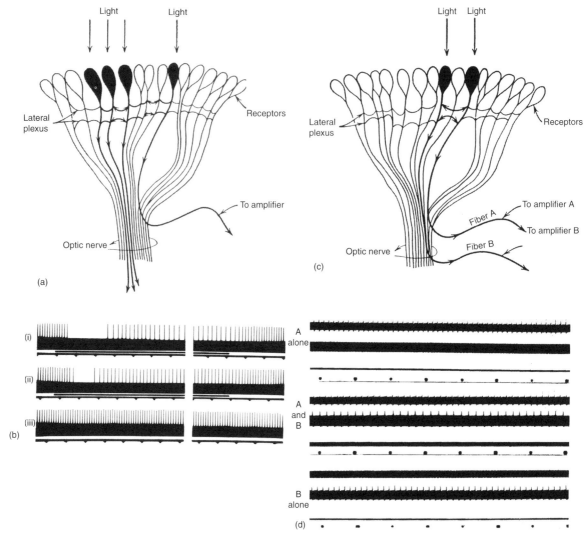

Figure 15.16 (a) Lateral inhibition in *Limulus* retina. Activity in the optic nerve fibre leading from a single ommatidium is recorded. (b) Oscillograph recordings of action potentials in nerve fibre. (i) When nearby ommatidia are strongly illuminated, activity is suppressed. The black bar above the time record (0.2 s marks) indicates the duration of illumination. (ii) In response to weaker illumination the inhibition still occurs but for a shorter period. (iii) Control when neighbouring ommatidia are unilluminated. (c) Pencil beams of light illuminate two nearby ommatidia. The result is shown in (d). When A is illuminated alone, a tattoo of impulses is induced in its optic nerve. When B is illuminated alone a similar tattoo of impulses can be recorded. When both are illuminated together, mutual inhibition reduces activity in both optic nerve fibres. From Hartline, H.K. (1959) Receptor mechanisms and the integration of sensory information in the eye, in *Biophysical Science – A Study Program* (ed. J.L. Oncley). Copyright © 1959, John Wiley & Sons.

above, that the individual ommatidia interact with each other before sending information to the brain. They act, in other words, interdependently as a primitive retina. The biological significance of the wiring is also clear. If the ommatidia are *all* subjected to

diffuse illumination, lateral inhibition will reduce the impulse traffic in all the optic nerve fibres. If, however, there is a sharp discontinuity in the illumination as, for example, when a shadow falls across the retina, then inhibition on the illuminated ommatidia will be reduced from those which are covered by the shadow. They will, in consequence, be disinhibited and fire with a greater frequency. The system thus serves to mark where the edges of shadows are falling across or moving across the retina – information which may clearly be of life and death importance to the King Crab.

15.2.6 The Advanced Ocellar Eyes of Jumping Spiders (Salticidae)

Spiders, although also members of the subphylum Chelicerata, are far removed from the ponderous armour plated King Crabs. Nevertheless, many spiders, especially web-building spiders, have rather poor eyesight, being largely nocturnal and relying on their tactile and, to a lesser extent, olfactory sense, to detect prey. On the other hand, excellent vision is vital for diurnal 'hunting' spiders belonging to the orders Lycosidae, Thomisidae and Salticidae. The largest eyes of all are, however, found in the Australian net-casting spider, *Dinopis*, where they reach a diameter of 1.4 mm. These eyes do not have particularly good resolution, although they are extremely sensitive. This is crucial for *Dinopis*, as it is a nocturnal spider which hunts in the dark and, when it senses a prey insect, literally throws a net over it. The principal eyes of the diurnal hunting spiders are much smaller than those of *Dinopis*, seldom exceeding 0.4 mm in diameter. The visual acuity in these spiders is, however, far greater than in the Dinopidae and we shall confine ourselves to a discussion of these spiders in this section, in particular, to members of the Salticidae, the jumping spiders (see Figure 15.17(a)).

The majority of spiders have eight eyes, a pair of principal eyes facing forward and known as anterior median eyes (AMEs), and three pairs of secondary eyes on the sides of the cephalothorax known, respectively, as the anterior lateral eyes (ALEs), posterior median eyes (PMEs) and posterior lateral eyes (PLEs) (Figure 15.17b).

Although the eyes of most spiders, especially the lateral eyes, are rather simple ocelli, the eyes of hunting spiders, especially the AMEs and ALEs are very highly evolved. The ALEs have moved to the anterior of the cephalothorax so that four of the eight eyes face forward (Figure 15.17d). Whereas the ALEs and PMEs function as movement detectors (compare the peripheral regions of mammalian retinae), the AMEs have evolved into very precise imaging devices. Seeing shape and form is vital to a hunting spider which has to identify its prey before it jumps. It is also important in the complex mating dances which hunting spiders have developed. It has been shown that the acuity of the AMEs of the African jumping spider, *Portia*, is about 0.04°, some ten times better than the best compound eye, that of the dragonfly, and only about five times worse that the human eye. With such a high acuity *Portia* is able to resolve objects 0.12 mm apart at a distance of 200 mm.

The structure of the salticid AME is shown diagrammatically in Figure 15.17c. Beneath the large corneal lens is a deep 'eye tube' containing a vitreous body ending in a rhabdomeric retina. The eye tube is formed so that light is focused once at the corneal lens and a second time towards the base of the tube (Figure 15.17c). The retina consists of four layers of rhabdoms. In layers I, II and III the photosensitive parts of the rhabdoms, the rhabdomeres (like those of the cephalopods), face outwards towards the incoming light. In layer IV, however, the rhabdomeres are aligned at right angles to the light and this may account for the spider's sensitivity to the plane of polarized light (Chapter 21).

It has been found that the retina is maximally sensitive to light at wavelengths 360 nm (ultraviolet), 480–500 nm (blue) and 580 nm (green) and it may be that each of the three 'bottom' retinal layers contain different visual pigments, allowing the spider to visualize different colours. Chromatic aberration by the corneal and secondary lenses ensures that the longer wavelengths, towards the green part of the spectrum, are preferentially focused on the bottommost layer (layer 1) and shorter wavelengths in the upper layers. That jumping spiders have colour vision has been confirmed by behavioural experiments.

The detailed organization of the AMEs, PLEs and PMEs in the prosoma of a jumping spider is shown in Figure 15.17d. The retinae of the AMEs have definite 'foveas', where the density of rhabdomeres is some ten times greater than at the periphery. This is not the case in the PLEs and PMEs. Here the retina is much more extensive and there is no specialized central fovea. Figure 15.17d also shows that, unlike the ALEs and PMEs, the AMEs have muscle bands which control the position of the eye tube. We noted in Section 15.1.3 that when the PLEs and PMEs

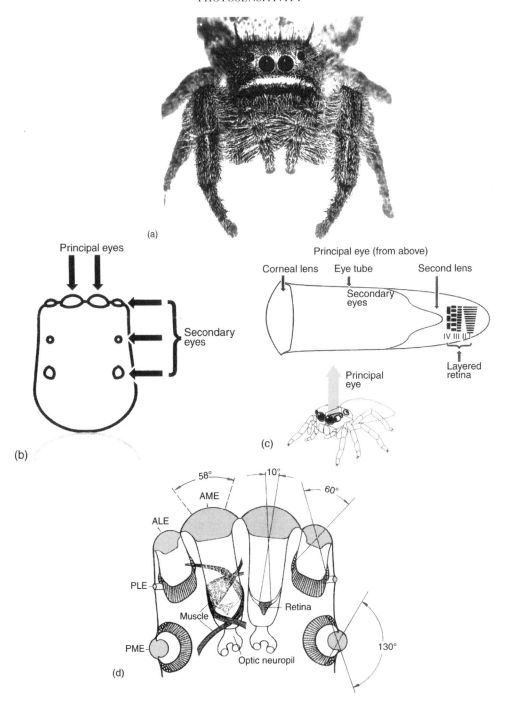

Figure 15.17 Ocellar eyes of Salticid spiders. (a): Head-on view of a salticid spider. A pair of anterior median eyes and a pair of anterior lateral eyes face forward. (b): Position of eyes on the cephalothorax of a salticid spider. (c). Internal structure of a salticid principal eye. For explanation see text. (d). Horizontal section of the prosoma of a salticid spider to show detail of the photoreceptor apparatus. The angle (58°) for the left AME is the maximum angle through which the eye muscles can swing the field of vision by moving the retina laterally. (a) From David Hill phidippus@uswest.net; (b) and (c) from Harland and Jackson (2000), Copyright © 2000, the National Museum of Namibia; (d) from Foelix (1982) *Biology of Spiders* Copyright © 1982, Harvard University Press.

catch sight of a movement, the spider turns to 'fix' whatever has caused the movement on the fovea of the AMEs. The eye-tube muscles now come into play. There are six of these and they allow the tube to be moved horizontally, vertically and rotated. Action of these muscles ensures that the fixation is maintained. The fixation is very precise. The image is focused on only a hundred or so foveal rhabdomeres. This allows the object to be identified. It has been suggested that the eye movements may allow the spider to search for particular identifiers in the visual image. If the search succeeds in finding these identifiers, perhaps those of a suitable prey insect, stalking behaviour is triggered. When the insect is brought to within about 2 cm, the final leap is made. The fact that the fields of vision of the ALEs overlap by about 40°, in contrast to the very narrow, nonoverlapping fields of the AMEs, suggests that this final feral leap may be guided by some stereoscopic depth perception. Moving images of salticid spiders can be found in the web pages prepared by David Edwin Hill.

In conclusion we can see that the ocellar type eye is capable of extraordinary development when appropriate evolutionary pressures are applied. In the jumping spiders the essentially ocellar foundation has been developed into an integrated **system** that allows hunting behaviour, which some have compared to that of *Felix domestica*, the domestic cat.

15.2.7 The Advanced Compound Eyes of Flies (Diptera)

As we saw in Section 15.1 above, the insects and crustacea have developed a wide variety of compound eyes. In this section we shall consider in detail just one type: the neural superposition eye of Dipteran flies (house flies, blowflies, fruit flies, gnats, mosquitoes and so on). The Dipteran compound eye is an apposition eye. The structure of apposition ommatidia was discussed in Section 15.1 (Figure 15.3) and little more need be said about it here. Figure 15.18 shows, however, a number of details and the light path through the system. Unlike the ommatidium of *Limulus,* the Dipteran ommatidium consists of a fixed number (six or seven) retinula cells and one or two further cells (perhaps related to *Limulus*' eccentric cell) towards the bottom of the system.

Each retinula cell develops a rich column of microvilli constituting a rhabdomere. The retinula cells

are set close together to form a cylinder and their rhabdomeres are closely adposed to each other (as can be seen in the electronmicrograph of the lacewing ommatidium (Figure 15.18b)) and together constitute the rhabdom. The visual pigment (rhodopsin) is located in the microvilli of the rhabdomeres. The rhabdom (about 1 μm in diameter and up to 100 μm in length) acts as light guide or optic fibre (Figure 15.18a). Pigment granules prevent light escaping into other parts of the retinula cells. Light therefore has the maximum opportunity of interacting with the rhodopsins in the rhabdomeres. Figure 15.18a also shows that the position of the pigment granules within the retinula cell varies over the diurnal cycle. During the day they are close to the microvilli of the rhabdomeres so that light is concentrated on the visual pigment. The daytime eye thus has high acuity. In dim illuminations, however, the pigment granules migrate away from the rhabdomeres so that, although acuity is lost, the system becomes more sensitive.

The response of the rhabdomere to illumination is a **depolarization**. Action potentials are not found in the fibres leading away from the base of the retinula cell. Information is transmitted by electrotonic conduction. Many insects have rhodopsins with differing λ_{max} in the different retinula cells. Light of different wavelengths will thus cause different patterns of response from an ommatidium. This accounts for the excellent colour vision of, especially, the flower-visiting insects.

The optic nerve fibres from the majority of the retinula cells run to the **optic lamina** directly beneath the compound eye. These are known as short visual fibres (SVFs). They terminate in narrow 'cartridges' where they synapse with second order fibres that carry this 'high resolution' data to the **medulla**. It is found that the SFVs from retinula cells having the same field of vision in different ommatidia run to the same cartridge. Thus, as mentioned in Section 15.1, although the fly's eye is of the apposition type with all the acuity which this gives, the neural wiring in the optic lamina ensures that a superpositioning of images occurs, with all the attendant sensitivity which that entails. The fibres from the deeper ('eccentric') retinula cells, however, pass straight through the lamina to terminate directly in the medulla (Figure 15.19a). These are the long visual fibres (LVFs). It can be seen from Figure 15.19a that both the second order fibres and the LFVs

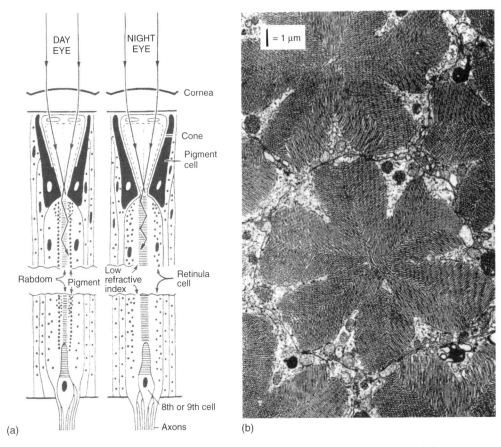

Figure 15.18 (a) Vertical sections of an ommatidium of a large diurnal insect. Explanation in text. (b) Transverse section of the ommatida of a nocturnal eye (*Chrysopa* (green lacewing)). Each ommatidium has six principal retinula cells and the microvilli of their large rhabdoms fill most of the electronmicrograph. A single ommatidium in cross section fills the centre of the picture. A 1 μm scale bar is shown in the top left corner of the picture. G.A.Horridge, 1991, in J.R. Cronly-Dillon & R.L. Gregory, *Vision and Visual Dysfunction, Vol 2*, p. 232, Fig 11.2, reproduced by permission of the author.

cross-over between the lamina and the medulla. But in both visual areas a retinotopic map is maintained; in other words the cells in these areas are arranged in columns corresponding to their points of origin in the eye. This retinotopic organization is retained after a further cross-over leads the visual information into the last stratum of the optic lobe, the **lobula**. In the fly this last stratum is divided into two parts: a posterior part – the lobula plate – and an anterior part – the lobula. The main projection from the medulla enters between these two parts and diverges into each (Figure 15.19b).

In addition to maintaining a retinotopic organization, there are many tangential fibres with extensive arborizations in all three subdivisions of the optic lobe. Cells in the deeper parts of the optic lobe (the medulla and lobula) have been shown to respond to colour, direction of motion, orientation of edges and so on. Object recognition appears to begin in the lobula. We shall find analogous mechanisms at work in the vertebrate visual cortex. Beyond the lobula the visual information is transmitted deep into the brain, where we will not presume to follow it. It should, moreover, be noted that Figure 15.19a is a highly generalized diagram to show the common features of most arthropod, from crustacean to insect, optic lobes. Figure 15.19b gives some impression of the full complexity of the 'wiring' in the fly's optic lobe and further detail may be found in the publications cited in the bibliography.

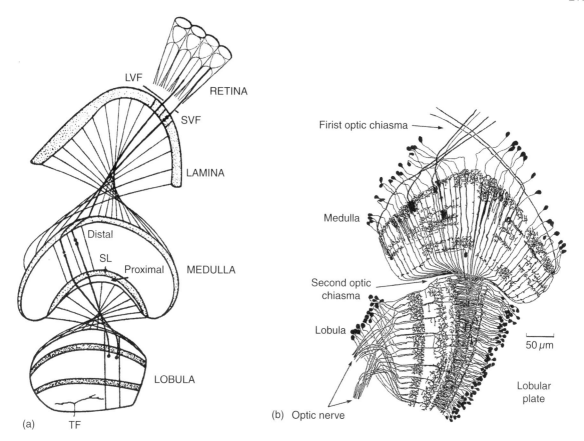

Figure 15.19 (a) Generalized arthropod optic lobe. The three major ganglia of the optic lobe – the lamina, medulla and lobula – are separated from each other by a cross over of fibres. LVF = long visual fibres; SL = serpentine layer; SVF = short visual fibres; TF = tangential fibre. Further explanation in text. From Osorio, 1991. From N.J. Strausfield (1976), *Atlas of an Insect Brain* p. 142, fig 7.13, reproduced by permission of Springer-Verlag GmbH. (b) The second and third synaptic regions of the fly's optic system. Fibres from the lamina (SVFs) and from the retina (LVFs) enter the top of the figure and synapse in the medulla. After a further cross over (second optic chiasma) further neurons make synapses in the lobule or lobular plate. Visual information is carried into the protocerebrum by fibres of the optic nerve at the bottom of the figure.

15.3 CONCLUDING REMARKS

The foregoing review has emphasized the huge variety of eye designs that have emerged over half a billion years of biological history. Of necessity only a few of the major and most successful types have been described. The precise distance information delivered by sense organs sensitive to electromagnetic radiation in the 'visible range' is evidently of surpassing value in the struggle for existence. How far do the invertebrates 'see' in the sense in which we 'see'? This, as Adrian Horridge remarks, is a difficult question

to answer. Human vision, as he says, is from the beginning full of meaning. Each object has its name, perhaps even an emotional resonance. We cannot escape this when we open our eyes and look. It would seem to be somewhat anthropocentric to suppose that the insect visual system, or even the belemnoid visual system, provides its owner with a similar experience, or even a 'whisper' of that experience. But, by definition, we cannot know. To know what their 'seeing' is like (to paraphrase Thomas Nagel), we would have to *be* an individual *Portia fimbriata, Musca domestica* or *Octopus vulgaris!*

16

THE HUMAN EYE

Vertebrate eye probably essentially unchanged since Precambrian period. Vision at centre of human life-style. **Overview** of 'vegetative' ocular anatomy and adnexa. **Embryology** - phylogenetic speculation - neurectoderm - tubular CNS - optic vesicle - inverted retina - induction of lens - aphakia, anophthalmia, micro-ophthalmia - coloboma - elimination of optic ventricle - differentiation of retina - differentiation of cornea and iris - formation of sclera and choroid. **Detailed anatomy and physiology**: **cornea**: anterior epithelium - Bowman's membrane - stroma, collagen fibres and their organisation - Descemet's membrane - endothelium - innervation; maintenance of transparency; **sclera**: shape of eye, myopia? **lens**: lens fibres - transparency - crystallins - heat shock proteins - accommodation - myopia, hypermetropia, astigmatism, presbyopia - cataract; **choroid**: four layers - vascular support for retina; **ciliary body**: histology - ciliary processes - secretion of aqueous humour - circulation - absorption - IOP - glaucoma; ciliary muscles - histology - innervation - lens accommodation; **Iris**: histology - physiology; **vitreous humour**: floaters. **Movements of eyeball**: vestibulo-ocular - optokinetic - pursuit - saccadic - vergence - efference copy. **Concluding remarks**: fitness for purpose of eye design.

The vertebrate eye has an immense history. We noted in Chapter 15 that it probably originated in the Precambrian period more than half a billion years ago. Fossils of *Pikaia*, identified as an early chordate, are found in the Burgess shale dating from 525 million years BP. Agnathan fish (the Anaspids) have left fossils, showing well-developed bilaterally-paired orbits, dating back to the Silurian period. Unlike the arthropod compound eye the vertebrate eye does not, however, lend itself to fossilization. We can only infer the 'soft' structure by examining the eyes of the only extant Anaspids – the Cyclostomata (hagfish and lampreys) – the most primitive living vertebrates. Although the hagfish eye is almost vestigial, resembling the pineal of nonmammalian vertebrates and probably having much the same function as that organ, lampreys possess well formed vesicular eyes which do not differ in any really major way from those found in other living vertebrates. Indeed, it is found that, except in details (Chapter 19), the vertebrate eye does not vary greatly in structure or functioning across the living vertebrates, from the jawless (agnathan) Cyclosotomes, through the jawed fish, amphibia, reptiles and birds to the mammals. In this it differs dramatically from the eyes of Mollusca which, as we noted in Chapter 15, show a full range from eyespots to the complex vesicular eye of the Belemnoidea. Because of this striking regularity, it is possible to describe the mammalian eye, indeed the human eye, as a type example. Moreover, so large is

Biology of Sensory Systems, Second Edition   C.U.M. Smith
© 2008 John Wiley & Sons, Ltd

the topic, we shall discuss only the non-neural parts, the so-called 'vegetative' aspects, of the eye in this chapter. We shall postpone a detailed discussion of the retina, the vital photosensory and neural tissue, until Chapter 17. Then, in Chapter 19, after considering the visual pathways and cortices in Chapter 18, we shall look at some variations on the theme by examining the eyes of some of the other vertebrates.

Humans are very visual creatures. Our mentality is permeated with visual imagery: we 'visualize' an outcome, we 'see' a solution. we 'outline' a plan; we fill in 'background'; we 'speculate', 'imagine' and 'foresee' and so on. This visual bias should not surprise us. All primates are very visual animals. For tens of millions of years our ancestors passed their lives in the canopies of tropical and subtropical forests. Good vision, good distance judgment, good discrimination of load-bearing branches from those liable to give way, good perception of routes through a complexity of foliage, good colour vision to detect ripe fruit, edible nuts, dangerous predators, all put a premium on evolution of an excellent visual system.

16.1 ANATOMY

In this section an overview will be presented. Subsequent sections will discuss each element in more detail. We shall begin with the eyeball, or 'globe', and then discuss the accessory structures, or **adnexa**.

16.1.1 Eyeball

An equatorial section through the eyeball is shown in Figure 16.1. The wall consists of three layers (= tunics). On the outside is a tough collagenous layer, the **sclera** or **sclerotic coat**. This forms the 'white' of the eye and its mechanical strength protects the eye's delicate interior and holds it in shape. Anteriorly it is continuous with the transparent **cornea**. Over the surface of the cornea is a layer of transparent epithelial cells continuous with the epidermis of the skin. This is the **conjunctiva**. Within the sclera is the **uveal tract**. The name comes from an ancient observation that it easily detaches from the sclera in the dissected eye when it clumps together rather like a bunch of grapes (uva (L) = grape). The uveal tract consists of three major parts: the **choroid** (a vascular and pigmented layer lining the major part of

eye's posterior chamber), the **ciliary body** from which **zonule fibres** (= suspensory ligaments) spring to hold the lens in place, and the **iris** which extends in front of the lens. Finally, the innermost layer is perhaps the most important of all, the **retina**.

As Figure 16.1 shows, the retina covers all the posterior part of the eyeball and extends forward to the ciliary body where it terminates at the **ora terminalis** (alternatively known, because of its serrated edge, as the **ora serrata**). In fact, it is only the photosensitive retina which finishes here, a nonphotosensitive epithelial continuation of the retina extends forward to cover the surface of the ciliary body and iris. At the back of the eye, where the visual axis intersects the retina, there is a depression, the **fovea**, populated by cones and responsible for daytime vision. Surrounding the fovea is a wider circle of retina known as the **area centralis**, or when pigmented, as in humans and other primates, as the **macula lutea (yellow spot)**. This is also adapted (though to a lesser extent) for high resolution photopic vision. This small area of tissue, 5–6 mm in diameter, has been said, size for size, to be the most important area in the human anatomy. Loss of function (macular degeneration) has disastrous and disabling consequences (Box 17.2). To the nasal side of the area centralis, and consequently off the optic axis, is the **optic disc**, where the optic nerve fibres gather to leave the retina as the optic nerve. This area is consequently devoid of photoreceptors and, being insensitive to light, is known as the '**blind spot**'. It is also a weak spot in the otherwise tough sclerotic coat. To strengthen this potential weakness the optic nerve fibres pass through a perforated collagenous plate, the **cribriform plate**, just beneath the disc.

The equatorial section of Figure 16.1 shows that the lens divides the internal cavity into two parts: the anterior and posterior chambers. The anterior chamber is filled with **aqueous humour**, a watery solution secreted (as we shall see) by the ciliary body, whilst the posterior chamber is filled with a jelly-like **vitreous (= glassy) humour**, secreted during the development of the eye by the retina. The vitreous humour helps to hold the eyeball in shape and its backward pressure assists in keeping the retina in place. The pressure exerted by the aqueous humour on the vitreous (and this pressure is, as we shall see, subject to pathological change) thus has an effect on the retina. If it should rise beyond normal bounds, the delicate retina and optic nerve are damaged and the individual suffers from the condition known as **glaucoma**

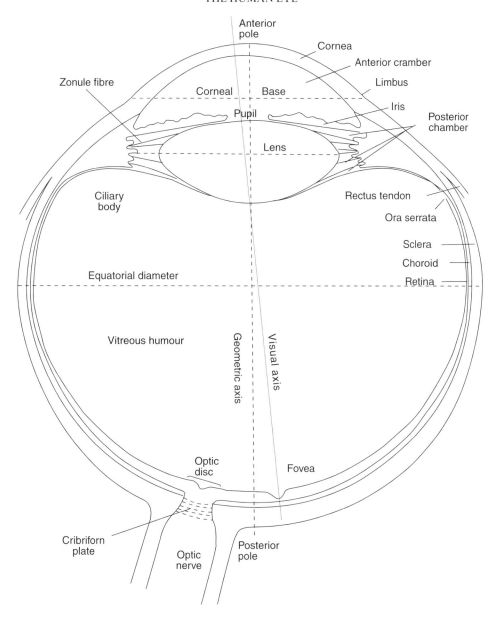

Figure 16.1 Equatorial section through human eye. Explanation in text.

leading (unless remedial measures are taken) to loss of sight.

16.1.2 Adnexa

Outside the eyeball are a number of accessory structures known collectively as the **ocular adnexa**: the extrinsic eye muscles, the eyelids and the lacrimal system.

16.1.2.1 Extrinsic (Extraocular) Eye Muscles

The eyeball, as we all know, is fully motile in its socket. This motility is due to the action of the six

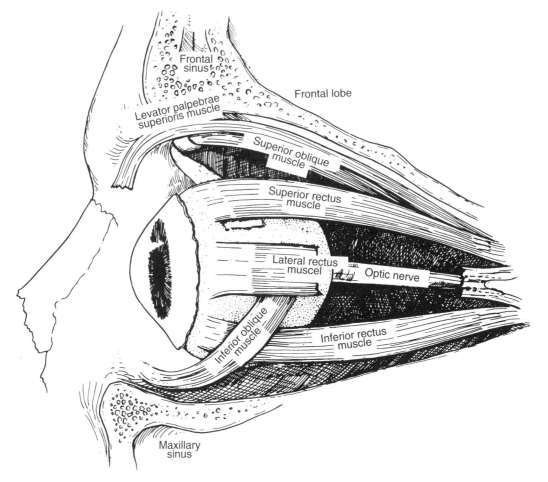

Figure 16.2 Extrinsic eye muscles. The inferior and superior oblique muscles are inserted behind the eyeball's equator. The superior oblique (as shown) passes through a loop of fibro-cartilage, the trochlea, before turning back to be inserted in the eyeball under the superior rectus muscle. The trochlea acts as a pulley. Only three rectus muscles are visible in the figure. The fourth, the medial rectus, runs parallel to the lateral plexus on the nasal side of the orbit. The lateral rectus is shown cut away to reveal the position of the optic nerve. Contraction of the levator palpebrae superioris muscle raises the upper eyelid. From F.W. Newell (1996) *Opthalmology: Principles and Concepts*, fig 1–36, Copyright © 1996 Elsevier.

extrinsic eye muscles: the **superior**, **inferior**, **lateral** and **medial rectus** muscles, and the **superior** and **inferior oblique** muscles. These muscles are shown in Figure 16.2. The superior, inferior and medial recti and the inferior oblique muscles are innervated by branches of cranial nerve three, the **oculomotor nerve**. The superior oblique is innervated by the fourth cranial nerve (**trochlear nerve**) and the lateral rectus by the sixth cranial (**abducens**) nerve. The tendon of the superior oblique muscle passes through a ring projecting from the lacrimal bone (one of the bones of

the orbit) known as the trochlea. The muscles all act in cooperation to rotate the eye in its boney orbit.

16.1.2.2 Eyelids

From the biological point of view, the eye presents a considerable challenge. Other parts of the body's surface are protected by a stratified epithelium. This cannot be appropriate for the eye. Transparency is of the essence and this transparency has to be maintained over, perhaps, a century. The solution, therefore, was to evolve what some have called retractile flaps of skin – the eyelids.

The eyelids form one of the most important elements of the eye's defences. By means of their lashes (cilia) they sense danger and screen it away; by means of their secretions they prevent dessication; by means of their constant motion up and down over the surface of the cornea they distribute secretions and the lacrimal fluid, which helps to remove any dangerous irritants.

Each lid consists of a wide fibrous tarsal plate that follows the curvature of the eyeball. The cilia (or eyelashes) are arranged in two rows on both the upper and lower lids. They grow from typical hair follicles. A nerve plexus with a very low threshold of excitation surrounds each follicle. Touching a cilium

is sufficient to excite one or more nerve fibres and elicit a reflex blink. Just behind the inner row of cilia are the openings of large sebaceous glands, the **Meibomian glands** (Figure 16.3). There are about thirty of these glands in each tarsal plate and they produce an oily secretion which forms an important part of the tear film covering the cornea. It functions to prevent too rapid an evaporation of tear fluid and also to prevent spillage of the tears at the lid margins. Figure 16.3 shows that the inner surface of the lids also contains a number of accessory lacrimal glands: the glands of **Krause** and **Wolfring**.

The ocular surface of the lids is covered by a mucous epithelium – the **conjunctiva** – which is continuous with the conjunctiva covering the bulbar surface of the eye. The bulbar conjunctiva is, in turn,

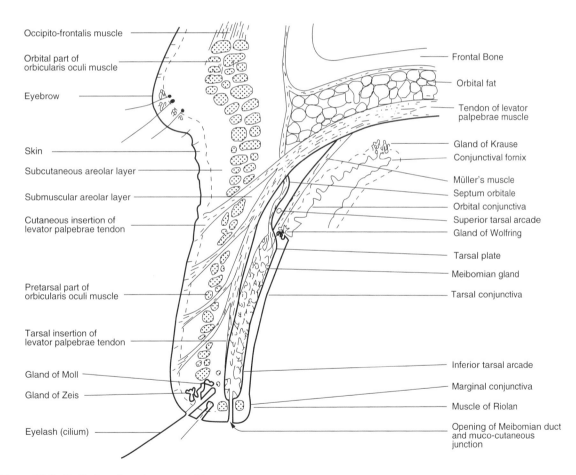

Figure 16.3   Vertical section of upper eyelid.

continuous with the corneal epithelium. The conjunctiva is richly provided with mucus-secreting goblet cells which, along with the glands mentioned above, also make their contribution to the constitution of the lacrimal fluid. The blinking activity of the lids distributes the quite complex lacrimal fluid over the surface of the cornea: it provides the essential living conditions for the cornea.

Each person has their own spontaneous rate of blinking. On average, the period between blinks is about 2.8 s in men and 4.0 s in women. It varies widely in nonhuman animals. The period for which the eye is closed during a blink is 0.3–0.4 s. The brain automatically compensates for these intervals of darkness; we are not aware of them, yet a darkening of the visual field of only 0.03 s (other than by automatic blinking) is fully perceptible.

Blinking is also a reflex response to danger. It may be induced by loud noises, by tactile stimuli to the vicinity of the eyes and by sudden strong lights. The tactile reflex is lost if there is a cortical lesion in the Rolandic area; the dazzle reflex disappears in response to certain lesions of the midbrain. Loss of blink reflexes is thus useful clinical signatures of specific brain damage.

16.1.2.3 The Lacrimal System

We have already noted some of the glands contributing to the lacrimal system in the previous paragraphs. The major source of lacrimal fluid is, however, the **lacrimal gland**, which is located in the superior-lateral corner of the orbit. It possesses 10–12 medium-sized ducts that open independently of each other into the conjunctival fornix. It secretes a watery fluid which is (except for the markedly higher concentrations of K^+ and Cl^-) not greatly dissimilar to the composition plasma minus most of the organics (Table 16.1). A number of enzymes are present, but the most important is **lysozyme,** which attacks bacteria by dissolving their cell walls. The lacrimal fluid is moved across the cornea by the action of blinking and is drained at the nasal corner of the eye by a system comprised of the lacrimal puncta, canaliculi, sac and nasolacrimal duct into the nasal cavity (Figure 16.4).

The tear film is largely composed of the aqueous secretion of the lacrimal gland but its surface consists of an oily layer derived from the Meibomian glands.

Table 16.1 Composition of lacrimal fluid

	Plasma	Tears
Electrolytes (mM)		
Na$^+$	137.5	135.0
K$^+$	4.3	36.0
Cl$^-$	108.5	131.0
HCO$_3$$^-$	27.0	27.0
Ca^{2+}	2.3	0.5
Mg^{2+}	0.2	0.36
Organics (mg/ml)		
Glucose	0.8	0.05
Lysozyme	—	2.1
Albumen	40–48	0.04

Data from Tiffany, 1997.

This, as mentioned above, is essential if the thin film of lacrimal fluid is not to dry up. The mucous secretions of the conjunctiva form the bottom-most layer of the tear film, which is held in position by a multitude of microvilli projecting from the corneal epithelium (Section 16.3.1). The tear film is well oxygenated as it is moved across the cornea by the blinking action of the eyelids, and uptake of oxygen from the film by the corneal epithelium is essential for the well being of the cornea.

Reflex secretion from the lacrimal gland is caused by irritation of the cornea, conjunctiva, nasal mucosa and also by thermal stimuli, bright lights and

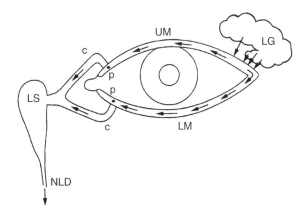

Figure 16.4 Lacrimal system. The tear fluid is moved across the eye in the direction of the arrows. c = canaliculi; LG = lacrimal gland; LM = lower meniscus; LS = lacrimal sac; NLD = nasolacrimal duct; p = lacrimal puncta; UM = upper meniscus. Further explanation in text. From Harding, 1997.

peppery foods applied to the mouth and tongue. It is also caused by emotional upset. Section of the trigeminal nerve (cranial V) removes all reflex weeping but leaves psychogenic weeping unaffected. Indeed, psychogenic weeping seems (like laughing) to be unique to humans. Parasympathetic innervation is also important. Fibres belonging to this system run in the facial nerve (cranial VII) to the gland, and parasympatheticomimetic drugs induce a large and prolonged increase in tear flow.

16.2 EMBRYOLOGY

Let us now return to the eye itself. There is no better way towards an understanding of its anatomy than to follow its origin in embryology. It may also be, if we allow Haeckel's biogenetic law some validity, that tracing its development (at least in its earliest stages) may provide us with some insight into its evolutionary origins. It will be seen that these origins are distinctively different from the invertebrate vesicular eyes we reviewed in Chapter 15 (but note the evidence for an **initial** commonality rehearsed in Box 15.2). It does not derive **straightforwardly**, as they do, by invagination of the surface epithelium. The retina originates in a circuitous manner, internally, from the central nervous system (CNS). We shall see that it is because of this convoluted route of origin that it is '**inverted**'. The photoreceptors end up facing away from the incoming light.

The vertebrate eye develops partly from mesodermal tissue and partly from ectodermal tissue. The ectodermal tissue forms the retina and the non-neural epithelial continuation of the retina which covers the ciliary body and the posterior of the iris. Ectoderm also forms the lens. Mesodermal tissue forms all the rest. It has often been said that the retina is a portion of the brain pushed to the exterior. We shall see the sense of this proposition when we follow its embryological origin.

The chordate central nervous system begins as a specialized strip of ectoderm – the **neurectoderm** – running longitudinally along the dorsal surface of the early embryo (Figure 16.5). In this respect it differs radically from the origin of invertebrate central nervous systems, which are always in the ventral position. Does this mean that our earliest ancestors, in contrast to the bottom-crawling invertebrates, were

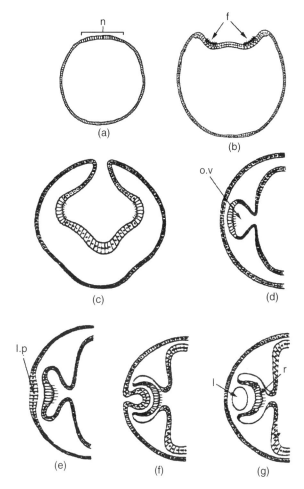

Figure 16.5 Series of transverse sections to show the embryological origin of retina and lens. (a) Early embryo (neurula) in which a strip of neurectoderm differentiates on the dorsal surface; (b) Neurectoderm sinks inwards and two hollows, the foveolae opticae, appear; (c) Neural tube beginning to form; (d) Evagination of optic vesicle; (e) Optic cup beginning to form and lens beginning to be induced from the overlying ectoderm. (f) Optic cup continuing to invaginate and lens continuing to form. (g) Optic cup almost fully formed; lens detached from overlying ectoderm. Note the position of the photoreceptor outersegments throughout. f = foveolae opticae; l = lens; l.p. = lens placode; n = neurectoderm; o.v = optic ventricle; r = photoreceptor outersegments.

free swimmers in the upper waters of the oceans, where light (and the shadows of predators and prey) would have come from above? However this may be, the primordial photoreceptor cells are believed to have been embedded in this strip of reactive tissue. At this point they are 'verted' (to use the ugly neologism coined by comparative anatomists of the visual system), that is, they face outwards towards the incoming light. Early in embryology, however, the neurectoderm sinks inward forming first a 'gutter' and then rolling up to form the tubular central nervous system – again a defining characteristic of chordate animals. As Figure 16.5 shows, this leaves the primordial photoreceptor cells facing inwards into the central canal of the CNS. It is interesting to note that the anterior eye of the cephalochordate, *Amphioxus*, consists of a pigmented eyespot beside a group of photoreceptor cells which do, indeed, face inwards into the cerebral vesicle (Figure 4.10). It is thought that these cells act as 'shadow detectors' warning the animal of the approach of predators from above. We have already noted (Section 4.7.8) that the anterior eye is believed to be the primordium of the lateral eyes of the vertebrates. During evolution it is obvious that this internal position could not be a long term solution. As chordates evolved, grew in size and bodily opacity, the evolution of lateral eyes ensured that photoreceptors necessarily assumed a more superficial position.

Figure 16.5 shows how this happens in vertebrate embryos. Even before the neural tube is formed, two small depressions, the primordia of the retinae, known as the **foveolae opticae**, become apparent in the neurectoderm of what is destined to be the forebrain. Is it possible to see these incipient depressions as analogous to the invaginations leading to invertebrate vesicular eyes (compare *Nautilus* and *Octopus* of Chapter 15)? As soon as the neurectoderm has rolled up to form a tube these dimples grow larger and push out toward the surface on each side of the forebrain. They quickly expand, as if inflated from within, to form the **optic vesicles**. They remain connected to the forebrain by **optic 'stalks'**. There are two important things to note at this stage. Firstly, the ciliary photoreceptors remain facing inwards, now into the so-called **optic ventricle**. Secondly, as soon as the optic vesicles come into contact with the overlying epidermis, a thickening and sinking in of the latter begins. This is the **lens placode** or **primordium**. It appears that some still unknown biochemical influence spreads from the optic vesicle to the overlying epidermis, inducing the formation of the lens. This is one of the earliest cases of **embryological induction** known,

still one of the most impressive and still, in spite of spectacular advances in molecular embryology, mysterious. If the optic vesicle is removed, the lens does not form; if the optic vesicle is implanted beneath the epidermis in some other part of the body, even the trunk, a lens will be induced in that position.

The lens rudiment is, as shown in Figure 16.6, at first a cup and then a hollow sphere of cells. Soon, however, the cells in the posterior wall of the sphere begin to elongate by growing into the cavity and it is not long before the hollow ball is transformed into a solid mass of cells. The long thin cells are known as **lens fibres**. This growth of originally cuboidal cells into long thin fibres continues throughout life in the region of the lens's equator. The lens comes to resemble an onion with layer upon layer of lens fibres, one outside the other. As the fibres are too short to stretch all the way round the lens, the growing tip of one fibre meets the growing tip of another and these points of juncture form the so-called **lens sutures**. We shall return to consider the mature lens in Section 16.3.3.

Faults in embryological development, if they occur, are most catastrophic if they occur at an early stage. Lens development is no exception to this rule. Thus if, right at the beginning of the process, the optic vesicle fails to contact the overlying epithelium a lens may not develop at all – a condition known as **aphakia**. Lack of a lens may in turn affect the development of the optic vesicle itself, leading to **anophthalmia**. If the lens–optic vesicle interaction is not totally lacking, a less dramatic though still distressing **micro-ophthalmia** may result.

Let us, however, turn from these embryological disasters to continue the story of the developing optic vesicle. As Figure 16.7 shows, it begins to collapse into itself. The ventricle within slowly disappears. But the process is not quite as simple as merely pushing in one side of a rubber ball. As Figure 16.8 shows, the vesicle is, to begin with, largely above the optic stalk. As development continues it grows round, ventrally, to form a deep groove whose lips eventually close to form a tunnel. If the lips of the optic cup fail to meet and fuse, the finished eye is said to show a **coloboma**. Fortunately, these are rare. Normally the lips fuse about six weeks after conception and a temporary artery, the **hyaloid artery**, which supplies the developing eye, begins to grow out in the resulting tunnel.

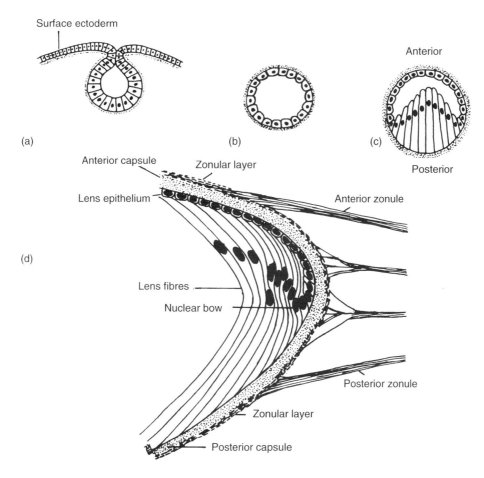

Figure 16.6 Embryological formation of the lens. (a) : Invagination from surface ectoderm along with basement membrane; (b): Separation from ectoderm as a hollow ball of cells; (c): Elongation of posterior cells which ultimately obliterate the internal cavity; (d) Equatorial section of the fully formed lens. The lengthy posterior cells (now known as lens fibres) have elongated so that they now completely fill the cavity and abut the anterior epithelium. Their nuclei form (as shown) a characteristic 'bow', the nuclear bow. The basement membrane becomes the lens capsule. Zonule fibres are inserted into this capsule and run to the ciliary body. From Davson, *The Eye, third edition,* vol 1, 1984, p. 223, fig 62, by permission of Academic Press Ltd.

This artery ultimately runs out into the optic cup, reaching as far as the posterior surface of the lens, and sends branches to all parts of the interior of the cup. When eye development is complete (in humans before birth) it atrophies back to the point where it emerges into what is now the vitreous-filled posterior chamber. Together with the remnant of the 'primary vitreous', which it was largely instrumental in supplying, it forms the **canal of Cloquet**, which remains visible in the adult eye. The proximal part of the hyaloid artery, meanwhile, is now known as the **central retinal artery**. It still runs along its old route, now associated with the optic nerve, and emerges into the retina at the optic nerve head (optic disc) and branches into the retina where, with the central retinal vein, it provides the principal blood supply.

The collapse of the original optic vesicle has another consequence. If we refer back to Figure 16.5, we can see that, as the original optic ventricle is eliminated, the wall of the optic cup becomes two layered. The outer layer of the cup is destined to form the retina's pigment epithelium, the inner layer comes

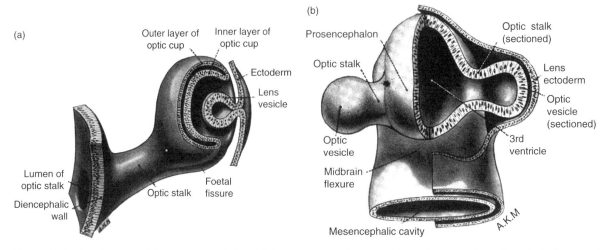

Figure 16.7   Development of the optic cup and lens (a) 4 mm human embryo; (b) 7.5 mm human embryo. From Duke-Elder and Cook, 1963.

to form the retina itself. Although the optic ventricle is nearly completely obliterated in the adult eye, the join between the retina and the pigment epithelium remains a point of weakness. In cases of **detached retina** this is where the disjunction occurs. Indeed, the retina is mainly held in position against the pigment cell layer by the pressure of the vitreous humour.

It remains for the layers of the retina to differentiate. The retina, as we have emphasized, is part of the brain pushed to the surface. It is thus only to be expected that its differentiation will be similar to that of other parts of the brain. The columnar epithelial cells lining the defunct optic ventricle become a **germinative layer**. Initially the number of cells in this layer is quite small. At about the fourth week, however, a rapid 'proliferative' stage begins and the number of cells increases dramatically. When this stage is complete, the cells begin to differentiate and move away from the 'optic vesicle' towards the vitreous humour. The first cells to differentiate are destined to form retinal **ganglion cells**. They begin to climb away from the germinative layer along the fibre guides provided by retinal glial cells, the **Müller cells**. As they climb away from the germinative layer, they develop axons that grow back as elements of the optic nerve, along the optic stalk, to the diencephalon.

After this first wave of cells, another type of cell differentiates from the germinative layer. These are the **amacrine cells**. This change in cell type appears to be due to the freshly differentiated ganglion cells secreting a factor which inhibits the differentiation of germinal cells into further ganglion cells. The amacrine cells, in their turn, migrate away from the germinative layer, following the ganglion cells toward the surface of the retina and secreting inhibitory substances, preventing the next set of cells becoming amacrines. Following behind the amacrines come successive waves of cells, destined to form **bipolar**, **horizontal** and **interplexiform cells**, all climbing towards the vitreous humour, away from the germinative layer and differentiating in an increasingly complex environment of inhibitory substances. Last of all, the photoreceptor cells, the **rods** and **cones**, differentiate. These, however, do not migrate, but remain next to the now only virtual optic ventricle, entangled with the processes put out by the pigment epithelial cells.

The cellular structure of the retina is now complete. It will be discussed in detail in Chapter 17. It is worth noting, however, that the retina does not all form at exactly the same time. Differentiation occurs first at the posterior pole of the optic cup (the **fundus**) and only occurs later (weeks later) at the periphery. It is likely (though this still remains controversial) that differential cell death is responsible for the great variation in the number of cells (especially ganglion cells) in different parts of the retina. There are, for instance, several hundred more ganglion cells per unit

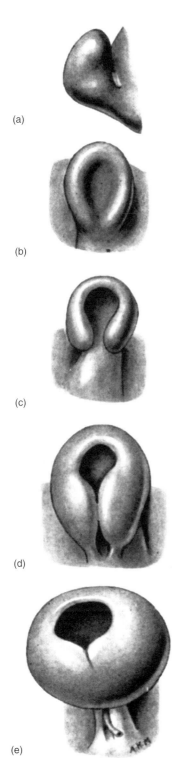

(a)

(b)

(c)

(d)

(e)

area of the fovea than per unit area of the peripheral retina. Finally, it is worth re-emphasizing that the whole intricate process leaves the photoreceptor cells facing inwards away from the incident light, and covered by several layers of neurons. This must remain a puzzle for those who, disdaining evolutionary explanations, would rather invoke the cunning of the President of the Immortals.

Whilst the retina and lens have been differentiating, other parts of the eye are also developing. In front of the lens three waves of mesoderm migrate under the corneal epithelium. The first wave is destined to form the corneal **endothelium**, the second wave, following about a week later, begins to form the **stroma** of the cornea, whilst the third grows beneath the other two but still in front of the lens to ultimately form anterior cell layers of the **iris** (Figure 16.9). Whilst all this is happening, the lens is continuing its development and, under this influence and the gradual build up of intraocular pressure due to the formation of the aqueous and vitreous humours, the cornea begins to bulge outwards. As Figure 16.1 shows this makes for a distinct corneoscleral junction, called the **limbus**.

The cornea continues its differentiation. The anterior epithelium develops three cell layers, the stroma begins to secrete mucopolysaccharides and collagen fibres, whilst the endothelium retains its single cell layer structure. As development proceeds, the collagen fibres begin to orientate themselves with extreme precision into a series of lamellae (Section 16.3.1). This does not happen in the sclera. As a consequence, the cornea gradually clears (becomes transparent), whilst the sclera, if anything, becomes more opaque. Meanwhile the mesodern around the optic cup is differentiating into the vascular choroid and the extraocular muscles begin to attach to the developing sclera. By about seven months after conception the eye is complete (though only some 10–14 mm in diameter), the retina, apart from the fovea, is fully developed and the hyaloid artery begins to atrophy leaving only the canal of Cloquet.

Figure 16.8 (*Opposite*) Three-dimensional views of the formation of the optic cup. The embryonic fissure is shown well in (c) and (d), and in (e) the hyaloid artery is shown entering the proximal end of the fissure. Further explanation in text. From Duke-Elder, 1958.

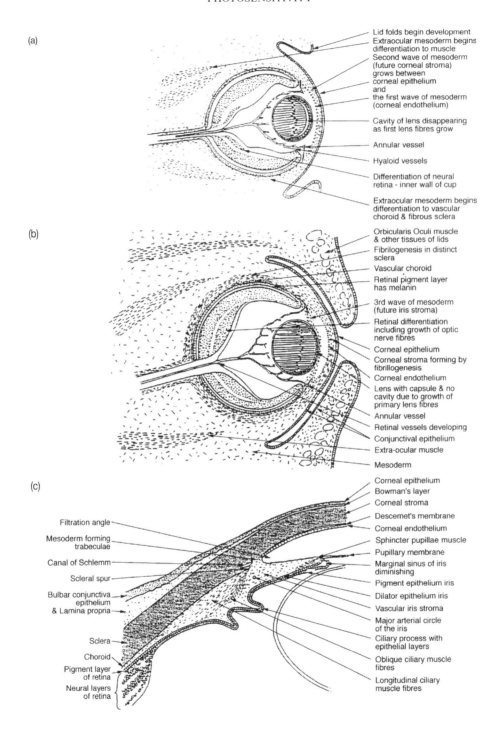

(a)

Lid folds begin development
Extraocular mesoderm begins differentiation to muscle
Second wave of mesoderm (future corneal stroma) grows between corneal epithelium and the first wave of mesoderm (corneal endothelium)
Cavity of lens disappearing as first lens fibres grow
Annular vessel
Hyaloid vessels
Differentiation of neural retina - inner wall of cup
Extraocular mesoderm begins differentiation to vascular choroid & fibrous sclera

(b)

Orbicularis Oculi muscle & other tissues of lids
Fibrilogenesis in distinct sclera
Vascular choroid
Retinal pigment layer has melanin
3rd wave of mesoderm (future iris stroma)
Retinal differentiation including growth of optic nerve fibres
Corneal epithelium
Corneal stroma forming by fibrillogenesis
Corneal endothelium
Lens with capsule & no cavity due to growth of primary lens fibres
Annular vessel
Retinal vessels developing
Conjunctival epithelium
Extra-ocular muscle
Mesoderm

(c)

Filtration angle
Mesoderm forming trabeculae
Canal of Schlemm
Scleral spur
Bulbar conjunctiva epithelium & Lamina propria
Sclera
Choroid
Pigment layer of retina
Neural layers of retina

Corneal epithelium
Bowman's layer
Corneal stroma
Descemet's membrane
Corneal endothelium
Sphincter pupillae muscle
Pupillary membrane
Marginal sinus of iris diminishing
Pigment epithelium iris
Dilator epithelium iris
Vascular iris stroma
Major arterial circle of the iris
Ciliary process with epithelial layers
Oblique ciliary muscle fibres
Longitudinal ciliary muscle fibres

Figure 16.9 This series of diagrammatic sections shows the progressive development of the eye from about five weeks to six months after conception. (a) Five weeks. Note development of cornea and lens. (b) Eight weeks. Note further development of cornea and lens. Iris and retina developing. (c) Six months. Eye nearly completely formed. Further explanation in text.

16.3 DETAILED ANATOMY AND PHYSIOLOGY

Having seen how the human eye develops let us now return to its adult structure and consider the anatomy and physiology of its parts in more detail.

16.3.1 Cornea

We saw in Section 16.2 that the cornea consists of three layers: the anterior epithelium, the stroma (or lamina propria) and the endothelium. Separating these three layers from each other are two 'membranes', *Bowman's layer* (between epithelium and stroma) and *Descemet's membrane* (between stroma and endothelium). This five-layered structure is shown in Figure 16.10.

16.3.1.1 Structure

The anterior epithelium consists of five or six layers of stratified noncornified epithelium. The innermost layer is a germinal layer, showing mitotic figures, and the cells replicate throughout life. As they move upwards to the surface they flatten and are finally lost to the lacrimal fluid. A few nonepithelial cells are present, including lymphocytes, macrophages and tall deeply staining cells of unknown significance,

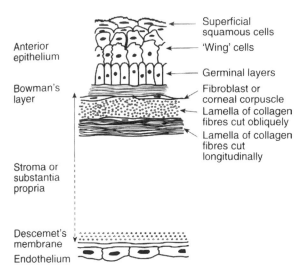

Figure 16.10 Transverse section through adult cornea. Explanation in text.

variously known as 'Langerhans', polygonal or dendritic cells.

The epithelial cells in the middle layers produce deep invaginations in their surface membranes into which the membranes of neighbouring cells fit. These cells are known as 'wing' cells and their tight interdigitations with each other ensure that they form a mechanically firm layer. At the surface the cells become flattened plates and lose their internal organelles but produce numerous microvilli, which project into and stabilize the lacrimal fluid (Section 16.1).

Bowman's layer lies beneath the anterior epithelium. Electron microscopy shows that it consists of numerous fine collagen fibres (25 nm in diameter) interwoven in a mucopolysaccharide matrix. The fact that it is secreted by the underlying stroma rather than the overlying epithelium means that it is better regarded as a layer than a membrane.

The **Stroma** or **lamina propria** is, perhaps, the most interesting, as it is also the thickest (about 480 nm, 88% of cornea), of all the layers of which the cornea is composed. It consists of **cells** (fibroblasts also known as **corneal corpuscles** and macrophages), **matrix** and **collagen fibres.** The matrix consists of proteoglycans, glycoproteins, inorganic salts and water.

Collagen is one of the most common proteins in the animal kingdom, from the Cnidaria to the Primates. It is found in all connective tissues, where it provides mechanical, especially tensile, strength. It is thus particularly important in the wall of the eye. In the cornea, however, there is a problem. Tensile strength is very necessary, but equally, if not more, necessary is transparency. This presents an intriguing design problem. Before we look at Nature's solution, let us briefly consider the nature of collagen.

As might be expected in so ancient and ubiquitous a molecule, collagen comes in a large number of different varieties (at least nineteen). Fortunately (for students), they all have a number of essential features in common. They all consist of amino acid chains but with a remarkably small variety of different amino acids. Glycine takes up every third position in the chain and proline and hydroxyproline are also exceedingly common. This unimaginative constitution is forced on collagen by its secondary structure. The amino acid chains are twisted round each other to form a compact three-stranded 'rope', each strand is hydrogen bonded to the others, and such a structure is not possible if the amino acid sequence is not very closely specified. The outcome, however, is a three-stranded fibrous molecule, known as **tropocollagen**, which has a very high tensile strength. Tropocollagen was given its name from 'tropos' (meaning 'turning into'), for the collagen fibres found in connective tissues (including the cornea) are formed by the lining up of tropocollagen molecules, head-to-tail and side-to-side (quarter staggered) (Figure 16.11). The hydroxyl groups in some of the lysine and hydroxylysine residues are oxidized as this happens, allowing cross-links to be formed between adjacent tropocollagens. In this way a tough, inextensible, collagen fibre is formed. It has been found that the fibroblasts (= corneal corpuscles) synthesize

the tropocollagen molecules and extrude them into the matrix. It is only here that the assemblage into collagen fibres occurs (Figure 16.11).

In physiological conditions, each collagen fibre in the human cornea has a diameter of 31 nm and the spacing between individual fibres is 55 nm. The fibres are embedded in a matrix composed of proteoglycans and glycoproteins. They form beautifully regular, indeed quasi-crystalline, arrays which make up layers or **lamellae** from 1.5 to 2.5 µm thick. There are about 200 of these lamellae in the stroma. Each lamella consists of fibres running at a large angle to those in the lamella above and below (Figure 16.12A). In each

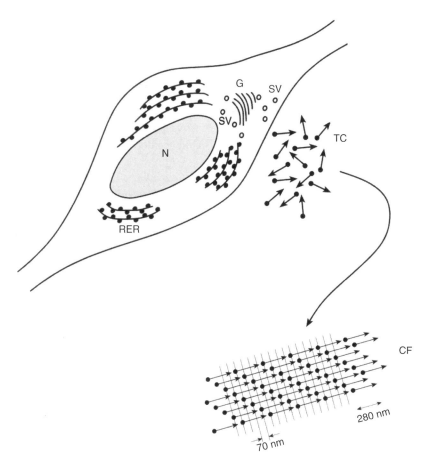

Figure 16.11 Formation of collagen fibres. Tropocollagen fibres are synthesized and wound into their triple stranded conformation in the endoplasmic reticulum and Golgi complex of a fibroblast (corneal corpuscle). They are secreted into the extracellular space where they are shown as linear structures with distinctive 'heads' (arrow head) and 'tails' (circle). In the extracellular space they line up head-to-tail and side-by-side (quarter staggered). As each tropocollagen molecule is about 280 nm in length this organization gives the collagen fibre a 70 nm banding, which can be detected in the electron microscope. These fibres then align themselves to form the higher order structure of the corneal stroma. CF = collagen fibre; G = Golgi complex; N = nucleus; RER = rough endoplasmic reticulum; SV = secretory vesicle; TC = tropocollagen.

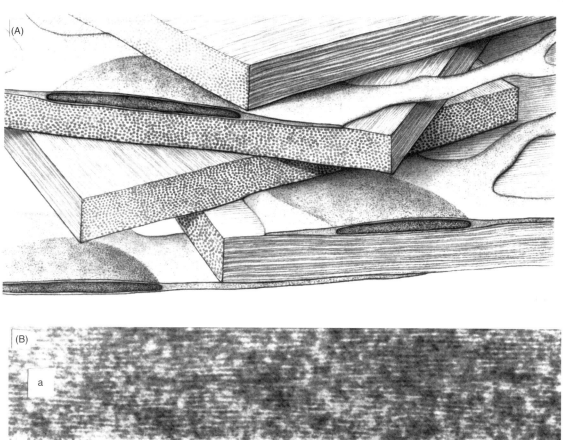

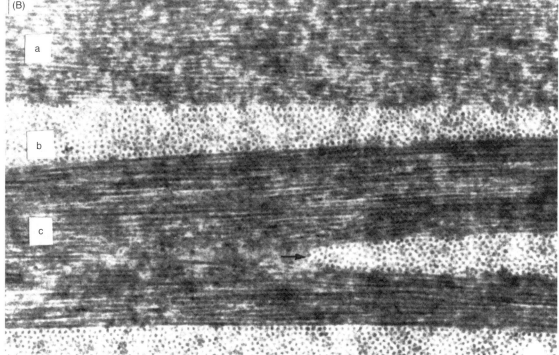

Figure 16.12 Collagen lamellae in cornea. (A) The orientation of collagen lamellae in the cornea. Three fibroblasts are shown between the lamellae. (B) Electronmicrograph (×28 000) of collagen fibres in the corneal stroma. Because of their orientation (see (a) above) the first collagen layer (a) is cut obliquely, the second (b) in transverse section and the third (c) longitudinally. The arrow indicates where the longitudinal lamella bifurcates into two. From Hogan, Alvarodo & Weddell (1971) *Histology of the Human Eye*, Fig 3.24A and Fig 3.26B. Copyright © 1971, Elsevier.

lamella the fibres run parallel to each other from limbus to limbus. This extraordinarily regular structure is essential to the transparency of the cornea. We shall see below that any disruption leads to corneal opacity.

Descemet's membrane bounds the inner surface of the collagen stroma. It is secreted by the endothelium (see below), and is thus a true basement membrane. It is some 10 μm thick and consists largely of collagen fibres.

The **endothelium** forms the inner surface of the cornea. It consists of flattened cells, some 5 μm high and 20 μm wide. Electron microscopy shows that they are filled with organelles – mitochondria, endoplasmic reticulum, golgi bodies and so on – indicative of a highly active metabolism. The cells do not replicate throughout life and are joined firmly together by tight junctions, preventing diffusion between them, and by gap junctions, which allow passage of materials laterally from cell to cell. Because the cells lack replicative ability, any extensive damage cannot be repaired and irreversible corneal oedema and, consequently, corneal opacity, results.

16.3.1.2 Innervation

The outer part of the stroma is richly innervated by branches of the ophthalmic division of the trigeminal nerve (cranial V). The cornea is consequently very sensitive although localization is poor.

16.3.1.3 Physiology

The essential objective of corneal physiology is to maintain transparency. This, as we have already seen, is crucially dependent on the regular organization of the collagen fibres. The collagen fibres, as again we have seen, are embedded in a matrix composed of proteoglycans, glycoproteins, inorganic salts and water. Of these constituents the **proteoglycans** are the most significant. They make up some 10% of the dry weight of the cornea. They consist of a so-called core protein (about 40 kDa) to which are attached one or more **glycosaminoglycan** (*GAG*) chains. There are a number of different GAGs but all are very bulky (up to 50 or 60 kDa), negatively charged polysaccharide chains composed of repeated disaccharide units. A common GAG, dermatan sulfate, is shown in Figure 16.13. One of the monosaccharides in

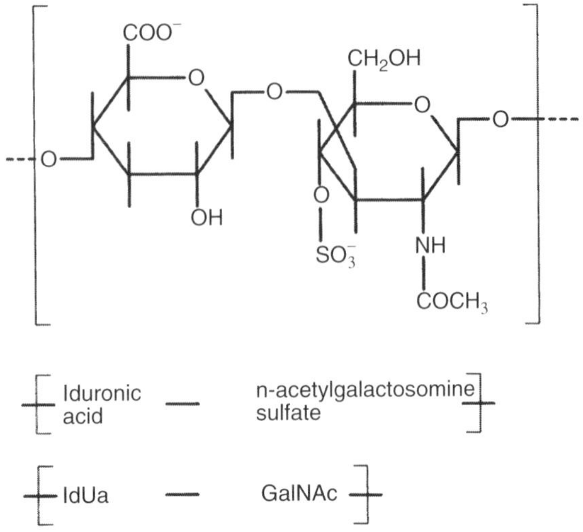

Figure 16.13 Repeat unit of dermatan sulfate (a glycosaminoglycan). The unit [IdUa-GalNAc] may be repeated up to a hundred times. Both the sulfate and the carboxylic acid groups bear negative charges.

each of the disaccharide repeats has an imino group attached.

There is more water (75–80%) in corneal stroma than in any other connective tissue. Yet it is avid for even more. This avidity is largely due to the cloud of negative charges on the GAG chains. This attracts the partial positive charges on the water molecule dipole (Figure 16.14; see also Figure 2.1 for water dipole structure). Hydration of GAG chains, however, increases their bulk and forces collagen fibres further apart from each other and out of alignment. Result: opacity.

Corneal metabolism is geared to prevent this happening. It can be shown first that osmosis can occur across both the corneal epithelium and the endothelium. If hypertonic solutions are applied to either surface, water leaves the cornea and it becomes thinner. Normally, both lacrimal fluid and the aqueous humour in the anterior chamber are isotonic with the corneal stroma, so these osmotic stresses do not happen. But this will not obviate the hygroscopic avidity of the GAGs. If both membranes are permeable to water, as the osmotic experiments show, water will be dragged into the stroma by clouds of positivity around the GAGs.

The answer, of course, is to pump out this unwanted water. The cornea thus has an active

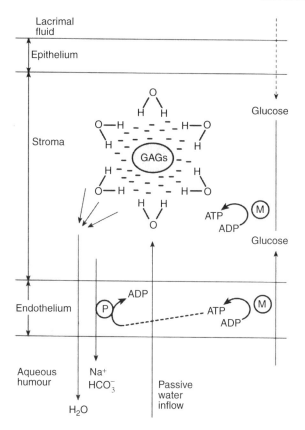

Figure 16.14 Schematic figure to show the biochemical mechanisms maintaining the state of hydration of the cornea. The glycosaminoglycans attract water molecules by their cloud of negative charge. Glucose enters, mostly via the endothelium, from the aqueous humour. A lesser flow of glucose enters via the epithelium from the tear film. The Krebs cycle enzymes and other forms of energy metabolism catabolize glucose and transfer the liberated energy into the energy-rich phosphate bonds of ATP. This energy store is, in turn, used for tissue maintenance and, most importantly, for energizing pumps which extrude HCO_3^- and Na^+ through the endothelium. Water follows passively along its osmotic gradient. GAGs = glycosaminoglycans; M = metabolism; P = pump. Further explanation in text.

glycolytic metabolism. Glucose is present in both the aqueous humour of the anterior chamber (see below) and in the lacrimal fluid (Table 16.1). Oxygen is also present in both the aqueous humour and the lacrimal fluid. The appropriate enzymes for the Krebs cycle, hexose monophosphate shunt and anaerobic glycolysis are all present. The majority of these enzymes are present in the endothelium which, as we noted above, shows all the ultrastructural signs of being a metabol-

ically highly active tissue. The energy derived from glucose breakdown is used to activate pumps that transport HCO_3^- and Na^+ across the endothelium from the stroma into the aqueous humour of the anterior chamber (Figure 16.14). Water molecules are carried along passively with the HCO_3^- and Na^+ ions. Hence, the endothelial pumps force any water pulled in by the avidity of the GAGs out again. The cornea is held in a state of dynamic equilibrium between the hygroscopic attraction of the GAGs and the pumping action of the endothelium. If oxygen supply falls or metabolic inhibitors are present and the pumps begin to fail, the GAG-induced inward flows of water will so disrupt the collagen organization that corneal opacity ensues.

16.3.2 Sclera

This consists of dense white connective tissue. Anteriorly it is continuous with the cornea and posteriorly it surrounds the optic disc and continues as the outer sheath of the optic nerve. In contrast with the regularity which is such a feature of the cornea, the collagen fibres in the cornea become quite irregularly arranged and vary markedly in diameter, one from another (Figure 16.15). In addition to collagen fibres, the sclera contains (like the cornea) proteoglycans but, unlike the cornea, it also contains a significant (about 2% dry weight) quantity of **elastin fibres**. A loose outer layer of the sclera, known as the **episclera**, contains blood vessels, which carry nutriment to the sclera and carry away wastes.

The principal function of the sclera is to provide a tough protective layer for the delicate retina within. It also helps to hold the eye in shape and may play a part in determining its axial length. If this is so, and there is some evidence from animal experimentation that it *is* so, defects may well contribute to the development of **myopia**.

16.3.3 Lens

The lens shares, with the cornea, the necessity of maximum transparency but it differs in also having, for the purposes of accommodation (focusing), to be highly flexible. We followed the development of the lens in Section 16.2 and we saw there that it came

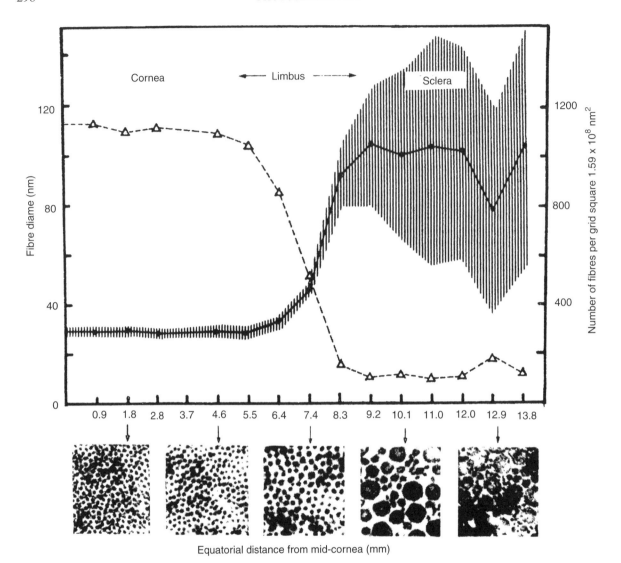

Figure 16.15 Variation in fibre diameter and number per unit area from mid-cornea to sclera. Triangles represent numbers; black dots represent mean diameter (nm). Scale is in mms from mid-cornea. Electronmicrographs (×33 000) show loss of regularity as distance from mid-cornea increases. From Harding, J.J. (ed.) (1997) *Biochemistry of the Eye*, with permission of Chapman and Hall.

to be composed of long (8–10 mm) thin ribbon-like cells, known as lens fibres. These cells are in fact hexagonal in cross section (Figure 16.16, see also Figure 16.6), seldom more than 8–12 µm across and 1–2 µm thick. As they develop, they lose their nuclei, mitochondria and all other intracellular organelles. They must survive throughout life (for they are not replaced) without benefit of protein synthesis or oxidative phosphorylation. The advantage gained is almost complete transparency. There are no organelles to scatter light. In the absence of a vascular supply, for this would impede transparency, nutritional support is provided by circulation of the aqueous fluid (Section 16.3.4).

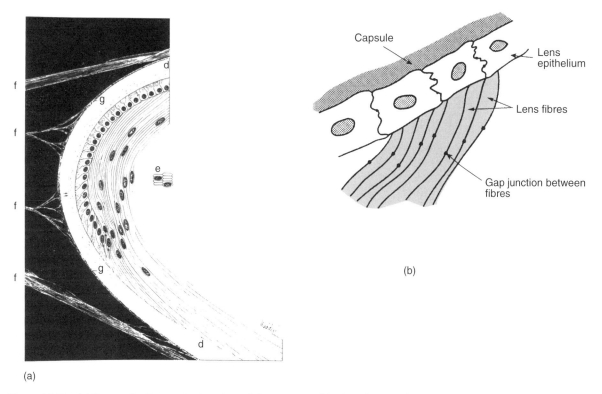

(a)

(b)

Figure 16.16   (a) Composite diagram to show the cellular structure of the lens, its capsule and its suspensory ligaments (zonules). d = lens capsule; e = lens fibres cut in transverse section; f = zonule fibre; g = pericapsular or zonular lamella (attachment of zonule fibres). From Hogan, Alvarodo & Weddell (1971) *Histology of the Human Eye*, Fig 4.1. Copyright © 1971, Elsevier. (b) Detail of attachment of lens fibres to anterior epithelium of the lens. The membranes of adjacent epithelial cells are highly irregular and bound together by tight junctions (dark spots) so that the tissue does not easily tear. The lens fibres are similarly bound together by gap junctions.

The lens fibres are held together by numerous **gap junctions** and there is very little intercellular space (Figure 16.16b). In addition to gap junctions, so-called 'thin junctions' also form between adjacent fibres. Whereas gap junctions allow the passage of ions, second messengers and small metabolites, thin junctions only allow the transfer of water molecules. The gap junctions also allow electrical coupling across the lens. Surrounding the entire lens is a tough capsule which, like Descement's membrane, is a basement membrane secreted by the epithelial cells and lens fibres. It varies in width, reaching 23 µm at the equator where the zonule fibres are inserted, and diminishing to 4 µm or less at the posterior pole. The anterior epithelial cells also vary in height, ranging from 5 to 8 µm in height at the anterior pole and increasing to 21 µm towards the equator, where they

begin to transform into the hugely elongated lens fibres. These variations are all in the cause of maintaining maximum transparency.

The transparency of the human lens is excellent. Most light with a wavelength between 450 and 700 nm is transmitted. Light with a wavelength above 720 nm is, however, not perceived. The human lens is almost colourless at birth but becomes yellowish with age. This seems to be a human phenomenon: it is not found in most laboratory or domestic mammals. The lens grows throughout life by the formation of new lens fibres that grow over and encase the older fibres. Careful inspection of the lens thus reveals an embryonic lens nucleus within a foetal nucleus, within an adult nucleus, which is itself enclosed in a cortex.

The lens owes its remarkable and long lasting resilience and transparency to the presence of soluble

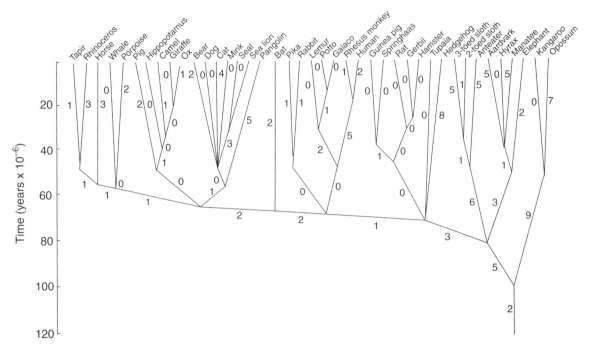

Figure 16.17 Phylogenetic tree of 41 mammalian αA crystallins. The numbers indicate nucleotide replacements for each branch. From de Jong, W.W. (1982) 'Eye lens proteins and vertebrate phylogeny' in Goldman, *Macromolecular Sequences in Systematic and Evolutionary Biology*, Copyright © 1982 Blackwell publishing.

proteins, the **crystallins**, within its fibres. The high concentration of these proteins in the fibres (90% of the dry weight of the lens) also creates the refractive index necessary to focus light on to the retina. The crystallins are classified into two major groups: alpha crystallins and beta/gamma crystallins.

Alpha crystallins are very large molecules, about 700 kDa, consisting of 35–40 subunits with M_r of about 20 kDa. There are two major types, αA and αB, derived by the duplication of an ancestral gene some 500 million years ago. The precise three-dimensional structure is still in dispute but all current models envisage the 20 kDa subunits grouped together to form a large globular structure some 16 nm in diameter. Such large molecules would be expected to scatter light; the fact that they do not and that the lens is as transparent as water implies that the α-crystallins are held in some form of short range quasi-crystalline order.

Finally, it is interesting to note that when the amino acid sequences of α-crystallins from many different animals were determined, the sequences showed only a slow change over geological time and, hence, have been useful in working out evolutionary relationships. A phylogenetic tree is shown in Figure 16.17. Pursuing this line of study, it turned out that the α-crystallins are related to the heat-shock proteins of *Drosophila*, the nematode *Caenorhabditis elegans* and several other animals. Heat shock proteins (hsps) are instances of so-called **molecular chaperons**. They are designed to prevent incorrect binding between the partially denatured proteins that accumulate in stressed cells. This has led to the recognition that the α-crystallins themselves act as molecular chaperones. It is not difficult to speculate that this chaperoning activity of the α-crystallins has, over evolutionary time, been made use of to prevent light-scattering protein aggregations growing in lens fibres.

The β- and γ-crystallins are smaller molecules than the α-crystallins. The β-crystallins are multimeric forms with M_rs ranging from 40 to 200 kDa whilst the γ-crystallins are monomers with M_r about 20 kDa. They are all related and form a large family of structural proteins. A number of other crystallins (δ, ε, ρ, τ, π and ξ) have been detected in nonmammalian vertebrates, and relatives have also been found in the lenses of belemnoid cephalopods.

Finally, we come to that other vitally important feature of the lens: accommodation. We shall see in the next section that the lens is held in position by zonule fibres originating in the ciliary body. It is not only held in position by these fibres but is also held under a certain degree of tension. This tension is opposed by the elasticity of the lens capsule. Hence, if the tension is reduced, the lens capsule tends to contract and the lens becomes more spherical. This is the essence of accommodation. By varying the tension on the zonule fibres, the lens can be made more or less convex. Eyes that are unable to focus distant objects are said to be **myopic** (short sighted) whilst those that are unable to focus near objects are defined as **hypermetropic** (long sighted). With age the lens capsule loses its elasticity. In consequence, its ability to focus near objects declines. On average the lens of a child of ten has a power of 14 D, which diminishes to 6 D at forty and 1 D at sixty (for definition of D (Dioptres) see the Introduction to Part Four).

A further type of focusing defect is **astigmatism**. In this case the optical system focuses a point not as a point but as a line. This is due to one (or both) of the refracting surfaces being cyclindrical in one dimension in addition to its overall spherical curvature. The surface responsible for this defect is almost always the cornea. Astigmatism, as with the optical deficiencies of the lens, can be corrected by a skilled optician.

We have noted that as the lens ages, its capsule becomes sclerosed and loses its elasticity. This does not only mean that its power declines but also that its ability to alter its focus diminishes. This loss of ability to focus is known as **presbyopia** (from L. **presbus**, old man + **ops**, eye). It is one of the misfortunes of life that we all tend to become presbyopic as we age. A final misfortune that often attacks the ageing eye is cataract.

Cataract is usually defined as an opacity of the lens leading to a reduction in vision. It is the major cause of blindness in both the developing and the developed world. In 1987 it was estimated that of the approximately 42 million blind people in the world about 40% suffer from cataract. Although cataract is mostly a disease of the elderly, increasing markedly after the age of fifty, it is found to a lesser extent in all age groups.

Cataract has many causes. These range from genetic (Box 16.1) through radiation (X-ray, UV, IR), to trauma (electric shock, cold), to nutritional (amino acids, trace elements), to causes secondary to uveitis and, most importantly, to diabetes. Surgical removal of the lens is at present (as it has been for the last 4000 years) the only treatment. This is nowadays followed by an intraocular implant. Fortunately, this is usually highly successful. Unfortunately, it requires skilled surgery and the waiting lists in the less developed parts of the world are sometimes endless.

Lens opacity is due (as in the case of the cornea) to the breakdown of its precise histological structure. The transparency of the lens depends on the regular alignment of the lens fibres and of the crystallins within them. Once this regularity is disrupted by, for example, aggregation of the crytallins into globular units or by the appearance of vacuoles, incoming light will be scattered and the lens becomes opaque. Disruption of the crystallins may be due to any and all of the insults mentioned in the previous paragraph and when this happens 'phase separation' often ensues. This means that the crystallins aggregate in one part of the lens fibre leaving other parts empty.

One of the commonest causes of cataract is, as noted above, as a side effect of **diabetes**. In this case it can be shown that increased quantities of galactose in the plasma diffuse, via the aqueous humour, into the lens. This triggers aldose reductase, which converts galactose into dulcitol. Dulcitol cannot diffuse out through the lens fibre membranes. The interior of the lens fibres thus increase in osmolarity and water moves into them down its osmotic gradient. This, in turn, causes swelling and disruption of the regular histological and molecular structure. Opacity ensues.

So far no similarly clear aetiology has been discovered for **age-related** cataract. It is likely to be a multifactorial condition. The many insults accumulated over a lengthy life eventually trigger the disease. There is probably also a genetic predisposition in some individuals. The great increase in our understanding of molecular genetics in recent years has allowed significant progress to be made in understanding this predisposition (Box 16.1). It appears that mutations in the genes coding for β- and γ-crystallins may be responsible for some of these hereditary cataracts.

BOX 16.1   GENETICS OF CATARACT

In Europe and the United States of America, inherited cataract has an incidence of about 1 in 10 000 (nongenetic cataract has, of course, a much higher incidence, especially amongst the elderly). The rapid advance of molecular genetics in recent years has uncovered a large number of genes (perhaps as many as 40) whose malfunction lead to this condition. The guilty genes either program the construction of the connexin subunits which form gap junctions between lens fibres or program the synthesis of the crystallins with which the fibres are packed.

Connexin Genes. The gap junctions (or connexons) between lens fibres consist of cylinders of six connexin subunits. The connexin subunits are large proteins (25–28 kDa) and each has four membrane spanning segments. The six connexin subunits that form the connexon are grouped around a hydrophilic pore which consequently penetrates the membrane. Two connexons, one in each adjacent lens fibre membrane, align themselves so that a continuous passage forms between the two fibres. Through this passage ions and small molecules pass and thus provide metabolic coupling between adjacent fibres. Two genes responsible for programming the connexin subunits have been implicated in cataract. The first, located on chromosome 1, programs the synthesis of **connexin 50** and the second, located on chromosome 13, encodes **connexin 46**. A transition at nucleotide 262 in the gene on chromosome 1 leads to C being replaced by T. This, in turn, leads to Proline being replaced by Serine at position 88 in connexin 50 ($pro_{88} \rightarrow ser$ or, to use the shorthand of molecular biology, P88S). The gene on chromosome 13 undergoes an A to G transition at nucleotide 188, which leads to the substitution of Serine for Asparagine at position 63 in connexin 46 ($asp_{63} \rightarrow ser$ or N63S). Another mutation in the latter gene, at nucleotide 1137, leads to a frame shift mutation after position 379 in the connexin protein and a consequent mistranslation of the C-terminal 56 amino acids. All three of these abnormal connexins upset the coherence of the lens fibre physiology and lead to the patchy, dust-like, lens opacities known as **pulverulent cataract**.

Crystallin Genes. Crystallins are encoded by genes located on chromosome 21 (α-crystallin), chromosome 22 (β-crystallin) and chromosome 2 (γ-crystallin). Mutations in all three of these genes have been identified. Mutation of the gene on chromosome 21 leads to substitution of Cys 116 by Arg ($cys_{116} \rightarrow arg$ or C116R) in α-crystallin. A mutation on chromosome 22 results in a stop codon appearing at position 155 and this results in the loss of 55 C-terminal amino acids from β-crystallin. Finally, a mutation in the promoter region of one of the six γ-crystallin genes leads to a 30% overproduction of a γ-crystallin fragment. All of these malfunctions result in abnormal crystallins in the lens fibres and thus to one or another form of cataract.

Galactose Metabolism Genes. As mentioned in the text galactosemic cataracts (usually associated with diabetes) are some of the most common. In addition to increased galactose due to diabetes, some cataracts are due to deficiencies in the enzymes responsible for galactose metabolism. When these deficiencies exist, galactose accumulates in the lens fibres with the result mentioned in the text. A variant of galactokinase, with a substitution of valine for alanine at position 198 in the amino acid chain (A198V), has been shown to be responsible for about 7% of Japanese and lower percentages of Korean and Chinese cataracts. Interestingly, this mutation appears to be confined to the Orient, suggesting that genetic contributions to cataract differ in different ethnic groups. Mutations in the aldose reductase gene have also been shown to increase susceptibility to cataract in Chinese type 2 diabetic patients.

The experimental study of cataract has been greatly helped by the development of a mouse 'model'. Almost 100 cataract mutants have been genetically engineered in this model. This has greatly helped in the task of understanding the genetic basis of the human pathology. It is satisfactory to note

(Continues)

(*Continued*)

that extensive regions of similarity (synteny) exist between the mouse and human genomes, so that mutations found in the mouse can provide strong clues as to where they might also be found in humans. Furthermore, with the exception of sugar-induced cataracts, the types of cataract displayed in mouse lenses are in many cases quite similar to those found in our own. The resistance of mice to sugar-induced cataracts is due to a very weak aldose reductase activity in the lenses of their eyes. However, mice engineered to express adequate quantities of aldose reductase readily develop cataracts. Mice, therefore, present very useful model organisms to study all aspects of human cataract.

REFERENCES

Francis, P.I. *et al.* (1999) Lens biology: development and human cataractogensis. *Trends in Genetics*, **15**, 191–6.
Hejtmancik, J.F. (1998) The genetics of cataract: our vision becomes clearer. *American Journal of Human Genetics*, **62**, 520–25.
Hejtmancik, J.F. and Kantorow, M. (2004) Molecular genetics of age-related cataract. *Experimental Eye Research*, **79**, 3–9.

But how do these changes in crystallin structure (and that of other lens proteins) lead to lens opacity? There are a number of possible biochemical mechanisms but the most important is probably oxidation. The mutated protein may not fold into its correct conformation and, consequently, leaves exposed sulfhydryl (SH) groups; or it may be that, unmutated protein, having to persist for a long period in the metabolically inactive lens fibre, begins to denature, which also exposes SH groups. In the presence of oxygen, neighbouring SH groups cross-link to form disulfide bonds, hence creating insoluble masses of protein (Figure 16.18). The exposed SH groups may also react with glutathione. Table 16.2 shows that this tripeptide is present in large quantities in the lens. Forming disulfide links with glutathione once again produces unnatural proteins, which can mass together and ultimately form opacities.

16.3.4 Uveal Tract

This consists, as we saw in Section 16.1, of the choroid, ciliary body and iris. The choroid lies between the sclera and the retina and is a highly vascular pigmented tissue. Anterior to the ora serrata, the uveal tract is covered with a double layer of ectoderm. This, as we saw above, is a non-neural continuation of the retina and pigment epithelium. In the ciliary body, as we shall see, this ectodermal layer is concerned with the production of aqueous humour. It continues forward to form the (usually) pigmented posterior surface of the iris. It also develops (most unusually for ectoderm) the sphincter and dilator muscles of the iris.

16.3.4.1 Choroid

This ranges from about 0.22 mm thick posteriorly to 0.1 mm thick anteriorly. There are four main layers (Figure 16.19):

1. **Suprachoroid (= lamina fusca)**. This consists of loose connective tissue containing many melanocytes (brown pigmentation) and a rich nerve supply.
2. **Stroma**. Once again this consists of loose connective tissue but it is far more richly vascularized than the suprachoroid. It is supplied by 15–20 short posterior ciliary arteries and the long posterior ciliary artery. It is drained by the four vortex veins into the inferior orbital vein.
3. **Choriocapillaris**. All the capillaries of the choroidal vessels are arranged in a single closely packed layer separated from the retinal pigment epithelium only by Bruch's membrane (= lamina vitrea). Whereas most of the body's capillaries are

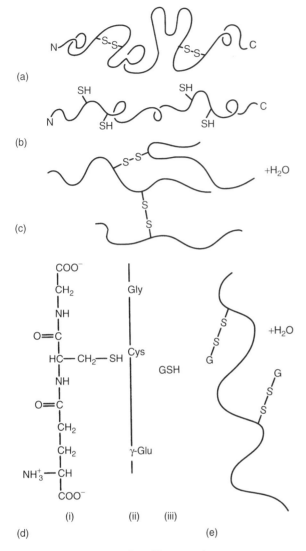

(a)

(b)

(c)

(d)

(i)   (ii)   (iii)

(e)

Figure 16.18 Denaturation of lens proteins causes cataract. (a) Native protein with three-dimensional conformation held in place by disulfide linkages. (b) Unfolded protein exposing sulfhydryl (-SH) groups (c) In presence of oxygen SH groups react together to form insoluble masses of protein. (d) Glutathione (i) molecular formula; (ii) amino acid constitution; (iii) abbreviation. (e) Reaction of GSH with exposed SH groups of denatured protein. Further explanation in text.

Table 16.2 Composition of lens

	Aqueous humour	Lens
Electrolytes (mEq/l)		
Na^+	142.0	20
K^+	4.0	125
Cl^-	131.0	18
Ca^{2+}	1.7	0.4
Organics (μmol/g)		
Glucose	3.3	1.0
Lactic acid	4.5	14.0
Glutathione	2.0	12.0
Ascorbic acid	1.1	0.6
Inositol	0.1	5.9
Amino acids	5.0	25.0
Protein	0.04%	33%

rior of the orbit to 1–2 µm anteriorly. It consists of (i) basement membranes of the capillaries of the choriocapillaris, (ii) an inner collagenous layer, (iii) an elastic layer, (iv) an outer collagenous layer and, finally, (v) the basement membranes of the retinal pigment cells. There is evidence that imbalances in the turnover of structural proteins in Bruch's membrane leads to one form of macular degeneration – Sorsby's fundus dystrophy (SFD) (Box 17.2).

The function of the choroid is to provide vascular support to the pigment epithelium and retina. The capillaries of the choriocapillaris and Bruch's membrane are permeable to large organic molecules. Both ferritin (500 kDa) and fluorescein (40 kDa) have been shown to pass from the choroid into the pigment epithelium. In physiological conditions it would, therefore, allow the passage of plasma proteins.

16.3.4.2 Ciliary Body

This part of the uveal tract reminded the ancients of eye lashes, hence they named it from 'cilium' meaning a hair. Figure 16.20 shows that it consists of two major parts, the **pars plana** (also known as the **obicularis ciliaris**) and the **pars plicata** (or **corona ciliaris**). The figure also shows that whilst the pars plana is smooth and contains the ciliary muscle the pars plicata is thrown out into about eighty **ciliary processes**.

8–10 µm in diameter, these are much wider, ranging from 18 to 50 µm.

4. **Bruch's membrane (= lamina vitrea).** A thin translucent membrane (hence the term 'lamina vitrea') varying from 2 to 4 µm wide in the poste-

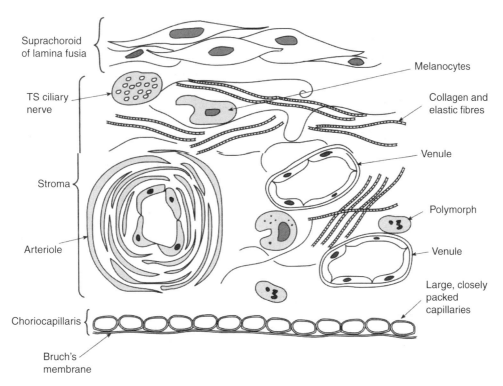

Figure 16.19 Transverse section of choroid. Explanation in text.

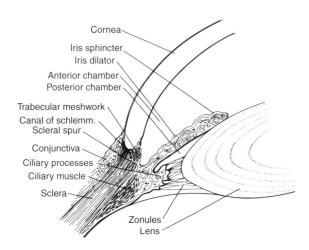

Figure 16.20 Ciliary body. The position of the ciliary body with respect to the lens, cornea and sclera is shown. It can also be seen that it is composed of two major parts, the pars plana containing the ciliary muscle and the pars plicata thrown out into ciliary processes, which are involved in the secretion of aqueous humour. From Harding (1997). Reproduced by permission of Chapman and Hall.

In addition some eighty of so **zonules** (or **suspensory ligaments**) connect the pars plicata to the lens. It can be seen why the anatomists of antiquity thought they had found a second set of eyelashes!

The ciliary body plays two vitally important roles in the physiology of the eye. The ciliary processes secrete aqueous humour and the ciliary muscle, via the zonules, is responsible for focusing the lens. Let us consider each in turn.

Ciliary Processes and the Production and Absorption of Aqueous Humour: This is continuous throughout life. Aqueous humour is secreted into the posterior chamber, just behind the iris, around which it circulates to the anterior chamber where most (75–95%) is absorbed at the **filtration angle** (Figure 16.21). A smaller quantity is absorbed via the **uveo-scleral** pathway. This pathway runs between the ciliary muscle bundles (Figure 16.24). The rates of production and absorption thus determine the pressure of aqueous fluid in the eye, known as the **intraocular pressure** (**IOP**). The circulation of aqueous fluid

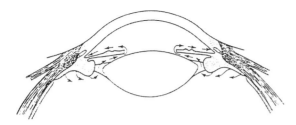

Figure 16.21 Circulation of the aqueous fluid. The fluid is secreted from the ciliary processes and flows through the posterior chamber between the iris and the lens and then through the pupil to be absorbed at the filtration angle eventually into the canal of Schlemm. From Cole, 1984.

supplies essential nutritional support for the lens. But it is a delicate process which can go awry. The IOP is an important parameter. Studies have shown that in healthy eyes it ranges between 10.5 and 20.5 mm Hg; if it should rise much above its maximum value the pressure on the vitreous humour in the posterior chamber also rises. This in turn increases the pressure on the delicate retina and optic nerve head which may sustain damage. Abnormally increased IOP is known as **glaucoma**. It can lead to blindness .

The aqueous humour is secreted at about $2.75 \pm 0.63 \, \mu l/min$. Its composition is shown in Table 16.3. It can be seen that it is very similar to blood plasma. It is derived from the very heavily vascularized stroma of the ciliary body. The capillaries in the stroma are of two types: 'continuous' and 'fenestrated'. The endothelial cells making up the walls of the 'continuous' capillaries are some $0.2–0.3 \, \mu m$ thick, whilst

Table 16.3 Composition of aqueous fluid

	Plasma	Aqueous
Electrolytes (mM)		
Na^+	137.5	142.0
K^+	4.3	4.0
Cl^-	108.5	131.0
Ca^{2+}	2.3	1.2
HCO_3^-	27.0	20.0
Organics (mM)		
Glucose	6.0	3.3
Glutathione	4.0	2.0
Lactate	0.65	4.5

Data from Abdel-Latif, 1997.

the walls of the fenestrated capillaries are unique in having circular areas (60–80 nm in diameter) that are only some $0.05–0.1 \, \mu m$ across. The walls of the endothelial cells are attached to each other by tight junctions. There is thus little possibility of material diffusing out into the stroma between the cells. Instead, electron microscopy reveals continuous lines of pinocytotic vesicles transversing the endothelial cells, especially in the fenestrated regions. Pinocytosis allows the passage of proteins and other macromolecules; hence it appears that the first stage in the formation of aqueous humour is the formation of a protein-rich intercellular fluid.

The capillaries in the stroma are, as Figure 16.22 shows, in very close contact with the pigmented cells of the outer epithelial layer of the ciliary processes. The basement membranes of the pigmented cells are extensively folded so that the surface area in contact with the stroma is large. Their cytosol contains sparse endoplasmic reticulum, mitochondria and plentiful melanosomes. There are no tight junctions between these cells, although there are numerous gap junctions. It is thus fully possible for the ultrafiltrate from the stromal blood vessels to percolate between them. But, in addition, there are a number of ion pumps in the membranes adjacent to the stroma so that an active uptake from the stromal ultrafiltrate can occur. The pigmented cells make large numbers of gap junctions with the nonpigmented cells. It is likely that metabolites and ions absorbed from the stroma are passed on to the latter cells.

The nonpigmented cells, in contrast to the pigmented cells, are welded together with numerous tight junctions and their surface membranes are thrown into a number of complex interdigitations. This prevents the protein-rich ultrafiltrate penetrating between them. These inner cells show, moreover, a richly developed ultrastructure of endoplasmic reticulum, mitochondria and so on. It can be shown that the Krebs tricarboxylic acid cycle is actively at work generating much ATP. It can also be shown that metabolic inhibitors which either uncouple the Krebs cycle from oxidative phosphorylation (for example dinitrophenol) and/or inhibitors, like fluoroacetate, which interfere with the cycle itself, reduce the quantity of aqueous fluid produced by 70–80%. Hence, there is good evidence that the final stage in the production of aqueous humour involves the passage of the ultrafiltrate into the nonpigmented

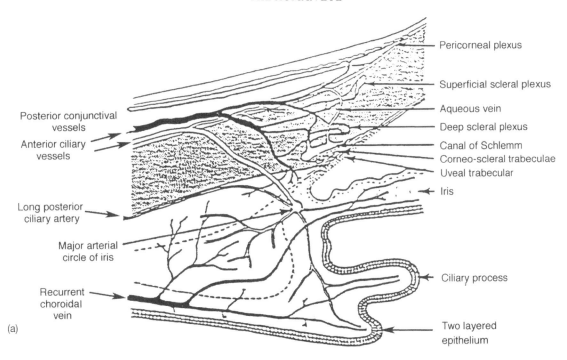

Pericorneal plexus

Superficial scleral plexus

Aqueous vein

Deep scleral plexus

Canal of Schlemm

Corneo-scleral trabeculae

Uveal trabecular

Iris

Posterior conjunctival vessels

Anterior ciliary vessels

Long posterior ciliary artery

Major arterial circle of iris

Recurrent choroidal vein

Ciliary process

Two layered epithelium

(a)

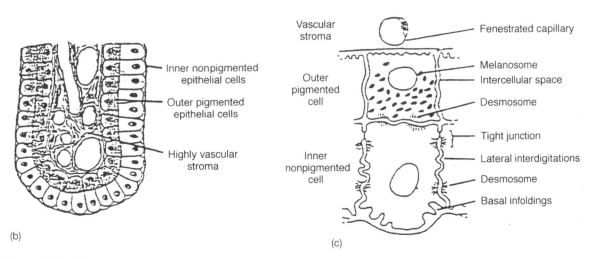

Inner nonpigmented epithelial cells

Outer pigmented epithelial cells

Highly vascular stroma

(b)

Vascular stroma

Outer pigmented cell

Inner nonpigmented cell

Fenestrated capillary

Melanosome

Intercellular space

Desmosome

Tight junction

Lateral interdigitations

Desmosome

Basal infoldings

(c)

Figure 16.22 Ciliary processes, ciliary epithelium and the secretion of aqueous humour. (a) Diagram to show the position of the ciliary processes, the filtration angle just above the iris and the intricate vascularization. (b) Diagram of part of a single ciliary process as seen by high power optical microscopy. (c) Diagram of the ciliary epithelium as shown by electron microscopy.

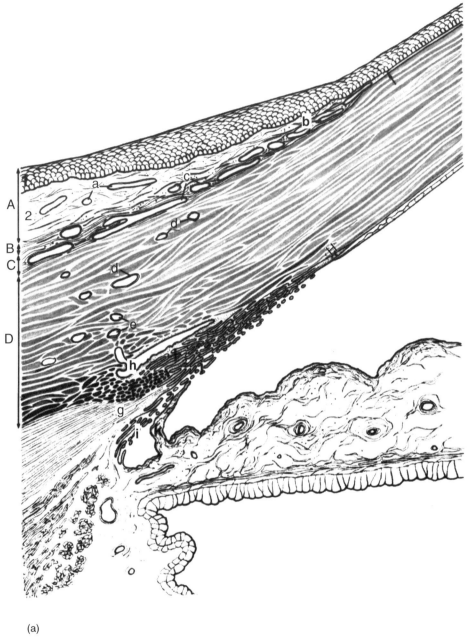

(a)

Figure 16.23 Histology of the filtration angle. (a) The delicate histology of the filtration angle is well shown in this micrograph. The limboscleral and corneo-limbal junctions (the commencement of Bowman's layer and the commencement of Descemet's membrane) are marked by arrows. A = limbal conjunctiva consisting of both (1) stratified epithelium and (2) loose aeolar connective tissue. B = Tenon's capsule. C = episclera. D = limbal stroma, continuous with the stroma of the cornea. a, b, c, d, e = blood vessels. f = scleral spur. g = ciliary muscle. h = Schlemm's canal. i = trabecular network. j = uveal trabeculae; k = process of iris which may join with the trabecular meshwork. From Hogan, Alvarodo and Weddell, 1971. (b) Diagram to show detail of the histology of the filtration angle to show the flow of aqueous fluid into Schlemm's canal. Further explanation in text.

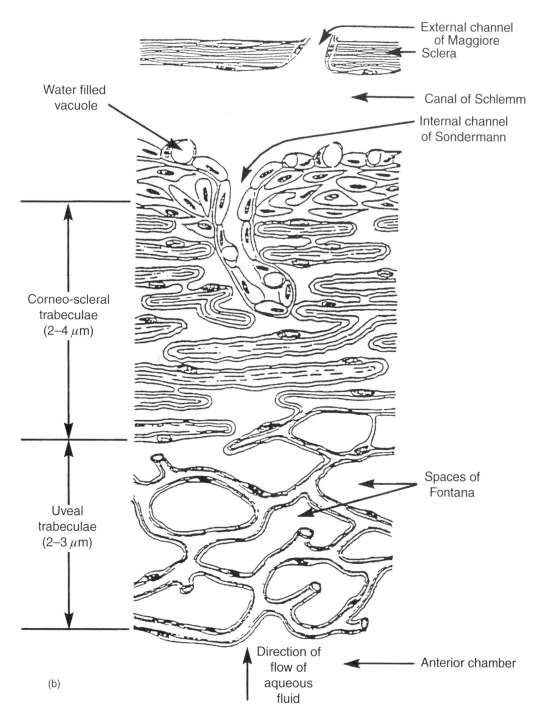

External channel
of Maggiore
Sclera

Canal of Schlemm

Internal channel
of Sondermann

Water filled
vacuole

Corneo-scleral
trabeculae
(2–4 μm)

Uveal
trabeculae
(2–3 μm)

Spaces of
Fontana

Direction of
flow of
aqueous
fluid

Anterior chamber

(b)

Figure 16.23 (*Continued*)

cells and the active pumping of the final solution across the boundary membrane into the posterior chamber.

We have already noted that an extraordinarily large number of gap junctions are made between the pigmented and nonpigmented cells. This suggests that the two layers of cells are coupled together both metabolically and electrically. Indeed, an electrical potential of some 10 mV (negative in the stroma) exists across the bilayer. This implies the transport of positively charged ions, probably Na^+. In support of this conclusion it can be shown that the glycoside **ouabain** reduces the production of aqueous fluid, the electrical potential and the quantity of Na^+ in the posterior chamber. Ouabain is a well known inhibitor of the $Na^+ + K^+$ pump. Vice versa, the hormone **aldosterone** which increases Na^+ transport, increases the IOP (aldosterone inhibitors, for example sprionolactone, which reduce Na^+ transport, reduce IOP). It seems, therefore, that the production of aqueous humour depends crucially on the active pumping of Na^+ (and also HCO_3^-), both of which carry water molecules along with them into the posterior chamber. In addition to this active transport there is also a passive flow through the bilayer of cells.

The aqueous humour is secreted from the ciliary processes behind the iris but in front of the jelly-like vitreous humour. It flows around the iris into the anterior chamber and is absorbed at the so-called 'filtration angle'. This is the angle which the cornea makes with the iris. Because the bulge of the cornea tends to flatten out at the limbus, the angle might be better termed an 'inlet' (Figure 16.23a). The histology is complex. Figure 16.23b shows that the aqueous fluid percolates first through **uveal trabeculae** and then into **corneo-scleral trabeculae**. Ultimately it finds its way via the **channels of Sondermann** into **Schlemm's canal**. Electron microscopy of the walls of the latter two ducts shows giant vacuoles containing fluid. These eventually burst into the lumens of the ducts. The aqueous fluid in the canal of Schlemm, which circles the limbus of the cornea, makes its way via the **external channels of Maggiore** to aqueous veins and from these to episcleral venous vessels, which ultimately discharge into the anterior ciliary veins and back into the venous system.

Between 5% and 25% of aqueous fluid is drained by a second route: the **uveo-scleral** or **accessory** route (Figure 16.24). In this pathway the fluid is absorbed between the muscle fibre bundles of the ciliary muscle into the suprachoroid and then into the veins of the sclera. The amount of drainage by this route depends on the state of contraction of the ciliary muscles. When the muscles are relaxed, up to 25% takes this route; when they are contracted, the muscle fibres squeeze the connective tissue channels and only about 5% escapes along this pathway.

The intraocular pressure (IOP) is clearly due to the balance between aqueous production and absorption. There is a diurnal variation, the IOP being highest in the morning and lowest in the evening. Abnormally high IOP (glaucoma) is usually due to defective absorption at the filtration angle. This is known as **'open angle' glaucoma** and is the most common form of the condition. It has been computed to affect some 33 million individuals worldwide. It develops slowly over time and may be due to a number of factors: either increased aqueous production by the ciliary processes or decreased absorbtion at the filtration angle. There is some hereditary component and accumulating evidence indicates that mutation of a gene, known as *optineurin* (**OPTN**), located on chromosome 10 (10p14), which encodes a protein, optineurin, expressed in the trabecular network (amongst other places), is causative in these cases. **Closed angle glaucoma**, where the filtration angle is narrowed, is a rarer condition; it usually affects just one eye and is characterized by a sudden and painful increase in IOP.

Ciliary Muscle and Lens Accommodation: The bulk of the ciliary body is composed of a mass of smooth muscle fibres, most of which take their origin from a projection of the sclera into the choroid known as the **scleral spur** (Figure 16.24). The muscle fibres run in three major directions: meridional, radial and circular. All these fibres working together pull the ciliary body upwards and, the circular fibres in particular, narrow the diameter of the ring formed by the ciliary body (Figure 16.25). This relaxes the tension on the zonule fibres, and the lens (providing the capsule retains its elasticity) becomes more spherical. Innervation is by parasympathetic fibres running in the oculomotor nerve (cranial III).

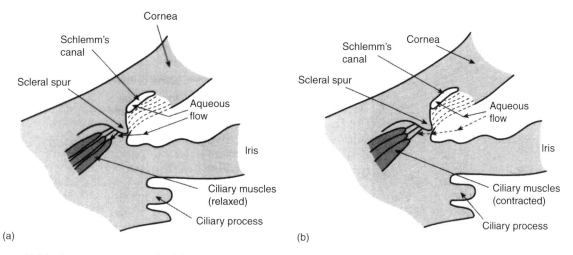

Figure 16.24   Accessory or uveo-scleral drainage route. (a): Ciliary muscles relaxed. Aqueous fluid makes its way between them into the episcleral veins. (b): Ciliary muscles contracted. Space between their fibres occluded. Scleral spur drawn back widens the spaces between the trabeculae, thus allowing an easier route for aqueous fluid into Schlemm's canal.

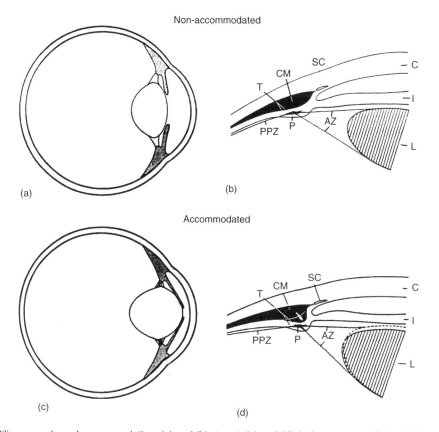

Figure 16.25   Ciliary muscle and accommodation. (a) and (b) at rest; (c) and (d) during accommodation. During accommodation the ciliary body moves in the direction of the white arrow and tension on the zonule fibres is relaxed. Because of the elasticity of its capsule the lens becomes more spherical (broken line). AZ = zonule fibres; C = cornea; CM = ciliary muscle; I = iris; L = lens; P = zonular plexus; SC = Schlemm's canal; T = tension fibre system. Modified from Hart, 1992.

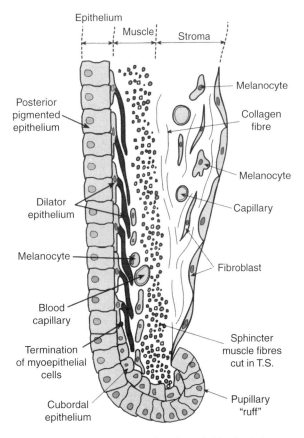

Figure 16.26 Transverse section through iris. Posterior epithelium faces the lens. Further explanation in text.

16.3.5 Iris

This is the most anterior part of the uveal tract. At its root in the ciliary body it is about 0.5 mm thick and it becomes slightly thicker (0.6 mm) at its tip. It can be treated as having five layers (Figure 16.26), although these are far from being sharply demarcated from each other. Outermost is the anterior border layer consisting of fibroblasts, collagen and melanocytes. Within this is the stroma, which is continuous and rather similar to the stroma of the ciliary body and choroids, though with far fewer blood vessels than the latter. Beneath this there is a thick layer of smooth muscle fibres. These fibres run around the iris to form a circular **sphincter muscle**. Very unusually these muscle fibres develop not from mesoderm but (as we noted above) from ectoderm. They are innervated by parasympathetic fibres from the oculomotor nerve

(cranial III) and have a dominant role in controlling the aperture of the iris. Next, continuous with the pigment epithelium of the retina and ciliary body, is a single layer of myoepithelial cells whose contractile regions together constitute the **dilator muscle**. Each cell consists of an apical epithelial portion and a basal muscular tail that extends into the stroma. These tails are innervated by sympathetic fibres. Finally, next to the lens, is the posterior pigmented epithelium, a layer of epithelial cells some 36–55 μm in height and 16–25 μm across, densely packed with melanin granules.

The sphincter and dilator muscles work together to vary the size of the pupil. The amount of light entering the eye is directly proportional to the area of the pupil. Hence, variation in pupil size is of great significance in controlling the quantity of light reaching the retina under different ambient illumination. Variation in pupil size also affects depth of focus. This is not important for distant objects but for near objects it becomes significant: the smaller the pupil size the more precise is the focus (Figure 16.27). Finally, the size of the pupil is important in limiting optical defects in the lens. In dim illumination optical perfection is not important: visual detail is anyway imperceptible. In daytime conditions, however, a constricted pupil ensures that only a small and optically optimal part of the lens is employed.

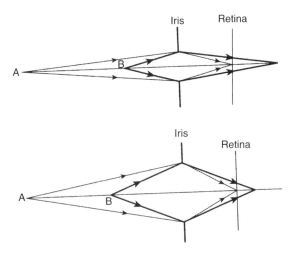

Figure 16.27 The size of the pupil affects depth of focus. The depth of focus (AB) is smaller with a large pupil (below) than with a small pupil (above). From Davson, 1963.

16.3.6 Vitreous Humour

The glassy vitreous humour is a jelly-like material occupying the posterior chamber of the eye. It consists of collagen fibres, hyaluronan, a few soluble proteins, especially glycoproteins, a few cells known as hyalocytes and 99% water. Hyaluronan is a very lengthy and massive molecule (M_r 3000 kDa in newborn calf; 500 kDa in adult cattle). Hyaluronan molecules form a network in the vitreous humour that binds water to form a 'jelly'. The whole is held in position by the collagen fibres passing into the basement membrane of Müller cells and into the inner limiting membrane of the retina. These bindings are strongest at the pars plana of the ciliary body and around the optic disc. The hyalocytes are confined to the cortex of the vitreous body and, again, are most numerous in the vicinity of the pars plana and the optic disc. This has led some to speculate that they are involved in the secretion of the hyaluronan acid. However, it is more likely that it is the pars plana itself which is involved in this process, whilst the hyalocytes play a scavenging role as macrophages. The vitreous humour, as we have already noted, is of great importance in holding the retina in place against the suprachoroid and may also provide some nutritional support for the neural layers against which it presses.

Degenerative changes of the vitreous humour are one of the major causes of retinal detachment. The vitreous humour is, however, seldom completely clear. Small mounts of debris left over from the eye's complex development often remain and are seen as 'floaters'. These tend to increase in number with age but are seldom very troublesome. With age, too, the vitreous tends to pull away from the retina and this may be seen as sudden flashing lights and be followed by an increase in floaters. However, if the flashing persists and becomes continuous and if there is an obscuration of vision, as if a grey curtain were being pulled across the eye, medical treatment should be urgently sought. These symptoms could indicate a tear in the retina or, at worst, a detachment of the retina from the underlying pigment epithelium and choroid.

16.4 MOVEMENTS OF THE EYEBALL

A great deal is known about the nervous mechanisms controlling the movement of the eyeball. This chapter is, however, already overlong and to provide a detailed account of the oculomotor system would take us too far into neurology and too far away from the biology of sensory systems. However, we cannot close without a brief description of the movements of the eyeball.

We have already noted the effectors which bring about this movement, the six extrinsic or extraocular muscles, and their innervation in Section 16.1 above. These muscles bring about five types of movement. Two of these movements stabilize the eyes when the head moves, whilst the other three fix the fovea on a visual target. Let us briefly consider each of these in turn.

The first of the stabilising movements is brought about by the **vestibulo-oculomotor reflex**. When the head begins to move in any direction (acceleration), the semicircular canals of the inner ear are stimulated (Chapter 9). The oculomotor system responds by causing the eyes to move with an equal velocity in the opposite direction. We looked at this reflex in Chapter 10 (Section 10.1) and saw that the characteristic ocular movements are defined as nystagmus. The influence of the semicircular canals is simple to demonstrate for oneself. If the fingers of the outstretched hand are waved rapidly in front of the eyes they blur into indistinctness. If, however, instead of waving the hand, the head is shaken from side to side with equal rapidity the fingers remain perfectly distinct. The influence of the pathway from the semicircular canals is plain. The second of these stabilizing reflexes is the **optokinetic reflex**. This reflex is actuated through the visual system itself. When the head rotates the stable features of the environment flow past the eyes in one direction or another. The optokinetic reflex causes the eyes to fixate on one of these stable features and hold it as long a possible and then flick back to pick up another and hold that as long as possible and so on. Unlike the vesitbulo-ocular reflex, the optokinetic reflex does not, for obvious reasons, operate in the dark.

There are three types of fixation movement. The first such movement, the **slow pursuit movement**, requires conscious attention. It keeps the fovea fixated on the object of interest as it, or the observer, moves. The movement of the eye can be quite rapid, up to $100°/s$. It is slowed by drugs, fatigue and alcohol. The second fixation movement is more rapid. It is known as a **saccade**. When an image moves away from the fovea, the eye remains stationary for about 200 ms and then flicks rapidly (about 900°/s) to bring it back on to the fovea once again. It may over or undershoot. If this is the case a microsaccade follows to centre the image on the fovea. One can look at these movements as a form of tuning. The oculomotor system restlessly gropes until maximum discharge from the fovea occurs.

Finally, there are **vergence** movements. In all the previous movements both eyes have moved in the same direction. These movements are consequently known as **conjugate**. In vergence movements this is not the case. As an object moves toward or away from the face the two eyes move in different directions. This is known as **disconjugate** movement. Vergence movements are driven by differences in the position of the image of an object on the two retinae, known as **retinal disparity**. Vergence movements are linked to lens accommodation. As an object varies in its distance from the face, the ciliary muscles controlling accommodation and the extrinsic eye muscles controlling vergence work in harmony, so that an image remains sharply focused on the foveae of both retinae.

Before finishing this section it is important to make reference to the important neurophysiological concept of '**efference copy**' or '**corollary discharge**'. Although saccadic movements are continuously occurring (see, also, Chapter 24), we do not perceive the world as trembling and flicking from one place to another. If, however, we jiggle the eye with a finger, the world jiggles too. How can this be explained? The conundrum was recognized by Helmholtz in the nineteenth century. He suggested that when the brain sends a signal to the extrinsic eye muscles to initiate a saccade, it also sends a copy to the visual areas of the brain. It is this which has subsequently been termed an 'efference copy' or a 'corollary discharge'. The brain can thus distinguish internally generated movements from those generated by the outside world (in our example, the finger) when no such copy is received. This notion of comparing a virtual world (the efference copy) with the real world is an important idea in neurophysiology and has been generalized, as we shall see, to other sensory systems.

16.5 CONCLUDING REMARKS

In this chapter we have reviewed the structure, development and functioning of the non-neural parts of the eye. Although, in Section 16.2, when referring to the back-to-front design of the retina, we saw the power of evolutionary over teleological explanations, we must nevertheless feel (with Charles Darwin) a sense of awe at the superb design of the eye, its fitness for purpose, from macroscopic anatomy down to submicroscopic molecular biology. We shall continue in this feeling of awe in the next chapter when we look in detail at the organization and operation of the retina.

17

THE RETINA

Retina in fact cerebral tissue. **Retinal pigment epithelium (RPE)**: outer wall of optic cup - cytology - ultrastructure - melanosomes - phagosomes - absorption of light - phagocytosis of outersegment membranes - re-isomerisation of retinal - control of flow of material into outer retina. **Retina**: duplex structure - foveation - histology - nine-layer 'vertical' structure - horizontal structure. **Rods and cones**: morphologies - numbers and distribution – light-capturing design - orientation of rhodopisn - photoisomerisation - transducins - cGMP-PDE - CNG Na^+-Ca^{2+} channels - dark current - light inhibits dark current - hyperpolarisation; transformation of cGMP to $5'$GMP causes CNG channel closure - recoverin disinhibited removal of Ca^{2+} - activates GC to synthesise cGMP - sensory adaptation - rhodopsin kinase and arrestin deactivate opsin - comparison between ciliary and rhabdomeric photoreceptors - details of photoisomerisation and retrieval of retinal; cones and cone opsins - evolutionary relationships. **Horizontal cells**: cytology - synaptology - biophysics. **Bipolar cells**: cytology - typology - synaptology - sign-inverting rod bipolars – sign-inverting and sign-conserving cone bipolars - biochemisty and biophysics - receptive fields (RFs) - wiring diagrams. **Müller cells** - ILM and OLM - function. **Interplexiform cells**: two types - efferent pathways. **Amacrine cells**: very diverse - synaptology. **Ganglion cells**: typology - action potentials - anatomical and physiological classification - number varies in different retinal regions - unmyelinated axons - concentric ON/OFF RFs - centre-surround antagonism - edge-detection. **Wiring diagrams**: cone and rod pathways - dark adaptation - inherent complexities - neurogenetics and the zebrafish retina. **Colour**: trichromaticity - opponent processes - RFs of ganglion cells - colour qualia sometimes called 'raw' feels are nevertheless in fact very thoroughly cooked. **Concluding remarks**: intricacy of the retina provides a foretaste of the intricacy of the brain.

In Chapter 16 we reviewed the non-neural parts of the human eye. These were all, in a sense, accessories. They were all concerned, had all evolved, in the service of the photosensory and neural tissue of the eye: the retina. It is to this that we turn in this chapter.

We saw in Section 16.2 that the retina originates as part of the brain. This is part of its fascination. It is a portion of the brain pushed to the exterior. It has long been the hope of students of the retina that an understanding of its structure and functioning will give us a lead into the structure and functioning of the brain itself. We noted also, in Section 16.3, that the outpushing from the brain consisted of two layers of cells, separated by a space, the optic ventricle, which soon disappears. The two layers were destined to form the pigment epithelium and the retina *sensu strictu*. In this chapter we shall, accordingly, start by considering the pigment epithelium and then move on to the retina, moving ever outwards towards the vitreous humour.

17.1 RETINAL PIGMENT EPITHELIUM (RPE)

We saw in Section 16.2 that the RPE is developed from the outer wall of the optic cup. The lumen of the optic ventricle disappears early in embryology and the RPE thereafter finds itself in very close association with the retina. Nevertheless, the RPE cells are more firmly attached to the choroid than they are to the retina. Indeed, the inner part (0.3 mm) of Bruch's membrane (Section 16.3.4) is secreted by the pigment epithelium as a basement membrane. Hence in cases of retinal detachment, the RPE is left attached to the choroid and the lumen of the optic ventricle reappears.

The adult eye possesses 4–6 million RPE cells. In transverse section they are hexagonal and are about 8 mm high and 16 mm in diameter. They are bound together by numerous tight junctions which prevent materials diffusing between the choroid and the retina via the intercellular space. Materials must enter or leave the retina through the RPE cytoplasm. To facilitate this, the bases of the RPE cells are thrown into complex folds and microvilli, which greatly increases the surface area. Their ultrastructure is also rich in endoplasmic reticulum and mitochondria, the latter being particularly numerous at the bases of the cells. The apical cell membrane is also evaginated into lengthy villi that envelope the rod and cone outersegments. Dark brown **melanosomes** are found in these microvilli and also in the apices of the cells. The cells also contain large inclusions known as **phagosomes** (Figure 17.1). These are composed of the ingested tips of rod and cone outersegments. Groups of between 30 and 40 discs are taken at a time. Each pigment cell is associated with some 30–45 photore-

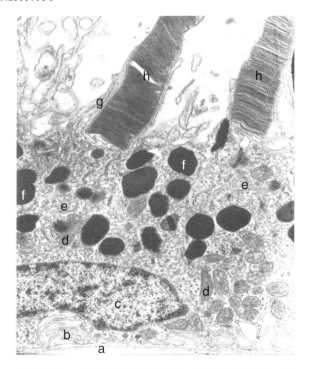

Figure 17.1 Electron micrograph (× 18 000) of retinal pigment epithelium. At the top of the micrograph, two rod cell outersegments (h) are shown encased in microvilli (g) extending from the RPE cell. a = basement membrane of pigment epithelium; b = infoldings of membrane of pigment epithelial cell, c = nucleus of RPE cell; d = mitochondrion; e = endoplasmic reticulum; f = pigment granule. From Hogan, Alvarado & Weddell (1971) *Histology of the Human Eye*, Fig 9.23. Copyright © 1971, Elsevier.

ceptor outersegments and digests 2000–4000 discs per day.

The RPE plays many important roles in the life of the retina. The brown melanin in the melanosomes absorbs light that has passed through the retina and the pigment in the microvilli isolates one outersegment from its neighbours, helping to increase visual acuity (compare compound eye, Section 15.1.2 (Figure 15.3)). In some animals (especially some fish) reflective crystals are present in the RPE which provide a vivid 'eyeshine' (Section 19.3). The microvilli also provide mechanical support for the delicate outersegments. Phagocytosis of outersegment discs is also, as we saw above, an important function. The pigment epithelial cells also take up photoisomerized visual pigments from the outersegments and transform them back to their original 11-cis form (Section 17.2.1 (Figure 17.14)). Finally, the RPE lying, as it does, between the choriocapillaris and the retina, regulates the passage of materials between these two layers. It can be shown that it actively pumps Na^+ from the choriocapillaris to the retina, creating a potential across the RPE of about 10 mV.

17.2 RETINA

We looked at the gross structure of the retina in Section 16.2. A more detailed depiction of its various regions and parts is given in Figure 17.2 (a, b and c). In Chapter 16 we noted that in the human retina, daytime vision was focused on to the fovea and within the fovea, the foveola. We saw that these regions were composed largely of cones. The peripheral parts of the retina, on the other hand, were composed largely of rods. The human retina is thus said to be **duplex**: it contains both rods and cones. Rods are much more sensitive than cones, but it is the cone population which provides our sense of colour and in the fovea, because of their close packing and individual wiring, our visual acuity. In dim light it is the rods which provide what vision we have. In daytime vision, objects, especially moving objects, seen out of the 'corner of the eye', sensed, in other words by the rods in the peripheral retina, initiate a reflex whereby the eye moves until the object is brought into the confines of the fovea, a process known as **foveation**. The human eye, like most mammalian eyes, is thus, in a sense, double. A comparison might also be made with the salticid visual system discussed in Section 15.2.6. Both parts of the mammalian retina have their parts to play. In this section we shall look at its structure and functioning in more detail.

There are six major types of neural cells and one type of glial cell, the Müller cell (Figure 17.3). Histologists have recognized well over fifty subtypes of these major classes. The major types of neural cells in the retina are, listing from the pigment cell layer towards the vitreous humour:

- photoreceptor cells (rods and cones)
- horizontal cells
- bipolar cells
- interplexiform cells
- amacrine cells
- ganglion cells.

These cells are conventionally regarded as organized into nine layers (Figure 17.3b): photoreceptor outersegments (OS); outer limiting membrane (OLM); outer nuclear layer (ONL); outer plexiform layer (OPL); inner nuclear layer (INL); inner plexiform layer (IPL); ganglion cell layer (GCL); optic fibre layer (OFL); inner limiting membrane (ILM). The Müller cells are squeezed in between the neural elements and span the whole width of the retina, their terminations, connected together by tight junctions, forming both the outer and inner limiting membranes (see also Figure 17.18).

The retina is organized in both vertical and horizontal dimensions Figure 17.3b). The vertical organization starts with the photoreceptor cells. The feet of these cells form intricate synapses with bipolar cells. This strip of synapses constitutes the outer plexiform layer, whilst the nuclei of the photoreceptors form the outer nuclear layer. The bipolar cells cross the middle segment of the retina and make synapses with dendrites of the ganglion cells. Their nuclei constitute the inner nuclear layer; their synapses ganglion cells the inner plexiform layer. The unmyelinated axons of the ganglion cells run along the front of the retina making up the nerve fibre layer. These fibres run to the optic disc (Figure 17.2) and then leave the retina as elements of the optic nerve. It may be remarked at this point that (with rare exceptions in amacrine cells) action potentials are not found in this 'vertical' pathway until we reach the ganglion cell axons (compare insect retinula cell output (Section 15.2.7)). In addition to this three cell vertical pathway, interplexiform cells extend across the retina connecting the two plexiform layers together. In fact, they transmit information against the major stream, conducting from the IPL to the OPL. Superimposed upon this vertical structure, two cells types, the horizontal and amacrine cells, run tangentially across the retina, connecting together populations of photoreceptors and bipolars and populations of bipolar, ganglion and interplexiform cells respectively. A simplified version of this intricate interconnexity is shown schematically in Figure 17.4.

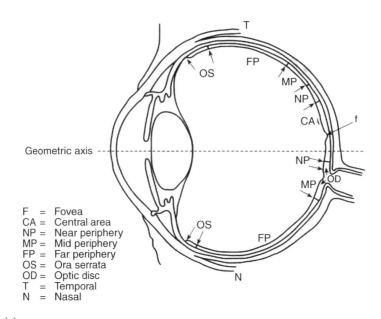

F = Fovea
CA = Central area
NP = Near periphery
MP = Mid periphery
FP = Far periphery
OS = Ora serrata
OD = Optic disc
T = Temporal
N = Nasal

(a)

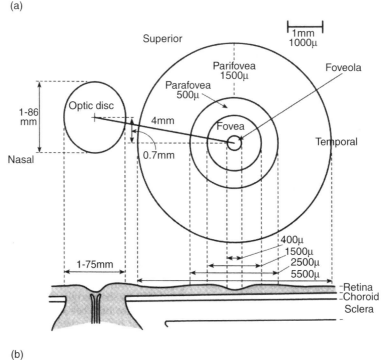

(b)

Figure 17.2 Regions of the human retina. (a) Horizontal section to show the different regions of the retina. T = temporal; N = nasal. As one proceeds towards the far periphery the number of bipolar and, especially, ganglion cells per unit area dramatically diminishes. There are, however, no sharp demarcations. (b) Surface and sectional views of the central region of the retina with (below) sectional view of same region. (*Continues overleaf*)

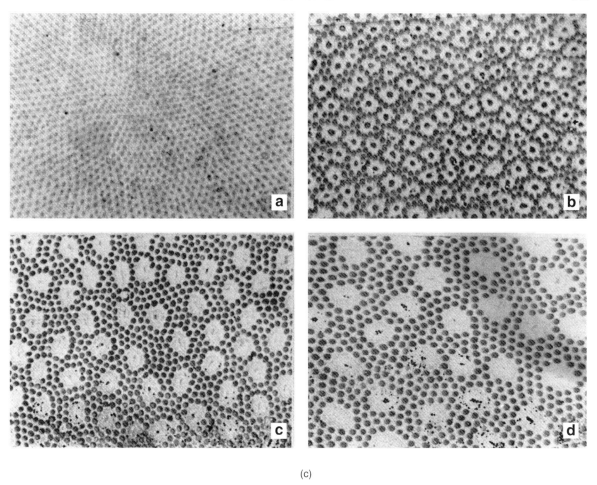

(c)

Figure 17.2 (*Continued*) (c) Tangential sections through different regions of rhesus monkey retina. The outersegments of the photoreceptor cells are cut in transverse section. (a) Fovea: note the densely packed, slender, cones. (b) Parafovea: the cone outersegments are surrounded by a white space. This is due to the large diameter of their inner segments. Surrounding the cones are rod outersegments. (c) Mid-periphery: the ratio of rods to cones has increased. (d) Far-periphery: the cones are markedly descreased in number. Reproduced with permission from *The Journal of Cell Biology*, 1971, **49**: 303–318. Copyright © 1971 The Rockefeller University Press.

17.2.1 Photoreceptor Cells

17.2.1.1 Morphology

Let us look first at the rod cell (Figure 17.5). It derives, as we have already noted, from a ciliated cell and traces of this origin remain throughout its life. During embryology the ciliary membrane becomes enormously expanded and invaginates to form large numbers of inpushings, which are ultimately 'nipped off' to form a stack of 'free-floating' discs (Figure 17.5a). This long membrane-enclosed pile of discs is known as the **outersegment**. In different vertebrates it varies from 10 to 200 mm in length and from 2 to 10 mm in diameter. The photosensitive pigment, rhodopsin, as we shall see more fully below, is concentrated in the disc membranes. In humans about 80% of disc membrane protein is rhodopsin. The outersegment is connected to the **inner segment** by a recognizable remnant of the original cilium, the so-called connecting cilium. The inner segment consists of an outer region termed the **ellipsoid** and an inner zone called the **myoid**. These regions are not sharply demarcated in mammalian rods and cones. The ellipsoid encloses large numbers of mitochondria, whilst the myoid shows a well developed endoplasmic reticulum and a prominent Golgi apparatus. These organelles are involved in a very active synthesis of new disc membrane. This is inserted at the base of the outersegment (Figure 17.5c) and the whole stack of discs is consequently forced upwards towards its tip. Discs are continuously removed from the tip and digested (as we saw in Section 17.1) by cells of the pigment epithelium. The cycle from disc synthesis to disc removal takes about ten days. Beneath this highly active region of the inner segment is the nucleus and then, after a more or less slender region, sometimes known as the axon or fibre, the cell expands once more to form the **foot, pedicle** or **spherule**. The spherule is filled with synaptic vesicles, containing l-**glutamate**, often organized on one or more **synaptic ribbons** and indented to form an intricate synaptic surface. This surface is both pre- and postsynaptic. Furthermore **gap junctions (= electrical synapses)** are made between rod spherules and adjacent cone pedicles. Rod–rod coupling has not, however, been shown to occur in mammals.

Cones (Figure 17.5b(ii)) are, in essentials, very similar to rods. The outersegments tend to be smaller, seldom more than 30 mm long and no more than 5 mm in diameter at their base. The discs are never pinched off from the boundary membrane and the intradisc space remains open to the extracellular environment. The inner segment is large and the ellipsoid is typically engorged with mitochondria. In many vertebrates (though not in eutherian mammals) it contains a prominent and sometimes coloured oil droplet (Section 19.2). Finally, the foot is typically much larger than that of rods and, moreover, has an even more complicated and usually multiple synaptic surface. As was the case with rods, this surface is both pre- and postsynaptic. In nonmammalian vertebrates it makes **gap junctions** with both adjacent cones and rods. In peripheral parts of the retina where photoreceptor density is low, the cone pedicle sometimes sends out lengthy processes to form these junctions with distant cone pedicles and rod spherules. The pedicle releases transmitter (**glutamate**) on to the dendritic endings of bipolar and horizontal cells and also receives input from horizontal

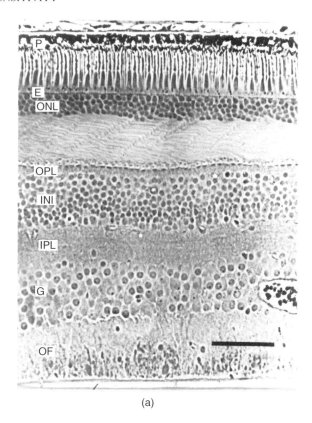

(a)

Figure 17.3 (a) (*caption overleaf*)

cells. It has been suggested that cones were the original receptor types from which rods have evolved. This, however, remains a matter of debate. Indeed, close examination of morphology and biochemistry reveals a continuum of intermediates between rods and cones.

17.2.1.2 Numbers and Distribution of Photoreceptors

Cones: In diurnal primates, such as humans, the density of cones reaches a maximum in the rod-free region at the centre of the fovea known as the **foveola**. In the human retina the foveola averages some 350 mm in diameter and the cone density ranges in different individuals from 100 000 to 324 000/mm^2. In plan view the cones in this region are arranged in a very regular triangular lattice with a center-to-centre spacing of 2.5–3.0 mm. The cone density falls off

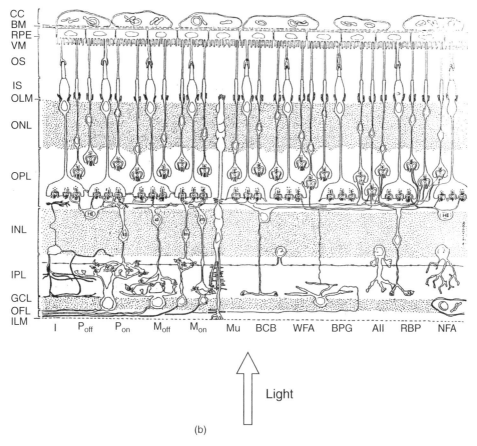

Light

(b)

Figure 17.3 Vertical section of primate retina (perifoveal region). (a) Micrograph. P = pigment epithelium; E = external limiting membrane; ONL = outer nuclear layer; OPL = outer plexiform layer; INL = inner nuclear layer; IPL = inner plexiform layer; G = ganglion cell layer, OF = optic nerve fibre layer. Scale bar = 75 μm. From Boycott and Dowling (1969), Organisation of the Primate Retina: Light Microscopy, *Phil Trans Roy Soc B*, **255**, p. 116, plate 32. Copyright © 1969, the Royal Society. (b) This figure frrom Rodieck, 1973, shows some of the complexity of the neural retina. Nevertheless, only a very few of the cells are shown. *Cells*: AII = AII amacrine; BCB = blue cone bipolar; BPG = biplexiform ganglion cell; H1 and H2 = two types of horizontal cell; I = interplexiform cell; id = diffuse bipolar cell; M_{off} = off-centre midget bipolar cell; M_{on} = on-centre midget bipolar cell; Mu = Müller cell; NFA = narrow field amacrine; P_{off} = off-centre parasol ganglion cell; P_{on} = on-centre parasol ganglion cell; RB = rod bipolar; WFA = wide-field amacrine cell. *Layers*: BM = Bruch's membrane; CC = choriocapillaris; GCL = ganglion cell layer; ILM = inner limiting membrane; INL = inner nuclear layer; IPL = inner plexiform layer; IS = inner segments; OFL = optic fibre layer; OLM = outer limiting membrane; ONL = outer nuclear layer; OPL = outer plexiform layer; OS = outersegments; RPE = retinal pigment epithelium. From Rodieck (1988) 'The Primate Retina' in Steklis and Erwin, *Neuroscience: Comparative Primate Biology*, by permission of the author.

very rapidly with distance from the foveola, reaching 10 000/mm² within 1 mm of the fovea and then falling away more slowly to a steady value of about 5000/mm² in the rest of the retina. In elevation, as Figure 17.2b shows, the retina in the region of the fovea and foveola falls away into a marked depression whose sides constitute the *clivus* (L: slope). This is due to the neural elements of the retina running nearly horizontally away from the cone pedicles (Figure 17.6), thus ensuring that the cones are not covered by layers of neurons and can receive maximal stimulation from incoming light. It can also be seen that the outersegments of the cones in this region are markedly elongated.

Rods: In the human retina rods outnumber cones by 20/1. They are absent from the foveola but reach a

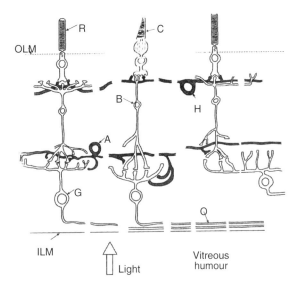

Figure 17.4 Simplified wiring diagram of retina (mid-periphery). Although not shown in the figure, there is considerable convergence. Many rods synapse with a single bipolar; many bipolars synapse with a single ganglion cell. A = amacrine cell; B = bipolar cell; C = cone; G = ganglion cell; H = horizontal cell; ILM = inner limiting membrane; O = optic nerve fibres; OLM = outer limiting membrane; R = rod.

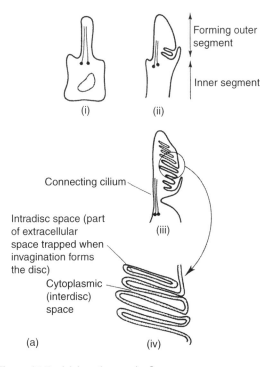

Figure 17.5   (a) (*caption overleaf*)

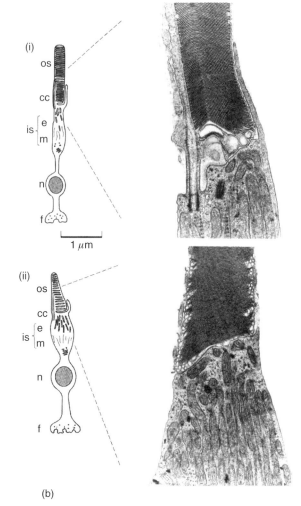

Figure 17.5   (b) (*caption opposite*)

maximum density of about 140 000 to 160 000/mm^2 in a ring about 5 mm away. The density then falls away to a steady state of about 70 000 to 80 000/mm^2 before diminishing abruptly towards the far periphery. This density distribution is shown in Figure 17.7.

17.2.1.3 Biophysics and Physiology

Let us start, once again, with rod cells. We have already noted that the visual pigment, rhodopsin, is located in outersegment disc membranes. It is highly concentrated. Indeed, it has been computed that no

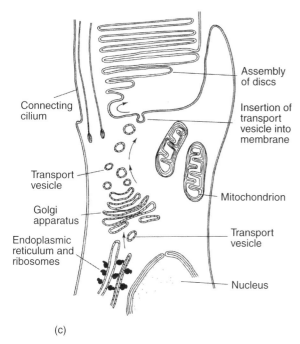

Connecting
cilium

Assembly
of discs

Insertion of
transport
vesicle into
membrane

Transport
vesicle

Golgi
apparatus

Endoplasmic
reticulum and
ribosomes

Mitochondrion

Transport
vesicle

Nucleus

(c)

Figure 17.5 Photoreceptor cells. (a) Embryological development. (i) Photoreceptor cells develop from ciliated cells lining the optic ventricle. Each cell bears a single cilium. (ii) The cilium grows and its membrane undergoes hypertrophy and begins to invaginate. (iii) Hypertophy of the ciliary membrane continues and invagination continues at the base of the forming outersegment. The original internal ultrastructure of the cilium remains in the 'connecting cilium' which connects the outer to the inner segment. (iv) Detail of (iii) to show how the invaginations of the ciliary membrane ultimately trap a small portion of the extracellular space as the intradisc space. The space between the discs is cytoplasmic. (b) (i) rod and (ii) cone cells. cc = connecting cilium; e = ellipsoid; f = foot or spherule; m = myoid; n = nuclear region; is = inner segment; os = outersegment. From Hogan, Alvarodo & Weddell (1971) *Histology of the Human Eye*, Fig 9.33. Copyright © 1971, Elsevier. (c) Disc membrane synthesis in rod and cone inner segments. The arrows indicate the direction in which new membrane material moves. Further explanation in text. After Besharse, 1986.

more than 20 nm separates one rhodopsin molecule from the next. It is evident that, like the rhabdomeric eye we considered in Chapter 15, the rod cell is an extremely good solution to the problem of detecting light. Incoming photons have to pass through a stack of perhaps 20 000 discs each with high photopigment concentration. Because of this stack of membrane discs, the refractive index within the outersegment is far greater than outside. It consequently

acts as a waveguide, channelling the light towards its tip (compare the insect rhabdom). This waveguide function also means that the outersegments are orientated so that, wherever they are, in the retina they are aligned towards the centre of the pupil. In some mammals, furthermore, (proverbially cats) reflecting pigment in the pigment epithelium gives any light getting that far a second chance of interacting with outersegment rhodopsin.

We looked at the structure of rhodopsin in the introduction to Part Four (Figure I4.3; Box I4.2). In rod outersegments it is orientated so that its carboxy terminal tail extends into the interdisc (= cytoplasmic) space. It holds 11-cis retinal by a Schiff base linkage to a lysine residue in the centre of its 'barrel of staves' (Figure 17.8a). When a photon of the appropriate wavelength (400–600 nm, λ_{max} 498 nm) interacts with 11-cis retinal, it provides the activation energy necessary to allow an intermolecular rearrangement to occur, producing the lower energy all-trans form. This is the crucial event in photoreception. All that follows depends on this photochemical change. The all-trans retinal is not acceptable to opsin and diffuses out of the 'barrel of staves', ultimately into the retinal pigment epithelium.

Lacking the 11-cis retinal in its centre, the opsin molecule undergoes a small conformational change. In this so-called 'activated' state it is able to react with a G-protein system in the outersegment membrane. These G-proteins are known as **transducins**, or T-proteins. The reaction of activated opsin with the alpha subunit of the T-protein is believed to be via its cytoplasmic loops (in the interdisc space). A typical collision–coupling biochemistry (Chapter 1) then ensues (Figure 17.9). There is, however, a difference. Instead of interacting with an adenylyl cyclase to generate cAMP (as is customarily the case) the alpha GTP subunit (G_α-GTP or T_α-GTP) acts on a large tetrameric enzyme: **cGMP-phosphodiesterase** (*cGMP-PDE*). This membrane-bound enzyme consists of an alpha, beta and two gamma subunits (λ, β, γ_2). When it comes into contact with a free T_α the two gamma subunits are displaced. This unveils the catalytic power of the alpha and beta subunits. These units are able to open the cGMP ring, transforming it into 5′GMP. Meanwhile, the two gamma subunits are at work catalysing the dephosphorylation of T_α-GTP to T_α-GDP. When this has happened, the T_α subunit detaches from the alpha and

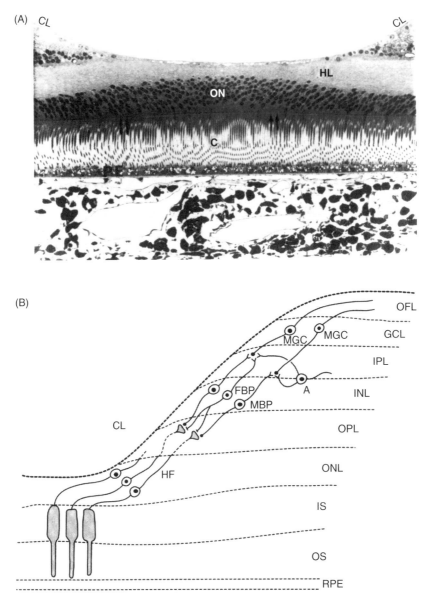

Figure 17.6 (a) Vertical section of human foveola. Although the photoreceptors in this area are exclusively cones (C) they develop long slender rod-like inner and outer segments. In consequence, many more can be packed into the limited space and the inner limiting membrane is bowed inwards (arrows) towards the aqueous humour. The outer nuclear layer (ON) is thickened because of the large number of cones and the cone fibres are elongated and project obliquely (Henle's fibres (HL) to form an inner plexiform layer and inner nuclear layer (INL) outside the bounds of the foveola. CL = clivus; PE = pigment epithelium. ×300. From Tripathi and Tripathi, 1984. (b) Diagram to show the organization of the neural elements in the region of the foveola. A = amacrine cell; CL = clivus; FBP = flat bipolar; HF = Henle's fibre; MBP = midget bipolar; MGC = midget ganglion cell. Other lettering as in Figure 17.3b.

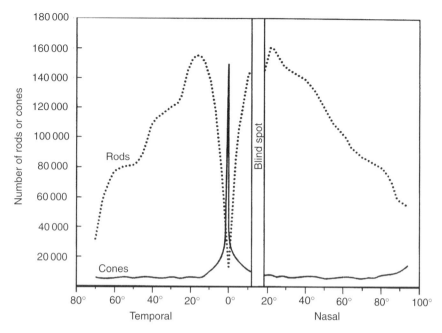

Figure 17.7 Distribution of rods and cones in the human retina. From Osterberg, 1935.

beta subunits of the cGMP-PDE and this allows the two gamma subunits to reattach. The catalytic activity of the enzyme ends.

So far, so good. But, the student may well ask, so what? To see the significance of this membrane biochemistry it has to be appreciated that cGMP plays a crucial role in the electrophysiology of the rod cell. It has been known for a good number of years that **in the dark** the rod cell is slightly depolarized. This is due the presence of Na^+ and Ca^{2+}-channels in the boundary membrane of the outersegment. Looking back to Chapter 2 it will be recalled that the electrical potential across a biomembrane is due to its differential permeability to small inorganic ions. We saw, indeed, that the potential is governed (to a first approximation) by the Goldman equation. Now if, for instance, we increase the sodium permeability, P_{Na}, fivefold to 5×10^{-7}cm/s, keeping the permeabilities of K^+ and Cl^- constant, and insert this value into the equation, we find that V_m works out at -20 mV (try it!). In the dark a current (known as the **dark current**), carried by Na^+ ions, flows from the inner segment through the extracellular space to enter the outersegment (Figure 17.10a). When a light is switched on, this dark current ceases and the rod cell loses its depolarization: in other words it **hyperpolarizes** (Figure 17.10b). But what, it will be asked, has all this to do with the collision–coupling biochemistry of the previous paragraph? The answer is obvious when we find that it is precisely cGMP that holds open the Na^+–Ca^{2+}-channels in the outersegment membrane. The collision–coupling biochemistry, as we saw, leads to the transformation of cGMP into straight chain 5′GMP. In other words, cGMP is removed, the Na^+–Ca^{2+}-channels close, the rod cell hyperpolarizes.

But the closure of the cyclic nucleotide gated (CNG) channels also has another consequence (Figure 17.11). In the interdisc (cytoplasmic) space is to be found a significant enzyme called **recoverin**. In the dark this enzyme is turned off by the presence of Ca^{2+}. When light is switched on, the Na^+–Ca^{2+}-channels close and the supply of Ca^{2+} is cut off. The enzyme is consequently disinhibited. It acts on another enzyme, **guanylyl cyclase** (*GC*), to synthesize cGMP from 5′GMP. The longer illumination persists, the more cGMP is synthesized by this route. This is a mechanism of **sensory adaptation**. The more cGMP, that is synthesized by GC the more it begins to outweigh its removal by the cGMP-PDE at the

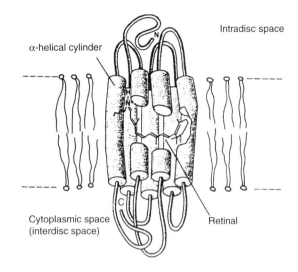

(a)

(b)

II-cis retinal₁

all-trans retinal₁

Figure 17.8 (a) 'Barrel of staves' conformation of rhodopsin in disc membrane. Note position of 11-cis retinal. (b) Schiff base linkage of retinal to lysine$_{296}$ residue in opsin. (c) Molecular structure of 11-cis and all-trans retinal$_1$.

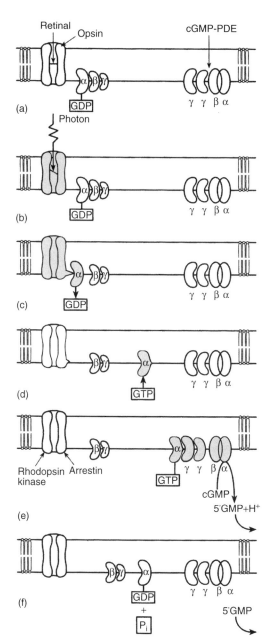

Figure 17.9 Collision–coupling in disc membrane. (a): resting condition. (b); On receipt of a photon of light retinal undergoes a cis-trans transformation. (c) and (d): 11-cis retinal diffuses out of the 'activated' opsin and the alpha subunit of T-protein is freed to accept GTP. (e): T_α-GTP activates cGMP-PDE and arrestin and rhodpsin kinase inactivate opsin. (f): GTP is de-phosphorylated and the action of T_α on cGMP-PDE is terminated. The system returns to rest. Stippling indicates activated state.

disc membrane. The more the Na^+–Ca^{2+}-channels begin to open, the more the rod cell begins to depolarize.

We have not finished with the biochemical subtleties of the rod outersegment yet! When opsin undergoes its conformational change on losing its chromophore, retinal, it unmasks attachment sites for two inhibitory proteins, **rhodopsin kinase** and **arrestin**. Rhodopsin kinase phosphorylates as many as nine serine and threonine residues on opsin's carboxy terminal chain (Figure I4.3). But full desensitization of opsin does not occur until arrestin attaches. This can only occur when opsin has been phosphorylated by rhodopsin kinase. When this has happened, arrestin attaches and alters the conformation of opsin in such a way that it can no longer interact with membrane-bound transducin. The collision–coupling mechanism is, in consequence, switched off. The cGMP-PDE returns to its inactive state; no further cGMPs are synthesized; the rod cell depolarizes.

Although the biochemistry and molecular biology outlined above may seem over-elaborate (and, no doubt, as research continues further complexities will be uncovered), the outcome is an extremely sensitive system for detecting photons. It has been computed that, when fully dark-adapted, a rod cell responds to a single photon. As with mechanoreceptive hair cells (Chapter 8), the system is as sensitive as physics allows. The response of the rhodopsin is multiplied by the transducin collision–coupling biochemistry (Figure 17.12) so that, in theory at least, a single photon could change the world.

17.2.1.4 Comparison Between Ciliary and Rhabdomeric Photoreceptors

We noted in Section 15.1 that the animal kingdom has evolved two major photoreceptor designs: the ciliary and the rhabdomeric (Figure 15.1). Having now discussed the ciliary type in some detail, it is time to look a little more closely at the comparison between the two. Although, as we shall see, they have many features in common, they are sufficiently different in their detailed molecular biology for us to recognize that they have both evolved on separate evolutionary tracks to near perfection for more that half a billion years.

We have already noted (Box 15.1) that both ciliary and rhabdomeric photoreceptors make use of opsins

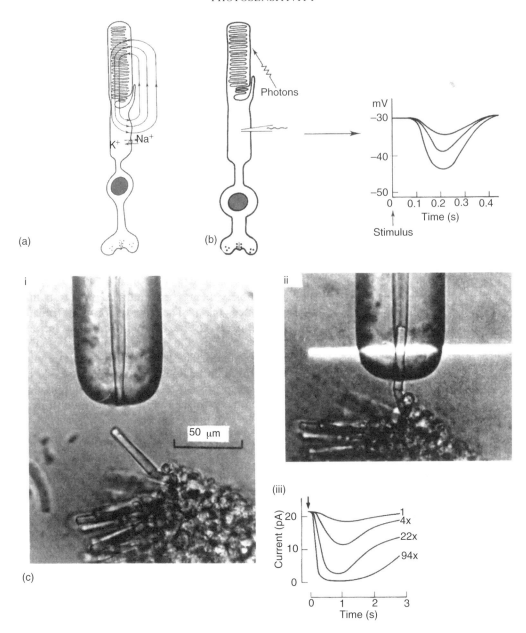

Figure 17.10 (a) Dark current. In the dark the boundary membrane of the outersegment possesses 'leak channels' which allows Na^+ to percolate inwards. They flow down their concentration gradient into the inner segment from whence they are extruded by a Na^+–K^+ pump. Hence, in the dark, a continuous current of Na^+ flows from the inner segment up to the outersegment. This is the 'dark' current. (b) If and when a photon of light is absorbed by the outersegment the Na^+-channels close and the rod cell hyperopolarizes. This hyperpolarization can be recorded by a microelectrode inserted into the cell. This hyperpolarization is shown by the graph on the right. After Penn and Hagins, 1969. (c) (i) A toad outersegment (much larger than a mammalian outersegment) is sucked into a glass pipette. Because it blocks the end of the pipette all the current which flows into or out of it is supplied from the interior of the pipette and can thus be measured. In the dark this current, as shown in the graph at (iii) is a little over 20 pA. (ii) A pencil beam of light is flashed through the pipette tip and the graph at (iii) shows the effect of this illumination starting at the point marked by the vertical arrow. The reduction in the dark current depends on the intensity of the flash. The bottom line of the graph shows the current when the flash intensity is $94\times$ as great as that responsible for the top line. From Baylor, Lamb and Yau, 1979, 'The membrane current of single rod outer segments' *J. Physiol*, **288**, p. 611, plate 1 by permission of Blackwell publishing.

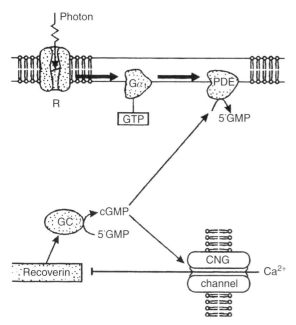

Figure 17.11 Biochemical mechanism responsible for adaptation in outersegment. When Na^+–Ca^{2+}-channels close due to illumination removing cGMP, the inflow of Ca^{2+} is reduced. Recoverin is consequently disinhibited and stimulates the activity of GC. Fresh supplies of cGMP are synthesized. This increases the open probability of the Na^+–Ca^{2+}-channels. Further explanation in text. Arrows symbolize activation; $\vdash$ = inhibition; $G\alpha_t$ = α-subunit of G-protein; GC = guanylyl cyclase; PDE = phosphodiesterase; R = rhodopsin.

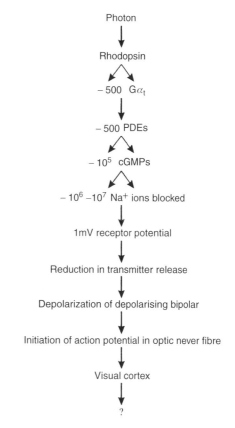

Figure 17.12 Amplification cascade in the visual system. Adapted from Alberts *et al.*, 2002, and Lamb and Pugh, 1992.

belonging to the same family of 7TM GPCRs. However, comparison of the amino acid sequences of the opsins of rhabdomeric and ciliary photoreceptors show that, although members of the same family, their common ancestor is very distant, some time in the mists of the Precambrian period before the origin of the bilateria. We have also noted that the design principle of both types of receptor is to display large concentrations of these photopigments in stacks of membranes arranged orthogonal to the incoming light. Clearly we have yet another case of 'evolution' coming up with a similar solution to the same problem, much as we have seen it did with Belemnite and vertebrate eyes. Which came first, the rhabdomeric or the ciliary design? Did both evolve independently? Or was there to begin with a 'bimodal' organ having features of both types, with one type being lost in the majority of protostomes and the other lost in

the deuterostomes? We have, of course, to remember the distinction is not quite clear cut. Ciliary photoreceptors, as we noted in Section 15.2.3, are also developed in Lamellibranch molluscs, and they have also been found in the polychaete worm, *Platynereis*, both members of the protostomata. It is also intriguing to find, as noted in Chapter 15, that *Amphioxus* develops photoreceptors of both types. At the time of writing the evolutionary origin of the two major types of photoreceptors remains of debate. But, whatever the outcome of this debate, it cannot be disputed that both types of receptor now show essentially the same design features (Figure 17.13).

When we come to look at the detailed molecular biology and biophysics of the two types of photoreceptor, we again find striking differences in an

BOX 17.1   RETINITIS PIGMENTOSA

The eye, like the ear (Chapter 8), is subject to a large number of genetic diseases. The genes responsible are distributed over nearly the whole of the human genome (20 out of the 23 chromosomes). This reflects the complexity of the eye's structure. Its development and maintenance involves the coordinated operation of many genes, any one of which may malfunction. The commonest form of inherited visual defect is *retinitis pigmentosa* (*RP*). The name, in fact, covers a very heterogeneous group of pathologies which, together, have an estimated prevalence of about 1/3000. The condition may be inherited as autosomal dominant (adRP), autosomal recessive (acRP), or linked to the X chromosome (xlRP). arRP is by far the most frequent form, being shown by at least half all families suffering from RP. The disease is caused by the (presently) irretrievable degeneration and death of rods and, to a much lesser extent, cones. The degenerating rod outersegments are scavenged and digested by the pigment epithelium, giving rise to a heavy pigmentation and hence the name, retinitis pigmentosa. The loss of rods leads to a cascade which ultimately effects cones and the retinal blood supply. Early indications are night blindness and abnormalities in the ERG. The end result, sooner or later, is blindness.

We have noted in this chapter some of the molecular and cellular elements of rod cells. All of these elements are open to mutational attack leading to misfunction and consequent visual impairment. Genetic analysis has implicated chromosomes 1, 3, 6, 7, 8 and the X chromosome. X chromosome-linked RP has been subjected to particularly intensive genetic analysis and the mutations responsible have been traced to two genes on the short arm of the chromosome. Neither gene has as yet been characterized or its biochemical effect determined.

Understanding is more advanced in some cases of autosomal dominant RP. The first mutation responsible for adRP to be tracked was located on chromosome 3. It was shown to lead to an amino acid substitution in rod opsin ($pro_{23} \rightarrow his$ or P23H). Since then more than thirty other mutations affecting the amino acid sequence of rod opsin have been detected. In some cases these mutations affect less essential regions of the molecule and hence the onset of RP is delayed and is less severe. The first mutation to lead to adRP (mentioned above) affects a large population of Irish origin in the Unites States and causes very early onset RP and major visual impairment by the second decade of life. The mutation seems to be restricted to the United States, where it accounts for over 15% of adRP patients. The fact that it is not found in Europe suggests that it is a case of 'founder effect' in the early Irish emigrant community. Another Unites States Irish pedigree, with a less severe adRP, causing impairment only in the fourth or later decades of life, was shown to be linked to mutation on chromosome 6. The candidate gene encodes a structural protein in rod outersegment discs. This protein is called **peripherin-RDS** (the RDS suffix indicates that it was first characterized in mice suffering from slow retinal degeneration).

Genetic analysis of arRP is not so far advanced. It has been difficult to establish sufficiently extensive genealogies to undertake decisive genetic analysis. Nevertheless, a $G \rightarrow T$ transversion has been discovered in codon 249 of one arRP kinship, leading to GAG being substituted by TAG. This is transcribed as UAG, which is a stop signal in translation at the ribosome. The resulting opsin would thus lose its sixth and seventh transmembrane segments. The homozygous patient had suffered night blindness for as long as she could remember although her heterozygous parents and sibling were normal. Another arRP has been shown to be due to a $G \rightarrow A$ transition at codon 150. This leads to a GAG triplet (glutamate) being changed to AAG (lysine). Once again the heterozygous kinship showed no ill effect whereas the homozygous patient suffered severe night blindness. Other work suggests that arRP is not confined to mutation on chromosome 3; it can be due to mutant genes on a number of different chromosomes. It is rapidly becoming possible to engineer transgenic mice which express some of these defective genes. The molecular biological defects underlying RP are thus slowly being unravelled. In one case of mouse

(Continues)

(*Continued*)

retinal degeneration (rd) it is, for instance, known that the pathology is due not to a defect in opsin but in the beta subunit of cGMP-PDE. This defect has also recently been identified in some cases of human arRP.

We have noted in this chapter that rhodopsin and cGMP-PDE are present in large quantities in outersegment discs and that rhodopsin (at least) forms part of their structure. It is not surprising, therefore, that genetic errors in the manufacture of these elements (and, of course, peripherin) should lead to loss of outersegment integrity. But it is not only the manufacture and integrity of rod discs which are at risk but also their removal. Rod discs, as we have noted, are scavenged and digested by the retinal pigment epithelium (RPE). This process is also under genetic control. Perhaps it is a developing imbalance between synthesis and degradation that is responsible for the slow development of most RPs.

Molecular neurobiology is just beginning to elucidate this complex of interacting processes and, as in other cases, it is leading to crucial insights into the underlying causes of a devastating human disease. Recent success in inserting normal genes into mice homozygous for *Rds* and *Rd*, resulting in blockage of photoreceptor degeneration, hopefully points the way to rational therapies.

REFERENCES

Armstrong, R.A. (1999) Ocular disease and the new genetics. *Ophthalmic and Physiological Optics*, **19**, 193–95.

Berson, E.L. (1993) Retinitis pigmentosa: the Friedenwald lecture. *Investigative Ophtalmology and Visual Science*, **34**, 1659–76.

Humphries, P., Kenna, P. and Farrar, G.J. (1992) On the molecular genetics of retinitis pigmentosa. *Science*, **256**, 804–8.

Milam, A.H. (1993) Strategies for the rescue of retinal photoreceptor cells. *Current Opinion in Neurobiology*, **3**, 797–804.

overall similarity (Figure 17.13). The same outcome, a coupling of opsin photo-isomerization to changes in membrane potential is achieved by analogous, but not homologous, biochemical cascades. Each of the two types of opsin has its own subgroup of G-proteins leading to biochemical cascades which involve (as we have seen) phospholipase C and a **depolarising** response in the rhabdomeric type (Figure 17.13a) and PDE and a **hyperpolarising** response in the ciliary type (Figure 17.13b)). Yet again there are puzzling exceptions. We shall see in Section 19.6 that vertebrate parietal and pineal eyes (where they exist) develop ciliary type photoreceptors that **depolarize** in response to photic stimulation! However, putting these awkward exceptions to one side we can complete our review of the overall similarities, yet differences in the detail, between the two major classes of photoreceptor by noting how the response is terminated in the two types. In both cases arrestins and rhodopsin kinases are involved, al-though it is found that the arrestin α and rhodopsin kinase of ciliary receptors are nonorthologous to the arrestin β and rhodopsin kinase of rhabdomeric receptors.

17.2.1.5 Photo-Isomerization and Retrieval of Retinal

Let us now return to the mammalian eye and the initial event of photoreception: the transformation of 11-cis to all-trans retinal. This takes place via a series of intermediates that can be detected by their different λ_{max}: rhodopsin (498 nm) → prelumirhodopsin (543 nm) → lumirhodopsin (497 nm) → metarhodopsin 1 (478 nm) → metarhodopsin 2 (380 nm) → metarhodpsin 3 (465 nm) → all-trans retinal (387 nm). This sequence of intramolecular rearrangements is very rapid: it is completed in less than a millisecond. The all-trans

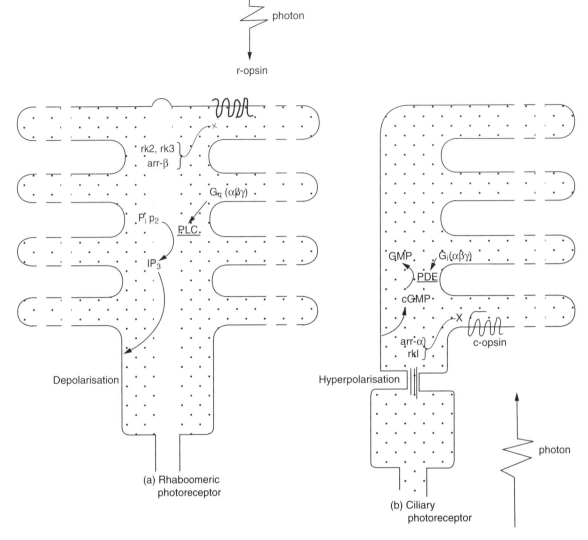

Figure 17.13 Comparison between (a) rhabdomeric and (b) ciliary type photoreceptor cells. arr-α = arrestin-α; arr-β = arrestin -β; Gq = rhabdomeric G-protein ($\alpha\beta\gamma$ subunits); Gi = ciliary G-protein ($\alpha\beta\gamma$ subunits); PDE = phosophodi-esterase; PLC = phospholipase C; rk1, rk2, rk3 = rhodopsin kinase 1,2,3; c-opsin = ciliary opsin; r-opsin = rhabdomeric opsin. Modified from Nilsson, 2004.

retinal (as we have already seen) detaches from the opsin. If it is displaced from a rod, it is transported into the retinal pigment epithelium (RPE) where rei-somerization occurs. The sequence of events is shown in Figures 17.14a and 17.14b. Figure 17.14a shows the sequence of biochemical changes; figure 17.14b

indicates where these reactions are occurring in the ultrastructure of the rod outersegment and the RPE.

The all-trans retinal is first reduced to the alco-hol form, all-trans retinol, by all-trans retinol de-hydrogenase (all-trans RDH) (Figure 17.14a). This is then transported across interphotoreceptor space

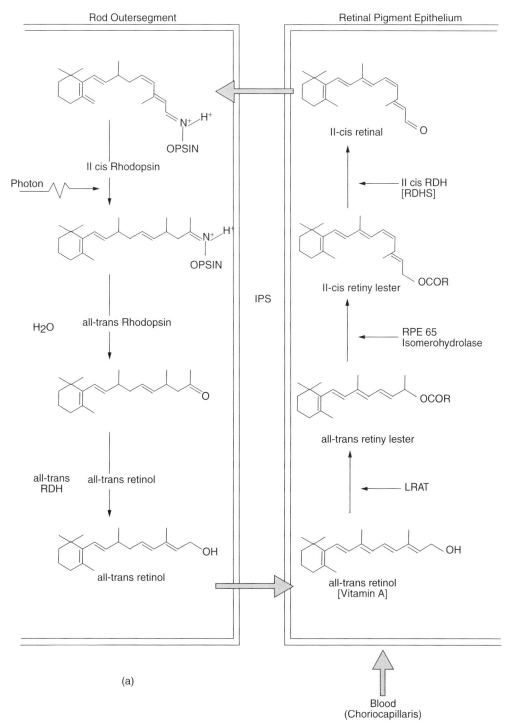

Rod Outersegment

Retinal Pigment Epithelium

ll cis Rhodopsin

Photon

all-trans Rhodopsin

H₂O

all-trans RDH · all-trans retinol

all-trans retinol

II-cis retinal

II cis RDH [RDHS]

II-cis retiny lester

RPE 65 Isomerohydrolase

all-trans retiny lester

LRAT

all-trans retinol [Vitamin A]

IPS

Blood (Choriocapillaris)

(a)

Figure 17.14 (a) (*(b) and caption overleaf*)

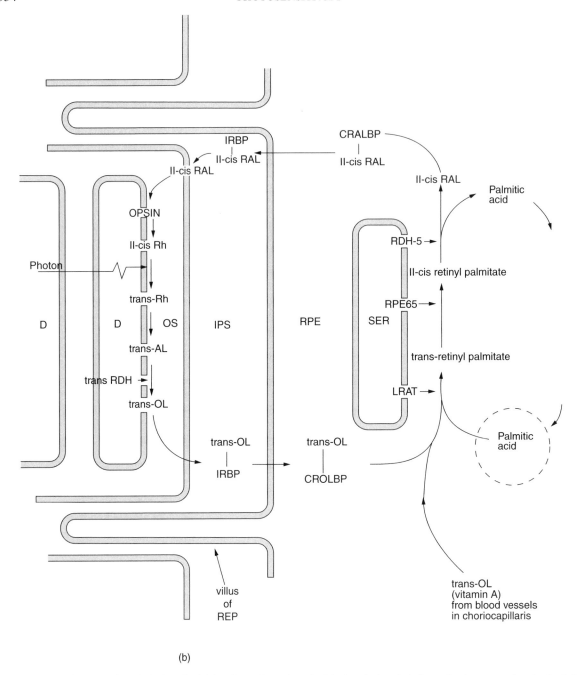

(b)

Figure 17.14   Regeneration of 11-cis retinal. (a): schematic to show the biochemical cycle in the rod outersegment and retinal pigment epithelium. Key: IPS = interphotoreceptor space; LRAT = lecithin retinol transferase; RDH = retinol dehydrogenase; RPE-65 =
retinal pigment epithelium 65 kDa protein. (b). Diagram showing the molecular biology of the regeneration cycle. Key: (i) *Anatomy*
D = outersegment disc; OS = outersegment; IPS = interphotoreceptor space; RPE = retinal pigment epithelium; SER = smooth
endoplasmic reticulum. (ii) *Molecular biology*: AL = retinal; CRALBP = cellular retinal binding protein; CROLBP = cellular retinol
binding protein; IRBP = interphotoreceptor retinoid binding protein (ABC retinoid transporter); OL = retinol; R = fatty acid (for
example palmitic acid); Rh = rhodopsin. Further explanation in text. A and B After Lamb, T.D. and Pugh, E.N. (2006).

(IPS) by a specific transport molecule, the interphotoreceptor retinoid binding protein (IRBP) (a member of the ABC transporter family) (Figure 17.14b). In the RPE, all-trans retinol is carried to the membranes of the smooth endoplasmic reticulum (SER) by another transport protein, cellular retinol binding protein (CROLBP). On the membrane of the SER it encounters another enzyme, lecithin retinol transferase (LRAT), which catalyses the formation of all-trans retinyl ester (retinyl palmitate) from a fatty acid (palmitic acid) derived from phosphatidyl choline (lecithin). Further supplies of all-trans retinol (vitamin A) are derived from blood vessels in the choriocapillaris. Next, a complex intramolecular transformation occurs in the retinyl palmitate that results in the all-trans retinal moiety being bent into the 11-cis conformation once again. This is catalysed by an enzyme associated with SER known as RPE65. The energy for this transformation appears to be derived from an intramolecular change in the palmitate moiety of the retinyl palmitate. The 11-cis retinyl palmitate may remain stored in the RPE or it may release 11-cis retinol which, with the assistance of 11-cis retinol dehydrogenase (RDH 5), is transformed to 11-cis-retinal, that is it is transported back to the RPE plasma membrane by cellular retinal binding proteins (CRALBP) and across the IPM by IRBP. Finally, the 11-cis retinal is released into the outersegment where it finds its way back into a vacant opsin molecule.

The regeneration of retinal from cones is not so well understood. It is believed to occur in the neural retina rather than the RPE. Recent work on the cone-dominated chicken retina suggests that an analogous cycle, perhaps substituting Müller cells for the RPE, exists. Whether Müller cells are also involved in duplex rod-dominated retinae, such as our own, has yet to be shown.

17.2.1.6 Consequences of Hyperpolarization

Finally, in this intricate story, let us draw back a little from the detailed biochemistry and consider the rod cell as a whole. We have seen that the absorption of a photon by a rhodopsin molecule ultimately leads to a hyperpolarization of the rod cell membrane. This hyperpolarization spreads throughout the cell down to, and including, the spherule. It will be known from first principles that release of transmitter molecules

from presynaptic endings occurs in response to a depolarization. It follows that a hyperpolarization will **inhibit** release of transmitter from the rod foot. We shall return to this below when we consider the synapse between rod and cone pedicles, horizontal and bipolar cells.

17.2.1.7 Cones

Before turning to horizontal and bipolar cells, however, let us give some consideration to those other photoreceptor cells, the **cones**. We looked at their structure in Section 17.2.1.1 above. Their biochemistry and biophysics is much the same as we have just described for rod cells. The major difference, of course, is that their visual pigments have three different absorption curves with λ_{max} in the short (S), medium (M) and long (L) wave regions of the visual spectrum. In the normal human retina, the three cone pigments display λ_{max} at 419 nm ('blue' or 'S'), 531 nm ('green' or 'M')) and 559 nm ('red' or 'L') (Figure 17.15). Each individual cone contains just one type of pigment (compare olfactory receptor cells). The pigments in the L and M cones are encoded by genes on the X chromosome, whilst the gene encoding the S pigment is located on chromosome 7

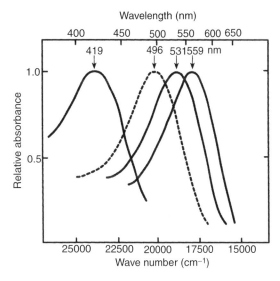

Figure 17.15 Absorbance curves for the three kinds of iodopsin (solid lines) and rhodopsin in the human retina. From Mollon, J.D. (1982) Colour vision and colour blindness, in *The Senses* (eds H.B. Barlow and J.D. Mollon), Copyright © 1982, Cambridge University Press.

(7q31.3-32). Defects in the X chromosome genes lead to the most common forms of colour blindness from which, for obvious reasons, males are most likely to suffer. The L gene is, moreover, highly polymorphic. It is consequently found that up to 10% of women have two slightly different L genes as well as the usual M and S genes. These 'tetrachromatic' women have almost an extra dimension in their colour sensitivity.

Differential stimulation of the three populations of cones is the first step in colour vision. We shall consider the subsequent steps which occur in the retina in Section 17.2.9 below. Further processing occurs in the cerebral cortex. Although differential stimulation of the three cone populations may be the first step, it is very far from being the last. Colour has sometimes been taken as the type example of a sensory qualia or 'raw feel'; we shall see that far from being 'raw' a very considerable neurophysiological 'cooking' occurs before we 'live through' a colour experience.

There has been some confusion over nomenclature. The pigment found in rods is (as we have seen) customarily termed rhodopsin whilst that in cones has been known as **iodopsin**. In both cases the photopigment consists of a 7TM protein (opsin) and a chromophore, retinal. The opsin found in rod outersegments is called **rod opsin** and that in cones, **cone opsin**. Clearly rod opsin should not be confused with rhodopsin.. The differences in absorption spectra (Figure 17.15) are not due to the chromophore but to differences in the amino acid sequences of the opsins (Table 17.1). In all cases,

retinal is attached to a lysine residue (lysine$_{296}$) by a Schiff base linkage. But the distribution of charged amino acid side chains in its immediate vicinity differs. It is likely that these differences and other subtle biochemical variations in the amino acid surroundings of retinal account for the differing absorption spectra. Indeed, it has been shown that three different amino acid substitutions can transform a green-sensitive into a red-sensitive opsin. These substitutions are alanine$_{180}$ → serine, phenylalanine$_{227}$ → trytophan and alanine$_{285}$ → threonine or, in the more compact terminology of molecular biology, A180S, F227W and A285T. It is salutary to reflect that the colour qualia which play so important a part in our subjective lives depend so crucially on which amino acid is incorporated at a particular position in the polypeptide chain of our cone opsins. Further discussion of the evolution of opsin may be found in Box 15.1.

Knowledge of the amino acid sequences of the rod and cone opsins gives an insight into their evolutionary relationships. It can be deduced from Table 17.1 that all the opsins form an evolutionarily related family. It can be further deduced that a single ancestral opsin gene duplicated twice at least 500 million years ago. One of the three resulting genes continued to code for rod opsin, the others evolved to code for the red and blue cone opsins. Comparatively recently, perhaps no more than 40 million years ago, the red cone opsin gene duplicated again. One of the two genes resulting from this duplication continued to code for a red opsin, the other evolved to code a green opsin. It is probable that this development proved of considerable evolutionary importance. It provided our primate ancestors with a means of distinguishing between green unripe fruit and sugar-laden red and orange coloured ripe fruit. In a rather minor way this resembles the coevolution of plants and insects seen in entomophilous plants. It may also be that, as we noted in Section 14.3, the development of colour vision provided an opportunity for the evolution of the vivid sexual colouration of some old-world primates.

But, it might be asked, would the intricate machinery of the brain be able to cope with the appearance of a 'green' opsin in the retina? We have been emphasizing throughout this chapter, and will continue to do so in the next, the hugely complex nature of

Table 17.1 Homologies of rod and cone opsins.

| | Percentage sequence homology | | | |
	Rod opsin	Blue opsin	Red opsin	Green opsin
Rod opsin	100	75	73	73
Blue opsin	42	100	79	79
Red opsin	40	43	100	99
Green opsin	41	44	96	100

Data from Nathans, 1987. Values below the 100% diagonal are percentage identical residues; values above the diagonal are percentage identical plus conservative substitutions mammalian visual systems. Would not the insertion of a new visual pigment at the periphery require the development of new 'wiring' in the visual centres of the brain? An answer to this question has recently been obtained by sophisticated genetic engineering, whereby a third visual pigment has been inserted into the normal dichromatic mouse retina. Mice, like most mammals, only possess 'S' and 'M' pigments in their cones. Genetic techniques allowed researchers to breed mice which expressed the human red (L) pigment in their retinae in addition to their normal 'S' and 'M' pigments. Extensive behavioural testing (tens of thousands of tests) showed that these genetically altered mice were indeed able to distinguish a 'trichromatic' colour world similar to that which we ourselves enjoy. This is remarkable. It seems to show that at one abrupt move a new set of 'qualia' can emerge. It shows, too, how such mutations can confer almost immediate selective advantage in the 'struggle for life'. Do such abrupt transitions occur in the other senses?

17.2.2 Horizontal Cells

These cells are large (100–400 mm) and, in the horizontal plane, star shaped. They extend their processes in the plane of the OPL, linking together groups of photoreceptor cell pedicles. No action potentials are developed and transmission of influence is by way of electrotonic conduction. Both pre- and postsynaptic contacts are made. In studies on the goldfish it has been found that, when the horizontal cell is postsynaptic to the photoreceptor cell, its response is 'sign conserving'. In other words, if the photoreceptor cell hyperpolarizes so does the horizontal cell; if the photoreceptor cell depolarizes so does the horizontal cell. On the other hand, if the horizontal cell is presynaptic to a photoreceptor cell, the response of the photoreceptor cell is 'sign inverting'. In other words, the horizontal cell produces the opposite effect in the photoreceptor cell, for example depolarization in response to hyperpolarization and so on. Finally, horizontal cells are linked to each other by gap junctions (= electrical synapses). This electrical coupling, which is always sign conserving, is controlled by the neurotransmitter, dopamine. Horizontal cells thus form an intricate transmitter-

controlled electrically-coupled web running tangentially through the OPL.

17.2.3 Bipolar Cells

These cells run between the OPL and the IPL. They transmit information from the photoreceptors to the ganglion and/or amacrine cells. In some cases this is done with great precision. In many cases in the primate retina bipolars, known as **midget bipolars**, synapse with a single cone (Figure 17.3b). A single midget bipolar in the primate retina has, for instance, been observed to contact a single foveal cone (with 25 dendritic processes) and run to a single ganglion cell. In other cases bipolars, called **diffuse bipolars**, contact many cone pedicles (Figure 17.3b). In peripheral parts of the retina, a bipolar cell may make synapses with up to 40 photoreceptor cells. Whereas there appears to be only one type of rod bipolar there seem to be a large number (up to ten in cat, six in primates) of different types of cone bipolars.

17.2.3.1 Rod Bipolars

These have a large cell body and usually an extensive dendritic tree, especially in the peripheral retina. The synapses which they make with rod pedicles are often complex, involving not only the bipolar cell synapses but also horizontal cells (Figure 17.16a). We noted (Section 17.2.1.3) that the 'dark current' ensures that in the dark rod cells slowly depolarize. When fully dark adapted (after about an hour) they reach a steady-state depolarization and at this stage the rod–cone gap junctions are believed to close. All activity in rod cells is thus directed exclusively to its bipolar cell. All rod bipolars are '**sign inverting**' (see below).

17.2.3.2 Cone Bipolars

We noted above that there are a number of different morphological types of cone bipolar. For the sake of simplicity we shall just mention two: **midget** bipolars which, as we have seen, may be monosynaptic and '**flat**' or '**brush**' bipolars which may make synapses with a number of cone pedicles. The synaptic junctions are again often very complex

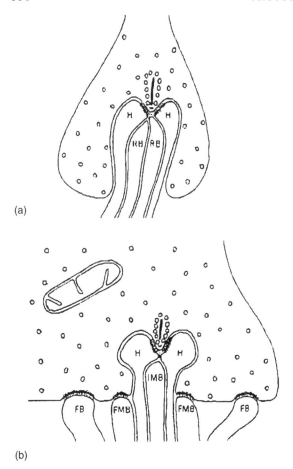

(a)

(b)

Figure 17.16 Synapses in primate outer plexiform layer. (a) Synaptic complex at rod spherule. H = horizontal cell; RB = rod bipolar dendrite. Note synaptic ribbon and synaptic vesicles. (b) Synapses and synaptic complexes at cone pedicle. Note the much greater size of the pedicle compared with the rod spherule. FB = flat bipolar; FMB = flat midget bipolar; IMB = invaginating midget bipolar; H = horizontal cell. IMBs frequently branch and often a single IMB makes multiple triadic synapses with a single cone pedicle. Cone pedicles and IMBs are thus in very firm synaptic contact. Reproduced from Dowling, J.E. (1987) *The Retina: An Approachable Part of the Brain*, Copyright © 1987, Harvard University Press.

believed to be glutamate. In the dark, when the photoreceptors are depolarized, this transmitter is continuously and slowly released. Probably the synaptic ribbons, which are such a characteristic feature of photoreceptor terminals, have to do with organizing this slow leakage. The presence of glutamate has different effects on the two types of bipolar dendrites (Figure 17.17). In one case it opens cation channels, allowing Na^+ ions to leak into the dendrite. The dendrite is consequently depolarized. When the photoreceptor cell hyperpolarizes, the release of glutamate

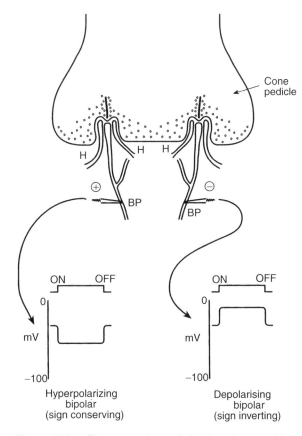

Figure 17.17 Sign conserving and sign inverting cone bipolar synapses. The lower part of the figure shows the response of the bipolar cells when the cone is illuminated. The hyperpolarizing (sign conserving) bipolar gives an 'OFF' response; the depolarizing (sign inverting) bipolars give an 'ON' response. These responses are greater the more intense the illumination. H = horizontal cell; BP = bipolar cell. Further explanation in text.

(Figure 17.16b). Cone bipolars, unlike rod bipolars, may be either '**sign inverting**' or '**sign conserving**'.

Next let us consider the neuropharmacology of 'sign conserving' and 'sign inverting' synapses. We have seen that both rod and cone synaptic terminals are filled with vesicles containing neurotransmitter, from its pedicle is cut off and the bipolar dendrite in consequence hyperpolarizes. This is the **sign conserving** bipolar. In the other case something analogous to the effect of light on the CNG channels of outersegments is thought to occur. Glutamate (like light on outersegments) appears to actuate a biochemical cascade which removes the cGMP that would otherwise keep Ca^{2+}–Na^+-channels open. Hence, in the dark, when glutamate is present in the synaptic cleft, these CNG channels are closed and the bipolar is in a relatively hyperpolarized state. When light is switched on, the photoreceptor cell hyperpolarizes, glutamate release is inhibited, the CNG channels open and the bipolar cells depolarizes. This is the **sign inverting** bipolar.

Although bipolar cells do not generate action potentials they can be shown to have what are known as centre–surround receptive fields and to give either '*ON*' or '*OFF*' responses. Let us see what is meant by this. Figure 17.17 shows a cone making synapses with sign conserving and sign inverting bipolars. When a light is switched ON, a depolarization can be detected in the sign inverting bipolar; vice versa, when

the light is switched OFF, a depolarization can be recorded in the sign conserving bipolar. In the majority of cases a bipolar cell will make synapses with a number of photoreceptor cells and will also receive input from horizontal cells. Consequently, it will be influenced by light on a small patch of retina. This is defined as its **receptive field** (**RF**). The synaptic interactions in the web of connections beneath the receptive field are, as we noted above, extremely difficult to analyse. Suffice it to say that, in general, a bipolar cell which generates an ON response when the centre of its RF is illuminated, gives an OFF response when the periphery of its RF is illuminated. Vice versa, when a bipolar gives an OFF response at the centre, stimulation of periphery generates ON responses. It is believed that it is principally the horizontal cells which are responsible for these antagonistic surrounds (Section 17.2.9).

One mechanism believed to be at work is shown in Figure 17.18. It has been shown that, in the dark, cone pedicles release glutamate on to the horizontal cells keeping them in a depolarized state. In this state they release an inhibitory transmitter onto

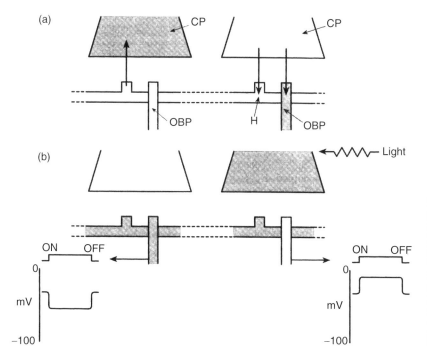

Figure 17.18 Centre–surround interaction. (a) In the dark. Horizontal cell inhibits central cone. Sign inverting bipolar is depolarized. (b) Illumination of peripheral cone leads to inhibition of horizontal cell and release from inhibition of central cone. Sign inverting (ON) bipolar hyperpolarizes. Explanation in text. unstippled = depolarization; stippled = hyperpolarization; CP = cone pedicle; H = horizontal cell; OBP = 'ON' bipolar.

neighbouring cone pedicles. This makes them less de-polarized than they otherwise would be in the dark. When a light is switched on at the periphery of the RF, release of glutamate from the peripheral cone pedicles is reduced, the horizontal cell hyperpolar-izes, the release of glutamate on to the centre cone pedicles is reduced and they consequently depolar-ize. The sign inverting (ON) bipolar is, consequently, inhibited by the release of extra amounts of gluta-mate from the pedicle. If both centre and periphery of the field are illuminated at the same time, similar arguments show that activity in both centre and pe-ripheral bipolars is reduced. This is an instance of **lateral inhibition** which, it will be remembered, we first met in the *Limulus* compound eye.

In general, though the division is not clear cut, the axons of bipolar cells with 'ON' responses ter-minate in the outer part of the IPL (sublamina 'b'), whilst those giving 'OFF' responses terminate in the inner part of the IPL (sublamina 'a') (Figure 17.3b). In both cases their terminals synapse with amacrine and ganglion cell dendrites. We shall return to a dis-cussion of RFs when we come to consider the elec-trophysiology of ganglion cells (Section 17.2.8).

17.2.4 Müller Cells

This is the place to describe the only type of glial cell present in the retina: the **Müller cell** (Figure 17.19). We have already seen that these cells play an important role in the embryology of the retina (Section 16.2). In the adult retina they remain impor-tant. They provide both structural and biochemical support. Their basal end feet, adjacent to the vitre-ous humour, are coupled by tight junctions to form the impenetrable inner limiting membrane (ILM). Their apices are similarly coupled with each other and with the inner segments of photoreceptors to form the outer limiting membrane (OLM). The neu-ral elements of the retina are thus isolated between these two membranes in a space sometimes called the **inner chamber**. The space between the outer limiting membrane and the pigment epithelium, which is con-sequently called the **outer chamber**, houses the inner and outer segments of the photoreceptors. The apices of the Müller cells, besides forming the OLM, are de-veloped into a multitude of microvilli, which greatly increase the surface area through which materials can

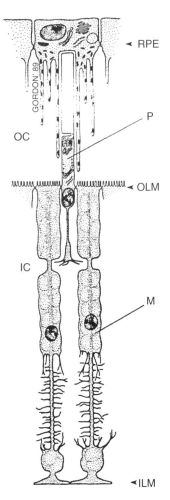

Figure 17.19 Müller cells and the inner and outer chambers of the retina. IC = inner chamber; ILM = inner limiting mem-brane; M = Müller cell; OC = outer chamber; OLM = outer limiting membrane; P = photoreceptor cell; RPE = retinal pig-ment epithelium. From Harding, J.J. (ed.) (1997) *Biochemistry of the Eye*, with permission of Chapman and Hall.

diffuse between the outersegments/RPE and neural retina. The Müller cells are thus believed to play important rôles in the biochemistry of the neural parts of the retina, controlling flows of nutriment, acting as sinks into which potassium extruded dur-ing electrophysiological activity can be taken up, and probably having a role (as noted in Section 17.2.1) in the transformation of all-trans retinol derived from cones back into 11-cis retinal.

17.2.5 Interplexiform Cells

These are the rarest and least diversified of all retinal cells. Only two subtypes are known: dopaminergic and glycerinergic. They transmit information outwards from the IPL to the OPL where they synapse with bipolars and horizontal cells. They are part of the efferent path by which the brain modulates the activity of the retina. They receive input from amacrine cells in the IPL and from efferent fibres from the brain.

17.2.6 Amacrine Cells

In contrast to the interplexiform cells, amacrine cells are the most diversified of all the retina's neurons. They are axon-less cells and are classified on the branching patterns of their dendritic trees. Forty three distinct subtypes have been identified in the roach (*Rutilus rutilus*) and at least 26 subtypes are recognized in the primate retina. Like the horizontal cells of the OPL, amacrine cells run in the plane of the IPL and form an extremely complex branching, interconnected (by gap junctions), network. They receive input from bipolar cells. It appears that bipolar cells either make two synaptic junctions on an amacrine or one junction on an amacrine and another on a ganglion cell. Amacrines deliver their output on to the dendritic trees of ganglion cells. Action potentials can occasionally be detected in amacrine cells.

17.2.7 Ganglion Cells

These are also a very diverse group of cells. Although the occasional action potential can be detected in amacrine cells, ganglion cells are the only cells in the retina where action potentials are always found. A classification into subtypes has been made on the basis of both their morphology and their physiology.

17.2.7.1 Histology

Histologists have described many different morphological types. Here we will mention just three: α or M, β or P and W cells. **Alpha or M (for magnocel-** lular) **cells** have large perikarya and large diameter axons and sparsely branched but widely spreading dendritic trees. **Beta or P (for parvocellular) cells** have medium sized perikarya and a more focused dendritic tree. *W cells* have small diameter axons but a wide spreading dendritic arborization.

The electrophysiologist finds that all three morphological types resemble bipolars in having **centre–surround receptive fields**. The large α **ganglion cells** correspond to cells which have, as might be expected, large centre–surround fields. In response to continuous illumination they give quick transient responses. These are known to electrophysiologists as **Y cells** and are believed to signal gross features of an object and, more importantly, its movement. The smaller β **cells** have narrower centre–surround fields and show a more sustained response to illumination. The electrophysiologist classifies these as **X cells**. They are considered to signal fine detail and colour. Finally the **W cells** have slowly-conducting axons and often do not have centre–surround fields at all but merely respond to contrast by increased or decreased firing rates.

The number of ganglion cells found in any unit area of the retina varies greatly. In the central region of the retina they are very numerous and are often piled one above the other to form several layers. Vice versa, the numbers fall off dramatically in the peripheral parts of the retina. This, of course, reflects the fact that whilst there may sometimes be a one-to-one relation between photoreceptor and ganglion cell in the fovea, there is huge convergence of photoreceptors and bipolars onto single ganglion cells at the periphery.

Finally, the axons of the ganglion cells run along the vitreal surface of the retina towards the optic disc. They remain unmyelinated in the interests of maintaining maximum transparency. At the optic disc they plunge inward, through the cribiform plate, to emerge on the other side as the optic nerve. At this point they develop myelin sheaths, which largely accounts for the dramatic increase in diameter of the optic nerve beneath the cribiform plate. Fibres from the lateral retina run to the ipsilateral lateral geniculate nucleus (LGN), with a few going to the superior colliculus; fibres from the nasal retina cross over at the optic chiasma and make their way to the contralateral LGN with, again, a few going to the colliculus (Figure 18.2).

BOX 17.2   MACULAR DEGENERATION

Macular degeneration is a disease that mainly affects the elderly, where it is known as age-related macular degeneration, *AMD*. Because there is a genetic component, it can also, though less frequently, affect younger individuals.

AMD is the leading cause of severe vision loss in those over 60. It affects about 1.5% of people of European descent over the age of 50 and about 10% of those over the age of 75. Epidemiological studies suggest that the principal causes are family history, age and cigarette smoking. The first of these causes shows the importance of genetics (AMD amongst monozygotic twins is 100% and the risk is doubled if AMD occurs in a first degree relative).

There are two major types: wet and dry. In the first type, **wet AMD**, blood vessels start to grow from the choroid beneath the macula. These vessels are very fragile and tend to leak blood and serum; this tends to prise the retina from the underlying chorea. Loss of central vision occurs rapidly. An early symptom is that straight lines begin to appear wavy. Treatment should be sought urgently. The second type, **dry AMD**, occurs when relatively discrete deposits, known as **drusen**, appear in the fundal RPE and gradually increase in numbers and/or fuse. Early signs are blurred vision and increased need of light for reading and so on.

Ophthalmoscopic examination of the fundus of patients suffering from dry AMD shows that the drusen, accumulations of protein and lipid, lie between Bruch's membrane and the RPE. In addition, nearly continuous deposits are laid down in Bruch's membrane itself. Associated with these deposits is the loss of photoreceptors. Whether the association of drusen and photoreceptor loss is causal seems likely, but is not yet proven. It is also not understood why the deposits should be associated with the macula lutea and not with other parts of the retina.

There are various types of early-onset macular degeneration: Stargardt macular degeneration; vitelliform macular degeneration (VMD or Best macular dystrophy); Sorsby's fundus dystrophy (SFD) and so on. The genetic basis for these conditions is now known.

Autosomal Recessive Stagardt Disease. This is the most common early-onset macular degeneration. The incidence is 1/10 000 and the age of onset is between 7 and 12 years. Fortunately, peripheral vision is retained throughout life. Ophthalmoscopic examination of the fundus shows numerous small yellow deposits in or beneath the RPE, which give the condition its alternative name: flavimaculatus. There are several varieties of the disease related to mutations on different genes. The most common form, Stargardt 1, is due to mutations on gene (*ABCR*) on chromosome 1 (1p21-p13) encoding an ABC retinoid transporter (Figure 17.14b). This transporter is located on the membranes of outersegments. It is not only involved in transporting all-trans retinal out of outersegments but also, with the help of retinal dehydrogenase, in facilitating the reduction of all-trans retinal to all-trans retinol. When this transporter is inactivated, two all-trans retinals condense with ethanolamine, derived from the common membrane phosopholipd, phosphatidyl ethanolamine, to form A2E a toxic compound (Figure A.1). In the presence of light, when 11-cis is being continuously transformed into all-trans retinal, A2E accumulates in the RPE. Because the RPE is so close to the highly vascular choroid (Section 16.3.4) there is an abundance of oxygen and this reacts with A2E to generate free radicals. These radicals attack the RPE cells in which A2E has accumulated and their loss leads, in turn, to loss of photoreceptor cells.

Vitelliform Macular Degeneration (VMD; Best Macular Dystrophy). This is caused by the mutation of a dominant gene (*VMD2*) on chromosome 11 (11q13). The age of onset varies from very early childhood to adolescence and later. The *VMD2* gene encodes a membrane protein known as bestrophin, which turns out to be an anion channel. The ophthalmoscope shows that large quantities of yellow

(*Continues*)

(*Continued*)

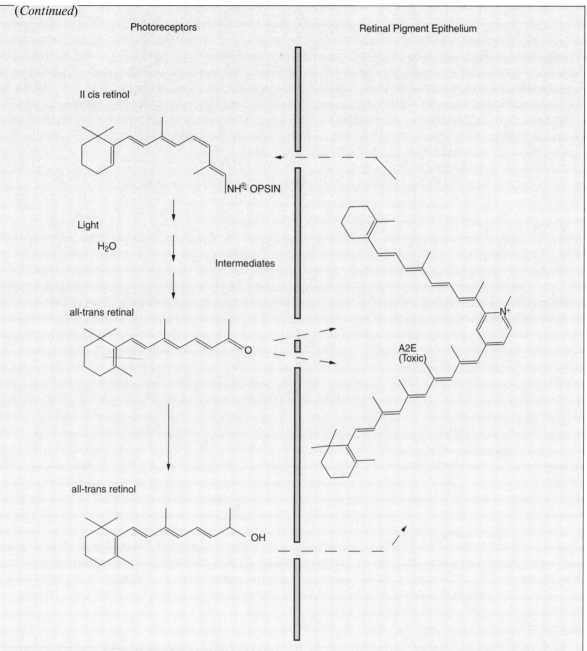

Figure A.1 Biochemical basis of Stagardt early onset macular degeneration. A mutation disrupts the reduction of all-trans retinal to all-trans retinol. All-trans retinal consequently accumulates in the RPE, where it condenses with ethanolamine to form A2E leading to the production of dangerous free radicals. Further explanation in text. Modified from Rattner and Nathans, 2006.

(*Continues*)

(*Continued*)

pigment accumulate in or just beneath the RPE centred on the macula, which is, again, associated with photoreceptor loss.

Sorsby's Fundus Dystrophy (SFD). The gene (*TIMP3*) on chromosome 22 (22q12-q13.2), which when mutated leads to SFD, normally codes for a metalloproteinase, which is important in regulating the extracellular matrix. The age of onset, from 13 to 40 years of age, is much later than in the previous two macular degenerations. The symptoms include a massive thickening of Bruch's membrane. This suggests that the defective metalloproteinase is normally concerned with the turnover of proteins in that membrane. The consequent thickening of Bruch's membrane might well prevent the diffusion of nutrients, especially Vitamin A, to the photoreceptor cells.

There are, as mentioned above, several other types of genetically induced macular degeneration and these are well described in the literature indicated below, especially Rattner and Nathans (2007).

Are there any treatments? Laser surgery has been used to destroy the fragile vessels of wet AMD and break up the drusen particles in dry AMD but these treatments only affect the symptoms and do not prevent a recurrence and further progress of the disease. Pharmacological interventions have also been developed. Drugs can either be injected systemically or directly into the eye that destroy the errant blood vessels of wet AMD and/or prevent their growth. The ingestion of Vitamin A has been found effective in early stages of Sorsby's dystrophy.

Fortunately, several genetically-engineered mouse 'models' now exist where conditions analogous to those found in humans can be studied. Additionally, a colony of Macaques has been identified which show early-onset macular degeneration histologically indistinguishable from that found in the human retina. Hopefully, studies of these animal models will assist neuroscientists in finding the underlying causes and thus suggest a therapy for what is a disheartening and disabling disease.

REFERENCES

National Eye Institute at http://www.nei.nih.gov/health/maculardegen/armd_facts.asp.

Rattner, A. and Nathans, J. (2006) Macular degeneration: recent advances and therapeutic opportunities. *Nature Reviews Neuroscience*, **7**, 860–72.

17.2.7.2 Physiology

The major physiological classification of ganglion cells in the Primate retina is, as we have already seen, into '**ON' centre**, '**OFF' centre** and '**ON/OFF' centre** types but there are several others and non-primate retinae sometimes show a great diversity. All three types pf receptive field (like those of bipolars) have **antagonistic centre–surround** organization. Switching a light ON at the centre of an ON field will generate a burst of activity in the ganglion cell. Conversely, switching a light ON at the periphery of the field will inhibit any random activity in the cell and only when the light is switched OFF is there a burst of action potentials. Vice versa, switching a light ON at the centre of an OFF field will inhibit any ongoing activity and only when it is switched off is there a tattoo of impulses; switching it ON at the periphery initiates a burst of activity. These characteristics are shown in Figure 17.20.

There are several points to note about this RF electrophysiology. Firstly, ganglion cells only fire in response to changing illumination. In constant conditions little activity is found in their axons. Secondly, the centre–surround antagonism ensures that, if light falls on both centre and surround, the ON and OFF responses tend to cancel each other out. Diffuse light falling equally all over the whole of one of these concentric fields thus causes very little activity in the cell.

The RFs are organized to detect change of illumination across the field: edges of shadows, boundaries of moving images and so on. We found the same design principle in the compound eye of *Limulus* and other arthropods discussed in Chapter 15.

Can we go further and account for these receptive field characteristics in terms of retinal 'wiring diagrams'? Before taking up this challenge we should note that another, and quite different, class of ganglion cells has recently come to light: the 'intrinsically photosensitive retinal ganglion cell' (ipRGC).

The discovery of this new class of ganglion cells emerged from studies of the entrainment of circadian rhythms. These rhythms are synchronized from a 'master clock' in the hypothalamus but this clock require information about photoperiod from the eyes. If this information is blocked, the master clock loses contact with the diurnal light–dark cycle and circadian rhythms soon run out of phase with sun-up and sun-down. But how does the retina communicate with the suprachiasmatic nucleus in the hypothalamus? Experiments with mice genetically-engineered to lack rods and cones show that these photoreceptors are not necessary for this communication. It was ultimately shown that a small group of ganglion cells, some 1–2%, are intrinsically light-sensitive, these are the 'intrinsically photosensitive retinal ganglion cells' or ipRGCs. They contain a light-absorbing pigment – melanopsin – which, when activated by light, leads to the depolarization of the ganglion cell membrane and hence a signal to the suprachiasmatic nucleus. As noted in Box 15.1, this, and the fact that melanopsin is more closely related to invertebrate opsins than to those found in the vertebrates, has suggested that ganglion cells originated as rhabdomeric photoreceptors.

Photic stimulation is, however, not the only way in which the ipRGCs are activated. It can be shown that elimination of melanopsin does not completely eliminate light-induced signals. Complete inhibition of the ipRGCs only occurs when both melanopsin and the rods and cones are eliminated. It turns out that ipRGCs can be subdivided into three types and that the first two types receive innervation from amacrine cells, whilst the third type is innervated by interplexiform cells. It seems, therefore, that the retinal signals which align circadian rhythms with photoperiod are generated by light acting directly on ipRGC melanopsin, supplemented by light-stimulated photoreceptors acting through amacrine and interplexiform cells.

17.2.8 Wiring Diagrams

Let us now return to the 'circuit diagrams' responsible for the different receptive fields of ganglion cells. There have been many attempts to understand the functioning of the retina in terms of its synaptic organization. These have become more sophisticated as more has become known of its synaptic interconnexity and pharmacology. We saw in Section 17.2.4, that whilst the bipolars synapsing with cone pedicles may be either sign inverting or sign conserving, those synapsing with rod spherules are always sign inverting. Yet both cones and rods induce centre–surround fields in underlying ganglion cells. Let us consider each case in turn and then conclude by putting them together to form a tentative retinal 'wiring diagram'.

17.2.8.1 *Cone Pathway*

The ON bipolars make glutaminergic synapses with the dendritic arbors of ON ganglion cells in the outer layer of the IPL (sublamina b). OFF bipolars make glutaminergic synapses with arbors of OFF ganglion cells distributed in the inner sublamina of the IPL (sublamina a). This organization has been shown to

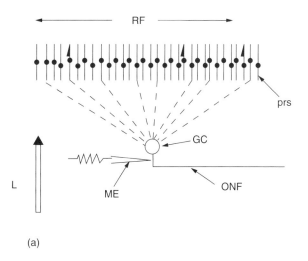

(a)

Figure 17.20   (a) (*caption opposite*)

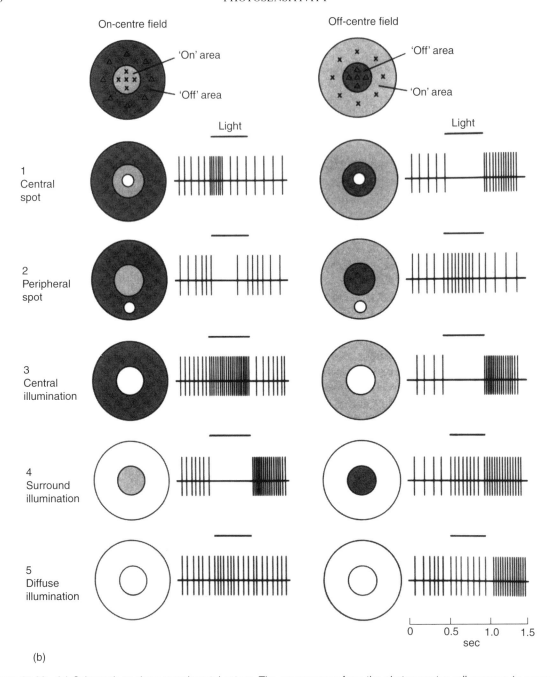

(b)

Figure 17.20 (a) Schematic to show experimental set up. The convergence from the photoreceptor cell array on to a ganglion cell is shown by the broken lines. GC = ganglion cell; L = light probe; ME = microelectrode; ONF = optic nerve fibre; prs = photoreceptor cells; RF = receptive field. (b) The characteristics of 'ON' and 'OFF' centre receptive fields. The white part of the RF signifies the illuminated area. To the right of each RF is the activity in the ganglion cell. The duration of the light stimulus is indiated by the bar. Note case 5 where, in both instances, diffuse illumination over entire field generates only a weak response in the ganglion cell. This is due to lateral inhibition (that is centre–surround antagonism). From Kandel, E.R., Schwartz, J.H. and Jessel, T.M. (eds) (1991) *Principles of Neuroscience*, with permission from Elsevier.

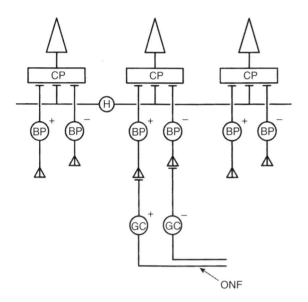

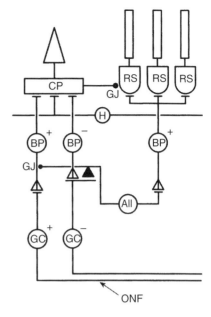

Figure 17.21 The characteristics of the 'ON' and 'OFF' ganglion cells are due to the action of the horizontal cells (Figure 17.18) on the cone pedicle. The ganglion cells share the centre–surround characteristics of their bipolars. BP^+ = ON bipolar; BP^- = OFF bipolar; CP = cone pedicle; GC^+ = ON centre ganglion cell; GC^- = OFF centre ganglion cell; ONF = optic nerve fibre.

Figure 17.22 Interconnections of rods, cones and ganglion cells. The rod bipolar does not communicate directly with the ganglion cell but via the AII amacrine cell and the cone bipolars. Note the gap junction made by the cone pedicle and the rod spherule and the inhibitory (black) synapse made by the AII amacrine on the GC^- dendrite. Explanation in text. AII = AII amacrine cell; BP^+ = ON bipolar; BP^- = OFF bipolar; CP = cone pedicle; GC^+ = ON centre ganglion cell; GC^- = OFF centre ganglion cell; GJ = gap junction; H = horizontal cell; ONF = optic nerve fibre; RS = rod spherule. After Schiller, P.H. (1992) and Nakanishi, S. (1995).

be highly regular. There have been several proposals for the antagonistic surround. The consensus is that this surround is due to the inhibitory activity of horizontal cells. We noted the synaptic characteristics of horizontal cells in Section 17.2.3. It follows from those characteristics that when an ON centre ganglion cell is stimulated, stimulation of its surround will be antagonistic; similarly with an OFF centre ganglion cell. A highly schematized diagram of the wiring is shown in Figure 17.21. It should be borne in mind that other wirings have been proposed and the situation in the retina is undoubtedly more complicated than the schematic shown in the figure.

17.2.8.2 Rod Pathway

Rods make glutaminergic synapses with (exclusively) sign inverting bipolars. Usually (especially in the peripheral retina) rod bipolars synapse with a comparatively large number of rod spherules. They do

not synapse directly with ganglion cells but with AII amacrine cells in the IPL (Figure 17.22). This synapse is sign conserving. The AII cells, in turn, make glycerinergic (that is inhibitory) synapses with OFF ganglion cells and gap junctions (excitatory electrical synapses) with ON bipolars. This organization ensures that (under dark adapted conditions when the cones are inoperative) increases in illumination will activate the ON ganglion cells and decreases in illumination will activate (or at any rate release from inhibition) the OFF ganglion cells. Once again the antagonistic surround is created by the activity of horizontal cells.

The pedicles of rod and cone cells make gap junctions (that is electrical synapses) with each other (Figure 17.22). It is found that signals generated by rod cells can be detected in cone cells. During prolonged dark adaptation these gap junctions close, thus confining any signal to the rod pathway. This has the effect of increasing the sensitivity of the retina, as the rod pathway (Figure 17.22) activates ON ganglion cells and inhibits OFF cells. In other words, signals from the inhibitory surround are switched off. The retina thus loses its ability to detect contrast and instead becomes extremely sensitive to general illumination. A fully dark-adapted retina can detect single photons.

The wiring diagrams of Figures 17.21 and 17.22 are huge oversimplifications of the true situation in the retina. It has already been mentioned that neuro-histologists recognize more than fifty different sub-types of cell in the neural retina and neurobiologists are coming to understand that each neuron is an individual with its own 'personality'. Most of the two dozen or so neurotransmitters and neuromodulators known to neuroscience have also been detected in the retina, as have a great and ever increasing variety of receptor molecules. Nevertheless, the diagrams given in this section show that the main outlines of the system are beginning to emerge through the overwhelming complexity of detail.

One of the most interesting new developments has been to use the full panoply of modern genetics to dissect and analyse the retina of the zebrafish, *Danio rerio*. We saw in Box 15.2 how genetics was throwing fascinating new light on the early stages in the development (and evolution) of vertebrate and other eyes. This application of the powerful techniques of genetics is somewhat different. The zebrafish is an ideal and much used organism in neurogenetics. It has a well developed retina with four types of cone in addition to rods. It is a far more visual animal than the mouse, the only other vertebrate whose genetics is similarly well understood. Zebrafish are easily kept, have a rapid generation time, transparent larvae and their 1.7Gb genome has been completely sequenced. Large numbers of mutants with different types of visual defect have been isolated and work is rapidly determining where and how the retina has been affected. The power of modern genetics strongly suggests that the retina of *Danio rerio* will be the first to be understood from molecule to totality. The interested student (and it is a fascinating subject, for the retina as we have already noted is a portion of the brain pushed to the exterior and for this reason

highly 'approachable') can find more detail in the references listed in the bibliography.

17.2.9 Colour

We saw in Section 17.2.1 that the discrimination between different wavelengths (the discrimination of colour) depends on the presence in the (human) retina of three different populations of cones: responding to blue (λ_{max}: 419 nm), green (λ_{max}: 531 nm) and red (λ_{max}: 559 nm). It might be thought (indeed was thought for many years) that the sensation of colour was created by the brain on receipt of information along these 'labelled lines'. However, it turns out the situation is very far from being that simple. Several features in our experience of colour cannot be explained by this simple idea.

First, it is found that certain colours cancel each other in such a way that a mixture is never experienced. For instance, although we can see mixtures of red and yellow (orange) well enough, or blue and green (cyan), mixtures of red and green can be so arranged that no remnant of either colour can be perceived and a pure yellow results. Similarly, yellow and blue can be mixed so that a pure white is seen. This is very peculiar and in order to explain it Ewald Hering proposed a theory of **opponent processes**. He suggested that the three primary colours are processed in the visual system as antagonistic or 'opponent' pairs: red/green; yellow/blue; white/black. Stimulation of one opponent induces excitation (or inhibition) whilst stimulation of the other opponent induces inhibition (or excitation). Hence, when the stimuli are properly balanced, when, for example, appropriate quantities of red and green light are provided, the different parts of that channel cancel out and the system engenders a yellow sensation. This processing probably starts in the retina but continues in the lateral geniculate bodies and in the visual cortex.

Restricting ourselves to the retina, it has been possible to demonstrate the presence of ganglion cells in the cat retina which have these colour opponent properties. In the instance shown in Figure 17.23, two ganglion cells are shown, one with a concentric RF with the centre giving ON responses to red and the surround giving OFF responses to green, and

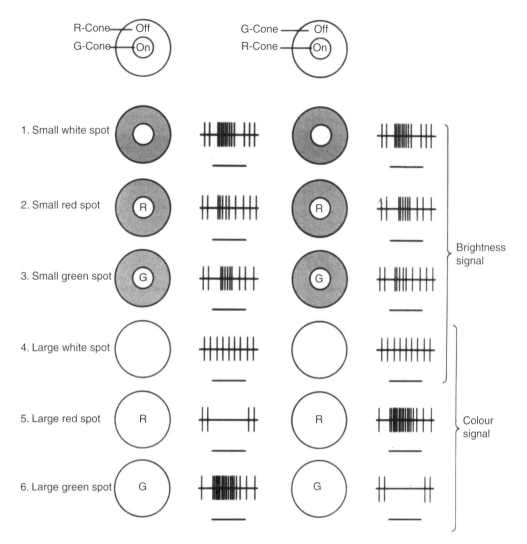

Figure 17.23 Receptive fields of single colour opponent cells in the cat's retina. Both types of cell are excited by small white spots in the centre of the field, The best responses to colour are given in cases 5 and 6 where large red or green spots cover the whole of the field. From Kandel, E.R., Schwartz, J.H. and Jessel, T.M. (eds) (1991) *Principles of Neuroscience*, with permission from Elsevier.

the other giving ON responses to green at the centre and OFF responses to red at the periphery. Cells of this type do not provide the brain with very reliable colour information. The brain would be hard put to discriminate between a small bright white spot at the centre of the RF and a large green spot covering the whole field (Figure 17.23).

The retinal pathways responsible for colour opponency such as that shown in Figure 17.23 are still being worked out. It is clear, however, that the sensation of colour, which seems so immediate and unchallengeable to us, is due to intricate interactions, not only in the retina, but at all levels in the visual system.

17.3 CONCLUDING REMARKS

The retina, as we noted at the outset of this chapter and in Section 16.2 of the last, is a portion of the brain pushed to the periphery. In this chapter we have looked at some of its intricacies, from the level of molecules to the level of 'wiring diagrams'. We have, indeed, seen that biologists are well advance in tracing its functioning all the way down to the molecular level. Although much remains to be understood, especially in the intricacies of its wiring and synaptology, we are well on the way to a seamless theory. If this research can be maintained, it will be the first part of the brain to yield up such a total understanding. The implications of such an ultimate theory are immense.

Yet the problem remains formidable. The retina is organized in both vertical and horizontal dimensions. Diffuse bipolar cells may contact and bring together activity in up to ten distinct cone pedicles and focus it on to a ganglion cell; midget bipolars, on the other hand, often provide a precise 1 : 1 pathway to a ganglion cell and thus an optic nerve fibre. Horizontal and amacrine cells cut across this vertical stream and modulate its transmissions. In this way the retina can be said to exhibit both parallel and hierarchical processing. This, at the periphery, is a foretaste of what occurs centrally. We shall see, in Chapter 18, that the more than two dozen extrastriate visual cortices in the primate are connected both 'upwards', 'downwards' and 'cross-ways'. In the retina we can study, a little, the intricate mixture of parallel and hierarchical processing which is a feature, on a much greater scale, of the brain itself.

The complexity does not, moreover, end there. Unlike the clean 'on'/'off' relays of computer hardware, the 'wetware' of the brain works with complex cocktails of neurochemicals. GABA, glutamate, ACh, dopamine, serotonin, somatostatin and so on are all present, and many more. Some are excitatory, some inhibitory, some modulatory. The receptors on which they operate are also many and various. The techniques of contemporary molecular biology have been applied to clone many of these receptor proteins and to show not only their structural variety but also the dynamic state of synthesis and degradation which perpetually varies their population profile and hence the receptivity of postsynaptic membranes to multi-ingredient cocktails of neurochemicals. This portion of the brain pushed to the periphery may be simple compared to the cererbral cortex but its complexity will provide a challenge to scientists for many years to come.

It must always be borne in mind, furthermore, that the human retina is just one instance amongst many. It is one instance of a primate retina (and these are very various) and primates are just one among the many orders of mammals (Chapter 4). Widening the focus still further, mammalian retinae form but a small subsection of the great range of vertebrate retina. We shall touch on some of these nonmammalian retinae in Chapter 19. There we shall see that the extremes represented by the deep-sea fish and predatory birds have evolved fascinating modifications on the comparatively unspecialized retinae that we and our fellow primates possess.

However, there is one feature in which primate retinae outperform other mammalian retinae (though not, it must be said, a number of nonmammalian vertebrates) and, that is colour vision. We saw in Section 17.2.9 that colour vision in the human retina depends (initially) on the presence of three distinct cone pigments. Primates are alone among mammals in having three pigments. All the rest develop only two. Roughly speaking they have a short wave pigment and a long wave pigment. The dog, for instance, a typical dichromat, has one cone pigment with a $\lambda_{max} = 450$ nm and another with $\lambda_{max} = 555$ nm. The domestic cat is also a dichromat, with a short wave and a long wave cone pigment. Unlike the dog, however, it has so far not proved possible to demonstrate colour vision in the cat by behavioural testing. Why should humans and the other primates share the lonely distinction of trichromaticity? The most plausible answer, as noted in Section 17.2.1, has to do with the pressing need, during their evolution in the forest canopies, to correctly evaluate the ripeness or otherwise of tropical fruits. We saw in Section 17.2.1 that the evolutionary event leading to the development of a green cone opsin, between the long wave red and the short wave blue opsins, is believed to have occurred some 40 million years ago when the early primates were accustoming themselves to a largely frugivorous arboreal life. Indeed, recent research indicates the presence of trichromaticity in some species of diurnal prosimians, the early ancestors of monkeys, apes and humans.

Although other mammalian retinae cannot compete with primate retinae in numbers of cone opsins, they are often specialized in other ways. In many cases, for instance the rabbit, and *a fortiori* in many nonmammalian vertebrates, far more information processing occurs in the retina than occurs in that of the primates. In the rabbit's retina it is possible to find ganglion cells responsive to a large variety of trigger stimuli, not merely the simple spots of light characteristic of primate and feline retinae.

Ganglion cells triggered by moving edges (local edge detectors), edges of specific orientations, moving in certain directions and ganglion cells, whose receptive fields are tuned to respond to other and often very specific trigger features, are to be found. In the primates and the cat, cells responding to these specialized trigger features are confined to the visual cortex. We shall discuss some instances in the next chapter. It is as if the rabbit needs to process quickly and simply the data which less hunted forms can consider more deliberately. However this may be, it is to the visual analysers in primate and feline cortices that we turn in the next chapter.

18

VISUAL PATHWAYS AND CORTICES

Advanced primates have more than two dozen interconnected visual cortices and three visual pathways. Evolutionary considerations. **Retino-tectal pathway**: partial decussation - superior colliculus - map of visual space - saccadic eye movements. **Retino-geniculo-striate (RGS) pathway**: optic disc - cribriform plate - optic nerve - partial decussation - optic tract - dorsal lateral geniculate nucleus (LGNd) - lamination, histology, cortifugal innervation - RFs of geniculate cells - M, P and W fibres - M motion sensitive, P colour sensitive - optic radiations - Meyer's loop - pathologies. **Primary visual (=striate) cortex (V1)**: location - magnitude - lamination - stripe of Gennari; micro-electrode recording - RFs of cortical cells - layer IVc circular - other layers edge detectors - putative 'wiring'; classification of RFs into simple, complex and 'end-stopped' (hypercomplex); biological significance; columnar organisation - deoxyglucose histology and edge detectors - cytochrome oxidase histology and blob/interblob organisation - colour sensitivity (blobs) - double-opponency; ocular dominance columns - stereopsis; hypercolumns and aggegate RFs (ARFs) - variation in size of ARFs - non-isomorphous map of retina in V1; population responses and disambiguation. Plasticity: sensitive periods - kitten - macaque, **Extrastriate cortices**: maps of different features of visual input - input from pulvinar as well as V1 - three information streams - cytochrome exidase staining of V2 - thick stripe (M-stream), thin stripe (P-stream) - large areas of primate cortex involved in vision. **Face recognition**: importance for social primates - macaque IT cortex - hand and face recognition cells - iconic patterns - columnar organisation - population response. **Prosopagnosia**: importance of face recognition for humans - neuroanatomy - prosopagnosiac symptoms. **Concluding remarks**: intricacy of cortical analysers - significance of vision - hopes for the future and for the present.

In this chapter we shall consider the way in which visual information from the retina is transmitted to the primary visual (= striate) cortex. We shall, as in the previous two chapters, concentrate our attention on the primate and, in particular, the human system. It must be emphasized at the outset that the primary visual cortex is not the only visual cortex in the primate brain. Studies of the macaque brain have shown there to be upwards of two dozen cortices devoted to various aspects of the analysis of vision. All of these cortices are, moreover, intricately interconnected both 'forward' and 'backward'. It is not possible to discuss the central analysis of vision without alluding to them; equally it is not possible in a book

Biology of Sensory Systems, Second Edition   C.U.M. Smith
© 2008 John Wiley & Sons, Ltd

of this nature to treat them all in detail. This chapter will take the story no further than the first cortex, the striate or primary visual cortex. Only brief accounts of some of the salient features of the extrastriate cortices will be included.

18.1 VISUAL PATHWAYS INTO THE BRAIN

The pathway to the striate cortex, the so-called **retino-geniculo-striate** (**RGS**) pathway, is not the only pathway from the retina into the brain in mammals. Two other less important pathways exist: a pathway from the retina directly via the optic chiasma to the superior colliculus (**retino-tectal** pathway) and a multisynaptic pathway via the hypothalamus and superior cervical ganglion to the **pineal**. The former pathway is more important in nonmammalian vertebrates. It will be discussed more fully in Chapter 19 but it is nevertheless appropriate here to sketch an appealing evolutionary scenario.

In the anamniotes – the fish and amphibia – the major visual area is developed in the midbrain, the mesencephalon. The roof of this part of the brain, the **tectum**, becomes strongly developed to analyse the visual information. It also receives input from other senses. This so-called retino-tectal or tectofugal pathway remains the predominant route in the reptiles (Chapter 19). In the mammals this part of the brain has a much reduced importance, being almost completely overshadowed by the hugely developed cerebral hemispheres. Four small swellings, the **superior and inferior colliculi**, are all that remains of the well developed tecta of the fish and amphibia. The tectofugal pathway is correspondingly reduced in importance.

Why have the mammals changed their visual system? The appealing evolutionary scenario mentioned above suggests that during the long age of the Mesozoic era when the early mammals shared the globe as somewhat downtrodden competitors of the 'ruling reptiles', especially the dinosaurs, they were forced into a hidden, crepuscular, almost subterranean existence. The visual sense took a very subsidiary place to olfaction, gustation and the auditory sense. The chemical senses, which remain redolent with emotional colouring in us today, run to the forebrain and thence into the limbic system. The suggestion is

that the forebrain consequently assumed enhanced importance. When, for whatever reason – meteoric impact, supernova explosion, global cooling – the ruling reptile fauna became extinct at the end of the Mesozoic era, the world opened to the long suffering proto-mammals. They radiated out into all the possible niches afforded by this freshly vacated environment. Vision once again became, for most, an all important sense. But, starting afresh, a new visual pathway could be constructed to what was now the most important part of the brain, the forebrain, expanding, as it was, to form the characteristically mammalian cerebral hemispheres. Whilst the retino-tectal pathway remained as a remnant of the old way, the retino-geniculo-striate pathway quickly became the most important route for visual information into the brain.

18.1.1 The Retino-Tectal Pathway

Although, as indicated above, this pathway is more significant in nonmammalian vertebrates and, as such, will be discussed more fully in Chapter 19, it is appropriate to outline its significance in the mammalian visual system at this point. Optic nerve fibres run from the retina in the optic nerves (Section 18.3) to the chiasma where, in primates, they undergo a partial decussation. Fibres from the nasal retina cross over to the contralateral colliculus, whilst those from the temporal retina run to the ipsilateral colliculus (Figure 18.1). In many nonprimate mammals, in contrast, there is either a complete or nearly complete decussation.

The superior colliculus is generally regarded as consisting of seven layers of cells. It is not only concerned with vision. Its evolutionary origin ensures that it also receives input from the other senses. This sensory input is organized into maps. There are three such maps – visual, somatosensory and auditory – one above the other. The visual map is derived partly from direct input from the retina and partly from input from the visual cortex (Section 18.3). The map has a different organizational principle from that found in the visual cortex. Instead of representing the retina in a nonisomorphous but topologically accurate manner, it represents visual space around the animal. The other sensory maps – somatosensory and auditory- are organized on the same principle

Complete decussation

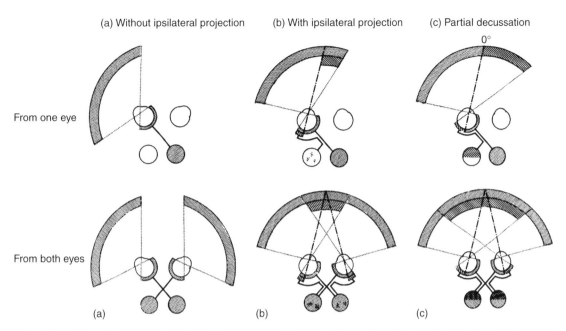

Figure 18.1 Schematic diagram to show three different types of decussation in the retino-tectal pathway in different mammals. In (a) there is complete decussation. This condition is found in the Microchiroptera. In (b) there is only a small ipsilateral component. This condition is found in a number of mammals including squirrels, cats, rabbits and so on. Finally (c), in primates (and Megachiropteran bats) the entire temporal hemifield of the retina runs to the ipsilateral superior colliculus. The stippled areas represent ipsilateral projections and the hatched areas contralateral projections. Modified from Henry and Vidyasgar (1991).

and lie, point for point, one below the other in the colliculus. An account of the intensively studied map of auditory space in the barn owl's inferior colliculus is given in Section 10.3. In the deepest layers of the colliculus lies yet another map: a motor map. The sensory maps feed into this motor map to control the **saccadic eye movements** which direct the gaze at significant features of the visual field. This highly important function is carried out in collaboration with a region of the frontal cortex known as the frontal eye field.

18.1.2 The Retino-Geniculo-Striate (RGS) Pathway

Let us now turn to and discuss in some detail the major visual pathway in mammals: the retino-geniculo-striate pathway. In Chapter 17 we left the optic nerve fibres (the axons of the ganglion cells) cours-

ing across the vitreal surface of the retina towards the optic disc. In the human retina the disc is a somewhat elliptical area with a vertical diameter of about 1.86 mm and a horizontal diameter of 1.75 mm. Its centre is about 4 mm medial and 0.8 mm superior to the foveola (Figure 17.2b). Although there is always a small depression, a 'physiological cup', this is much increased in cases of glaucoma, where the intraocular pressure (IOP) is above normal (Chapter 16). In these cases the ophthalmoscope shows that the disc is markedly depressed inwards towards the optic nerve. This so-called 'cupping', a diagnostic feature of a raised IOP, shows that the disc is a weak spot in the eyeball's design. If not treated, the optic nerve is damaged. When the IOP is normal, this mechanical weakness is counteracted by a mesh of collagen fibres, the **cribriform plate**, which grows from the sclera just beneath the disc. The optic nerve fibres gathered in the optic disc plunge inwards through the cribriform plate to form the optic nerve.

18.1.2.1 *Optic Nerve*

Once through the cribriform plate, oligodendrocytes wind myelin sheaths around the optic nerve fibres. Other glial cells and connective tissue cells form septa between groups of optic nerve fibres, collecting them into fasciculi. Numerous blood vessels from the pia run through these septa bringing nutriment to the optic nerve fibres. Myelination of the fibres and the presence of connective tissue septa markedly increase the size of the optic nerve so that it averages about 3 mm in diameter compared with the approximately 1.8 mm of the disc. To begin with, the fibres are distributed in the optic nerve much as they are in the retina. The foveal fibres which form about a third of the optic nerve fibres are at first laterally placed but, as they approach the chiasma, they move to a central position. At the chiasma, in primates, there is a **partial decussation** (Figure 18.2). The fibres from the nasal half of the retina, including those from the nasal half of the fovea, cross the midline and proceed to the **dorsal** part of the contralateral **lateral geniculate nucleus (LGNd)**. Those from the temporal half of the retina, including those from the lateral half of the fovea, stay on the same side and proceed to the dorsal part of the ipsilateral lateral geniculate nucleus.

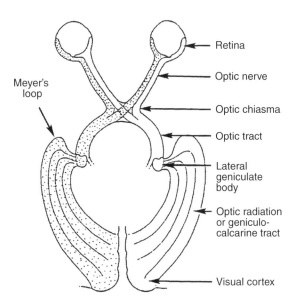

Figure 18.2   Visual pathway. Note the partial decussation at the chiasma.

From the chiasma to the LGNd the visual pathway is known as the **optic tract**. As it proceeds towards the lateral geniculate nucleus it undergoes a 90° twist so that fibres from the upper retinal quadrants pass to the medial side and those from the lower retinal quadrants move to the lateral side. It is here that fibres from corresponding parts of each of the two retinae become associated with each other. The two optic tracts terminate in the lateral geniculate nuclei.

18.1.2.2 *Lateral Geniculate Nuclei*

These nuclei (or bodies) are located in the posterior part of the thalamus. Their dorsal parts (LGNd) have a distinctive laminated structure (Figure 18.3). This has often been likened to a stack of hats, one inside the other. In primates there are six layers of cells separated by bands of fibres. It is here that the optic nerve fibres (the axons, it will be remembered, of the retinal ganglion cells) terminate. Because of the partial decussation described above (Figure 18.2), nerve fibres come from the temporal half of the ipsilateral eye and the nasal half of the contralateral eye. The LGNd maintains a strict segregation of these fibres. The fibres from the contralateral eye terminate in layers 1, 4 and 6, whilst those from the ipsilateral eye terminate in layers 2, 3 and 5. The fibres make synapses with a second set of neurons which, forming the **optic radiations**, carry the visual information on to the primary visual cortex.

How precise the connectivity is remains a matter of debate. It is known, however, that optic nerve fibres divide into up to six branches, making synapses with six separate neurons in the **same layer** of the LGNd. One geniculate neuron, vice versa, may synapse with more than one incoming optic nerve fibre. Connector neurons are also present running between neurons in a single lamina. The separation of the input from the two eyes is, however, maintained. Finally, there is a significant innervation from the visual cortex (**corticofugal innervation**). This has a powerful feedback function. The LGNd cannot, therefore, be considered a simple junction box.

Let us now return to the fibres in the optic nerve and tract. We noted in Section 17.2.8 that these fibres could be classified into two major and one minor group: magnocellular (M) fibres, parvocellular (P) fibres and W fibres. The M pathway, which carries information mostly pertaining to movement of

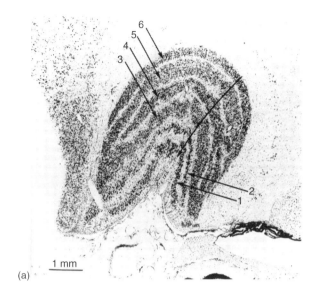

(a)

1 mm

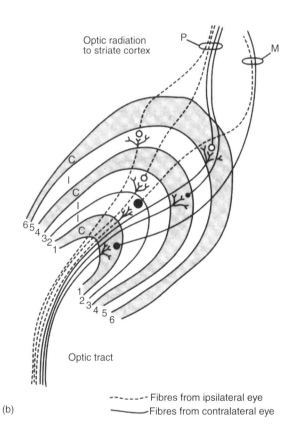

Optic radiation
to striate cortex

P

M

C

I

C

I

I

C

6 5 4 3 2 1

1 2 3 4 5 6

Optic tract

(b)

- - - - - Fibres from ipsilateral eye
———— Fibres from contralateral eye

the visual image, terminates in layers 1 and 2 of the LGNd (the magnocellular layers) whilst the P pathway, mostly concerned with colour information, terminates in layers 3, 4, 5 and 6 (the parvocellular layers). These cells can be investigated by microelectrode recording. As would be expected, they respond to illumination of appropriate patches of the retina. These patches are consequently said to constitute the **receptive fields** of the geniculate cells. In layers 1 and 2 the receptive fields have a 'colour blind' centre–surround organization similar to the centre–surround fields of alpha ganglion cells. These cells are highly sensitive to motion in their RFs. Receptive fields with similar characteristics can, indeed, be found throughout the LGNd's six layers. But in the upper layers, as would be expected from the parvocellular input, the cells are mostly responsive to colour. Layers 3 and 4 are dominated by OFF-centre blue/yellow (or, better, blue/red + green) opponent cells, whereas in layers 5 and 6 ON-centre red/green opponent cells predominate. The narrow diameter slowly-conducting axons of the W cells project to the parvocellular layers.

18.1.2.3 Optic Radiation (= Geniculo-Calcarine Tract)

Fibres originating in the lateral geniculate nuclei run to the primary visual cortex, which occupies the calcarine sulcus in the medial surface of the occipital lobe. Neurons in the lateral part of the LGNd (receiving input from the inferior retinal quadrants (superior quandrants of the visual field)) send their axons out laterally around the anterior tip of the temporal horn of the lateral ventricle to form **Meyer's loop**.

Figure 18.3 (*Opposite*) Dorsal lateral geniculate nucleus of primate. (a) The six layers of the primate LGN are well shown in this micrograph. The arrow from layer 6 to layer 1 shows the position of the layered retinotopic maps in the LGN. Cells along the line of this arrow have RFs in the same position in visual space. (b) Diagram to show the 'wiring' of the primate LGN. The six layers are numbered. The first two layers contain cells with large perikarya. They are known as the magnocellular layers. The remaining layers with smaller cells are known as the parvocellular layers. Note the segregation of the orptic tract fibres from contralateral and ipsilateral eyes. Further explanation in text. C = contralateral; I = ipsilateral; M = magnocellular; P = parvocellular.

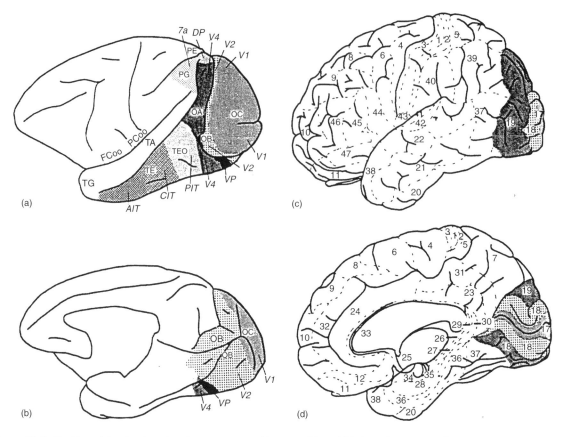

Figure 18.4 Position of the visual cortices in macaques and humans. (a) and (b) show the position of the cortices on the lateral (a) and medial (b) surfaces of the macaque brain. (c) and (d) show the positions of the lateral (c) and medial (d) surfaces of the human brain. The relative sizes of the macaque and human brains are not to scale. The numbers on the human brain are the Brodmann numbers. Seventeen is the primary visual cortex (V1); 18 is the secondary visual cortex (V2). Reprinted, with permission, from the Annual Review of Neuroscience, Volume 19 © 1996 by Annual Reviews www.annualreviews.org.

Geniculate cells which receive their input from the fovea are not much involved in Meyer's loop. They pass almost directly back to the calcarine fissure. These different routes have obvious implications for pathology. Whichever route they take, all the fibres of the optic radiation ultimately terminate in the primary visual cortex.

18.2 PRIMARY VISUAL CORTEX

18.2.1 Structure

In humans the primary visual cortex (Brodmann area 17, V1 or striate cortex) occupies the walls of the deep calcarine fissure in the medial surface of the posterior part of the occipital lobe (Figure 18.4d). It extends posteriorly along the walls of this fissure and a small portion continues on to the postero-lateral aspect of the occipital lobe (Figure 18.4c). Its total area in humans averages about 3000 mm^2.

Clearly it is unethical to carry out experimental investigation of human visual cortices. Most experimental work has consequently been carried out on the Macaque or the domestic cat, *Felis domestica*. Fortunately, in both these animals the visual cortex is far more accessible. The visual cortex of the monkey is mostly located on the surface of the posterior pole of the occipital lobe (Figures 18.4a and 18.4b). In the cat it is in much the same position. In the

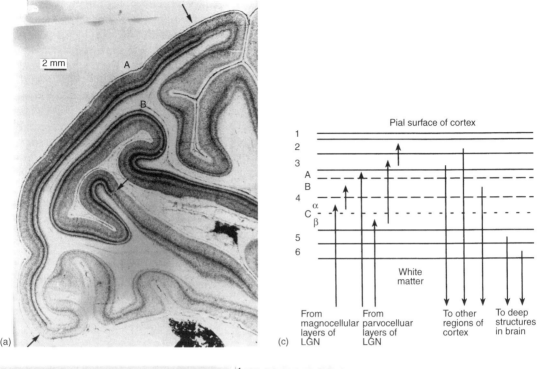

(a)

(c)

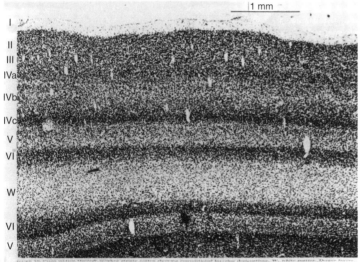

(b)

Figure 18.5 (a) Low power parasagittal section of primary visual cortex. Nissl stain. The arrows indicate the extremities of area 17, the striate or primary visual cortex. This cortex is defined by the presence of the stripe of Gennari (the darkly stained strip). 'A' marks the outer surface of the brain, 'B' indicates a buried fold. (b) Transverse section through striate cortex at a higher magnification. Cresyl violet stain. Layers are numbered on the left. W = white matter. From Hubel and Wiesel, 1977. (c) Input–output connections of the primary visual cortex. Explanation in text. B and C from Hubel, D.H. and Wiesel, T. (1977) Functional architecture of macaque monkey visual cortex. Proceedings of the Royal Society, B, 198, 1–59, with permission from The Royal Society.

monkey it extends over some $1400\,mm^2$ and in the cat about $380\,mm^2$.

Like other parts of the neocortex, the visual cortex is some 2 mm thick and is conventionally considered to consist of six layers of cells. The layers are numbered from the pial surface inwards. Layer 4 is usually subdivided into sublayers 4A, 4B and 4C. Sublayer 4C is subdivided yet again into α and β (Figure 18.5b). The primary visual cortex is, however, distinguished from other parts of the neocortex by the presence of a strongly developed strip of myelinated fibres running parallel to the pial surface in layer 4 known as the **stripe of Gennari** (hence the name, **striate cortex**).

If we trace the input from the LGNd, we find that the magnocellular fibres terminate in layer 4Cα and the parvocellular fibres in 4A and 4Cβ. The visual information is carried on from these layers to other layers of the cortex (Figure 18.5c). We shall see below that there is considerable branching of the neurons after the first synaptic contact has been made and considerable synaptic interaction. The lateral spread is, however, seldom more than a few millimeters. We shall see the significance of this below. Instead, lateral communication between more distant areas of the cortex is made by fibres which run out of the cortex altogether and traverse the white matter before re-entering the cortex at that distant point.

18.2.2 Functioning

There are many ways to investigate the physiology of the cortex. We shall touch on a number below. Historically the most important has been the use of microelectrodes to examine the activity of single cortical cells. In this technique a contact lens is placed in the eye of an anaesthetized animal and a microelectrode inserted into the visual cortex. Activity from a cortical cell is observed as the retina is exposed to visual stimuli. Once the activity has been recorded, the microelectrode can be moved to another cell and the procedure repeated. At the end of the session the animal is sacrificed and histological preparations made of the cortex. The track of the microelectrode can be discerned and the cells from which the recordings were made identified.

Once again the concept of a **receptive field (RF)** is fundamental. The RF of a cortical cell can be defined as that patch of the retina which, on being stimulated, generates a change in the activity of the cell. The receptive fields of cells in the primary visual cortex have been the subject of intense investigation. As would be expected, most of the cells in layer 4c have RFs with a centre–surround architecture similar to those of cells in the LGNd. There has, after all, been no opportunity to process the incoming information between the LGNd and these layers of the striate cortex. They can be excited by probing

the retina with small spots of light, just as was done when investigating the RFs of retinal ganglion cells or geniculate cells. But this was by no means the case with cells in the other layers of the cortex. For many years their 'trigger stimuli' remained a mystery.

As Hubel and Wiesel tell the story (and they were later to be awarded a Nobel prize for their work), the discovery of the physiology of the cells in the primary visual cortex was the outcome of serendipidity-serendipidity, it must be emphasized, in the hands of careful and highly attentive investigators. After much time spent attempting to excite the cells with black and white dots mounted on glass slides had ended in failure, they suddenly noticed that a faint response was being given to the edge of the slide as they slid it into the slide holder. This was the breakthrough. They soon showed that when a bar stimulus, or an edge, at **a particular orientation**, was either flashed on or swept across an appropriate part of the retina, the cortical cell would respond with a burst of activity (Figure 18.6).

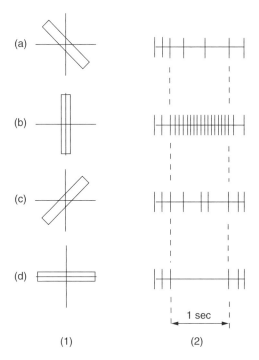

Figure 18.6 Response of orientation detector cell in the striate cortex. In the column on the left a bar stimulus is flashed to the retina (one second). In the column on the right the response of the cortical cell is shown.

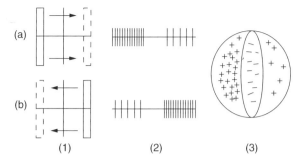

Figure 18.7 Direction selectivity. (a) Movement from left to right; (b) movement from right to left. The response of the cortical cell is shown in column (2) and the deduced 'architecture' of the field in column (3). The strengths of the excitatory parts of the field are indicated by density of the crosses and the inhibitory central area by minus signs.

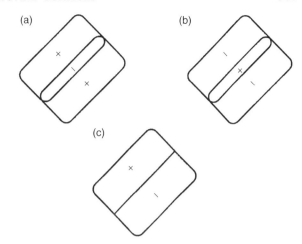

Figure 18.8 Common RF architectures of 'simple' cells in the striate cortex. + = 'ON' response; − = 'OFF' response. Further explanation in text.

Further work showed that, in the macaque striate cortex, some 70–80% of all the cells have this orientation specificity. Note that it is only movement of the bar stimulus across the field which elicits a response. Stationary stimuli have little effect. It was also found that in some 30% of the cells, the direction in which the bar was swept was significant. A large response could be elicited to one direction, little or nothing to the other (Figure 18.7).

In Figure 18.7 the deduced 'architecture' of the RF is shown. This can be checked by the usual technique of illuminating the appropriate part of the retina with small spots of light. The cortical cell responds with an ON or an OFF response. As in the retina, there is antagonism between the ON and OFF areas; unlike ganglion cell RFs, however, the design is not 'target-like' but rectanglar. There is either a slit-like ON or OFF centre, flanked on each side by the opposite areas with the opposite characteristic; or there may simply be two adjacent rectangles, one inducing an ON response, the other an OFF response (Figure 18.8).

There have been many attempts to work out 'wiring diagrams' to account for these receptive field properties since Hubel and Wiesel first discovered them in the late 1950s. We have already noted how difficult it has been to elucidate the wiring diagram of the retina (Section 17.2.9) and we are still far from a full understanding, so it is not surprising that wiring diagrams in the far more complex cortex are still under discussion. It may be, however, that Hubel and Wiesel's original suggestion that the architectures of

orientation selector RFs are created by the lining up of a number of concentric centre–surround fields will turn out to have been not too far off the mark (Figure 18.9).

The orientation selector cells described in the preceding paragraphs are known as '**simple cells**'. They are in fact in the minority of orientation detectors in the primary visual cortex. The majority of such cells, perhaps 75%, have rather different response characteristics. They are known as '**complex cells**'. They differ from simple cells in that their RFs are not subdivided into ON and OFF regions nor can they be excited by single spots of light; instead an **appropriately orientated edge** or **bar** of light flashed at any point or swept over the **entire field** will elicit a strong response from the cell (Figure 18.10).

The response is not induced by stimulation of a small subdivision of the field, as in simple cells, but from the whole field. Complex fields, however, resemble simple fields in that they are often sensitive to the direction in which the slit stimulus is moved. It is interesting to note that in some of the so-called 'lower' mammals, in particular the rabbit, directional selectivity is a feature of the RFs of some retinal ganglion cells. Ganglion cells with this RF property do not appear to be present in the monkey retina. Instead, the processing for directionality is carried out in the brain. Does the rabbit need to respond more rapidly to threats in the environment? Our common

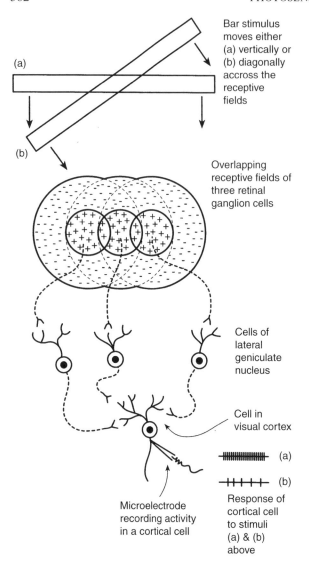

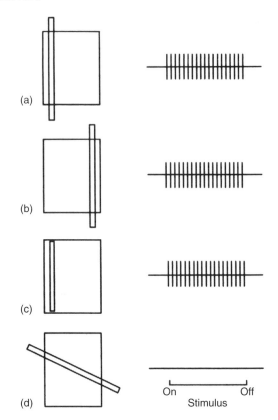

Figure 18.10 Response characteristics of a cortical cell with a complex field. A correctly orientated bar stimulus flashed to any part of the field elicits a strong response from the cell.

Figure 18.9 Possible 'wiring' responsible for orientation detector characteristics of cortical cells. A number of ganglion cells with overlapping centre–surround concentric fields ultimately feed on to a to a single cortical cell. The cortical cell accordingly responds maximally to a bar of light in the correct orientation in the correct place on the retina.

observation does suggest that rabbits are always timorously on the *qui vive*.

A further type of orientation selector cell is also present in the primary visual cortex. Hubel and Wiesel originally defined this type as '**hypercomplex**', believing that their receptive fields were derived from the input of many complex cells. This is not nowadays thought (always) to be the case so the term 'hypercomplex' has tended to drop out of the literature. This type of cell does, however, differ significantly from complex cells in that, to induce maximum response, the ends of the line stimulus must lie within the receptive field (Figure 18.11). Hence these cells are nowadays known by the less theory-laden term of '**end stopped**'. It may be that these cells have evolved to detect curved or wrinkled edges.

But why? Why should the primary visual cortex be filled with cells responding to the orientation of edges and lines? The most likely explanation is that the world is simply full of edges and lines – the outlines of objects moving across the field of vision; the vertical and diagonal lines of tree trunks and branches as the eye scans them; the wrinkled edges of leaves and the uneven contours of boulders; the long grasses of the savannah; the line of the distant horizon showing the conjunction of earth and sky.

There is more. The orientation selector cells are not distributed randomly throughout the primary visual cortex. Microelectrode studies have shown that there is a very precise, some have said almost quasi-crystalline, organization. We saw in Chapter 6, when discussing the somaesthetic cortex, that it was organized into vertical columns of activity. It is the same with the visual cortex. It turns out that, when a microelectrode is driven down the length of a column, it penetrates one cell after another, all with receptive fields responsive to the same orientation. One can speak not merely of an orientation detector cell but also of an orientation detector column. It turns out that, in general, end stopped cells are located in layers 2 and 3; layer 4 contains either concentric centre–surround cells (see above) or simple orientation detector cells; layers 5 and 6 contain complex cells.

If the microelectrode is inserted somewhat diagonally so that it escapes from one column and enters the next, it is found that the cells there respond to a slightly different orientation. There is a remarkable regularity (Figure 18.12). As the microelectrode penetrates column after column of cells, the preferred

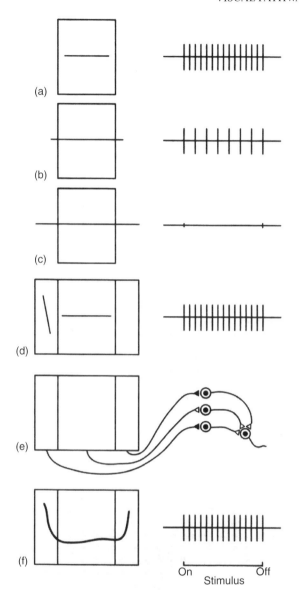

Figure 18.11 Cortical cell tuned to respond to 'end-stopped' bar stimuli. (a) The correctly orientated bar stimuli is completely within the field. The cortical cell gives a strong response. (b) The bar stimulus overflows the field. The response in the cell is reduced. (c) A yet longer bar stimulus causes no response in the cortical cell. (d) A short bar stimulus plus another such stimulus at a different orientation just outside the field generates maximal response in the cell. (e) Conceptual wiring diagram to account for case (d). The area just outside the RF is tuned to give responses to diagonal or vertical bars and to be inhibited by horizontal bar stimuli. (f) Possible biological significance of end stopped RFs in detecting curves or wrinkled edges. After Hubel, D.H. (1988).

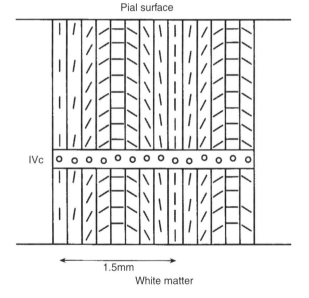

Figure 18.12 Orientation columns in the striate cortex. The optimal orientation of a bar stimulus varies regularly from one column to the next. Orientation selectivity is not shown by cells in layer IVc where input fibres from the LGN terminate; cells in this layer have circular receptive fields.

orientation varies in a regular fashion. It proceeds through a complete 180° in a tangential distance of about 1.5 mm. This astonishing regularity is occasionally broken by a sharp discontinuity known as a **fracture**. The regular sequence of small changes is interrupted by a sudden column-to-column change of 45 to 90°. Then the regular sequence of small changes reasserts itself.

So far, we have described the structure of the primary visual cortex in terms of microelectrode recording. The histological reality of this physiology can, however, be demonstrated by cunning histochemical techniques. One of the most impressive has involved the use of **deoxyglucose**. This chemical is mistaken for glucose by active cells and taken up into their cytoplasm. Only the first steps of glycolytic breakdown occur and the metabolite then merely accumulates in the cell. Being lipid insoluble, it cannot leak out of the cells. The principle of the technique is to attach a radioisotope (usually tritium, ^{3}H) to the molecule and then, after injection, to show a pattern of stripes (over a period of up to 45 min) to the anaesthetized animal. It was reasoned that the deoxyglucose would be taken up preferentially by activated cells. The animal was then sacrificed, histological sections cut of the visual cortex and autoradiographs prepared. The procedure was brilliantly successful; orientation detector columns could be clearly seen (Figure 18.13) and, moreover, a continuous band of radioactive darken-

ing stretched through layer 4C. This layer, it will be remembered, is activated whatever the orientation of the stimulus.

The deoxyglucose technique was applied to confirm (or, at the least, complement) the electrophysiological work. In contrast, a somewhat similar technique showed up something quite unexpected, something that had not been inferred by the electrophysiologist's probing microelectrode. In 1978, Margaret Wong-Riley stained the striate cortex with an agent to detect the enzyme **cytochrome oxidase**. To everyone's surprise, cytochrome oxidase appeared to be localized in a regular series of '**blobs**', which are particularly obvious in layers 2 and 3 of the striate cortex. These blobs are about 0.5 mm in diameter, separated from each by so-called '**interblob**' regions about 0.25 mm across. For some years no one took much notice of this unexpected finding. Then, in 1981, Hubel and Livingstone examined the blobs with the microelectrode. It was found that, far from being composed of orientation selector cells, the blobs consisted of cells with concentric centre–surround fields responsive to **colour**.

The RFs of the colour cells in the blobs are, like those in the LGNd, divided into two classes: red/green and blue/yellow (where yellow, as before, stands for input from red and green in parallel). But there is a difference. It was found that they did not respond to large white spots and, furthermore, both

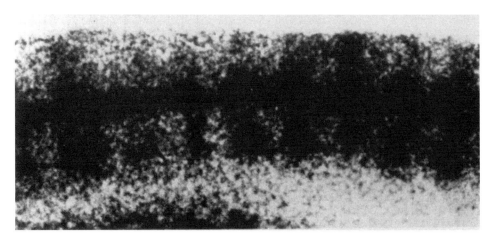

Figure 18.13 Orientation columns. Vertical section through the striate cortex of a monkey using the 2-deoxyglucose technique (see text). A pattern of vertical stripes was shown to the animal and the columns clearly evident in the section indicate where vertical orientation detector cells are located. From Hubel, D.H., Wiesel T. and Stryker (1977), Proceedings of the Royal Society, B, 198, with permission from The Royal Society.

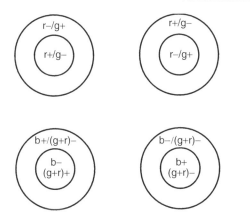

Figure 18.14 Concentric double opponent cells. The top pair respond to red/green contrasts; the bottom pair to blue/yellow contrasts. Double opponent receptive fields are not always circular. Orientation selector double opponent RFs have also been found in the striate cortex.

centre and surround seemed to consist of opponent pairs of colours. To take the simplest case, the red/green case, the centre gave an ON response to red, an OFF response to green (that is r+/g−) and the surround an OFF response to red and an ON response to green (that is r−/g+). This type of response characteristic is termed **double opponency** (Figure 18.14).

These double opponent cells seem designed to emphasize colour contrast at a border. That they do not respond to diffuse illumination again suggests that they are 'looking at' edges in the visual image.

It will be remembered that colour information is carried by the P fibre system. It is this system that terminates in the blobs. P fibres also innervate the interblob regions. Here, however, the cortical cells, in addition to colour sensitivity, also respond to edges. The edge detectors are slowly adapting and thus, rather than reporting movement are more concerned with the position and orientation of stationary edges. The interblob subdivision of the P fibre system thus supplements the form detection capability of the M system we discussed above.

There is one final organizational principle at work in the striate cortex. This is an organization into **ocular dominance columns**. It is found that, as a microelectrode penetrates vertically into the cortex, it finds one cell after another which is preferentially 'driven' by one eye. Again a diagonal penetration will encounter cells preferentially driven by the other eye and so on. Once again a very regular organization is revealed: an alternation of columns of cells driven first by one eye, then the other (Figure 18.15a).

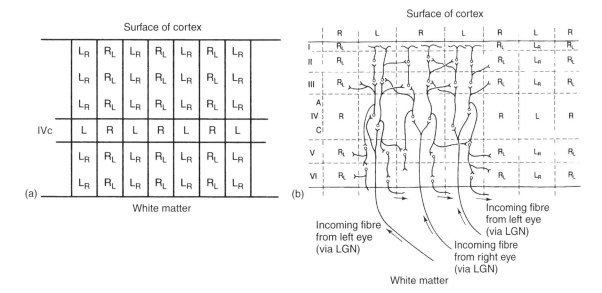

Figure 18.15 (a) Ocular dominance columns in the striate cortex of monkey. L = left eye drive; L_R = left eye dominant, some drive also from the right eye; R = right eye drive; R_L = right eye dominant, some drive from the left eye. (b) 'Wiring' responsible for the physiological characteristics of ocular dominance columns.

The dominance is complete in layer 4C (Figure 18.15). This is only to be expected, as this is the layer where input fibres from the LGNd terminate. It will be recalled that optic nerve fibres from each eye are strictly segregated in the LGNd (Section 18.2). Above and below layer 4C, however, subsequent neurons branch laterally so that some input from the opposite eye is asserted on the dominant input (Figure 18.15b). Clever staining techniques have once again revealed the histological reality of these alternating columns. It has been found that ocular dominance columns are present in animals with excellent binocular vision: cats, monkeys, chimpanzees and humans. They have, however, not yet been demonstrated in other mammals, for instance in the common laboratory rodents: rats, mice and guinea pigs. This suggests that the dominance columns are important in stereopsis. There has, recently, been a certain sceptical reaction to this conclusion (see below and Box 18.1).

Each cortical column, or macrocolumn, has a diameter of about 300 µm and contains some 7500 to 8000 neurons. Macrocolumns are made of about 80 minicolumns each consisting of some 100 or so neurons. This organization, and magnitude, remains remarkably constant from mouse to man. In the visual cortex Hubel and Wiesel suggested that the organization resembled nothing so much as a refrigerator's ice tray. One complete set of orientation columns, a set of colour detector blobs and a set of left and right ocular dominance columns forms the 'physiological unit' (Figure 18.16a). This unit has been called either a '**hypercolumn**' or a '**module**'. It 'looks' at a particular patch of each retina. Although the receptive fields of each orientation selector cell in a hypercolumn will have a different size, they will all be superimposed on each other in nearly the same place in the retina (Figure 18.16b). Together they make up the **aggregate receptive field** of the hypercolumn. The aggregate receptive fields will vary in spatial dimension in different parts of the retina, being smallest in the fovea and largest at the periphery.

Before leaving this account of what Szentagothai called the 'quasi-crystalline structure' of the cerebral cortex, some important caveats must be entered. Recent investigations have questioned the reality of this so-called 'ice tray' model of the visual cortex. This work and this scepticism is outlined in Box 18.1. However, although the 'rigid' architecture of the cortex implied by Szentagothai and by Hubel and Wiesel's 'ice tray' is certainly inappropriate, the overall evidence for a vertical columnar organization is too strong and wide ranging to be dismissed. The consensus is that, in some less inflexible form, it must exist.

After this brief sceptical excursus, let us return to our discussion of orientation or 'edge' detectors. It may already have occurred to the attentive student that there is a difficulty. Consider Figure 18.17. It shows three possible ways of stimulating the RF of an edge detector. In Figure 18.17a a sharp edge falls over the detector. None of the inhibitory area is exposed and all of the excitatory area is exposed to illumination. A strong response is generated in the cortical cell. In Figure 18.17b a less abrupt discontinuity in illumination falls over the RF. The inhibitory area will be weakly excited and the excitatory area less strongly excited than in the case in Figure 18.17a. It follows that the cortical cell will show a lower frequency response than in the first case. Finally, in the case of Figure 18.17c, a sharp diagonal discontinuity in illumination falls across the RF. This can be arranged so that part of the inhibitory area is fully illuminated as well as part of the excitatory area. The response from the cortical cell could be indistinguishable from that of the case in Figure 18.17b. How does the cortex cope with this ambiguity?

The short answer to this question is that as yet we do not know. But one attractive answer has been popularized by the neuropsychologist John Frisby. He suggests that we should not be looking so much at the activity of single edge detectors but at the activity of the whole population of edge detectors within the hypercolumn. Consider Figure 18.18. Once again we have the two visual stimuli, one a sharp diagonal discontinuity in illumination, the other a weaker vertical discontinuity. If these two stimuli fall across the aggregate receptive field of a hypercolumn, it is obvious that the **pattern** of edge detector cells excited in the hypercolumn will be significantly different. By looking at this pattern the visual system can readily discriminate between the two stimuli as, of course, we are well aware that we can.

This, of course, and Frisby is the first to acknowledge it, begs a supremely important question. What is it, and where is it, that 'looks' at the pattern of excitation in a hypercolumn? As of the time of writing we have no answer to this question. This, and questions like it, present one of the major challenges of the

BOX 18.1   THE REALITY OF CORTICAL COLUMNS

The search for 'units' of cortical activity stretches back for well over two centuries. At the beginning of the nineteenth century Franz Joseph Gall and his disciple John Spurzheim subdivided the brain into between forty and fifty different regions which, they argued, provided the anatomical basis of different mental characteristics: benevolence, acquisitiveness and so on. This early attempt to localize personality traits in brain areas, known as **phrenology**, was quickly shown to be fraudulent and soon dismissed as such. But the desire to key mental features into brain structure persisted, especially in hospitals concerned with mental disorders, and reappeared in the **cytoarchitectonics** of Korbinian Brodmann and others at the beginning of the twentieth century. Architectonicists also recognized some forty or fifty different cortical areas characterized by different microscopical structure. Architectonics again proved difficult to verify, although Brodmann's numbering of different brain areas retains its value, and was largely discarded by the mid-twentieth century. It was in a continuing attempt to tie brain structure to function that first Mountcastle, Berman and Davies (1955), working on the somaesthetic cortex (Chapter 8) and then Hubel and Wiesel (1962) working on the visual cortex (Chapter 18), developed the concept of **cortical columns**.

Does history repeat itself? The analytical urge to understand the structure and function of complex entities – and what more complex entity is there than the cerebral cortex? – in terms of the interaction of underlying units is strong. There is a great temptation to 'see' neat compartments, 'abrupt' demarcations. We have seen in Chapters 17 and 18 how the visual system has been 'selected' over evolutionary time to detect edges and borders, indeed, as many visual illusions demonstrate, to interpolate edges where no edges in reality exist.

It is thus worth noting that, after their early reports of regular sets of orientation columns in the visual cortex, Hubel and Wiesel themselves drew back a little, as it became clear that a more continuous orientation selectivity occurred across the cortex. Powell and Mountcastle, also, in their pioneering paper on the somaesthetic cortex in 1959, concluded that their work 'should not be interpreted to mean that only this pattern of functional organization exists, for cortical cells must certainly be grouped into various patterns subserving higher orders of cortical functioning, patterns of activity about which at present nothing is known'.

In more recent years it has been pointed out that the same cell may be part of different columns during an animal's life and/or in different states of its brain's activity and that, furthermore, the experimental techniques employed tend to eliminate the significance of 'context'. This scepticism has been reinforced by histological studies which show that injection of a tracer at any point in the cortex leads to a diffuse 'cloud' of local connections about 500 μm in diameter, the diameter of a macrocolumn. Finally, several investigators have reported that there seems to be little or no correlation between the presence of ocular dominance columns and visual performance in different species. Indeed, Horton and Adams (2005) report that their presence varies in different individuals of the same species with no noticeable affect on visual behaviour. 'Their expression,' they write, 'at least in spider monkeys, appears whimsical'. Other investigators have shown that, at least in the squirrel, the 'wiring' required for orientation detector cells appears not to involve an organization of macrocolumns.

So, does history repeat itself? Will columns go the same way as the phrenologist's bumps and protruberances, as the architectonicist's multiplicity of cortical areas cut off from each other by 'hair sharp' boundaries? Was George Santanyana right in believing that 'those who know no history are condemned to repeat it'?

Well yes and no. Szentagothai's concept of a 'quasi-crystalline' cortex is probably just too, well, 'crystalline', to reflect cortical reality. But the strong and varied evidence that the cortex has an important

(Continues)

(Continued)

'vertical' organization cannot be denied. It may well be that this vertical organization is built around the 'minicolumns' which, in turn, are most likely to be 'ontogenetic units' derived during embryology from the cortical plate. How far these units are built into **permanent** rather than transient macrocolumns, and these into similarly permanent hypercolumns, is at the time of writing very much a matter of debate. Horton and Adams (2003) suggest we might profitably make use of the concept of a 'spandrel'. The biologists Gould and Lewontin borrowed this term from architecture and applied it in their discussions of evolutionary theory. A spandrel is a necessary but structurally unimportant outcome of building with arches. Gothic architects often filled these spaces with elaborate decoration. Horton and Adams suggest that cortical columns might be regarded as somewhat the same, the consequence of some quite different and as yet unknown architecture. Time and further research will tell.

REFERENCES

Hubel, T. and Wiesel, D.H. (1962) Receptive fields of single neurons in the cat's cerebral cortex. *Journal of Physiology*, **160**, 106–54.

Powell, T.P.S. and Mountcastle, V.B. (1959) Some aspects of the functional organization of the cortex of the postcentral gyrus of the monkey: a correlation of the findings obtained in a single unit analysis with cytoarchitecture. *Bulletin of the Johns Hopkins Hospital*, **105**, 133–62.

Horton, J.C. and Adams, D.L. (2003) Capricious expression of cortical columns in the primate brain. *Nature Neuroscience*, **6**, 113–4.

Horton, J.C. and Adams, D.L. (2005) The cortical column: a structure without a function. *Proceedings of the Royal Society B*, **360**, 837–62.

Mountcastle, V.B., Berman, A.L. and Davies, P.W. (1955) Topographical organization and modality representation in the first somatic areas of the cat's cerebral cortex by single unit analysis. *American Journal of Physiology*, **183**, 646–7.

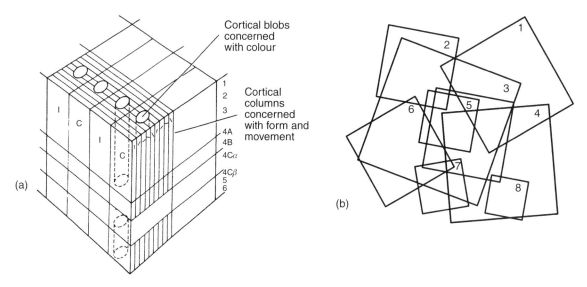

Figure 18.16   (a) Schematic figure to show the organization of the striate cortex. A hypercolumn is regarded as consisting of one complete set of orientation columns and two (left and right) ocular dominance columns. In addition, a 'peg-like' blob structure contains colour sensitive cells. It must be emphasized that the figure is highly schematic and the true histological situation is far less clear cut. C = contralateral: I = ipsilateral. From Kandel, E.R., Schwartz, J.H. and Jessel, T.M. (eds) (1991) *Principles of Neuroscience*, with permission from Elsevier. (b) Aggregate receptive field of a hypercolumn. The figure shows eight overlapping receptive fields making up the aggregate. In fact there would in most cases be many more.

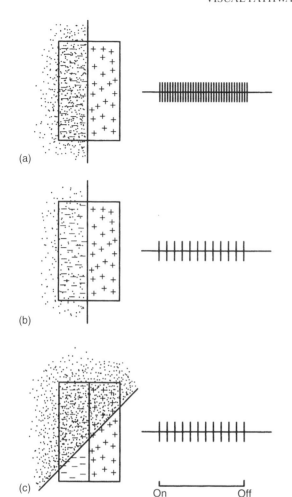

Figure 18.17 (a) A sharp luminant discontinuity falls at the inhibitory/excitatory boundary of an edge detector receptive field. The response of the cortical cell is shown on the right. (b) A weaker luminant discontinuity falls on the RFs inhibitory/excitatory boundary. A weaker response is generated in the cortical cell. (c) A sharp but diagonal luminant discontinuity falls across the the field. The response from the cortical cell is indistinguishable from case (b). How does the brain disambiguate these two signals? After Frisby, J.P. (1979).

Before turning to these extrastriate cortices, it is important to remind ourselves that, as in the other sensory systems considered in this book, the sensory surface, in this case the retina, is displayed as a non-isomorphous map in the sensory cortex, in this case the primary visual cortex. This map is shown in Figure 18.19. As noted above, the aggregate receptive fields in the fovea are the smallest in extent, hence far more of the visual cortex is devoted to them than to other parts of the retina. It can be seen from the figure that the upper parts of the retina are mapped in the lower bank of the calcarine fissure and vice versa. It must be remembered that, because of the optics of the eye, the upper part of the retina corresponds to the lower part of the visual field and vice versa. The cortex devoted to the fovea is almost as large as all the rest (Figure 18.19) and, indeed, extends out on to posterior surface of the occipital lobe. It is from this map that fibres carrying processed information about the visual scene are directed onwards to the extrastriate cortices.

18.2.3 Plasticity

In Chapter 8 (Section 8.5) we saw how the somaesthetic cortex was open to 'environmental' moulding. The same plasticity has been demonstrated in the primary visual cortex. This plasticity is, however, largely restricted to the so-called sensitive (or critical) period in the mammal's development. This period, during which the brain is undergoing rapid maturation, lasts about six weeks in kittens and for perhaps eighteen months in infant humans. The sensitive periods of different brain systems have different durations and onset and offset times.

Kittens are born with their eyes closed and they do not open for about ten days. Even after that period they remain cloudy for another couple of weeks and there is little sign of accurate visuo-motor coordination. This, in conjunction with immaturity of the muscular system, ensures that they do not stray too far from home. During this early stage, electrophysiological recording from their visual cortices shows little of the structure of orientation and ocular dominance columns described above. It is only when visuo-motor co-ordination becomes established and the kitten begins to play at being an adult, that the cortex assumes its highly organized structure.

twenty-first century brain science. This, of course, is not to say that we have no knowledge of where the output from the primary visual cortex is directed. We do, and it may be that it is in these extrastriate areas that the disambiguation of the visual input occurs. Or it may be that the hypercolumn, with its quarter million cells, is able to compute the answer within itself.

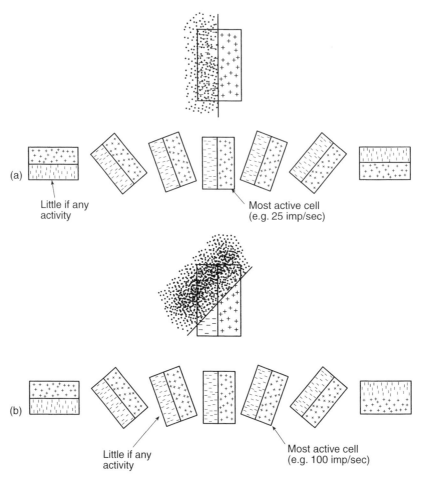

Figure 18.18 (a) Comparable to Figure 18.17b. The strongest response in the hypercolumn is given from the column containing cells tuned to vertical orientations. (b) Comparable to Figure 18.17c. The strongest response in the hypercolumn is given by the column containing cells tuned to diagonal orientations. The figure shows that the pattern of responses in the hypercolumn is distinctively different in cases (a) and (b). Further explanation in text. After Frisby, J.P. (1979).

This postnatal cortical development provides valuable opportunities for experimental investigation. Kittens reared in the dark show little sign of orientation selector cells in their primary visual cortices. Kittens reared in visual environments consisting of only vertical stripes will show a preponderance of cells responding to vertical bar stimuli; those reared amongst horizontal stripes a preponderance of cells responding to horizontal bar stimuli. Similarly, if before the eyes open one is patched and the patch maintained throughout the sensitive period, the primary visual cortex of the resulting cat is markedly deficient in cells driven from that eye. Few messages from the patched eye (which is now, of course, uncovered) make it through to the binocular columns of the primary visual cortex. If, however, both eyes are patched, the ocular dominance columns in the visual cortex are not very different from normal. It appears that the neural wiring responsible for binocular drive is genetically specified but is open to 'environmental' moulding. Furthermore, if the patched eye is unpatched during the third or fourth week after birth and the unpatched eye patched, the wiring is reversed. Binocular drive is lost from the originally

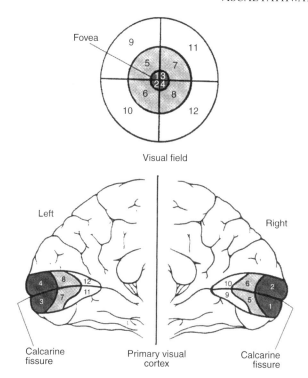

Visual field

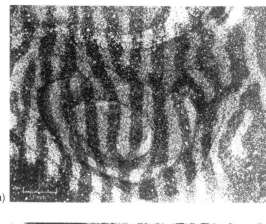

(a)

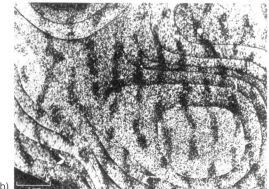

(b)

Figure 18.19 The upper part of the figure shows the visual field. The lower part shows a *medial* view of the occipital lobe. The two hemispheres, in other words, have been separated and splayed out so that the medial surfaces of each displayed. The visual cortex lies above and below the calcarine fissure. Further explanation in text. The numbers in the upper figure correspond to those in the lower. From Kandel, E.R., Schwartz, J.H. and Jessel, T.M. (eds) (1991) *Principles of Neuroscience*, with permission from Elsevier.

Figure 18.20 (a) Tangential section through radiolabelled ocular dominance columns. The light stripes show where the radiolabelled proline has accumulated. It can be seen that the light stripes (representing input from the labelled eye) and the dark stripes (representing input from the unlabelled eye) are of approximately equal width. (b) Tangential section through radiolabelled ocular dominance columns after patching one eye during the sensitive period. It is clear that the ocular dominance columns connected to the unpatched eye (light colour) have expanded greatly at the expense of the formerly patched eye. From Hubel, Wiesel and Le Vay, 1977: reproduced by kind permission of the Royal Society.

unpatched eye and restored to the originally patched eye. During this early period of the kitten's life, pathways can not only be reduced and enhanced but also reconstructed.

These electrophysiological experiments have been complemented with histochemical investigations. Radiolabelled proline is injected into the retina of an experimental animal (in this case a macaque). After about ten days the animal is sacrificed, its primary visual cortex prepared for microscopy, sectioned and autoradiographs prepared. The result is shown in Figure 18.20a. The light stripes show where the radioactivity has accumulated. It can be seen that ocular dominance columns of approximately equal width alternate in the way expected. If, however, one eye had been patched during the sensitive period and,

after unpatching, radiolabelled proline injected into the unpatched retina and the experiment repeated, the autoradiograph shown in Figure 18.20b results. It can be seen that the light stripes, representing the input from the unpatched eye, have greatly expanded at the expense of the input from the patched eye. This provides spectacular confirmation of the electrophysiological evidence for the plasticity of the primary visual cortex during the sensitive period.

18.3 EXTRASTRIATE CORTICES

Up until the early 1950s it was believed that the sense organs fed into rather closely circumscribed sensory areas leaving the major part of the cortex free for 'association'. Whether this concept had been imposed by the powerful influence of association psychology is an interesting historical question. Since the 1950s, however, it has become clear that this understanding is seriously at fault. In the case of the visual system, the cortical area devoted to its analysis is very far from being confined to the striate cortex or visual area 1. Indeed, in visual mammals such as the higher primates, large parts of the occipital and temporal lobes are devoted to vision. Between two dozen and thirty distinct 'extrastriate' visual areas have been identified in the macaque. Frequently, these areas contain maps of the visual field specializing in different features. The concept of 'association cortex' has been displaced (though not entirely) by the view that the cortex consists of layer upon layer of sensory maps.

In Section 18.1.2 above, we saw how the retinogeniculate pathway led into the primary visual cortex. After processing in this cortex, the information is passed on to the extrastriate cortices. But, as noted in Section 18.1.1, this is not the only route from the retina into the brain. A less important route runs to the superior colliculus. We saw that the visual maps generated in the superior colliculus play a crucial role in controlling eye movement and the direction of gaze. Fibres from the superior colliculus also run via the pulvinar nucleus to the extrastriate visual cortex. The **pulvinar nucleus** is a large and intricately subdivided nuclear mass forming the posterior and postero-lateral part of the thalamus, just anterior (superior) to the superior colliculus. Not only does it direct fibres onwards towards wide areas of the extrastriate cortex but it also receives (like the lateral geniculate nuclei) afferent fibres from the cortex. The extrastriate cortex thus receives overlapping input from the striate cortex and the pulvinar nuclei. Although the visual system takes up large volumes of the primate brain, it is interconnected in intricate ways which ensure that it all works together as a coherent unit.

Let us return, however, to the output from the striate cortex. We have seen how, from the retina onwards, the input along the geniculostriate pathway has been segregated into magnocellular fibres (largely carrying information about motion and form) and parvocellular fibres (carrying information about colour and also some information about form). We saw that this information remained segregated in the striate cortex. The M fibres leading to the edge detector cells and the P fibres running to the 'blobs' and 'interblobs'. We see here the outlines of a 'three-stream' system: one stream carrying information about form, motion and stereopsis; another about colour; a third about all four features of the visual scene (Figure 18.21b).

The three streams of visual information continue on into the extrastriate cortex, first into visual area 2 and then into visual area 3 (both parts of Brodmann area 18). Cytochrome oxidase staining showed that visual area 2 is also differentiated, this time into **thick stripe**, **thin stripe** and **interstripe** areas. Figure 18.21b shows that the M stream from V1 projects into the thick stripes, the P stream from the blobs goes to the thin stripes and the P stream from the interblobs is directed to the interstripes.

We shall not follow the transmission of visual information further into the brain. Interested readers should consult one of the texts listed in the bibliography. Suffice it to say that visual pathways have been traced 'upwards' to the middle temporal (MT) and superior temporal gyri (Brodmann area 19, comprising visual areas 4 and 5) and then into many other parts of the cortex, especially regions of the parietal and temporal cortices (Figure 18.21b). It should not be thought, though, that the transmission is all one way. As mentioned at the beginning of this chapter, the monkey visual system consists of more than two dozen cortical areas connected 'downwards' as well as 'upwards'. Furthermore, as we also saw above, the geniculostriate pathway is not the only visual input to the brain. Important contributions come from the pulvinar, the superior colliculus and elsewhere. Nor is the cerebral cortex the only 'end station'; visual information makes its way to many other parts of the brain including the diencephalon and the basal nuclei. In highly visual animals, such as the primates, most parts of the brain have some involvement in vision.

18.4 FACE RECOGNITION

Although it would take us too far afield to follow the detailed neuroanatomy of the numerous primate

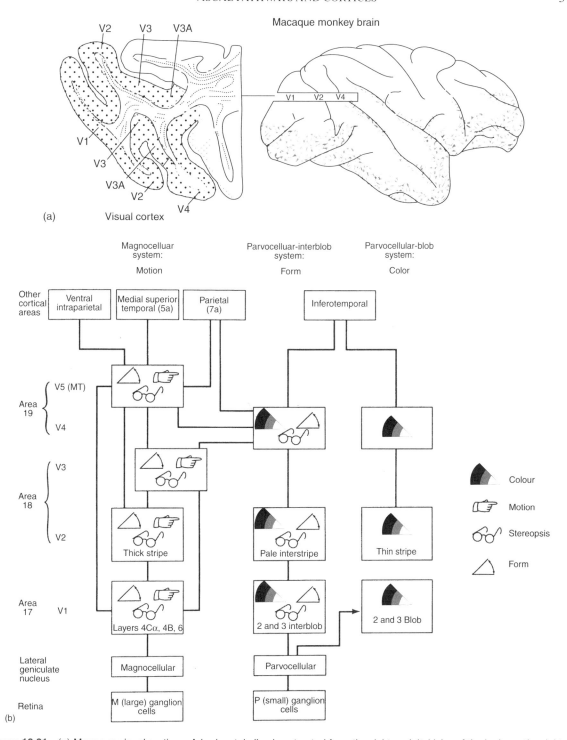

Figure 18.21 (a) Macaque visual cortices. A horizontal slice is extracted from the right occipital lobe of the brain on the right of the figure, rotated through ninety degrees and displayed on the left side of the figure. The position of the visual cortices – V1, V2, V3, V4 and V5 (MT) – is shown. (b) Schematic to show the three-stream visual system of primates. Explanation in text. B from Kandel, E.R., Schwartz, J.H. and Jessel, T.M. (eds) (1991) *Principles of Neuroscience*, with permission from Elsevier.

BOX 18.2   BLINDSIGHT

Like the 'unconscious mind', 'blindsight' is seemingly an oxymoron. But, again like the 'unconscious mind', the concept has proved useful. Indeed, the two concepts have more in common than mere usefulness. They both point to the fact that we know more than we think we do. Much of our knowledge of the world is, as Polyani long ago pointed out, 'tacit'.

The first accounts of blindsight derived from experiments and observations on monkeys missing their striate cortices. These experiments were first carried out in the late nineteenth century. They appeared to show that, if carefully nurtured, the monkeys recovered useful sight. They were able to navigate spaces crowded with obstacles and grasp small objects. But they appeared unable to judge the nature of the objects they grasped and manipulated. These experiments were taken up again in the early 1970s with a monkey whose striate cortices had been surgically removed. At first, as Nicholas Humphrey writes (for he was the experimenter), the monkey seemed, as expected, totally blind. But after close personal supervision over a period of seven years, sight of some kind seemed to have returned. The macaque was able to navigate through a room full of obstacles and pick up tiny objects, such as currants, from the floor. Yet, says Humphrey, the overwhelming impression he gained was that the monkey still did not 'see' in the normal sense of that term, but merely 'guessed', merely hazarded actions which would formerly have been full of meaning. How was this possible without a striate cortex? We have to remember, as we have seen in this chapter, that the RGS pathway is not the only input route for visual information. It may be that the monkey was using the older retino-tectal pathway or some other nonstriate pathway and learning how to use this to generate visually guided behaviour.

It is difficult to be sure of the quality of a monkey's subjectivity. This is less so with members of our own species and 'blindsight' (obviously not experimentally caused) also occurs in humans. It presents itself to neurologists when patients, for whatever reason, have suffered extensive damage to cortical area 17, the primary visual cortex on one side. These hemianopic patients insist that they have no visual sensation in the blind hemifield. Yet it can be demonstrated that some visually guided functions remain. The best known experiments have made use of pointing behaviour. The patient was asked to point to a target flashed up for two seconds or less in the blind hemifield. This he succeeded in doing with significantly more than random success. Yet he insisted that he had no visual awareness and was merely guessing.

These experiments were continued by testing for discrimination between a grating and a diffuse homogeneous field of equal luminance, for ability to detect the orientation of a bar stimulus, and for the ability to recognize whether a letter X or O was being shown. In all cases the patient performed at better than chance levels, but in all cases maintained that he saw nothing and was simply hazarding a guess. Nicholas Humphrey summarizes the patient's attitude as, 'I don't know anything at all – but if you tell me I'm getting it right, I have to take your word for it'.

Blindsight has been subjected to detailed and exhaustive criticism. Is the patient detecting stray light? Is the striate cortex only incompletely destroyed? But the consensus is building that it is a genuine phenomenon. That, in other words, the visual information is reaching the decision centres in the brain via pathways other than the RGS pathway and never affecting consciousness. The patient sees but does not see. He perceives, but is unconscious of perceiving. Does this have any implications for the nature of 'seeing' in the 'lower' vertebrates and invertebrates?

REFERENCES

Campion, J., Latto, R. and Smith, Y.M. (1983) Is blindsight an effect of scattered light, spared cortex, and near threshold vision? *Behavioural and Brain Sciences*, **6**, 423–86.

Humphrey, N. (1992) *A History of the Mind*, Vintage, London.

(Continues)

(*Continued*)

Luciani, L. (1884) On the sensorial localisations in the cortex cerebri. *Brain*, **7**, 145–60.

Polyani, M. (1966) *The Tacit Dimension*, Doubleday, New York.

Weiszkrantz, L. (1986) *Blindsight: A Case Study and Implications*, Oxford University Press, Oxford.

visual cortices and their interconnections, we cannot finish this chapter without some allusion to one of the most important of primate visual abilities: face recognition. This ability is of considerable importance in those primates which have evolved towards sociality. This has happened in several groups, including the macaques, baboons, most of the great apes and, of course, the hominidae. Numerous ethological studies have shown that the social groups of infrahuman primates are held together by dominance hierarchies. Strife is avoided amongst members of a troop by each knowing his or her place in the pecking order. For such hierarchies to work, the members must be able to recognize each other. No doubt this recognition is of many individual characteristics – gait, colour, size, voice, odour and so on – but certainly one of these characteristics is the face

and its expressions. It is thus no surprise to find that an area of macaque visual system is specialized to respond to faces.

The macaque face recognition area is far up in the sequence of visual cortices in the **infero-temporal (IT) cortex**. It receives input from V4 (visual area 4) and the vast majority of its cells respond to the foveal region of the retina. They have large RFs, commonly measuring about 25° of the visual field . Sometimes they are so large that they include the whole visual field. Unlike the cells lower in the sequence of visual areas, there is no retinotopic organization. They respond to a number of very specific trigger stimuli. About 10% are triggered by images of hands and faces. A cell which gives maximal response to the image of an upwardly pointing hand is shown in Figure 18.22b. It is found that maximal response

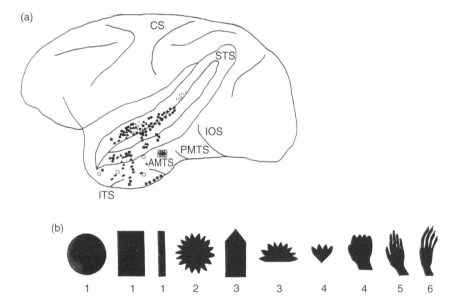

Figure 18.22 Feature detection in the Macaque brain. (a) Location of cells sensitive to faces in the macaque brain. AMTS = anterior medial temporal suclus; CS = central sulcus; IOS = inferior occipital sulcus; ITS = inferior temporal sulcus; PMTS = posterior medial temporal sulcus. The differently shaped symbols refer to the results of different investigators. From Perrett *et al.*, (1992), Copyright © 1992, The Royal Society. (b) Response of an inferior temporal cell to differently shaped stimuli. The stimuli are arranged from left to right in order of increasing ability to drive the cell from none (1) or little (2 and 3) to maximum (6). From Gross, C.G., Rocha-Miranda, C.E. and Bender, D.B. (1972) with permission of The American Physiological Society.

is given when the fingers of the hand are individually discriminable. In other words, the overall shape of the hand provides only a very suboptimal trigger stimulus.

In addition to cells triggered by images of hands, there are others which are triggered by images of monkey (and human) faces. Some cells respond best to full face images, others to side view profiles. Yet other cells are responsive to facial expression. Finally, there is evidence that some cells are more affected by some faces than others. There is evidence, for example, that very familiar faces, such as the experimenter's face, are more effective at triggering some of these cells than the faces of strangers. It seems as if the notion of a grandmother's face recognition cell may not be so far off the mark after all!

Nevertheless, we have to be cautious. Faces and other real world objects are built from a very large number of elementary features. Painstaking investigations of just which of these features induce maximum response in an IT cell have been carried out. The conclusions from this work have to remain provisional, as it is not possible to test all conceivable elementary or combinations of elementary features. It turns out, however, that colinear bars (e.g. eyebrows), T's (e.g. eyebrows and nose), ovoids (e.g. full face) and so on as well as complete faces engender maximal responses in different cells (Figure 18.23a). It turns out, further, that these so-called 'iconic patterns' are grouped into columns (Figure 18.23b). They are, in short, organized in the same way as we have seen features in other parts of the sensory cortex are organized. Tangential microelectrode penetrations found groups of cells with similar (though not identical) iconic preferences clustered into $500 \mu m$ diameter columns, followed by areas where no response could be triggered by that icon. After a further tangential penetration of about 1 mm, cells responding to the original icon were once again encountered.

The outcome of this laborious electrophysiology is in line with the upshot of the orientation detector investigations described in Section 18.2.2. There, we saw that it was not just the response of a single column of cells which represented the orientation of an edge but that of a whole group of columns; similarly with the recognition of complex objects and images in the infero-temporal cortex. It is the response of the array of columns made up of cells triggered by different image elements or 'partials' which represent the object. The 'discovery' of 'experimenter's 'or 'grandmother's face' recognition cells once again seems premature and likely misconceived.

Furthermore, the research is as yet far from over. There is evidence that the response of at least some ITC cells to an iconic 'partial' varies according to whether or not other elements are present in its receptive field. There is also evidence that the cells in an iconic column differ slightly in their selectivity, angle of presentation, illumination and so on. This ensures that the output from the column and group of columns does not vary greatly when an object or a face is viewed in different illuminations or from different angles. The population response acts as a buffer to absorb changes. The recognition of 'grandmother's face' turns out to be not the responsibility of one cell but, as had long been suspected, the outcome of activity in an intricate population of cells spread over several columns in the infero-temporal cortex.

18.5 PROSOPAGNOSIA

Face recognition is not only of importance to infrahuman primates but is also of very considerable significance to humans. During the million generations of the Palaeolithic, most humans lived in bands of between 50 and 100 individuals. Face signals then, as now, must have formed an important channel of nonverbal communication. It must have been important to be able to recognize friend and foe, to distinguish members of the band from foreigners. Indeed, the whole process of reciprocal altruism and the deontic codes which hold humans together in communities depends on the ability to recognize and remember other individuals. As with the other primates, it is therefore no surprise to find that an area of the brain, in the human case a remarkably large area, is dedicated to face recognition.

This area of the brain is located (bilaterally) in the infero-medial part of the occipito-temporal lobes (Figure 18.24). Endocasts of human skulls suggest that this region (in contrast to some of the linguistic areas (Chapter 10, Section 6)) was well developed in *Homo habilis* and *Homo erectus*. This goes some way to suggesting that nonverbal communication by way of facial expression preceded sophisticated

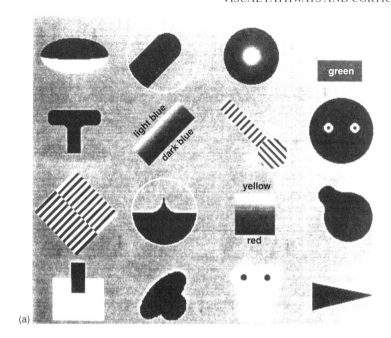

(a)

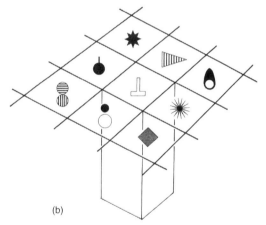

(b)

Figure 18.23 (a) Examples of trigger features of some of the cells in the anterior inferior temporal cortex (ITC). (b) Schematic to show the columnar organization of feature recognition cells in ITC. Explanation in text. From Tanaka, K. (1996) Inferotemporal cortex and object vision. *Annual Review of Neuroscience*, **19**, 109–39 with permission from Annual Reviews.

linguistic ability. This suspicion is supported by the observation that several facial signals – the eyebrow 'flash', the smile and so on – are (unlike language) universally understood. A connection might be made here with the mirror-neuron system, which will be discussed in Section 23.8. We shall see there that neurons which fire empathically in response to facial movements made by others in a social situation exist in both monkey and human brains. There is also some evidence that the mechanisms of this facial recognition area of the brain are also called into

play when other objects which have 'physiognomic' properties – animal faces, cars, furniture, crockery and so on – are recognized.

The loss of the ability to recognize the faces of people otherwise well-known is known as **prosopagnosia**. The condition has been recognized since the mid-nineteenth century and has been popularized by Oliver Sacks in his strikingly titled book, *The Man who Mistook his Wife for a Hat*. Prosopagnosia is caused by damage, either by the growth of a tumour or, more usually, by vascular damage, to the face

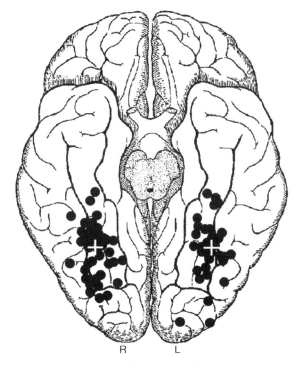

Figure 18.24 Location of regions sensitive to faces in the human brain. The black dots represent sites on the inferior surface of the brain where evoked potentials were detected in response to the presentation of faces. There is a slight preponderance in the right hemisphere (41) compared with the left hemisphere (34) and significantly more sites in the infero-temporal lobe (53) compared with the infero-occipital lobe (25). From Allison, T., Puce, A., Spencer, D.D. and McCarthy, G. (1999) with permission from Oxford University Press.

recognition area, especially on the right side. Individuals suffering from the condition often find it more difficult to recognize those closest to them than more distant and infrequently seen relatives and friends. This strange conjunction is sometimes brought to an extreme in the prosopagnosiac's inability to recognize him or herself in a mirror. Other aspects of the prosopagnosiac's recognition system usually remain intact. Friends and relatives can be recognized by their voice, or by their clothes, or by their manner-

isms. Only the face recognition system is impaired. The condition is, nevertheless, socially disabling. A patient never knows whether the person approaching is friend or stranger (unless the clothes or walk are recognized) and never knows whether to stop, smile and enter into conversation or to pass coldly by. Unless the friend or relative knows about the pathology, social intercourse may be abruptly terminated. Few forgive a snub. The social exclusion suffered by undiagnosed prosopagnosiacs points up the great significance of face recognition in both modern and, perhaps even more, in primitive societies.

18.6 CONCLUDING REMARKS

This chapter, although it has done no more than scratch the surface of a vast subject, has shown that primate central visual analysers have evolved into massively sophisticated systems. The more than two dozen currently recognized visual areas are interconnected both 'upward' and 'downward', and in both a hierarchical and parallel manner. We touched on the evolutionary reasons for this huge complexity at the beginning of the chapter. Vision is for us, as it is for all primates, the imperial sense. The human world, with the proliferation of modern electronic media, is becoming ever more dominated by the visual sense. Our literary and philosophic vocabulary has long been marinated in visual metaphor. Martin Heidegger points out that the original sense of the Greek word for knowledge was 'seeing'. It has, furthermore, been suggested that our ever-increasing understanding of the neuroscience of vision provides the least worst chance of bridging the gap between brain and mind. That remains a hope for the future. For the present we can hope that neuroscientific principles discovered in the visual brain can be of help in understanding the workings of less intensively studied areas. We can also hope, with David Marr, that these principles and these insights may be of value in the design of the brain's silicon rivals.

19

OTHER VERTEBRATE VISUAL SYSTEMS

Visual pigments: rhodopsin, porphyropsin - adaptation to aquatic life? **Photoreceptors**: oil droplets - colour filters - paraboloids; double and triple cones - fish; double rods - reptiles - amphibia; photomechanical movements. **Tapeta**: choroidal - various types - occlusibility; retinal - fish - occlusibility - prey-detection. **Retina**: multiply banked of deep sea fish; Anuran: RFs - ON, OFF, ON/OFF - sustained contrast - 'bug' detector; mammals, birds: convexiclivate foveae - multiple areae centrales and foveae - visual streak - pecten. **Dioptric apparatus**: retinal area and resolving power - tubular or 'telescope' eyes - 'four-eyed' fish - focusing by cornea and lens - cornea predominates in aerial vertebrates - corneal 'spectacle' in some reptiles - lens predominates in fish - Mathiesson's ratio - 'discovered' by eight groups of aquatic animals. **Median eyes**: parietal and pineal - histology - evolution - reproductive cycles etc. - synthesis and release of melatonin. **Visual pathways**: tectofugal pathway dominant in non-mammals - Newton-Muller-Gudden law for RGS pathway - complete chiasmatic decussation in tectofugal pathway - partial decussation elsewhere. **Visual centres**: Amphibia: optic tectum - histology - physiology - RFs - 'newness' and 'sameness' RFs; Reptilia - tectofugal and thalamofugal pathways - optic tectum - dorsoventricular ridge (DVR) - comparisons with mammalian primary visual cortex; Aves - great variety of visual systems - thalamofugal and tectofugal pathways; thalamfugal wulst - comparable to mammalian primary visual cortex - four cell layers - RFs - binocular drive; tectofugal contralateral tectum - retinotopic organisation - RFs; nucleus rotundus - RFs - movement - optic flow - comparison to mammalian extratriate cortices - feedback and feedforward connections. **Concluding remarks**: huge variety of vertebrate visual systems - antidote to anthropocentrism.

We started Chapter 16 with some remarks about the great antiquity of the vertebrate eye. We saw that it can be traced in its essentials back five hundred million years to the beginning of the Cambrian period. The vast stretch of time since that period has seen the vertebrates radiate into a huge number of different habitats and develop a multitude of different styles of life. Although, as we noted, the vertebrate eye has remained essentially unchanged through this radiation, it has obviously undergone many modifications to fit it (or rather fit its owners) for their particular stations in life. In this chapter we shall look at some of the major adaptations.

Biology of Sensory Systems, Second Edition   C.U.M. Smith
© 2008 John Wiley & Sons, Ltd

19.1 VISUAL PIGMENTS

We saw in the Introduction to Part Four that animal visual pigments consisted of opsins attached, via a Schiff's base linkage, to chromophores derived from Vitamin A. In Box 15.1 the evolution of the opsins were reviewed and we saw that they all belong to one great superfamily of 7TM proteins. Also in the Introduction to this Part, we noted that vertebrate chromophores were of two types, $retinal_1$ and $retinal_2$ (3,4 dehydroretinal). When opsin is attached to $retinal_1$ the resulting photopigment is called **rhodopsin**; when it is attached to $retinal_2$ it is called **porphyropsin**.

Rhodopsin and porphyropsin differ in their λ_{max}. On average the λ_{max} of porphyropsin is 'red-shifted' some 20 nm from the λ_{max} of rhodopsin. At one time it was believed that this reflected an adaptation to life in somewhat murky waters where the shorter wavelengths of white light are preferentially scattered. This is often the case in freshwater rivers and streams or in ponds and lakes into which run-off from the surroundings drain. It is perhaps for this reason that porphyropsins are mostly restricted to the rod cells of freshwater fish, although they are also found in a few marine species. It is satisfactory to find that bottom dwelling fish tend to have porphyropsin, whilst those that feed at the surface have predominantly rhodopsin systems. However, the ecological relationship is by no means clear cut. The dependence of photopigment sensitivity on λ_{max} is very small; it has been calculated that only about a 10% increased sensitivity is gained from a pigment with λ_{max} at 480 nm compared with λ_{max} at 500 nm. Furthermore, many deep sea fish develop red-shifted rhodopsins rather than porphyropsins. Both elasmobranchs and teleosts have evolved rhodopsins with λ_{max} between 470 nm and 480 nm.

It is interesting to note that fish, such as the European and North American eel, *Anguilla* sp., which spend part of their life in freshwater and other parts in the deeper waters of the ocean, change their pigment to suit their different environments. The eel spends most of its life in freshwater, using a predominantly porphyropsin system but before it migrates to its spawning grounds, 400 m deep in the Sargasso sea, it undergoes a major metamorphosis. This includes a change from a porphyropsin system, λ_{max} 520 nm, to a rhodopsin system with λ_{max} at about 500 nm. On the other hand, the lamprey, *Petromyzon marinus*, which spawns in freshwater streams and migrates to the ocean, has rhodopsin on the way down but returns with porphyropsin. It can be seen that the situation is difficult to rationalize. It may be that the distribution of porphyropsin and rhodopsin photo pigment owes more to chance and happenstance than to habitat or evolutionary ancestry. Or it may have some biochemical significance which confers a yet undiscovered selective advantage.

19.2 PHOTORECEPTORS

We have already noted that vertebrate photoreceptors are of two main types: rods and cones. Although rods do not vary greatly throughout the vertebrates there are many different types of cone. Some of these are shown in Figure 19.1. We described the structure of the mammalian cone in Chapter 17. Cones in other vertebrates often develop **oil droplets** in the ellipsoid. These droplets have not been reported in vertebrates 'lower' than the amphibia. They usually contain carotenoids which give them a distinctive colour. In diurnal birds they are generally red, orange, yellow or green; in nocturnal species they are either colourless or pale yellow. In the budgerigar, for instance, there are four classes of cone pigment with λ_{max} at 565, 507, 445–430 and 380–360 nm respectively. The three longer wavelength classes contain oil droplets with upper cut offs at about 570, 520–500 and 445 nm, whilst the short wavelength (ultraviolet) cone has a transparent droplet. In general, the droplets selectively filter incident light so that discrimination between different colours is enhanced and they also help to focus light on cone outer segments.

Whilst the oil droplet normally develops in the ellipsoid, another dioptric organelle, the **paraboloid**, sometimes develops in the myoid (Figure 19.1). Unlike the droplet, the paraboloid is not coloured and instead of carotenoids it contains a high concentration of glycogen. Having a considerably higher refractive index than the surroundings, it too plays a significant role in focusing light on to the outersegment.

Another feature of many vertebrate retinae is the presence of **double and sometimes triple cones** (Figure 19.1c). They occur in fish, amphibia, reptiles, birds, one monetreme (the platypus) and marsupials.

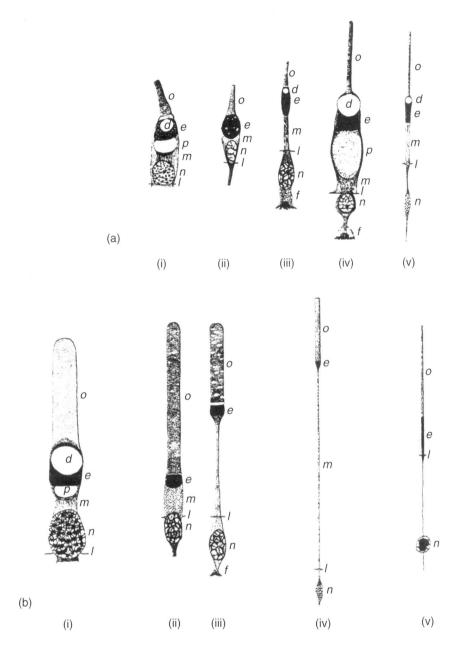

Figure 19.1   Vertebrate photoreceptor cells. (a) Cones (×1000). (i) Cone of *Acipenser fulvescens*, the sturgeon. (ii) Light adapted cone of *Carassius auratus* (myoid contracted). Note that the cone nucleus, as in other fish, lies outside the external limiting membrane. (iii) Dark adapted cone of *Rana pipiens*, a frog (myoid elongated). (iv) Cone from *Chelydra serpentina*, the snapping turtle. (v) Cone from the circumfoveal eminence of *Circus hudsonius*, the marsh hawk. Note the slender structure and the long thin outersegement. (b) Rods (×1000). (i) Rod of *Protopterus ethiopicus*, a lungfish, unusual in that it contains an oil droplet which implies origination from a cone. (ii) Dark adapted red rod of *Rana pipiens* (myoid contracted) (iii) Light adapted green rod of *Rana pipiens* (myoid relaxed). (iv) Light adapted rod of *Carassius auratus*, the goldfish. During light adaptation the myoid (as shown) is greatly elongated; in the dark it contracts. (v) Filamentous rod of *Glaucomys volans volans*, the flying squirrel. This long thin rod is characteristic of many nocturnal and crepuscular animals. (*Continues overleaf*)

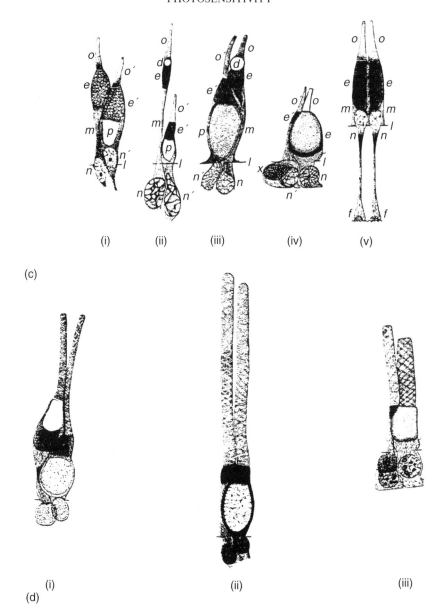

Figure 19.1 (*Continued*) (c) Double cones (×1000). (i) Double cone of *Amia calva*, a holostean fish; (ii) Dark adapted double cone of *Rana pipiens* (myoid of chief cone elongated). (iii) Double cone of *Chrysemys picta marginata*, a turtle. (iv) Double cone of *Natrix natrix*, grass snake; (v) Light adapted double cone of *Lepomis macrochirus*, the bluegill, a teleost fish. The fused myoids are contracted. (d) Double rods (×1000). (i) Double rod of *Xantusia riversiana*, Rivers' night lizard. The photoreceptor is intermediate between rod and cone. Although structurally rod-like they contain no rhodopsin and are low-threshold. (ii) Double rod from the retina of *Coleonyx variegatus*, the banded gecko. (iii) The double rod of *Hypsiglena ochrorhynchus*, the spotted night snake. c = 'clear' area; d = oil droplet; e = ellipsoid (ellipsoid of chief); e' = ellipsoid of accessory; f = foot; l = external limiting membrane; m = myoid; n' = nucleus (nucleus of chief); n = nucleus of accessory; o = outersegment (outersegment of chief); o' = outersegment of accessory; p = paraboloid. From Walls, G.L. (1963) with permission from Hafner, and from Crescitelli, F. (1977) with permission from Springer-Verlag.

For some as yet unknown reason they have not yet been shown to occur in eutherian mammals. Double cones usually consist of two very unlike cones fused together at their myoids. The two fused cones normally differ greatly in size; the major (or principal) cone often has an oil droplet and the minor cone a very large paraboloid. But this is not always the case, and all combinations of size and structure have been found. In some cases, for instance the various species of snapper (*Lutjanus* sp.) found on Australian Great Barrier Reef, the double cones contain different photopigments. It has also been suggested that double cones may be involved in the detection of the plane of polarization of incident sunlight. Finally, in many fish retinae the cones form a very regular mosaic with four double cones forming a rectangle around a single cone.

In addition to double cones, many teleostean fish retinae develop **twin cones**. Unlike double cones, the two members of a twin cone are (at least structurally) equal partners. They are fused throughout their length (Figure 19.1c (v)) but have separate pedicles. Whether twin cones are evolutionarily related to double cones or can, indeed, be sharply distinguished from them in the inevitable continuous spectrum of forms in the biological world, remains a debateable point. Indeed, some fish possess retinae with all four varieties of cone. The retinae of the common barbel (*Barbus barbus*), for instance, contain short single cones, long single cones, twin cones and unequal double cones distributed throughout the retina in no particular order.

Cones are not unique in doubling up. Double rods are frequently found in the lacertilian retina, especially in those of snakes and geckoes (Figure 19.1d). The Geckoes have been particularly well studied. They are a family of mainly insectivorous lizards found in a variety of habitats in the warmer parts of the world. Many of them are nocturnal or crepuscular but diurnal forms also exist. Their eyes are large and well developed. In diurnal forms double cones are well represented. In the nocturnal and crepuscular forms the outersegment is long and cylindrical so that the photoreceptor is better termed a double rod (Figure 19.1d). The Tokay Gecko (*G. gekko*) has two photopigments with λ_{max} at 521 and 467 nm. In some cases both members of the rod pair contain the same pigment, in others one member contains the 521 pigment and the other the 467 pigment.

Rods, also, have various shapes and forms. Perhaps the best known dimorphism is shown in the frog retina, where the rods are of two major types: red rods and green rods. Figure 19.1b (ii) and (iii) shows that they have very different structures, the green rod (containing a 432 nm pigment) having a long thin myoid whilst the red rod (with a 502 nm pigment) has hardly a myoid at all. This brings us to the last feature of many nonmammalian photoreceptor cells: their **photomechanical movements**. These movements are brought about by actin filaments in the myoid. In bright light the **rod** myoid relaxes and the outersegment moves towards the pigment epithelium. Vice versa the **cone** myoids contract and bring their outersegments towards the source of the light. In the case of double cones the major member may show photomechanical movement but the minor member is usually unaffected and remains in position. Photomechanical movements are quite slow, to be measured in minutes (birds) to tens of minutes (fish). These mechanical movements of the photoreceptors are complemented by similarly slow movement of pigment granules in the microvilli of the pigment epithelial cells. The granules move into the microvilli to shield the rods and increase the acuity of the cones in bright light and move back towards the RPE in dim illuminations. It has been said that animals with well developed photomechanical mechanisms effectively have two retinae, one for dim and one for bright light.

It is clear from the foregoing that, compared with the retinae of other vertebrates, the human retina, which has been the focus of so much research, is remarkably impoverished in photoreceptor types.

19.3 TAPETA

The retinal pigment epithelium and choroid in humans contains large quantities of melanin, which absorb any light that escapes absorption in either the neural or photoreceptor layers of the retina. This is important as reflections might well confuse the image. However, in dim illumination it can be of great advantage to allow any light falling on the retina a second chance, through reflection, to interact with the visual pigment in the outersegments. Hence, as every motorist knows, the eyes of many hedgerow animals reflect the car headlights as the driver sweeps through country lanes. We would be very surprised (indeed alarmed) if the eyes of humans also reflected the headlights as we drive through urban areas. The layer which reflects light in many nocturnal and crepuscular animals is called the **tapetum**, or, more precisely, the **tapetum lucidum** (literally 'bright carpet'). In some cases it has an almost mirror-like quality (compare *Pecten* in Chapter 15), in others, probably the majority, the reflected light is scattered and diffuse. The tapetum is either formed in the **choroid** or (less often) in the **retinal pigment epithelium**.

Choroidal tapeta are of three types: '**fibrosum**', '**cellulosum**' and '**guaninum**'. The **fibrosum** type (tapetum fibrosum) is found in many hooved animals. It is formed of a dense deposition of white collagen fibres in the choroid just behind the choriocapillaris. This provides a good, though not excellent, reflective layer. The **cellulosum** type (tapetum cellulosum) provides a more effective mirror. It is developed in nocturnal prosimian primates and also in the carnivores – animals which have a proverbially vivid eyeshine – especially the domestic cat. A tapetum cellulosum is also found in seals. This type of tapetum, as its name suggests, is formed not of collagen fibres but of cells. Endothelial cells just beyond the choriocapillaris have proliferated and formed a close-set multilayered 'tiling'. These cells are packed with highly refractile threads which criss-cross to form mirror-like mesh. Finally, the **guaninum** type (tapetum guaninum) is found in a number of fish, both elasmobranchs and teleosts. Here, as in the case of the cellulosum type, a close-set multilayered tiling of cells develops just behind the choriocapillaris, but in this case, instead of fibres, the cells are filled with plates of guanine crystals. In some fish, especially some elasmobranchs (for example *Squalus acanthias*; *Mustelus mustelus*), this brilliantly reflective layer is **occlusible** (Figure 19.2). In dim light, pigment granules are concentrated in the centres of the choroidal cells and light penetrating to the tapetum has maximum chance of reflection from the layered guanine crystals; in bright light, on the other hand, the granules migrate out into the main body and processes of the choroidal cells and obscure the mirror.

Retinal tapeta are particularly well known in fish. Here, once again, guanine crystals form the reflective layer, though this time in the pigment epithelium. There it forms a bright silvery reflector. In some cyprinid fish, for instance *Abramis brama*, which live in the shallow turbid waters of Lake Balaton (west-

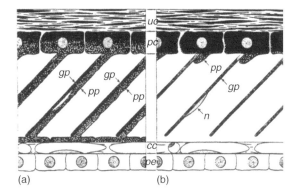

Figure 19.2 Vertical sections through the occlusible tapetum of *Mustelus.*, a dogfish. (a) Light adapted. Pigment granules have migrated between the guanine crystal plates diminishing the reflectivity. (b) Dark adapted. The pigment granules have withdrawn towards the pigment epithelum layer and the guanine crystals now form a brilliantly reflective layer behind the photoreceptor outersegements. cc = choriocapillaris; gp = guanine plate; pc = layer of migratory pigment cells in the choroid; pe = pigment epithelium of retina (devoid of pigment); pp = pigmented process; uc = unmodified choroid. From Walls, G.L. (1963) with permission from Hafner.

ern Hungary), the tapetum, like that in the elasmobranch tapetum guaninum described above, is 'occlusible'. In dim, uncertain, light the bright silvery mirror in the pigment epithelium reflects back almost all the light which strikes it. In brighter light pigment granules, which are also present in the RPE cells, migrate out into the processes of the cells and in front of the guanine crystal layer. In this state hardly any light is reflected back on to the photoreceptors to confuse the image. It is likely that the very variable turbidity of the shallow lake waters in which *Abramis brama* and its relatives have been confined is responsible for this valuable adaptation; the majority of fish with retinal tapeta are unable to control its reflectivity.

Reflecting tapeta have developed in many specialized ways, especially in vertebrates living in regions of low light intensity. This, of course, is especially the case with deep sea fish. Here any device which increases the sensitivity of the eye is valuable, even if the image quality is degraded. Some deep sea fish, for instance, emit light and search for reflections from suitable prey. One such fish, *Pachystomias*, emits a shaft of red light which is preferentially reflected back from red crustacean zooplankton. This fish has a red tapetum which is well adapted to scatter any such reflected light and thus increase the likelihood of the crustacean being detected. Many other similarly interesting tapetal adaptations have been found; all help to fit the eye to its owner's lifestyle.

19.4 RETINAE

The human 'duplex' retina was discussed in some detail in Chapter 17. We noted there that, although there are many modifications, the basic structure remains remarkably similar throughout the vertebrates. In this section we shall consider just a few of the variations on this retinal theme. In particular, we shall look at modifications of the **area centralis** in mammals and birds. Before doing so, however, it is worth noting, once again, the adaptations of the retinae of deep sea fish to dim illumination and the physiological adaptation of the frog's retina to its way of life.

19.4.1 Deep Sea Fish

In addition to the development of tapeta of various sorts (Section 19.3), deep sea fish develop not only rod cells with abnormally long outersegments but also (in many cases) **multiple banked retinae**. In one deep sea fish, *Diretmus argenteus*, the outersegments in a retina 900 μm thick are 600 μm in length! In many other species the outersegments are stacked one above the other to form a multiple bank. The outermost outersegments in these banks (there may be up to six or seven layers) are connected to their nuclei by long slender myoids (Figure 19.3).

In addition to these specializations, the retinae of many deep sea fish show several other adaptations to maximize sensitivity. These include regions of high ganglion cell density, bands of increased rod and cone density, accessory retinae and retinal diverticula and so on.

19.4.2 Frog

No account of vertebrate retinae would be complete without mention of the pioneering work of H.K. Hartline on the physiology of frog retinae. As early as 1938, Hartline had succeeded in dissecting out bundles, and in some cases single fibres, from the surface of the bullfrog retina (*Rana catesbiana*) and

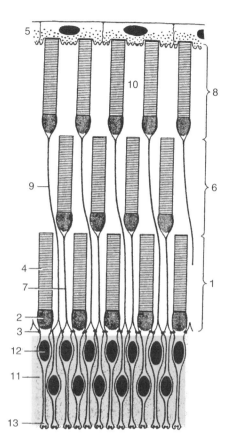

Figure 19.3 Diagram of a multibank retina. 1 = innermost (vitread) rods; 2 = ellipsoids of innermost rods; 3 = outer limiting membrane; 4 = outersegments of innermost rods; 5 = pigment epithelium; 6 = middle bank of rod outersegments; 7 = slender filamentous myoid of middle bank of outersegments; 8 = outer bank of outersegements; 9 = long filamentous myoid of outer outersegments; 10 = optic ventricle in which the outersegments of the middle and outer banks lie; 11 = rod fibre; 12 = rod nuclei; 13 = rod spherules. From Locket, N.A. (1977) with permission from Springer-Verlag.

recording from them by means of a wick electrode. He was able to detect three types of receptive field: **ON**, **OFF** and **ON/OFF** (Figure 19.4). The RFs were found to be roughly circular and up to 1 mm in diameter. When it is remembered that the entire eye of the frog measures only about 8 mm in diameter, the extraordinarily large size of these RFs can be appreciated. Hartline's work was later confirmed by microelectrode techniques. It was found that whereas ON and OFF units responded to brightening or

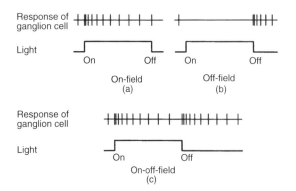

Figure 19.4 Physiological characteristics of frog ganglion cells with the commonest types of retinal receptive fields. Further explanation in text.

dimming of light wherever it fell on the field, ON/OFF units responded differently to diffuse and focused illumination. It was shown that the response to light falling on the centre of the field is much reduced if, at the same time, light is switched on at the periphery. A similar interaction is found if, vice versa, lights are switched off at the centre and the periphery. ON/OFF units, in other words, show some of lateral inhibition characteristics we met when we considered mammalian concentric receptive fields (Section 17.2.8). They respond most vigorously to edges and other discontinuities in illumination.

Further electrophysiological work on the frog retina showed the presence of two other types of receptive field. The first generates a sustained output whenever an edge is present in the field. For obvious reasons this is called a '**sustained contrast detector**' (sometimes class 1 unit). The second responds to moving small dark objects crossing the field. A straight edge fails to stimulate the ganglion cell. This second type of cell is called a '**net convexity detector**' (class 2 unit) or, more colloquially, a 'bug detector'.

In the absence of movement or changes in light intensity, there will be little activity in frog optic nerve fibres except from those originating in the sustained contrast detectors. It is appealing (and probably not too far from the truth) to imagine the frog sitting on its lily pad with just the sustained contrast detectors signalling the horizon and other significant edges and all else in the retina silent. A change in illumination, a sudden darkening as of a predatory duck or a sudden increase in illumination, will actuate the ON, OFF and ON/OFF fields. But, and most importantly, the incursion of a small dark object, an insect, will trigger the ON/OFF and, particularly, the net convexity detectors. The frog will bestir itself and shoot out its tongue.

The anuran visual system has been a favourite preparation for vision scientists. We shall return to consider the analysis of the visual information in the optic tectum in Section 19.8. The system has also lent itself to important investigations in developmental neurobiology. The student will find references listed in the bibliography. Let us now, however, turn our attention to the specializations which have evolved in the retinae of mammals and birds.

19.4.3 Areae Centrales of Mammals and Birds

This region of the retina is somewhat difficult to define. It is not necessarily at the centre of the retina. Nor is it always (or even frequently) impregnated with the yellow pigment which is so diagnostic a feature of the human area centralis, justifying the name **macula lutea** or yellow spot (Section 16.1.1). Some retinae, as we shall see, have more than one area. It is perhaps best to define it somewhat loosely as that part (or parts) of the retina which provides the best resolving power. In human retinae, as we saw in Chapters 16 and 17, it surrounds a small depression, the **fovea**. Far from all areae have a fovea.

Defining the area as that part of the retina possessing maximum resolving power immediately implies that it is the part which has the closest packing of photoreceptor cells. In the human case the cones are particularly long and thin. This is also the case with other retinae. In order to retain resolving power the cone/bipolar/ganglion cell ratio should approach 1/1/1. This has an unfortunate consequence. It means that a high density of cones is accompanied by a high density of all the other elements of the retina. This would make for comparative opacity. The solution (as noted in Chapter 17) is to route the bipolars diagonally away from the area centralis (Figure 17.6). Their cell bodies, IPL connections, amacrines and ganglion cells can thus be displaced to one side of the area. This displacement of the neural elements of the retina leads to a thinning of the retina in this position. This depression is the fovea. It is surrounded by a raised 'crater-like' rim which is created by the displaced neural elements.

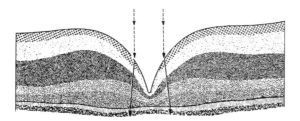

Figure 19.5 Convexiclivate fovea of an avian predator such as *Astur palumbarius*. Arrows indicate the direction of incident light which is refracted laterally to give an enlargement of the image. From Meyer, D.B. (1977) with permission from Springer-Verlag.

Most retinae possessing areae with high resolving power develop fovea. In many cases these foveae are far deeper than that of the human retina. These deep foveae are termed **convexiclivate** to distinguish them from the shallower and more irregular **concaviclivate** fovea of the human retinae. Do convexiclivate foveae have a function other than the histological function described above? This has been the source of much argument. Some have thought that the steep convex sides of the foveal pit magnify the image (Figure 19.5). Others have argued that an image falling on the sides of the pit will be distorted and only when it is centred will it be isomorphous with the object. They have argued that this provides a signal, aiding accurate aim in predatory and highly active animals. In support of this interpretation, strongly convexiclivate foveae are found in both birds of prey, such as the hawk, and also in predatory deep sea fish. On the other hand, the same argument would apply if convexiclivate foveae acted as magnifiers. This would also be of selective advantage to swiftly moving predators. Maybe both features have been selected. The jury is still out.

It has already been mentioned that some retinae possess more than one area and sometimes more than one fovea. Multiple areae and foveae are best known in the retinae of birds. Although a more or less central area centralis and fovea are found in most bird retinae, a number of alternatives have long been known, including the total absence of a fovea. The best established case of an afoveate avian retina is that of the Californian Valley Quail (*Lophortyx californicus vallicola*). Some of the other variants are shown in Figure 19.6. It can be seen that the 'area centralis' is sometimes central, sometimes lateral, sometimes contains a fovea and sometimes not. In some cases there are two areae each with a fovea. This condition is characteristic of birds which obtain their

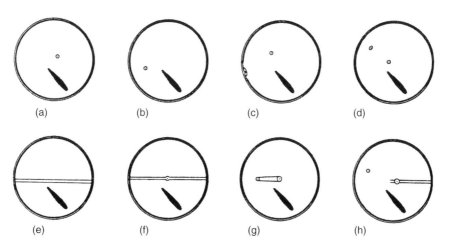

Figure 19.6 Retinal areae and foveae in some birds. The black ovoid represents the position of the pecten. (a) Central fovea (e.g. *Cyanocitta stelleris*, the Steller jay). (b) Lateral fovea (e.g. owls and swifts). (c) Bifoveate retina of the kingfisher, *Alcedo ispida*. Note highly eccentric lateral fovea. (d) Bifoveate retina of bittern, *Botaurus lentigenosus*. Note superior position of lateral fovea. (e) Linear afoveate area. This type of retina is found in some sea birds, for example Manx shearwater (*Puffinis puffinis*) and the fulmar petrel (*Fulmaris glacialis*). (f) Linear area with an enclosed central area containing the fovea, for example the American coot, *Fulica americana*. (g) Linear area stretching between a lateral and central area, both containing a fovea, for example sparrow hawk, *Falco sparverius*. (h) Linear area with enclosed centra area including a fovea and a separate lateral area and fovea, for example the tern, *Sterna hirundo*. From Meyer, D.B. (1977) with permission from Springer-Verlag.

food whilst flying: many passerines (songbirds and so on), kingfishers, hummingbirds. Evidently these birds require very precise perception of distance and speed. In many birds the area is not circular but a strip running across all or part of the retina. This organization is most often found in birds which inhabit open spaces and whose head bobs back and forth when walking on the ground. It is consequently thought that these ribbon-like areae have to do with the perception of the horizontal. Finally, perhaps the most highly developed retinae are those of diurnal birds of prey – eagles, hawks, buzzards, falcons – which have a combination of circular and ribbon areae with deep convexiclivate fovea in each. This organization provides a superb combination of visual acuity and distance perception.

Although ribbon-like areae are not so obvious in mammalian retinae, there is nevertheless evidence for a strip of enhanced visual acuity, known as the **visual streak**, in the great majority of mammals. Anatomically this shows itself in increased photoreceptor density, increased ganglion cell density, decreased convergence from photoreceptors on to ganglion cells and absence of overlying blood vessels. The streak is usually produced in the horizontal plane and is especially well developed in mammals living in open terrains. It is, for instance, prominent in the retinae of rabbits and hares, in the savannah-dwelling chetah and the greyhound, which is a domesticated form of the desert hunting dog, but is not well developed in small nocturnal species such as the mouse and hedgehog. Although the matter is still controversial, the consensus is that, like the ribbon areae of birds, the visual streak of mammals is an adaptation to assist alignment with the horizontal planes of open country.

Before ending this section one final striking retinal feature must be mentioned: this is the **pecten** (from Latin-pecten, a comb). This large structure is a feature of the avian eye. It grows from the elongated site of exit of the optic nerve and projects into the vitreous (Figure 19.7). It consists almost entirely of rather outsize capillaries and a few pigmented cells. Although its existence has been known since Perrault described it in 1676. and it has been subjected to a great deal of painstaking research, its function remains controversial. Its form and size varies in different birds – conical, vaned, pleated – but in all cases its one invariant characteristic is

its intense vascularization. Hence, in spite of ingenious theories giving it a part to play in avian visual physiology, its most probable role is its most obvious role: that of providing nutritional exchange for the vitreous humour and the neural layers of the retina. Its position over the bird retina's elongated 'blind spot' ensures that there is minimal obstruction of vision.

19.5 DIOPTRIC APPARATUS

The minimum diameter of rod and cone outersegments is limited by the physical characteristics of electromagnetic radiation in the visible spectrum. They cannot be less than about $2\,\mu m$ in width (see the Introduction to Part Four). It follows that to resolve fine detail the retina must be fairly extensive. A small retina cannot pack in sufficient outersegments to discriminate fine detail in the image. Hence, animals with good vision have large eyes, not simply relative to their body size, but on an absolute scale. This is evident if we examine the eyes of small passerine birds, such as hedge sparrows or chaffinches. To achieve excellent vision their eyes are far larger than their brains. The relatively small eyes of nocturnal and crepuscular rodents, rats and mice, indicate that their visual acuity is poor.

Turning from the absolute size of the eye to its overall shape, we find a number of adaptations to fit it to different habitats and lifestyles. Some of the most striking of these adaptations are found in deep sea fish. The best known of these adaptations are the tubular eyes of a number of genera, for example *Scopelarchus*, *Argyropelecus* and so on (Figure 19.8a). Here, to discriminate as much detail as possible, the eyeball is not increased in diameter (it would not fit into the skull) but deepened along one dimension. Hence an older name, the 'telescope' eye. There is an enormous lens and a long tubular eye cup with a well developed retina at the bottom. An accessory retina extends up the wall of the tube. Although the lens is under some degree of focusing control, the optics suggest that the eye is always myopic. It has been suggested that the accessory retinae permit the formation of images of distant objects; more recent work, however, suggests that this is unlikely. It is probable that the accessory retina is largely concerned with the detection of diffuse illumination,

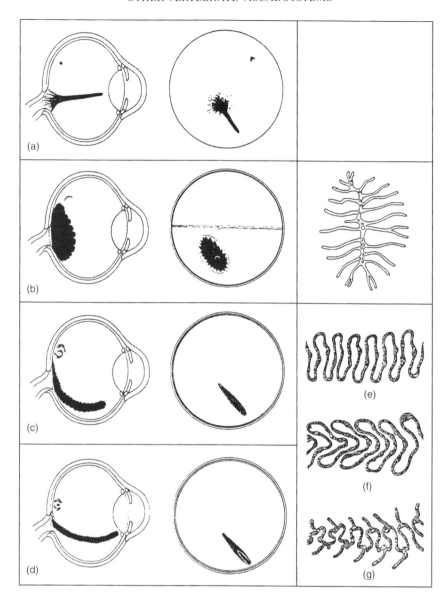

Figure 19.7 Various types of avian pecten. The left column shows lateral views, the middle column plan views and the right column transverse sections of the pecten. (a) Conical pecten of kiwi (*Apteryx mantelli*). (b) Vaned pecten of ostrich (*Struthio camellus*). (c) Pleated pecten of wood pigeon (*Columba palumbus*). (d) Pleated pecten of the Wonga Wonga dove (*Leucosarcia picata*). (e), (f) and (g) illustrate three types of pleated pecten, (e) and (f) being the most common. From Meyer, D.B. (1977) with permission from Springer-Verlag.

perhaps provided by the photophores of other denizens of the deep sea.

Another interesting piscean eye is that of the South American species, *Anableps tetrophthalmus* (four-eyed fish) (figure 19.8b), which swims with its eyes half in and half out of the water. This eye has interested scientists since the times of Artedi (1758) and Soemerring (1818). It possesses a lens shaped so that it focuses light from above (the atmosphere) on to one segment of the retina and light from below (the

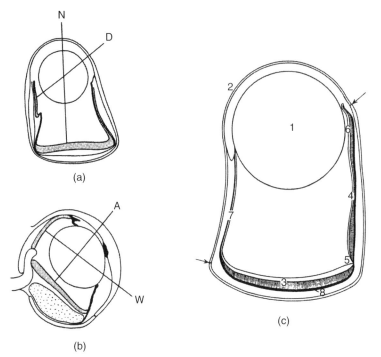

Figure 19.8 Fish eyes. (a) Tubular eye of deep sea fish showing the two retinae: N, for myopic vision and D, for hypermetropic vision. (b) Eye of *Anableps*. The pyriform shape of the lens and the possession of two pupils allows the fish to see in both air and water. Aerial vision uses the upper pupil and the lower retina (A); aquatic vision uses the lower pupil and the upper retina (W). From Walls, 1963. (c) Detail of the tubular eye of a deep sea fish. 1 = large lens; 2 = thin but very extensive cornea, its limits being marked by the arrows; 3 = retina; 4 = accessory retina which extends between the points marked 5 and 6; 7 = lateral wall of eye vesicle, formed by iris; 8 = choroid lies just behind both main and accessory retinae. From Locket, N.A. (1977) with permission from Springer-Verlag.

aquatic environment) on to another segment. The cornea is similarly specialized to focus light onto the different segments of the retina. In effect, *Anableps* has two optical systems in each eye and well deserves its specific name of tetrophthalmus (Figure 19.8b).

It will have been noticed in the preceding paragraphs (and in Figure 19.8) that the lens of the fish's eye, when compared with that of humans, is both comparatively huge and spherical. This is because most of the focusing in the fish eye (and in aquatic eyes in general) is carried out by the lens. In an aquatic environment the contribution made by the cornea is minimal. This is in sharp contrast to the aerial eye, such as our own, where some two thirds of the optical power resides in the cornea (Figure 19.9c). In the latter eyes the lens is only used to make adjustments to the focus. An additional complication in some aerial eyes is the presence of a 'spectacle' in front of the cornea. This develops by fusion of the eyelids in some lizards and snakes. Its major and probably original function is to protect the cornea from abrasion but in some species it has evolved to play a significant refractive role. The fish cornea, in

contrast, is so unimportant to the optics that it is often highly irregular, a condition which would be fatal to the clear vision of a terrestrial vertebrate such as ourselves. The fish lens, moreover, generally lies close up behind the cornea, seldom giving room for an anterior chamber, so that it can both obtain maximal focal length from the retina and also achieve a measure of all round vision.

The insignificance of the fish cornea is due to the difference in refractive index between it and the environing water being insufficient to refract light to focus an image on the retina. This is almost entirely the job of the lens. In 1877, Matthiessen noticed that the retina is almost always about 2.5 lens radii behind the centre of the lens. This ratio of focal length to lens radius is known as **Matthiessen's ratio**. But there's a snag. If the lens were optically homogeneous, its refractive index would have to be about 1.66 if light were to be focussed on a retina 2.5 lens radii away. But a refractive index of 1.66 is not achievable with the materials at the fish's (or any other animal's) disposal. Matthiessen showed that the answer to this conundrum lies in the inhomogeneity of the lens. He showed that the refractive index varies from about 1.52 at the centre to less than 1.4 at the periphery.

The effect of a Matthiessen gradient in refractive index from centre to periphery is twofold. Firstly, the focal length is reduced, which allows the pupil aperture to be increased and, consequently, to garner more light. Secondly, the correct gradient of refractive index across the lens eliminates spherical aberration. A spherical lens without this gradient would be virtually useless in forming an image (Figure 19.9a). By measuring the focal length and the radii of lenses it is easy to determine whether an animal has 'discovered' how to make a Matthiessen lens. It has been found that this has been achieved at least eight separate and independent times: fish, belemnoid molluscs, four times amongst the gastropod molluscs, in a family of annelid worms (the Alciopidae) and in the copepod crustacean *Labidocera*. As Land and Fernald point out, this list includes all aquatic eyes of any size: there is, they say, 'only one right way of producing such lenses and ... natural selection always finds it'.

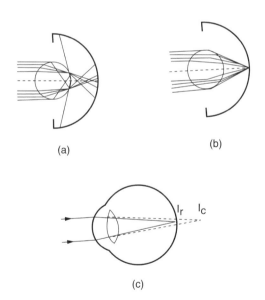

(a)

(b)

(c)

Figure 19.9 Optics of some vertebrate eyes. (a) Homogeneous spherical lens. (b) Inhomogeneous 'Matthiessen' lens (c) Human eye. Ic = image formed by cornea; Ir = image formed by cornea + lens. Explanation in text. After Land, M.F. and Fernald, R.D. (1992).

19.6 MEDIAN EYES

We noted in Section 4.7.8 that the lamellar body of the protochordate, *Amphioxus*, is believed to be the primordium of the vertebrate median eye. There is also good evidence from fossilized skulls that early vertebrates possessed a median eye. Many skulls from the palaeozoic and mesozoic eras show a parietal foramen. This is often quite large, being sometimes the same size as the foramen magnum. No living vertebrates develop such large median eyes. Nevertheless, the median eye in the most primitive of living vertebrates, the cyclostomata, is remarkably well developed.

Median eyes develop from the posterior roof of the diencephalon. In their most elaborate form they take the form of two outpushings, an anterior **parietal** (or **parapineal**) organ and a more posterior *pineal* organ, or **epiphysis**. The dual structure is best seen in cyclostomes such as the lamprey (Figure 19.10). In these forms both parietal and pineal organs develop retinae with cone like photoreceptors. Action potentials have been recorded in the dark and this activity is inhibited by illumination. The spectral sensitivity curve peaks at 525 nm. The biological significance of the system varies in different species. It can be shown by ablation experiments that, at least in *Lampetra planeri*, the median eye controls diurnal body colour changes. Chondrichthyan fish, such as the dogfish, possess well developed pineal photoreceptors with ciliary type photoreceptors (Figure 19.10).

The adaptive radiation of the median eye is shown in Figure 19.11. The pineal organ is found in an intracranial position in all classes of vertebrates. The parietal organ, on the other hand, is found intracranially in lampreys and some teleosts but rises to an extracranial position in frogs and lizards. The photoreceptors of both pineal and parietal organs resemble the cones of the lateral eyes in many ways. As Figure 19.10b shows, they develop stacks of membranes by invagination, thus displaying the visual pigment to light from above. They also possess characteristic synaptic ribbons in their synaptic terminals. It must be noted, however, that (in many but not all) cases the retina is 'verted', that is the photoreceptor outersegments face towards the light. It should also be noted that, at least in parietal eye

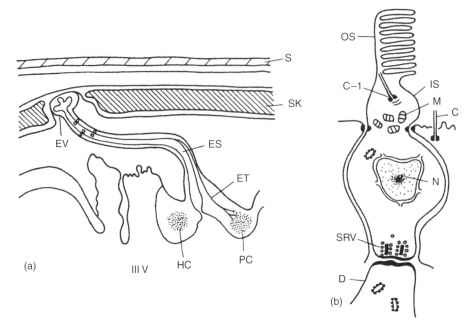

Figure 19.10 Pineal system of a Chondrichthyan fish such as a dogfish. (a) Schematic drawing of a midsagittal section through brain; (b) schematic drawing of a photoreceptor and ganglion cell. C = cilium; C-1 = centriole; D = dendrite of underlying ganglion cell; E = pineal (= epiphysis); ES = pineal (epiphyseal) stalk; ET = pineal (epiphyseal) tract; EV = pineal (epiphyseal) vesicle; HC = habenular commissure; IS = inner segment; M = mitochondrion; N = nucleus; OS = outersegment; PC = posterior commissure; S = skin; SK = skull (cartilage); SRV = synaptic ribbon and vesicles; III V = third ventricle. From Hamasaki, D.I. and Elder, D.J. (1977), with permision from Springer-Verlag.

photoreceptors, the response to light is not a hyper-polarization but a depolarization.

The median eye starts out in the stem vertebrates as a photoreceptor. It retains this function in both bony and cartilaginous fish (chondrichthyes) and in the amphibia, although, in some cases, only in the latter's tadpole stage. It reaches a climax as a photoreceptor (so far as living vertebrates are concerned) in the reptiles and especially in the tuatara lizard, *Sphenodon*. Here the parietal organ develops a retina consisting of several thousand photoreceptors facing towards the incoming light, which is focused by a cellular lens. This third eye is only functional in hatchlings. In the adult it is covered by the scaly skin. In both amphibia and reptiles the median eye plays a role in controlling colour change and certain behavioural (especially reproductive) cycles. It is known that the epiphysis synthesizes **melatonin** in all these vertebrates and it may be that this hormone is involved in the biological responses initiated by variations in illumination.

In birds and mammals only the epiphysis (pineal) develops and it never penetrates the meninges. It is thus intracranial, and being covered not only by the dura but also by the parietal bone of the skull is not directly exposed to illumination. Although some remnant of photoreceptor ultrastructure remains, the so-called **pinealocytes** no longer develop outersegments or contain visual pigments. Nevertheless, in both birds and mammals a multisynaptic nerve pathway from the lateral eyes provides it with information about photoperiod. The origins of this pathway in the intrinsically photosensitive ganglion cells, ipRGCs, of the retina were noted in Section 17.2.7. This pathway is important as in both birds and mammals the pineal, although losing its photoreceptor function, retains its ability to synthesize and release melatonin. In many birds and mammals this hormone is important in regulating reproductive cycles. The visual input from the lateral eyes thus ensures that these cycles are related to day length and thus season of the year.

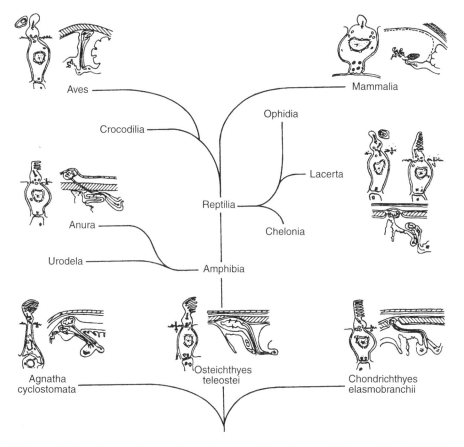

Figure 19.11 Adaptive radiation of the median eye. Explanation in text. From Hamasaki, D.I. and Elder, D.J. (1977), with permision from Springer-Verlag.

19.7 VISUAL PATHWAYS

The primate visual pathways were described in Chapter 18. We saw that the major flow of visual information was transmitted from the retina through the LGNd to the striate cortex. Less significant pathways run to other areas, including the superior colliculus, the pulvinar nucleus, the pretectum and the pineal gland. In nonmammalian vertebrates the same pathways are to be found but the pathway leading from the LGNd to the telencephalon is far less important. Instead, pathways leading to midbrain nuclei and, especially, the **tectofugal** pathway to the optic tectum are far more significant. We looked at a popular theory which accounts for this difference between the mammals and the rest of the vertebrates in Chapter 18. It is certainly not the case that a geniculostri-

ate system is crucial to excellent vision. The birds disprove this supposition every day.

In all nonmammalian vertebrates the optic nerves show complete decussation. The partial decussation and laminar organization of the LGNd in mammals is related to binocular vision and stereopsis. Indeed, in mammals the relative number of uncrossed fibres is roughy proportional to the frontality of the eyes. This proportionality is known as the **Newton–Muller–Gudden** law. In primates almost 50% of optic nerve fibres do not cross over, in the rat only about 20% and in the rabbit only 1 or 2%. This is not to say that no nonmammalian vertebrate possesses stereoscopic vision. Many birds have excellent binocularity, as their lifestyle demands. Here, however, the partial decussation does not occur at the optic chiasm but in the thalamo-telencephalic pathway (see below). Many fish also have frontal eyes providing binocular depth perception and it is believed, once again, that the partial decussation occurs in the thalamo-telencephalic connections.

19.8 VISUAL CENTRES IN THE BRAIN

19.8.1 Amphibia

The major features of frog retinal physiology were outlined in Section 19.4. After complete decussation, the optic nerve fibres run to the optic tectum in the roof of the midbrain (Figure 19.12). Here the fibres terminate in dense arborizations in four distinct layers. Each layer is organized into a complete map of the retina. These maps have been likened to four maps of a countryside laid one above the other. One might be a map of the contours, another of mineral deposits, another of population density and a fourth of vegetation. In the case of the anuran optic tectum, the uppermost map is innervated by fibres from the sustained contrast detectors, whilst the lower maps contain the terminals of the net convexity detectors, the ON/OFF (or moving edge) detectors, and the ON and OFF detectors in that order. It is tempting to believe that these maps, especially perhaps the net convexity (or bug) detector map, feed directly into the motor output system of the frog's brain.

In addition to the terminal arborization of the retinal ganglion cell fibres, the anuran optic tectum contains several other types of neuron. Two significant varieties have been described: so-called '**newness**' and '**sameness**' neurons. The 'newness' neurons have large receptive fields which respond to objects moving in particular directions. They quickly adapt to movements in this direction. If, however, the movement is altered through $90°$, the response is again vigorous until it, too, disappears through adaptation. The 'sameness' neurons also have large receptive fields and are characterized by 'attentiveness'; that is they respond to a small stimulus moving in one part of the their field and totally fail to respond to a second stimulus inserted into another part of the field. Neurons with several other types of receptive field have been detected in the tectum. In most cases the RFs are very large, sometimes equivalent to the entire field of the eye and their properties are often difficult to interpret.

19.8.2 Reptiles

In reptiles the major pathway from the retina is, like that of the amphibia, the **tectofugal** pathway carrying information to the optic tectum and then via a major thalamic nucleus, the nucleus rotundus, to the telencephalon. Other less important visual pathways from the retina also exist. In particular, optic nerve fibres run to the pretectum and also to the ventral subdivision of the lateral geniculate nucleus (LGNv) and (less importantly) to the LGNd in the thalamus. This latter route, which is homologous with the mammalian RGS route is known as the **thalamofugal** pathway. The optic tectum itself is fully equal in complexity to the amphibian tectum considered above. It

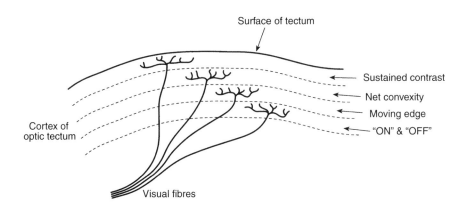

Figure 19.12 Schematic figure to show the organized termination of optic nerve fibres carrying different information about the visual scene in the frog optic tectum. Further explanation in text.

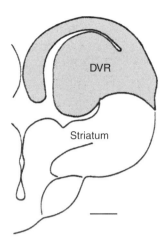

Figure 19.13 Transverse section through the telencephalon of a reptile to show the dorsoventricular ridge (DVR). Scale bar = 1 mm. From Shimizu, T. and Karten, H.J. (1991) Central visual pathways in reptiles and birds: evolution of the visual system, in *Vison and Visual Dysfunction, Vol. 2* (eds J.R. Cronly-Dillon and R.L. Gregory), copyright © 1991 Macmillan Press.

is generally considered to consist of six layers of cells, although other schematics visualize fourteen layers. The tectum projects via the nucleus rotundus to an area in the telencephalon known as the **dorsoventricular ridge (DVR)**. The DVR is a region equal in neuroanatomical complexity to the mammalian visual cortex. It receives input not only from the tectum but also from the thalamus and from other areas of the telencephalon. Figure 19.13 shows that it develops in the lateral wall of the telencephalon and bulges into the ventricle. Unlike the visual cortex of mammals, it is a massive rather than sheet-like structure.

The DVR receives input from all the major sense modalities. The visual input terminates in the lateral area but as yet no retinotopic organzation has been detected. Neurons in this region have large receptive fields and are sensitive to movement, especially the direction of movement. Finally, fibres project forward from the DVR to the dorsal wall of the telencephalon, a region which becomes the neocortex in mammals and the visual wulst in birds.

19.8.3 Birds

Birds are among the most 'visual' of all animals. Nevertheless, as would be expected in such a large and diverse group, there are many differences in the organization of their visual systems. One significant difference is found between birds which develop frontal eyes with large binocular fields such as owls, and those with lateral eyes and restricted binocularity, for instance pigeons, finches and so on. In the first case, the thalamofugal pathway is strongly developed, in the second the tectofugal pathway is more prominent. Both ultimately project forward into the telencephalon.

The optic nerve fibres in the **thalamofugal** pathway show complete decussation and terminate in a group of nuclei in the dorsal thalamus known, collectively, as the principal optic nucleus of the thalamus (OPT). This group of nuclei are regarded as analogous to the LGNd of reptiles and mammals. From the OPT, fibres project forward to an area of the dorsoventricular ridge known as the **wulst** (from German: 'bulge'). In birds with good binocular vision, the anterior fibres cross over to the contralateral wulst, whilst those from the posterior parts of the OPT project to the ipsilateral side. The wulst, as Figure 19.14 shows, is a swelling in the parasagittal region of the avian DVR. It is regarded as consisting of two regions: a medial part, which has been compared to the mammalian hippocampus (**wulst regio hippocampalis (Whc)**), and a lateral region comparable to the mammalian neocortex (**wulst regio hyperstriatica (Whs)**). The posterior part of the Whs

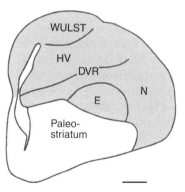

Figure 19.14 The avian wulst. Transverse section through telencephalon of pigeon. A comparison with Figure 19.13 shows that the wulst develops as a swelling on the surface of the DVR. E = ectostriatum; HV = hyperstriatum ventrale; N = neostriatum. Scale bar = 1 mm. From Shimizu, T. and Karten, H.J. (1991) Central visual pathways in reptiles and birds: evolution of the visual system, in *Vison and Visual Dysfunction, Vol. 2* (eds J.R. Cronly-Dillon and R.L. Gregory), copyright © 1991 Macmillan Press.

is comparable to the mammalian primary visual cortex. It has a laminar organization which is conventionally regarded as consisting of four layers of cells. There is evidence that the cells are retinotopically organized, although the maps vary in different birds. In the owls there are many binocularly driven neurons; this is much less evident in pigeons, where only a few neurons show responses to ipsilateral stimuli.

Optic nerve fibres in the **tectofugal** pathway terminate in the contralateral optic tectum. The superficial layers of the tectum are retinotopically organized and the cells have rather small RFs (less than $4°$ of arc) and respond to movement and direction of movement. Cells in deeper laminae have larger RFs but are not so precise in their directional selectivity. Cells in these deeper laminae send their output to the **nucleus rotundus**. The nucleus rotundus has been subdivided into cytoarchitectonic regions by histochemical staining for acetylcholinesterase. Many of its neurons have extremely large RFs (often over $100°$ of arc) and are sensitive to movement. Neurons have also been found which respond to expansion or contraction of the visual image thus providing information about 'optic flow'. The output from the nucleus rotundus is directed to a region in the central mass of the DVR known as the **ecostriatum**. From the **ecostriatum** there are further projections to other regions of the DVR (Figure 19.15). This series of sequential projections has been likened to the sequential projections through the mammalian striate and extrastriate cortices.

The thalamofugal and tectofugal pathways interact at many places, especially in the wulst and ecostriatum. There is also powerful feedback into the tectum and connections are made to the hypothalamus and backwards to the nuclei of the OPT and last, but far from least, to the retina itself. The central analysis of the visual information in the bird telencephalon–thalamencephalon–mesencephalon is probably fully as intricate, though far less well understood, as that which occurs in the mammal.

19.9 CONCLUDING REMARKS

This chapter has revealed something of the extraordinary variety of visual systems developed by the vertebrates. Even so, it has hardly done more than scratch the surface of an immense topic. It serves as

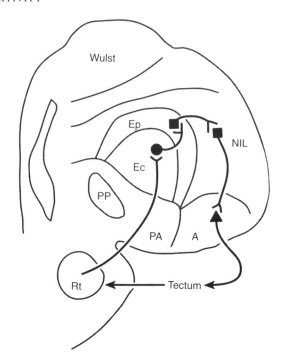

Figure 19.15 Transverse secition through avian telencephalon to show neural circuits of the tectofugal pathway. A = archistriatum; Ec = ectostriatum; Ep = periectostriatal belt; NIV = neostriatum intermedium ventrale; PA = palaeostriatum augmentatum (equivalent of mammalian caudate-putamen); PP = palaeostriatum primitivum (equivalent of mammalian globus pallidus); Rt = nucleus rotundis. From Shimizu, T. and Karten, H.J. (1991) Central visual pathways in reptiles and birds: evolution of the visual system, in *Vison and Visual Dysfunction, Vol. 2* (eds J.R. Cronly-Dillon and R.L. Gregory), copyright © 1991 Macmillan Press.

an antidote to the easy temptations of anthropocentricity. The human eye and visual system, although for obvious reasons the best known, is far from the only design in the phylum Chordata, let alone the animal kingdom. Although much is known of vertebrate visual systems, much remains unknown. This has been particularly brought out in the last section of this chapter, where we have seen how little is in fact known of the cerebral analysis of visual input in those most visual of animals: the birds. As always in zoology we are driven to see ourselves as just one species amongst many; we are driven to an intuition of the strangeness in similarity of other life forms. As always we come back to Nagel's famous question, what is it like to be a bat, what is it like to be a bird?

PART IV: SELF ASSESSMENT

The following questions are designed both to help you assess your understanding of the topics covered in the text and to direct your attention to significant aspects of the subject matter. The sequence of questions follows the sequence in which the subject matter is presented in the text. It is thus easy to refer back to the appropriate page or pages. After reading each chapter and/or each section you should look through these questions and make sure you know the answers and the issues involved.

CHAPTER 15: INVERTEBRATE VISION

15.1 Which wavelengths of the electromagnetic spectrum affect the human visual system?

15.2 Describe the two major types of photoreceptor cell. With which two major groups of animals are these types associated? Are there any exceptions to this association? If so, name them.

15.3 Name the two major types of multicellular eye which have evolved in the animal kingdom. In which phyla have they reached a climax of development?

15.4 Referring to specific examples, explain how the highly developed vesicular eyes of molluscs and vertebrates may have evolved.

15.5 What is a retinula cell and what is an ommatidium?

15.6 Draw a rough diagram to show the structure of an apposition and of a superposition ommatidium. Which type is found in diurnal and which in nocturnal insects?

15.7 Indicate the difference between a rhabdomere and a rhabdom.

15.8 What is the difference between a superposition and a neural superposition compound eye? What advantage does the latter design confer?

15.9 In addition to apposition, superposition and neural superposition eyes, what other types of compound eye have been evolved in the arthropods?

15.10 Describe some examples of scanning eyes.

15.11 Describe the *Chlamydomonas* eyespot. How is photoreception linked to locomotion? Is there any similarity to bacterial chemotaxis (refer to Chapter 11)?

15.12 Describe the eye of *Nautilus pompilius*. Which type of photoreceptor cell is found in its retinae?

15.13 Where are the eyes of *Pecten* located?

15.14 On which of *Pecten's* two retinae is the image formed? In which retina are ciliary type photoreceptors found? Is the biophysics of these photoreceptors different from that of vertebrate rods and cones?

15.15 To which of the three cephalopod subclasses do the squids and octopi belong?

15.16 Describe the similarities and differences between belemnoid and vertebrate eyes.

15.17 How is light focused on a belemnoid retina?

15.18 Where is the deep retina of *Octopus* located?

15.19 Compare *Octopus* retina with that of a typical vertebrate (see Chapters 16 and 17).

15.20 To which subphylum does *Limulus* belong?

15.21 What is the physiological significance of the lateral plexus beneath the ommatidia of *Limulus* compound eye?

15.22 What role do the eccentric cells play in *Limulus* retina?

Biology of Sensory Systems, Second Edition   C.U.M. Smith
© 2008 John Wiley & Sons, Ltd

15.23 What is the biological significance of lateral inhibition in *Limulus* compound eye?

15.24 How many eyes have the majority of spiders? Where are they located in the Salticidae?

15.25 How many layers of photosensitive rhadoms are found in a Salticid spider's AME?

15.26 How does a Salticid spider's combination of AMEs, PLEs and PMEs resemble a mammalian or bird foveate retina?

15.27 What structure acts as an optic fibre or light guide in the Dipteran compound eye?

15.28 How does the fly's eye combine acuity with sensitivity?

15.29 Describe the pathway optic nerve fibres take in the fly from the ommatidia to the lobula.

CHAPTER 16: THE HUMAN EYE

16.1 What does the term 'adnexa' denote?

16.2 Name the three layers or 'tunics' that consti-tute the wall of the eyeball.

16.3 Itemize the parts of the uveal tract. What is the origin of the name?

16.4 What is the area centralis (or macula lutea)?

16.5 Why is the optic disc also known as the 'blind spot'?

16.6 What is the cause of glaucoma?

16.7 Which cranial nerves innervate which extrinsic eye muscles?

16.8 What is the trochlea and what part does it play in the muscular control of eye movement?

16.9 What are the functions of the eyelids?

16.10 Referring to Figure 16.4 describe the movement of the tear fluid across the eye.

16.11 What prevents the tear fluid drying?

16.12 Explain why all vertebrates have 'inverted' retinae.

16.13 What role does the optic vesicle play in the formation of the lens?

16.14 How is the ventricle within the lens obliterated?

16.15 What defects are found in the conditions known as aphakia and coloboma?

16.16 What is the canal of Cloquet and how is it formed?

16.17 What happens to the optic ventricle? Does its existence still have importance in some ophthalmic pathologies?

16.18 What sequence of cell movements underlies the formation of the retina? What role is played by Müller cells?

16.19 What is the limbus?

16.20 Draw a diagram of the cornea in transverse section, labelling the three principal layers and the two membranes.

16.21 Which two functions does the collagen of the corneal stroma serve?

16.22 In addition to collagen, which other biological molecules are present in the stroma? Write down the structure of a typical GAG.

16.23 Why is the hygroscopic character of GAGs so important in corneal transparency?

16.24 How does the organization of collagen in the sclera differ from that of the cornea?

16.25 Do lens fibres possess mitochondria and other intracellular organelles? If not, why not?

16.26 Which proteins form the major constituents of lens fibres? To which other proteins are they related?

16.27 Define 'myopia', 'hypermetropia', 'astigmatism', 'presbyopia' and 'cataract'.

16.28 Describe some of the biochemical processes responsible for cataract.

16.29 How do the iris sphincter and dilator muscles differ from other muscles?

16.30 Describe the histological structure of the choriocapillaris and relate this structure to its function.

16.31 Which two functions does the ciliary body serve?

16.32 Where and how is aqueous fluid secreted? Provide evidence to show that at least some part of this secretion is an active process.

16.33 By which two routes is aqueous fluid absorbed? When the eye is focused on a near object which route is taken by 25% of the aqueous fluid?

16.34 Distinguish between open and closed angle glaucoma. Which is the commonest?

16.35 What role does the scleral spur play in lens accommodation? What part does the elasticity of the lens capsule play?

16.36 How do the dilator and sphincter muscles of the iris control the quantity of light reaching the retina? Explain how variation in pupil size affects depth of focus.

16.37 Discuss the role of hyalocytes in the vitreous humour.

16.38 Describe some of the age-related degenerative changes which affect the vitreous fluid.

16.39 Distinguish between the vestibulo-oculomotor and the optikinetc reflex. Which of these two reflexes is not present in the dark? Why?

16.40 Which eye movements are driven by retinal disparity?

16.41 Explain what is meant by 'efference copy' and give a simple instance which supports the idea.

CHAPTER 17: THE RETINA

17.1 Is the RPE more firmly attached to the retina or to the choroid?

17.2 Distinguish between melanosomes and phagosomes.

17.3 Enumerate four significant functions of the RPE.

17.4 Why is the human retina known as a 'duplex' retina?

17.5 What is foveation?

17.6 List the nine layers of the retina.

17.7 Name the retinal cells which run parallel to the vitreal surface.

17.8 Name the retinal cells which extend across the two plexiform layers. What rôle do Müller cells play in the embryology of the retina (refer to Chapter 16)?

17.9 Draw a diagram of a rod cell and label its different parts. How do cones differ from this structure?

17.10 What and where is the foveola?

17.11 Explain how the rod outersegment acts as a waveguide. Compare with the insect rhabdom.

17.12 Distinguish between retinol and retinal. How is retinal attached to opsin?

17.13 What intramolecular change occurs when a photon of the appropriate wavelength interacts with rhodopsin?

17.14 How does the detachment of retinal from opsin lead to the transformation of cGMP into 5′-GMP?

17.15 What is responsible for the 'dark current' in rod and cone cells?

17.16 Do rod and cone cells depolarize or hyperpolarize in the light?

17.17 How does recoverin cause sensory adaptation in vertebrate photoreceptors?

17.18 Which acts first on opsin's carboxyterminal chain: rhodopsin kinase or arrestin?

17.19 Compare and contrast the anatomy, biochemistry and biophysics of rhabdomeric and ciliary photoreceptors.

17.20 List the sequence of intermediates between rhodopsin and all-trans retinal when a photon is absorbed. Which is the high energy form: 11-cis or all-trans retinal?

17.21 List the sequence of steps by which all-trans retinal is converted back to 11-cis retinal showing the relevant enzymes for each step.

17.22 By means of a diagram show the series of transformations occurring in the RPE that transform all-trans retinol into 11-cis retinal. What part does palmitic acid play in this process?

17.23 How is malfunction of this regeneration process implicated in certain forms of macular degeneration (refer to Box 17.2)?

17.24 What rôle does the choriocapillaris play in the regeneration of 11-cis retinal? How are all-trans retinol and Vitamin A related?

17.25 Does exposure to light inhibit or trigger the release of neurotransmitter from photoreceptors?

17.26 Are the differences in the absorption spectra of rod and cone pigments due to the chromophore or to the opsin?

17.27 Does the so-called 'central dogma of olfactory biology' also apply to the visual system?

17.28 Why are men more likely to suffer colour blindness than women? Why are some women tetrachromatic?

17.29 Which is the most recently evolved of the visual pigments? What evolutionary imperatives drove the evolution of colour vision in primates?

17.30 With reference back to Section 14.3, discuss how the evolution of colour vision in old world primates may be associated with reduced development of the vomeronasal organ.

17.31 Explain what is meant by 'sign conserving' and 'sign inverting'. Are electrical synapses sign conserving or inverting?

17.32 Do diffuse bipolar cells synapse with more than one cone pedicle?

17.33 Draw a diagram to show the synaptic complex made by horizontal and bipolar cells with rod cell spherules.

17.34 Are rod bipolars sign inverting or conserving?

17.35 Explain the molecular biology of the sign inverting synapse. Is there a similarity with the response to light of outersegments?

17.36 Explain what is meant by 'receptive field' of a bipolar cell. What physiological characteristics do these fields have? Which retinal cells are largely responsible for these characteristics?

17.37 Do the receptive fields of bipolar cells share significant characteristics with the optic nerve fibres of *Limulus* compound eye?

17.38 List some of the functions of Müller cells.

17.39 Do interplexiform cells transmit from inner to outer plexiform layers or vice versa?

17.40 How are amacrine cells classified?

17.41 Describe the three major types of ganglion cell.

17.42 Describe the typical organization of the receptive fields of primate ganglion cells.

17.43 Which type of ganglion cell is sensitive to movement and which to colour?

17.44 Which ganglion cells are believed to control circadian rhythms and which photopigment do they contain?

17.45 Do ganglion cells respond best to small focused spots of light in their receptive fields or to wide diffuse illumination?

17.46 Draw diagrams to show the possible neural 'wiring' responsible for the receptive fields of ganglion cells.

17.47 How is the sensitivity of the retina increased by the closure of gap junctions between rod and cone cells?

17.48 Explain what is meant by the 'opponent processes' theory.

17.49 Explain why (in some cases) the output from ganglion cells with colour opponent RFs needs disambiguation.

17.50 Show how the higher level properties of a retinal receptive field may be derived from molecular and biophysical first principles. What remains to be done before we can say that we have a complete scientific understanding of the retina?

17.51 How are studies of the zebrafish (*D.rerio*) assisting an understanding of the retina?

17.52 Describe how mammalian retinae are adapted to their lifestyles.

CHAPTER 18: VISUAL PATHWAYS AND CORTICES

18.1 Name three visual pathways in a mammal.

18.2 Is there a possible evolutionary reason for the predominance of the RGS pathway in mammals? If so, give a brief account.

18.3 Describe the RT pathway. What form does the decussation take in primates?

18.4 Describe the physiological organization of the superior colliculus. What type of eye movement does it control?

18.5 Why is 'cupping' of the optic disc observed in the glaucomatous eye?

18.6 Do optic nerve fibres from the lateral part of the human retina show complete decussation, partial decussation or no decussation at the optic chiasma?

18.7 How many layers of cells are found in the primate LGN? Is the pathway from each retina kept separate?

18.8 Which layers of the LGN receive input from parvocellular fibres?

18.9 Which layers of the LGN contain cells responsive to movement in their RFs but are blind to colour?

18.10 Which layers of the LGN receive input from W fibres?

18.11 What is Meyer's loop?

18.12 Where is the primary visual cortex located in humans? Where is it in monkeys?

18.13 What and where is the stripe of Gennari?

18.14 In which layers of the primary visual cortex do parvocellular fibres from the LGN terminate?

18.15 Describe the experimental technique used to investigate the receptive fields of cells in the visual cortex.

18.16 What types of stimuli trigger responses in cells of the primary visual cortex?

18.17 Show how the RF properties of orientation selector cells may be derived from a combination of concentric fields.

18.18 Define the difference between 'simple' and 'complex' RFs.

18.19 Describe the properties of an 'end stopped' RF. What is the possible biological significance of this type of field?

18.20 How does the preferred orientation of the RFs of cells in the striate cortex vary as an electrode proceeds tangentially through the tissue?

18.21 What is the deoxyglucose technique and how has it been applied to investigate the histology of the visual cortex?

18.22 In what histological structures are colour-sensitive cells concentrated?

18.23 Sketch a possible 'wiring' diagram to account for the pattern of ocular dominance columns found in the primary visual cortex.

18.24 Distinguish between a mini and a macro-column.

18.25 Define a 'hypercolumn' and an 'aggregate receptive field'.

18.26 What is the 'ice tray' model of visual cortex organization? Provide some evidence for and against this model (see also Box 18.1).

18.27 Do orientation detectors give an ambiguous signal to higher centres? If so, how can this signal be disambiguated?

18.28 What are sensitive periods? Describe some experiments which show that early visual experience plays a significant role in moulding the 'wiring' of the visual system.

18.29 What and where is the pulvinar nucleus? What role does it play in processing visual information?

18.30 What is the 'three stream' system of visual processing? What information about the visual input does each of the three streams carry?

18.31 What type of differentiation does cytochrome oxidase reveal in visual area 2 (Brodmann area 18)? How does this organization relate to the blob–interblob differentiation of the primary visual cortex?

18.32 Why is face recognition important in social primates?

18.33 In what area of the macaque's brain are face recognition cells found?

18.34 Discuss the concept of a 'grandmother's face recognition cell'.

18.35 What are 'iconic patterns'? How are cells responsive to iconic patterns grouped in the inferotemporal cortex?

18.36 Where is the face recognition area located in human brains?

18.37 What is prosopagnosia? Give some examples of the condition.

CHAPTER 19: OTHER VERTEBRATE VISUAL SYSTEMS

19.1 What is the chemical difference between rhodpsin and porphyropsin?

19.2 Which of rhodopsin and porphyropsin has its λ_{max} further towards the red end of the spectrum?

19.3 In which fish (freshwater or seawater) are porphyropsins mostly found?

19.4 In which vertebrate classes are photoreceptors with oil droplets found? What is the function of these droplets?

19.5 What other dioptic organelle is often found in vertebrate photoreceptors? In which part of the cell is it developed?

19.6 What is the function of double cones and in which vertebrate groups are they found? How do double cones differ from twin cones?

19.7 In which vertebrate groups are double rods most well known?

19.8   Do cone myoids contract or relax in response to light? Rod myoids?

19.9   Do pigment granules in the RPE also show photomechanical movements? If so, in which direction do they move in the light? How does this compare with the migration of pigment in the belemnoid eye (Chapter 15)?

19.10   In what layers of the eye do some animals develop reflecting tapeta?

19.11   Describe the three types of choroidal tapeta.

19.12   What is meant by an 'occlusible tapetum', in which animals is it found and how does it operate?

19.13   What is a 'multiple banked retina'? In which animals is it found and for what purpose?

19.14   Describe the physiological characteristics of the five major types of receptive field in the frog's retina. How do these characteristics reflect the frog's way of life?

19.15   Define the area centralis.

19.16   Distinguish convexiclivate from concaviclivate foveae.

19.17   Discuss the functional advantages of convexiclivate foveae.

19.18   Review the types of areae found in the retinae of birds and relate them (as far as possible) to the lifestyle of their owners.

19.19   What is the visual streak ? In which mammals is it found?

19.20   What is the pecten and what is believed to be its function?

19.21   Describe the tubular eye of deep sea fish. What is the significance of the two retinae?

19.22   What is a 'spectacle', how is it formed and in which vertebrates is it found?

19.23   What is Matthiesen's ratio?

19.24   How are the lenses of animal eyes adapted to conform to Matthiessen's ratio?

19.25   Which two photoreceptor structures develop from the posterior roof of the diencephalon?

19.26   What is the principal physiological role of the vertebrate median eye?

19.27   Which reptile possesses a well developed parietal eye?

19.28   Which hormone is synthesized by the pineal?

19.29   What is the Newton–Muller–Gudden law?

19.30   Describe the physiological organization of the frog's optic tectum. What are 'sameness' and 'newness' neurons?

19.31   Describe the major visual pathway in reptiles.

19.32   What is the dorsoventricular ridge and where is it found?

19.33   In which birds is the thalamofugal pathway strongly developed?

19.34   Which group of nuclei in the avian optic pathway is regarded as analogous to the mammalian LGNd?

19.35   Is there complete, incomplete or no decussation in the thalamofugal pathway?

19.36   What is the avian 'wulst' and how is it related to the reptilian DVR?

19.37   Which part of the wulst is regarded as analogous to the mammalian primary visual cortex? How many layers of cell are present in this part of the wulst?

19.38   In which part of the avian brain do fibres of the tectofugal pathway terminate? What and where is the nucleus rotundus and what are the physiological characteristics of its neurons?

19.39   How similar and how different are the visual systems of birds and mammals?

PART IV: NOTES, REFERENCES AND BIBLIOGRAPHY

INTRODUCTION

David Hume (1711–76) was born in Edinburgh and is commonly regarded as the greatest philosopher of the first part of the eighteenth century. A draft of the *Dialogues concerning Natural Religion* existed in 1751 but it was not published until 1779, three years after its author's death. Charles Darwin's struggles with the eye's apparent implication that a foresightful designer must exist are to be found in his letter to Asa Gray (February, 1860): 'The eye to this day gives me a cold shudder, but when I think of the fine known gradations, my reason tells me I ought to conquer the cold shudder'. Later, in April of the same year he wrote again to Gray putting his queasiness into the past tense: 'I remember well the time when the thought of the eye made me cold all over, but I have got over this stage of the complaint...' (Darwin, 1860). Indeed, a modern analysis suggests that only a few hundred thousand years, a moment in the life's three and half billion year tenure of the planet, should be sufficient to evolve a recognisable eye (Nilsson and Pelger, 1994). Lamb, Collin and Pugh (2007) provide a detailed account of the origin and early evolution of the vertebrate eye, emphasizing that the major developments which created its 'ground plan' occurred before or during the Precambrian revolution some 500 Ma ago.

Details of the structure and relationships of opsin from the melanocyte pigment of frog skin (*Xenopus*) can be found in Provencio *et al.* (1998). These workers show that it more closely resembles invertebrate than vertebrate opsins. They also suggest that it may be related to pigments responsible for circadian rhythms and photoperiod responses of many nonmammalian vertebrates. A valuable account of the optical principles and evolution of image-forming eyes is given by Goldsmith (1990). Fernald (1997) discusses the evolution of animal eyes with particular references to molecular genetics (see also Box 15.1) and Wolken (1995) gives an authoritative overview of eyes and other light detectors in the biological world. Further material on geometrical optics is to be found in textbooks of classical physics.

Darwin, C.R. (1860) *The Correspondence of Charles Darwin*, Vol. **8**, Cambridge University Press, Cambridge.

Fernald, R.D. (1997) The evolution of eyes. *Brain, Behaviour and Evolution*, **50**, 253–59.

Goldsmith, T.H. (1990) Optimisation, constraint, and history in the evolution of eyes. *The Quarterly Review of Biology*, **65**, 281–322.

Lamb, T.D., Collin, S.P. and Pugh, E.N. (2007) Evolution of the vertebrate eye: opsins, photoreceptors, retina and eye cup. *Nature Reviews Neuroscience*, **8**, 960–75.

Nilsson, D.-E. and Pelger, S. (1994) A pessimistic estimate of the time required for an eye to evolve. *Proceedings of the Royal Society B*, **256**, 53–8.

Provencio, I. *et al.* (1998) Melanopsin: An opsin in melanophores, brain and eye. *Proceedings of the National Academy of Sciences USA*, **95**, 340–45.

Wolken, J.J. (1995) *Light Detectors, Photoreceptors, and Imaging Systems in Nature*, Oxford University Press, Oxford.

CHAPTER 15: INVERTEBRATE VISION

The subject of invertebrate vision is, of course, huge. Only a brief glimpse is given in this chapter. Comprehensive treatments are to be found in Alvi (1984), whilst Duke-Elder (1958) provides an easily accessible overview. Collections of authoritative and often highly detailed chapters are presented in the edited volumes of Autrum (1979, 1981) and Cronly-Dillon and Gregory (1991). Dodge (1991) provides a comprehensive account of algal eyespots covering a large number of different types and Foster and Smyth (1980) do the same for protistan eyespots. Harz, Nonnegasser and Hegemann (1992) discuss the biophysics and physiology of the eyespot in *Chlamydomonas* in detail. Accounts of the compound eye are to be found in the references noted above and also in Wigglesworth (1972) and Milne and Milne (1959), whilst Exner (1891) is the foundation work in the field and a mine of information: it is still a primary source of data about the compound eye over a century after its original publication. Land and Fernald (1992) discuss evolutionary issues, Lamb, Collin and Pugh (2007) review the early evolution of the vertebrate vesicular eye, paying particular attention to its early representation in the hagfish and Lacalli (2008) provides an up-to-date account of the photoreceptor systems in the 'urchordate' *Amphioxus*. Nilsson (1988) describes the optics of the compound eye of the swimming crab, *Portunus puber*. An insightful review of the eyes and visual behaviour of jumping spiders is provided by Harland and Jackson (2000). The publications by Horridge (1991), Osorio (1991), Strausfield (1976) and Strausfield and Nassel (1981) provide comprehensive, but advanced, accounts of the eyes and visual systems of Dipteran insects – not for the faint-hearted. Conway Morris (1998) gives a valuable discussion of the fossil forms of 525 million years ago and the evolutionary constraints, or 'morphospaces', conditioning their subsequent evolution.

Alvi, M.A. (ed.) (1984) *Photoreception and Vision in Invertebrates*, Plenum, New York.

Autrum, H. (ed.) (1979) Comparative physiology and evolution of vision in invertebrates, A: invertebrate photoreceptors, in *Handbook of Sensory Physiology*, Vol. **VII/6A** (ed. H. Autrum), Springer-Verlag, Berlin.

Autrum, H. (ed.) (1981) Comparative physiology and evolution of vision in invertebrates, B: invertebrate visual centers and behaviour, in *Handbook of Sensory Physiology*, Vol. **VII/6B** (ed. H. Autrum), Springer-Verlag, Berlin.

Autrum, H. (ed.) (1981) Comparative physiology and evolution of vision in invertebrates, C: invertebrate visual centres and behaviour II, in *Handbook of Sensory Physiology*, Vol. **VII/6C** (eds H. Autrum *et al.*), Springer-Verlag, Berlin.

Cronly-Dillon, J.R. and Gregory, R.L. (eds) (1991) *Vision and Visual Dysfunction, Evolution of the Eye and Visual System*, Vol. **2**, Macmillan Press, Houndmills.

Duke-Elder, S. (1958) *System of Ophthalmology: The Eye in Evolution*, Vol 1, Kimpton, London.

Exner, S. (1891) (edited and translated R.C. Hardie, 1988) *The Physiology of the Compound Eyes of Insects and Crustacea*, Springer-Verlag, Berlin.

Lacalli, T.C. (2008) Basic features of the ancestral chordate brain: a protochordate perspective. *Brain Research Bulletin* **75**, 319–23 doi: 10.1016/j.brainresbull.2007.10.038.

Lamb, T.D., Collin, S.P. and Pugh, E.N. (2007) Evolution of the vertebrate eye: opsins, photoreceptors, retina and eye cup. *Nature Reviews Neuroscience*, **8**, 960–75.

Land, M.F. and Fernald, R.D. (1992) The evolution of eyes. *Annual Review of Neurosciences*, **15**, 1–30.

Milne, L.J. and Milne, M. (1959) Photosensitivity in invertebrates, in *Neurophysiology*, Vol. **1** (ed. H.W. Magoun), in *Handbook of Physiology* (ed. J. Field), American Physiological Society, Washington, DC.

Morris, S.C. (1998) *The Crucible of Creation: The Burgess Shale and the Rise of the Animals*, Oxford University Press, Oxford.

Wigglesworth, V.B. (1972) *The Principles of Insect Physiology*, Chapman and Hall, London.

Design of Eyes

Eakin, R.M. (1968) Evolution of photoreceptors, in *Evolutionary Biology*, Vol. **2** (eds T. Dobzhansky, M.K. Hecht and W.C. Steere), Appleton-Century-Crofts, New York.

Land, M.F. (1991) Optics of the eyes of the animal kingdom, in *Vision and Visual Dysfunction, Evolution of the Eye and Visual System*, Vol. **2** (eds J.R. Cronly-Dillon and R.L. Gregory), Macmillan Press, Houndmills.

Compound Eyes

Land, M.F. (1984) The resolving power of diurnal superposition eyes measured with an ophthalmoscope. *Journal of Comparative Physiology, A*, **154**, 515–33.

Land, M.F. and Fernald, R.D. (1992) The evolution of eyes. *Annual Review of Neurosciences*, **15**, 1–30.

Nilsson, D.E. (1988) A new type of imaging optics in compound eyes. *Nature*, **332**, 76–8.

Scanning Eyes

Gregory, R.L. (1991) Origins of eyes – speculations on scanning eyes, in *Vision and Visual Dysfunction, Evolution of the Eye and Visual System*, Vol. **2** (eds J.R. Cronly-Dillon and R.L. Gregory), Macmillan Press, Houndmills.

Land, M.F and Fernald, R.D. (1992) The evolution of eyes. *Annual Review of Neurosciences*, **15**, 1–30.

Protistan Eyespots

Diehn, B. (1979) Photic responses and sensory transduction in protists, in Comparative physiology and evolution of vision in invertebrates, A: invertebrate photoreceptors, in *Handbook of Senory Physiology*, Vol. **VII/6A** (ed. H. Autrum), Springer-Verlag, Berlin.

Dodge, J.D. (1991) Photosensory systems in eukaryotic algae, in *Vision and Visual Dysfunction, Evolution of the Eye and Visual System*, Vol. **2** (eds J.R. Cronly-Dillon and R.L. Gregory), Macmillan Press, Houndmills.

Foster, K.W. and Smyth, R.D. (1980) Light antennae in phototactic algae. *Microbiological Reviews*, **44**, 572–630.

Harz, H., Nonnegasser, C. and Hewgemann, P. (1992) The photoreceptor current of the green alga. *Chlamydomonas' Philosophical Transactions of the Royal Society B*, **338**, 39–52.

Nautilus Pinhole Eye

Messenger, J.B. (1991) Photoreception and vision in molluscs, in *Vision and Visual Dysfunction, Evolution of the Eye and Visual System*, Vol. **2** (eds J.R. Cronly-Dillon and R.L. Gregory), Macmillan Press, Houndmills.

Young, J.Z. (1965) The central nervous system of *Nautilus. Philosophical Transdactions of the Royal Society, B*, **249**, 1–25.

Pecten Mirror Eye

Borradaile, L.A., Potts, F.A., Eastham, L.E.S. and Saunders, J.T. (1951) *The Invertebrata*, Cambridge University Press, Cambridge.

Dakin, W.J. (1928) The eyes of *Pecten, Spondylus, Amussium* and allied lamellibranchs, with a short discussion on their evolution. *Proceedings of the Royal Society, B*, **103**, 355–65.

Land, M.F. (1965) Image formation by a concave reflector in the eye of the scallop *Pecten maximus. Journal of Physiology*, **179**, 138–53.

Messenger, J.B. (1991) *Vision and Visual Dysfunction, Evolution of the Eye and Visual System*, Vol. **2** (eds J.R. Cronly-Dillon and R.L. Gregory), Macmillan Press, Houndmills.

Octopus Vesicular Eye

Messenger, J.B. (1991) Photoreception and vision in molluscs, in *Vision and Visual Dysfunction, Evolution of the Eye and Visual System*, Vol. **2** (eds J.R. Cronly-Dillon and R.L. Gregory), Macmillan Press, Houndmills.

Saibil, H. and Hewat, E. (1987) Ordered transmembrane and extracellular structure in squid photoreceptor microvilli. *Journal of Cell Biology*, **105**, 19–28.

Young, J.Z. (1962a) The retina of cephalopods and its degeneration after optic nerve section. *Philosophical Transactions of Royal Society, B*, **245**, 1–18.

Young, J.Z. (1962b) The optic lobes of Octopus vulgaris. *Philosophical Transactions of the Royal Society*, **245**, 19–58.

Limulus Compound Eye

Hartline, H.K. (1959) Receptor mechanisms and the integration of sensory information in the eye, in *Biophysical Science – A Study Program* (ed. J.L. Oncley), John Wiley & Sons, Inc., New York.

Laughlin, S. (1981) Neural principles in the peripheral visual systems of invertebrates, in *Handbook of Sensory Physiology*, Vol. **VII/6B** (ed. H. Autrum), Springer-Verlag, Berlin.

Meinertzhagen, I.A. (1991) Evolution of the cellular organisation of the arthropod compound eye and optic lobe, in *Vision and Visual Dysfunction, Evolution of the Eye and Visual System*, Vol. **2** (eds J.R. Cronly-Dillon and R.L. Gregory), Macmillan Press, Houndmills.

Spider Ocellar Eye

Foelix, R.F. (1982) *Biology of Spiders*, Harvard University Press, Cambidge Mass.

Harland, D.P. and Jackson, R.R. (2000) 'Eight-legged cats' and how they see: a review of recent research on jumping spiders (Araneae, Salticidae). *Cimbebasia*, **16**, 231–40.

Land, M.F. (1969) Movements of the retinae in jumping spiders (Salticidae: Dendryphantidae) in response to visual stimuli. *Journal of Experimental Biology*, **51**, 471–93.

Nakamura, T. and Yamashita, S. (2000) Learning and discrimination of colored papers in jumping spiders (Araneae, Salticidae). *Journal of Comparative Physiology A*, **186**, 897–901.

Dipteran Compound Eye

Horridge, G.A. (1991) Evolution of visual processing, in *Vision and Visual Dysfunction, Evolution of the Eye and Visual System*, Vol. **2** (eds J.R. Cronly-Dillon and R.L. Gregory), Macmillan Press, Houndmills.

Osorio, D. (1991) Patterns of function and evolution in the arthropod optic lobe, in *Vision and Visual Dysfunction, Evolution of the Eye and Visual System*, Vol. **2** (eds J.R. Cronly-Dillon and R.L. Gregory), Macmillan Press, Houndmills.

Strausfield, N.J. (1976) *An Atlas of an Insect Brain*, Springer, Berlin.

Strausfield, N.J. and Nassel, D.R. (1981) Neuroarchitecture of brain regions that subserve the compound eye of crustacea and insects, in *Handbook of Sensory Physiology*, Vol. **VII/6B** (ed. H. Autrum), Springer-Verlag, Berlin.

CHAPTER 16: THE HUMAN EYE

A comprehensive account of the human eye's embryology is given by Sir Stewart Duke-Elder and Cook (1963) in volume 3 of his magisterial *System of Ophthalmology*. Accounts of the eye's anatomy are given in many texts of ophthalmology and optometry, for instance Bron, Tripathi and Tripathi (1997), Hart (1992), Davson (1984), Duke-Elder and Wybar (1961), Newell (1996) and so on. Harding (1997) provides a recent treatment of ocular biochemistry and a comprehensive description of the eye's fine structure is to be found in Hogan, Alvarado and Weddell (1971). Harding (1984) provides a comprehensive account of lens development and metabolism with special reference to cataract. de Jong (1982) discusses the evolution of lens crystallins. Cataracts and their development are given monograph-length treatment by Harding (1991) and Jaffe and Horowitz (1992) include excellent full colour illustrations of histology and anatomy of the cataractous lens. The seminal book by Arbib (1989) provides (amongst much else) a useful engineering account of the feedback systems (including a discussion of efference copy) which control saccadic eye movements.

Abdel-Latif, A.A. (1997) Iris-ciliary body, aqueous humour and trabecular meshwork, in *Biochemistry of the Eye* (ed. J.J. Harding), Chapman and Hall, London.

Arbib, M.A. (1989) *The Metaphorical Brain*, Vol. **2**, John Wiley & Sons, Inc., New York.

Bron, A.J., Tripathi, R.C. and Tripathi, B.J. (1997) *Wolff's Anatomy of the Eye and Orbit*, 8th edn, Chapman and Hall, London.

Cole, D.F. (1984) Ocular fluids, in *The Eye. Vegetative Physiology and Biochemistry*, Vol. **1a** (ed. H. Davson), Academic Press, Orlando.

Davson, H. (1963) *The Physiology of the Eye*, 2nd edn, Churchill, London.

Davson, H. (ed.) (1984) *The Eye. Vegetative Physiology and Biochemistry*, Vol. **1a**, Academic Press, Orlando.

de Jong, W.W. (1982) Eye lens proteins and vertebrate phylogeny, in *Macromolecular Sequences in Systematic and Evolutionary Biology* (ed. M. Goldman), Plenum, New York.

Duke-Elder, S. and Wybar, K.C. (1961) *System of Ophthalmology The Anatomy of the Visual System*, Vol. **2**, Henry Kimpton, London.

Duke-Elder, S and Cook, C. (1963) *System of Ophthalmology Embryology*, Vol. **3**, part 1, Henry Kimpton, London.

Hart, W.M. (1992) *Adler's Physiology of the Eye*, 9th edn, Mosby, St Louis.

Harding, J.J. (1984) The lens: development, proteins, metabolism and cataract, in *The Eye*, Vol. **1b** (ed. H. Davson), Academic Press, Orlando.

Harding, J.J. (1991) *Cataract: Biochemistry, Epidemiology and Pharmacology*, Chapman and Hall, London.

Harding, J.J. (ed.) (1997) *Biochemistry of the Eye*, Chapman and Hall, London.

Hogan, M.J., Alvarado, J.A. and Weddell, J.E. (1971) *Histology of the Human Eye*, Saunders, Philadelphia.

Hyman, L. (1987) Epidemiology of eye diseases in the elderly. *Eye*, **1**, 330–41.

Jaffe, N.S. and Horwitz, J. (1992) *Lens and Cataract*, Gower Medical Publishing, New York.

Newell, F. (1996) *Ophthalmology: Principles and Concepts*, 8th edn, Mosby, St Louis.

Tiffany, J.M. (1997) Tears and conjunctiva, in *Biochemistry of the Eye* (ed. J.J. Harding), Chapman and Hall, London.

CHAPTER 17: THE RETINA

The retina has fascinated neuroscientists since at least the time of Ramon and Cajal who pioneered our modern understanding of its structure in a series of masterly publications (see Cajal, 1909, 1911). Modern accounts are to be found in Dowling (1987) and, in considerably greater histological detail, in the older publications of Polyak (1941) and Rodieck (1988). Geoffrey Walls' (1963) account of comparative anatomy, although published nearly half a century ago, remains an indispensable introduction to the topic, whilst the multivolume series edited by Cronly-Dillon (1991) provides more up to date information. Photoreceptor cells have been the object of intense investigation at the biophysical, biochemical and molecular biological levels. Harding (1997) gives a detailed overview, Lamb, Collin and Pugh (2007) discuss the origins and evolutionary relationships of ciliary and rhabdomeric photoreceptors and discuss the possible rhabdomeric origin of ganglion cells. The publications by Nathans and coworkers provide detail on the structure and evolution of visual pigments. Jacobs et al. (2007) describe the engineering of mice retinae to express a human cone photopigment. Yokoyama (1995) discusses the evolution of vertebrate visual pigments and presents a phylogenetic tree relating the opsins of 28 different species based on their amino acid sequences, whilst Conway (2007) describes genetic modification of mouse retina, allowing the animal to distinguish colours never before seen by mice. Odermatt and Lagnado (2007) and Viney et al. (2007) describe work on melanopsin and circadian rhythms, whilst Lamb and Pugh (2006) review the regeneration of rhodopsin in the pigment epithelium. The original work on visual receptive fields was carried out on frog retinae by Hartline (1938) and on mammalian retinae by Kuffler (1953); the rabbit's retina is described by Levick (1967). Wiring diagrams in the retina remain controversial but both Schiller (1992) and Nakanishi (1995) give valuable summary reviews and Odermatt and Lagnado (2007) discuss recent insights. Brockeroff, Dowling and Hurley (1998) describe the highly promising line of attack through the genetic analysis of the zebrafish retinae and Yazulla et al. (2002) have edited a comprehensive (though expensive) account of its neurochemical anatomy.

General

Alberts, B., Johnson, A., Lewis, J. et al. (2002) *Molecular Biology of the Cell*, 4th edn, Garland Press, New York.

Arendt, D. and Wittbrodt, J. (2001) Reconstructing the eyes of Urbilateralia. *Proceedings of the Royal Society B*, **356**, 1545–63.

Berson, E.L. (1993) Retinitis pigmentosa: the Friedenwald lecture. *Investigative Ophtalmology and Visual Science*, **34**, 1659–76.

Cajal, R. (1909, 1911) *Histologie du Système Nerveux de l'Homme et des Veretébrés*, Vol. **2** (trs. L. Azoulay), Maloine, Paris.

Cronly-Dillon, J.R. (1991) general editor, *Vision and Visual Dysfunction*, **17** vols., CRC Press, Boca Raton.

Dowling, J.E. (1987) *The Retina: An Approachable Part of the Brain*, Harvard University Press, Cambridge, MA.

Hartline, H.K. (1938) Responses of single optic nerve fibres of the vertebrate eye to illumination of the retina. *American Journal of Physiology*, **121**, 400–15.

Kandel, E.R., Schwartz, J.H. and Jessel, T.M. (eds) (1991) *Principles of Neuroscience*, Elsevier, New York.

Kuffler, S.W. (1953) Discharge patterns and functional organisation of the mammalian retina. *Journal of Neurophysiology*, **16**, 37–68.

Osterberg, G.A. (1935) Topography of the layer of rods and cones in the human retina. *Acta Ophthalmologica*, **13** (6), 1–102.

Nilsson, D.-E. (2004) Eye evolution: a question of genetic promiscuity. *Current Opinion in Neurobiology*, **14**, 407–14.

Polyak, S.L. (1941) *The Retina*, University of Chicago Press, Chicago.

Rodieck, R.W. (1973) *The Vertebrate Retina*, Freeman, San Francisco.

Tripathi, R.C. and Tripathi, B.J. (1984) Anatomy, orbit and Adnexa of the human eye, in *The Eye*, 3rd edn (ed. H. Davson), Academic Press, Orlando, Fla.

Walls, G.L. (1963) *The Vertebrate Eye and its Adaptive Radiation*, Hafner, New York.

Retinal Structure

Besharse, J.C. (1986) Photosensitive membrane turnover: differentiated membrane domains and cell-cell interaction, in *The Retina: A Model for Cell Biology Studies* (eds R. Adler and D. Farber), Academic Press, Orlando.

Boycott, B.B. and Dowling, J.E. (1969) Organisation of the primate retina: light microscopy. *Philosophical Transactions of the Royal Society, B*, **225**, 109–84.

Dowling, J.E. (1987) *The Retina: An Approachable Part of the Brain*, Harvard University Press, Cambridge, MA.

Gordon, W.C. and Bazan, N.G. (1997) Retina, in *Biochemistry of the Eye* (ed. J.J. Harding), Chapman and Hall, London.

Hogan, M.J., Alvarado, J.A. and Weddell, J.E. (1971) *Histology of the Human Eye*, Saunders, Philadelphia.

Rodieck, R.W. (1973) *The Vertebrate Retina*, Freeman, San Francisco.

Rodieck, R.W. (1988) The primate retina. *Comparative Primate Biology*, **4**, 203–78.

Rowe, M.H. (1991) Functional organisation of the retina, in *Vision and Visual Dysfunction: Neuroanatomy of the Visual Pathways and their Development*, Vol. **3** (ed. J. Cronly-Dillon), Macmillan, London.

Young, R.W. (1971) The renewal of rod and cone outer segments in the rhesus monkey. *Journal of Cell Biology*, **42**, 392–403.

Photoreceptor Cells

Baylor, D.A., Lamb, T.D. and Yau, K.-W. (1979) The membrane current of single rod outer segments. *Journal of Physiology*, **289**, 589–611.

Conway, B.R. (2007) Color vision: mice see hue too. *Current Biology*, **17**, R459.

Moiseyev, G., Chen, Y., Takahashi, Y. *et al.* (2005) RPE65 is the isomerohydrolase in the retinoid visual cycle. *Proceedings of the National Academy of Science*, **102**, 12413–18.

Harding, J.J. (ed.) (1997) *Biochemistry of the Eye*, Chapman and Hall, London.

Jacobs, G.H., Williams, G.A., Cahill, H. and Nathans, J. (2007) Emergence of novel color vision in mice engineered to express a human cone photopigment. *Science*, **315**, 1723–5.

Lamb, T.D. and Pugh, E.N. (1992) G-protein cascades: gain and kinetics. *Trends in Neurosciences*, **15**, 291–8.

Lamb, T.D. and Pugh, E.N. (2006) Photoreduction, dark adaptation, and rhodopsin regeneration: the proctor lecture. *Investigative Ophthalmology and Visual Science*, **47**, 5138–52.

Lamb, T.D., Collin, S.P. and Pugh, E.N. (2007) Evolution of the vertebrate eye: opsins, photoreceptors, retina and eye cup. *Nature Reviews Neuroscience*, **8**, 960–75.

Mollon, J.D. (1982) Colour vision and colour blindness, in *The Senses* (eds H.B. Barlow and J.D. Mollon), Cambridge University Press, Cambridge.

Muniz, A. *et al.* (2007) A novel cone visual cycle in cone-dominated retinae. *Experimental Eye Research*, **85**, 175–84.

Nathans, J., Thomas, D. and Hogness, D. (1986) Molecular genetics of human colour vision: the genes encoding blue, green and red pigments. *Science*, **232**, 193–202.

Nathans, J. (1987) Molecular biology of visual pigments. *Annual Review of Neuroscience*, **10**, 163–94.

Nathans, J. (1994) In the eye of the beholder: Visual pigments and inherited variations in human vision. *Cell*, **78**, 357–60.

Odermatt, B. and Lagnado, L. (2007) Retinal circuits: tracing new connections. *Current Biology*, **17**, R608.

Penn, R.D. and Hagins, W.A. (1969) Signal transmission along retinal rods and the origin of the electroretinographic a-wave. *Nature*, **223**, 201–5.

Viney, T.J. *et al.* (2007) Local retina circuits of melanopsin-containing ganglion cells identified by trans-synaptic viral tracing. *Current Biology*, **17**, 981–8.

Yokoyama, S. (1995) Amino acid replacements and wavelength absorption of visual pigments in vertebrates. *Molecular Biology and Evolution*, **12**, 53–61.

Physiology and Wiring Diagrams

Brockeroff, S.E., Dowling, J.E. and Hurley, J.B. (1998) Zebrafish retinal mutants. *Vision Research*, **38**, 1335–39.

Daw, N.W., Jensen, R.J. and Brunken, W.J. (1990) Rod pathways in mammalian retinae. *Trends in Neurosciences*, **13**, 110–5.

Levick, W..R. (1967) Receptive fields and trigger features in the visual streak of the rabbit's retina. *Journal of Physiology*, **188**, 285–307.

Nakanishi, S. (1995) Second-order neurones and receptor mechanisms in visual and olfactory information processing. *Trends in Neurosciences*, **18**, 359–64.

Schiller, P.H. (1992) The ON and OFF channels of the visual system. *Trends in Neurosciences*, **15**, 86–92.

Wassle, H. and Boycott, B.B. (1991) Functional architecture of the mammalian retina. *Physiological Reviews*, **71**, 447–80.

Yazulla, S., Studholme, K.M., Marc, R.E. and Cameron, D. (eds) (2002) *Chemical Anatomy of the Zebrafish Retina*, Kluwer Academic Publishers, Norwell, MA.

CHAPTER 18: VISUAL PATHWAYS AND CORTICES

The student is somewhat spoilt for choice in the number of excellent accounts of mammalian visual pathways and cortices. Most texts of neurophysiology and/or neuroscience include chapters. The following publications are merely a selection of what is available. Hubel (1988) provides an extremely clear, well illustrated, account of visual neurophysiology and Zeki (1993) provides a detailed and philosophically-aware text. The series edited by Cronly-Dillon (1991) contains chapters with much up-to-date and expert material. Peters and Jones (1984) provide detail of the visual cortices of mouse, rat, cat and several primates. Neri, Morrone and Burr (1999) show that the human visual cortices are adapted to picking up *biological* motion and a useful discussion of plasticity in the mammalian visual cortex is to be found in Barlow (1975). The topic of object and face recognition is under intensive research at the time of writing. An overview may be found in the symposium organised by Bruce *et al.* (1992). Although most work is (and has been) done on primates, Kendrick and Baldwin (1987) have shown that other social mammals have neurons responsive to similar trigger stimuli. Logothetis and Sheinberg (1996) and Tanaka (1996) review the response of IT cells to the presentation of not only faces but also other complex objects in the visual field. Prosopagnosia has attracted much attention and, in addition to the technical references listed below, Oliver Sacks' (1985) fascinating popular account is also very much to be recommended. A pioneering account of the analogies between animal and computer visual systems is given by David Marr (1981).

General

Campion, J., Latto, R. and Smith, Y.M. (1983) Is blind-sight an effect of scattered light, spared cortex, and near threshold vision. *Behavioural and Brain Sciences*, **6**, 423–86.

Frisby, J.P. (1979) *Seeing: Illusion, Brain and Mind*. Oxford University Press, Oxford.

Hubel, D.H. (1988) *Eye, Brain, and Vision*, Freeman, Scientific American Library, New York.

Humphrey, N. (1992) *A History of the Mind*, Vintage, London.

McIlwain, T.T. (1996) *An Introduction to the Biology of Vision*, Cambridge University Press, Cambridge.

Neri, P., Morrone, C. and Burr, D.C. (1999) Seeing biological motion. *Nature*, **395**, 894–900.

Smith, C.U.M. (1970) *The Brain: Towards an Understanding*, Faber, London.

Zeki, S. (1993) *A Vision of the Brain*, Blackwell Scientific Publications, Oxford.

Visual Pathways

Visual Pathways into the Brain

Dreher, B. and Robinson, S.R. (eds) (1991) Neuroanatomy of the visual pathways and their development, in *Vision and Visual Dysfunction*, Vol. **3** (ed. J.R. Cronly-Dillon), Macmillan, London.

Duke-Elder, S. and Wybar, K.C. (1961) *System of Ophthalmology: The Anatomy of the Visual System*, Vol. **2**, Henry Kimpton, London.

Hart, W.M. (1992) *Adler's Physiology of the Eye*, 9th edn, Mosby, St Louis.

The Retino-Tectal Pathway

Henry, G.H. and Vidyasgar, T.R. (1991) Evolution of mammalian visual pathways, in *Vision and Visual Dysfunction*, Vol. **3** (eds J.R. Cronly-Dillon and R. Gregory), Macmillan, London.

The Retino–Geniculo–Striate (RGS) Pathway

Duke-Elder, S. and Wybar, K.C. (1961) *System of Ophthalmology: The Anatomy of the Visual System*, Vol. **2**, Henry Kimpton, London.

Hubel, D.H. and Wiesel, T. (1977) Functional architecture of macaque monkey visual cortex. *Proceedings of the Royal Society, B*, **198**, 1–59.

Primary Visual Cortex

Structure

Brindmann, L. and Lippold, O. (1980) *The Neurophysiology of the Cerebral Cortex*, Edward Arnold, London.

Peters, A. and Jones, L. (eds) (1984) *Cerebral Cortex: Visual Cortex*, Vol. **3**, Plenum, New York.

Szentagothai, J. (1975) The "module concept" in cerebral cortex architecture. *Brain Research*, **95**, 475–96.

Functioning

Hubel, D.H. and Wiesel, T. (1977) Functional architecture of macaque monkey visual cortex. *Proceedings of the Royal Society, B*, **198**, 1–59.

Livingstone, M.S. and Hubel, D.H. (1984) Anatomy and physiology of a color system in the the primate visual cortex. *Journal of Neuroscience*, **4**, 309–56.

Plasticity

Barlow, H.B. (1975) Visual experience and cortical development. *Nature*, **258**, 199–204.
Hubel, D.H., Wiesel, T.N. and Le Vay, S. (1977) Plasticity of ocular dominance columns in monkey striate cortex. *Philosophical Transactions of the Royal Society, B*, **278**, 377–4.

Extrastriate Cortices

Felleman, D.J. and van Essen, D. (1991) Distributed hierarchical processing in the primate cerebral cortex. *Cerebral Cortex*, **1**, 1–47.
Logothetis, N.K. and Sheinberg, D.L. (1996) Visual object recognition. *Annual Review of Neuroscience*, **19**, 577–621.

Face Recognition

Bruce, V. *et al.* (1992) Processing the facial image. *Philosophical Transactions of the Royal Society, B*, **335**, 1–128.
Gross, C.G., Rocha-Miranda, C.E. and Bender, D.B. (1972) Visual properties of neurons in the inferotemporal cortex of the macaque. *Journal of Neurophysiology*, **35**, 96–111.
Grusser, O.-J. and Landis, T. (1991) Man as social partner in the visual world: perception and recognition of faces and facial expression, in *Visual Agnosias and Other Disturbances of Visual Perception and Cognition*, Vol. **12** (eds O.-J. Grusser and T. Landis), of *Vision and Visual Dysfunction* (ed. J. Cronly-Dillon), Macmillan Press, London.
Kendrick, K.M. and Baldwin, B.A. (1987) Cells in temporal cortex of conscious sheep can respond preferentially to the sight of faces. *Science*, **236**, 448–50.
Perrett, D.I., Mistlin, A.J. and Chitty, A.J. (1987) Visual neurons responsive to faces. *Trends in Neurosciences*, **10**, 358–64.
Perrett, D.I. *et al.* (1992) Organisation and functions of cells responsive to faces in the temporal cortex. *Philosophical Transactions of the Royal Society B*, **335**, 23–30.
Tanaka, K. (1996) Inferotemporal cortex and object vision. *Annual Review of Neuroscience*, **19**, 109–39.

Young, M.P. (1995) Open questions about the neural mechanisms of visual pattern recognition, in *The Cognitive Neurosciences* (ed. M.S. Gazzaniga), MIT Press, Cambridge, Mass.

Prospagnosia

Allison, T., Puce, A., Spencer, D.D. and McCarthy, G. (1999) Electrophysiological studies of human face perception, 1: potentials generated in occipitotemporal cortex by face and nonface stimuli. *Cerebral Cortex*, **30**, 415–30.
Grusser, O.-J. and Landis, T. (1991) Faces lost: prospagnosia, in *Visual Agnosias and Other Disturbances of Visual Perception and Cognition* Vol. **12** (eds O.-J. Grusser and T. Landis), of *Vision and Visual Dysfunction* (ed. J. Cronly-Dillon), Macmillan Press, London.
Sacks, O. (1985) *The Man who Mistook his Wife for a Hat*, Harper Collins, New York.

Conclusion

Marr, D. (1981) *Vision*, W.H. Freeman, San Francisco

CHAPTER 19: OTHER VERTEBRATE VISUAL SYSTEMS

There are four comprehensive sources for the comparative anatomy of vertebrate visual systems: Sir Stewart Duke-Elder's *System of Ophthalmology*; volume 1; G.L. Wall's *Vertebrate Eye and its adaptive radiation*. J.R. Cronly-Dillon's *Vision and Visual Dysfunction*, and H. Autrum *et al.*'s *Handbook of Sensory Physiology*. The latter two edited volumes contain numerous detailed chapters on particular animal groups. These publications and chapters contained therein are cited several times in the following bibliography. The adaptive values of rhodopsin and porphyropsin are reviewed in Goldsmith (1990) and Prosser and Brown's text (1961), although compiled many years ago, still provides much useful comparative information, often in the form of tables.

General

Charman, W.N. (1991) The vertebrate dioptric apparatus, in *Evolution of the Eye and Visual System* (eds J.R. Cronly-Dillon and R.L. Gregory), in *Vision and Visual*

Dysfunction, Vol. **2** (ed. J. Cronly-Dillon), Macmillan, London.

Crescitelli, F. (ed.) (1977) *Handbook of Sensory Physiology: The Visual system in Vertebrates*, Vol. **VII/5**, Springer-Verlag, New York.

Duke-Elder, S. (1958) *System of Ophthalmology: The Eye in Evolution*, Vol. **1**, Kimpton, London.

Land, M.F. and Fernald, R.D. (1992) Evolution of eyes. *Annual Review of Neuroscience*, **15**, 1–29.

Walls, G.L. (1963) *The Vertebrate Eye and its Adaptive Radiation*, Hefner, New York.

Visual Pigments

Goldsmith, T.H. (1990) Optimisation, constraint and history in the evolution of eyes. *Quarterly Review of Biology*, **65**, 281–322.

Prosser, C.L. and Brown, F.A. (1961) *Comparative Animal Physiology*, Saunders, Philadelphia.

Photoreceptors

Crescitelli, F. (1977) The visual pigments of Geckoes and other vertebrates: an essay in comparative biology, in *Handbook of Sensory Physiology*, Vol. **VII/5** (eds H. Autrum *et al.*), *The Visual System in Vertebrates* (ed. F. Crescitelli), Springer-Verlag, New York.

Vorobyev, M. (2003) Coloured oil droplets enhance colour discrimination. *Proceedings of the Royal Society B*, **270**, 1255–61.

Walls, G.L. (1963) *The Vertebrate Eye and its Adaptive Radiation*, Hefner, New York.

Tapeta

Locket, N.A. (1977) Adaptations to the deep-sea environment, in *Handbook of Sensory Physiology*, Vol. **VII/5** (eds H. Autrum et al.), *The Visual System in Vertebrates* (ed. F. Crescitelli), Springer-Verlag, New York.

Walls, G.L. (1963) *The Vertebrate Eye and its Adaptive Radiation*, Hefner, New York.

Retinae

Barlow, H.B. (1953) Summation and inhibition in the frog's retina. *Journal of Physiology*, **119**, 69–88.

Collin, S.P., Hoskins, R.V. and Partridge, J.C. (1997) Tubular eyes of deep sea fishes: a comparative study of retinal topography. *Brain, Behaviour and Evolution*, **50**, 335–57.

Collin, S.P.R., Hoskins, R.V. and Partrige, J.C. (1998) Seven retinal specializations in the tubular eye of the deep sea Pearleye, *Scopelarchus michaelsarsi*: a case stduy in visual optimisation. *Brain, Behaviour and Evolution*, **51**, 291–314.

Hartline, H.K. (1938) Responses of single optic nerve fibres of the vertebrate eye to illumination of the retina. *American Journal of Physiology*, **121**, 400–15.

Locket, N.A. (1977) Adaptations to the deep-sea environment, in *Handbook of Sensory Physiology*, Vol. **VII/5** (eds H. Autrum et al.), *The Visual System in Vertebrates* (ed. F. Crescitelli), Springer-Verlag, New York.

Meyer, D.B. (1977) The avian eye and its adaptations, in *Handbook of Sensory Physiology: The Visual system in Vertebrates*, Vol. **VII/5**, Springer-Verlag, New York.

Dioptric Apparatus

Artedi, P. (1758) *Rerum Naturalium Thesauri Descriptione (quoted in System of Ophthalmology: The Eye in Evolution*, Vol. **1** (Duke-Elder, S., 1958), Kimpton, London.

Charman, W.N. (1991) The vertebrate dioptric apparatus, in *Evolutionof the Eye and Visual System* (eds J.R. Cronly-Dillon and R.L. Gregory), in *Vision and Visual Dysfunction*, Vol. **2** (ed. J. Cronly-Dillon), Macmillan, London.

Collin, S.P., Hoskins, R.V. and Partridge, J.C. (1997) Tubular eyes of deep sea fishes: a comparative study of retinal topography. *Brain, Behaviour and Evolution*, **50**, 335–57.

Duke-Elder, S. (1958) *System of Ophthalmology: The Eye in Evolution*, Vol. **1**, Kimpton, London.

Land, M.F. and Fernald, R.D. (1992) Evolution of eyes. *Annual Review of Neuroscience*, **15**, 1–29.

Locket, N.A. (1977) Adaptations to the deep-sea environment in *Handbook of Sensory Physiology*, Vol. **VII/5** (eds H. Autrum *et al.*), *The Visual System in Vertebrates* (ed. F. Crescitelli), Springer-Verlag, New York.

Soemmering, D.W. (1818) *De Oculorum Hominis Animaliumque sectione Horizontali Commentatio*, Vandenhoeck and Ruprect, Goettingen.

Median Eyes

Duke-Elder, S. (1958) *System of Ophthalmology: The Eye in Evolution*, Vol. **1**, Kimpton, London.

Hamasaki, D.I. and Elder, D.J. (1977) Adaptive radiation of the pineal system, in *Handbook of Sensory Physiology*, Vol. **VII/5** (eds H. Autrum et al.), *The Visual System in Vertebrates* (ed. F. Crescitelli), Springer-Verlag, New York.

Xiong, W.-H., Solessio, E.C. and Yau, K.-W. (1998) An unusual cGMP pathway underlying depolarizing light response of the vertebrate parietal-eye photoreceptor. *Nature Neuroscience*, **1**, 359–65.

Visual Pathways

Henry, G.H. and Vidyasgar, T.R. (1991) Evolution of mammalian visual pathways, in *Vision and Visual Dysfunction*, Vol. 3 (eds J.R. Cronly-Dillon and R. Gregory), Macmillan, London.

Visual Centres in the Brain

Muntz, W.R.A. (1977) The visual world of amphibia, in *Handbook of Sensory Physiology*, Vol. **VII/5** (eds H. Autrum et al.), *The Visual System in Vertebrates* (ed. F. Crescitelli), Springer-Verlag, New York.

Shimizu, T. and Karten, H.J. (1991) Central visual pathways in reptiles and birds: evolution of the visual system, in *Vison and Visual Dysfunction*, Vol. **2** (eds J.R. Cronly-Dillon and R.L. Gregory), Macmillan, London.

Sivar, J.G. (1977) The role of the spectacle in the visual optics of the snake. *Vision Research*, **17**, 293–8.

PART V: OTHER SENSES

'If a lion could talk, we could not understand him'

Ludwig Wittgenstein: *Philosophical Investigations*, trs. G.E.M.Anscombe, Oxford: Blackwell, 1958: p. 223e

So far in this book we have discussed the major senses which the vast majority of animals – if not all animals – possess. In this penultimate section we consider first, in Chapter 20, one final major sense: that of temperature. This, although widespread throughout the animal kingdom, has (except in the infrared detectors of ophidians) evolved no intricate sense organs such as eye or ear or nose. Rather thermal sense endings are distributed over the whole surface of the body.

Next, in Chapter 21, we turn to some of the 'minority' senses: those which are found in only a small group of animals. We are not aware of electric or magnetic fields, although in our technological civilization it might have conferred considerable advantage if we had been. We are not aware of infrared radiation or of the plane of polarized light. Some animals have developed sense organs which can detect these features of the environment. It is difficult for us to enter into the life-worlds of animals so endowed. Wittgenstein's lion would be almost intelligible compared with them. Humans, of course, precisely through the technological civilization mentioned above, nowadays out-compete all other animals in their ability to detect and analyse all forms of environmental energy. Our military is well accustomed to infrared night-sights, our electrical engineers are well able to detect electric and magnetic fields, the makers of spectacles and windows of stretch limousines are fully informed of the nature of polarized light. Cultural evolution has far outpaced organic evolution in the fashioning of detectors of all forms of environmental energy. All these energies can be transformed by our technology into our customary sensory modalities.

One thing, however, our technology cannot do: it cannot manufacture what Patrick Wall has called a 'dolorimeter': a device for detecting and measuring pain. Here we move towards the end of our book. Pain has sometimes been called 'the existential sense'. We cannot shut our eyes, figuratively speaking, to the pain of a raging toothache. It follows us, it is us, wherever we are, whatever we are doing. But it is private, no one else can see it. They may see our grimaces, our behaviour, hear our groans and complaints, but they cannot feel our pain, gauge the subjectivity. How far through the animal kingdom does it spread? Birds, fish, cephalopods? We can only be sure of it in ourselves and the other mammals. We shall accordingly restrict ourselves to mammalian physiology when we discuss its biology in the third chapter of this Part, Chapter 22. We shall, however, return to some of the wider implications of this very private sense in the last chapter of the book, Chapter 24.

Biology of Sensory Systems, Second Edition   C.U.M. Smith
© 2008 John Wiley & Sons, Ltd

20

THERMOSENSITIVITY

Temperature range for life. Poikilotherms and homeotherms. Both need thermosensors. **Molecular biology**: dorsal root ganglion (DRG) cells - responsive to temperature change - Ca^{2+}-induced inward current - potentiated by both bradykinin and prostaglandin E; *C. elegans* - thermotactic mutants, tax 2 and tax 4 - protein products resemble CNG units of rod outersegments. **Poikilotherms**: fish lateral line? - insect sensilla - thermoreceptors grouped with hygroreceptors - biological roles. **Homeotherms**: evolution of homeothermy; homeothermy in Homo sapiens - locations of receptors: **skin** - warm and cold spots - paradoxical cold - Weber's illusion - histology - bare nerve endings - Aδ fibres (warmth), C-fibres (cold) - RFs - dynamic and static responses - spinothalamic and trigeminothalamic tracts to thalamus; **deep receptors**: spinal cord, abdominal viscera, great veins, interior of gut - guard against hypothermia - nasal mucosa; **hypothalamus**: pre-optic region - posterior hypothalamus - homeostatic control. **Concluding remarks**: homeothermy provides another instance of the body's need to maintain stability of the internal environment.

Until recent years it had been thought that the temperature range within which animal life could exist was rather limited: about 0–40 °C (or 273–313 K). Discoveries of large marine 'tube worms' living near deep water fumaroles at near 100 °C has placed question marks against the sharpness of the upper temperature limit. Nevertheless, the inescapable facts of chemistry seem to militate against any major departure from the 0–40 °C range. Below 0 °C the aqueous medium that constitutes more than 90% of any living organism undergoes a phase change which makes active metabolic processes sluggish at best (if some form of organic antifreeze can be evolved) and frozen solid at worst. Beyond about 40 °C thermal agitation tends to disrupt the delicate hydrophobic forces and other 'weak' chemical bonds which hold the structure of globular proteins in place.

Without this delicate and precise structure the biological function, especially the enzymatic function, of these great molecules is lost. Furthermore, biological membranes are also very sensitive to temperature. The phosopholipid bilayer tends to gel at low temperatures and break up into micelles at high temperatures. Every beginning student of biology knows that denaturation occurs beyond about 40 °C; every beginning microbiologist knows that boiling sterilizes. Yet, as we have seen, some tube worms can tolerate 100 °C and some hyperthermophilic bacteria continue growing at up to 113 °C in hot springs. We are still not sure how this is accomplished.

With respect to temperature, animals may be divided into two great groups: **poikilotherms** and **homeotherms**. The first group have no way other than behaviour to control their body temperature;

Biology of Sensory Systems, Second Edition   C.U.M. Smith
© 2008 John Wiley & Sons, Ltd

the second have evolved mechanisms to maintain the temperature of the internal environment constant no matter what (within limits) may be happening to the temperature outside in the external environment. Both groups, however, need some means of detecting the circumambient temperature. This is particularly important for small animals. Unless they are homeothermic, they will quickly assume the temperature of their surroundings; if they are homeotherms, their homeostatic mechanisms will have to operate quickly and effectively to prevent body temperature rising or falling to match that of the environment.

20.1 MOLECULAR BIOLOGY

Three approaches to the basic molecular biology of thermosensitivity have recently been made. The first depends on genetic analysis of thermotactic mutants in *C. elegans*, the second on the biophysical analysis of cells isolated from mammalian dorsal root ganglia (DRG) and the third on genetic manipulation of the thermosensory neurons in mouse. Let us consider each in turn.

20.1.1 *Caenorhabditis Elegans*

Temperature is obviously of great significance to small poikilothermic animals. In order to test the worm's thermal sensitivity, a radial maze was devised. A small vial of frozen ammonium acetate (melting temperature 17 °C) was placed at the centre of a petri dish lined with a thin agar film. The dish was then moved to a hotplate set at 25 °C. This created a thermal gradient from the centre (17 °C) to the periphery (25 °C). It was then shown that worms fed at a certain temperature would afterwards seek that temperature and track around that temperature zone in the dish. It was further shown that worms were able to detect the correct temperature to within 0.1 °C. If the major thermosensory nerve (AFD) was ablated, most of the animals lost all ability to detect the thermal gradient, moving randomly over the agar. Further experiments excluded the possibility that this was due to loss of 'memory'.

It has been known since the 1970s that genetic mutations eliminated this thermosensivity. Ultimately it was shown that mutations in two genes, *tax-2* and

tax-4, caused this loss of thermotactic behaviour. It is fascinating to find that the protein products of these genes are homologous to the α and β subunits of the cGMP-gated channels of vertebrate rod and cone cells (Chapter 17). When these two proteins are expressed in cell culture they can be shown to form a channel which (like its vertebrate homologue) is activated by cGMP applied to its intracellular face. Finally, tagging the proteins with a green fluorescent dye enabled the location of the channels to be determined. They were found to be expressed in the appropriate sensory neurons and endings in the worm's nervous system. Quite recently a third gene, *cng-3*, which also encodes another cyclic-nucleotide-gated channel, has been shown to be critical for the worm's ability to tolerate elevated temperatures

Let us turn from the thermosensitivity of *C. elegans* to that of more complex organisms. In general it seems that, instead of cyclic-nucleotide-gated channels, the thermosensitive neurons in the 'higher' invertebrates and vertebrates use members of the ubiquitous TRP superfamily.

20.1.2 Dorsal Root Ganglia (DRG)

These ganglia contain the cell bodies of sensory neurons. It is known that the membrane of each neuron is uniquely different from that of any other. In other words, each neuron inserts its own peculiar array of proteins in its boundary lipid bilayer. Thus cells responsive to ACh will incorporate acetylcholine receptors into their membranes, cells responsive to 5HT will incorporate one or other (or, perhaps, a unique cocktail of) 5HT receptors and so on. These receptors will, of course, be most concentrated in postsynaptic membranes and (in the case of thermosensory cells) 'bare' dendritic nerve endings, but will be present in smaller quantities in the membranes of the perikarya and so on. One approach to the investigation of the molecular biology of thermosensitivity made use of this fact.

Mammalian DRG cells are of many shapes and sizes. It is known, however, that the fibres responsible for thermosensitivity are of small diameter (Section 20.3.1) and it follows that it is the smallest cells in DRGs which are associated with thermosensitivity. It was thus satisfactory to find that, when dissociated DRG cells were exposed to rapid changes in temperature, a group of small neurons responded with large inward currents. Pharmacological analysis showed that these small cells were not sympathetic perikarya. Further analysis showed that they responded to variation in temperature in a 'dose-dependent' manner: the greater the temperature stimulus the greater the inward current. The inward current depended on the opening of nonselective cation channels. It appears that heat stimuli cause the release of Ca^{2+} from intracellular stores and it may be that increased levels of this cation trigger the opening of the channels. We shall see in Chapter 22 that heat-activated nociceptive fibres have the same characteristics.

20.1.3 Mouse Thermosensory Neurons

Investigations of mouse thermosensory neurons showed that heat-activated channels are members of the **TPRV** family of receptors. Ultimately it turned out that six members of the TRP family are involved, opening in response to different temperature thresholds: TRPV1 $\geq$ 42 °C; TRPV2 $\geq$ 52 °C; TRPV3 $\geq$ 33 °C; TRPV4 ~27–42 °C; the other two TRPs open in response to cold: TRPM8 $\leq$ 25 °C; TRPA1 $\leq$ 17 °C. The warmth receptor, TRPV3, is also expressed in epidermal skin cells. TRPV3 receptors pass a signal to sensory nerve endings by some as yet unknown mechanism. Another temperature receptor, TRPM5, is expressed in taste receptor cells and may be responsible for the fact that temperature has an affect on taste perception. Putting all this together it is easy to see that the TRP family of cation channels, located in the thermosensitive endings of narrow gauge thermosensory fibres and neighbouring epidermal cells, provides a sophisticated system for detecting temperature variations. Behavioural experiments confirm the molecular biology. It can be shown, for instance, that mice engineered to lack TRM8 show a marked (though not complete) insensitivity to cold, finding it difficult to discriminate between warm and cold surfaces and a marked insensitivity to evaporative cooling.

As a bonus to this molecular analysis, some light is also thrown on why tissue damage frequently elicits a burning sensation. Amongst the many biochemicals released when tissue is damaged are **prostaglandins** and **bradykinin**. Both prostaglandin

E and bradykinin are found to act on TRP channels in thermosensory nerve endings, increasing the amplitude of the heat sensitive current leading to generator potentials and thus action potentials. Other naturally occurring chemicals also affect the thermosensitive channels: capsaicin (found in chilli peppers) activates the TPRV1 (hot) channel, whilst cinnamon activates the TPRA1 (cool) channel. Indeed, it is found that many foodstuffs also affect one or several thermosensory receptors in addition to their action on the gustatory and olfactory receptors.

In conclusion, it should be said that it seems unlikely that the work on *C. elegans* and mammalian thermosensory systems can be combined into a large and coherent picture of the molecular biology of thermosensitivity. Mammalian (and invertebrate) thermoreceptors are members of the TRP family of cation channels whilst those of *C. elegans* are not. This makes it unlikely that the *C. elegans* work will throw much light on the molecular biology of thermosensitivity in mammals. Nevertheless, the development of these powerful experimental systems increases the possibility of understanding the fundamentals of the temperature sense at the same level as that of the senses we have discussed in the parts of this book.

20.2 POIKILOTHERMS

Poikilothermic animals are adapted to different optimal environmental temperatures. Aquatic animals adapted to low water temperatures may, for instance, have upper lethal temperatures below the lower lethal temperatures of animals adapted to higher temperatures. Such animals have low and high temperature sensors in their body surfaces which signal the need to take avoiding action should it be necessary. These sensors often take the form of **free nerve endings**. In fish and amphibian tadpoles, however, there is some evidence (though somewhat conflicting) that, in addition to subcutaneous afferents, the **lateral line system** is involved. This system, as we saw in Chapter 9, is primarily a system of mechanoreceptors evolved to detect pressure changes in the circumambient water, but it seems that it is also capable of detecting both steady temperature and temperature change in this water. In the Chondrichthyes, elaborations of the lateral line system on the surface of the head, the

ampullae of Lorenzini, although primarily (as we shall see in Chapter 21) electroreceptors, also respond to steady temperature and to change in temperature, especially to cooling.

Insects, as small animals, are especially sensitive to environmental temperature. In experimental conditions they respond to changes in temperature by moving to as near an optimal temperature as is provided. Investigators have shown that, in most cases, the thermoreceptors are located on the **antennae**. In the majority of species investigated these appear to be cold receptors, although in some cases heat receptors are also present. Cold receptors are defined as those which increase their firing frequency in response to falling temperature; heat receptors increase their activity when temperatures rise. In the stick insect, *Carausius*, for instance, there is a linear response to decrease in temperature below 20 °C. Thermoreceptor sensilla are often multimodal, containing one or more chemoreceptor and/or hygroreceptor neurosensory cells in addition to the thermoreceptor. As the combination of atmospheric temperature and humidity is often critical, it is not surprising that combinations of thermoreceptor and hygroreceptor cells are housed in one sensilla. The sensilla, as is customary in the insects, take many shapes and sizes, though most thermoreceptors are simple pegs which may be either aporous or multiporous.

Insect thermoreceptors are used in many ways in addition to sensing temperature and/or temperature change of the atmosphere. Cold sensors on the antennae of caterpillars can detect the **evaporative cooling** induced by moisture escaping from the cut ends of leaves. Thermoreceptors on the wing veins of some groups of butterfly are activated by the sun's warmth and reflexly cause the closing of the insect's wings. Voracious blood-sucking hemipteran bugs of the genus *Triatoma* have a specialized warmth receptor on their antennae. This structure is lacking in their nonblood-sucking cousins. It has clearly evolved for **host detection**. *Triatoma megista* is the main insect vector for *Trypanosoma cruzi* and is thus deeply implicated in human trypanosomiasis in South America. Other members of the genus may be involved in the transmission of Kal-azar. The mosquito, *Aedes aegyptii*, also depends on finding warm-blooded prey. It has two peg-like thermoreceptors at the tip of its antennae. One of these is a heat detector and the other a cold detector, The

heat receptor is activated by a rise in temperature and is tuned to give a maximum response between 25 and 28 °C. The cold receptor is similarly tuned to give maximum responses to falls in temperature in this range. Atmospheric convection currents caused by the warmth of a human arm can be detected at a distance of 40 cm by these receptors. They play an important role in directing the mosquito to an unclothed part of the human anatomy.

20.3 HOMEOTHERMS

Only the birds and mammals are true homeotherms and the condition seems to have evolved independently in both groups. Mammals evolved alongside the ruling reptiles, including the dinosaurs, in the Triassic period some 200 million years ago. Whether these early 'mammal-like reptiles' were homeothermic is, like the related question of whether some of the dinosaurs were homeothermic, a matter of dispute. Similarly, the birds may be traced back at least to the Jurassic period when *Archaeopteryx* (145 Ma BP) may or may not have been homeothermic. Whereas all birds are true homeotherms (some of them regulating their body temperatures at a set point as high as 42 °C), only the 'higher' eutherians amongst the mammals can be classified as such. The primitive mammals, the prototheria, can at best be said to be heterothermic and many of the metatheria are only inaccurately homeothermic as, indeed, are the more primitive orders of the eutheria, such as the Insectivora.

Let us, however, turn our attention to the human condition. Here homeothermy is well developed. The temperature of the body's 'core' is held constant at about 37 °C. The homeostatic mechanisms consist, in essence, of a balance between heat production and heat loss. Both sides of the equation can be varied but the fine control is on heat loss. This can be controlled by changing the amounts of heat lost by evaporation, radiation and convection. Physiology texts describe the effectors by which this control is exerted: the arrector pili muscles of the hair follicles, the sudorific glands, the vascular plexi in the dermis of the skin and so on. Here we shall concentrate only on the sensory systems that detect the temperature variations which demand the homeostatic response. These variations are sensed at the **periphery** (the skin); **deep** within the body, mainly in the spinal cord, abdominal viscera and in and around the great veins; and last, but perhaps most important of all, by temperature sensitive cells in the **hypothalamus**.

20.3.1 Thermoreceptors in the Skin

When the skin temperature is within the range 32–42 °C, no thermal sensations are felt. This, of course, is not to say that changes in temperature within this range cannot be detected. In fact, as we shall see below, the skin is exquisitely sensitive to sudden variations in temperature within this range. But when the temperature remains constant within these limits, little activity occurs in the thermoreceptors. This range is consequently known as the **neutral range**. Outside this range sensations of cold or warmth are experienced. At temperatures below about 18 °C the sensation of cold merges into that of cold-pain and, similarly, above about 45 °C warmth merges into heat-pain. Both 'warm' and 'cold' receptors are located in the **dermis**. It has been known for many years that they form a mosaic of 'warm' and 'cold' spots, each about 1 mm in diameter. This can be established by using a **thermode**: a small, needle-like, instrument which can be heated electrically or by the passage of water. The highest density of these thermosensitive spots is found in some regions of the face. The lips, for instance, develop 16–19 cold spots per cm^2, the nose 8–13/cm^2 and the forehead 5–8/cm^2. In contrast, the palm of the hand possesses only 1–5/cm^2 and the fingers only 2–4/cm^2. Warm spots are less frequent; the fingers possess about 1.7/cm^2 and the palm of the hand 0.4/cm^2. In many areas of the body they are quite sparse.

It can be shown that the thermosensitive endings responsive to cold are located in the upper part of the dermis (about 0.17 mm beneath the skin's surface), whilst those responding to warmth are located somewhat deeper (about 0.3 mm below the surface). It is interesting to note that when an excessive stimulus, such as a 45 °C thermode, is applied precisely on to a cold spot it is experienced as cold. This illusion, known as **paradoxical cold**, emphasizes the dependence of the central nervous system (CNS) on interpreting the input from labelled lines (Chapter 3). Another well authenticated illusion, **Weber's illusion**, is due to the fact that cutaneous mechanoreceptors are weakly activated by cold. Hence, as Weber pointed out, objects seem to weigh more in cold than in neutral or warm conditions.

Identification of the sensory endings in the skin that are responsive to warmth and cold has not proved easy. In general, it is believed that there are no dedicated histological structures but that bare nerve endings interweaving, but not anastomosing, at all levels in the dermis are responsible. These fibres are of small diameter (1.5–3 μm) and are classified as **Aδ fibres (cold)** and **C fibres (warm)**. There is considerable summation of the output, as it can be shown that the subjective threshold for stimulation of a large area of skin is significantly lower than that for stimulation of single fibres. About 50 or so warm or cold fibres have to be activated before a conscious sensation results. But these subjective thresholds are very sensitive. Humans are capable of detecting decreases of as little as 0.02–0.05 °C.

Both warm and cold receptor afferents can be examined with the techniques of electrophysiology. Each fibre responds to stimulation of one (sometimes more than one) spot. The magnitude of the receptive field varies with the intensity of the thermal stimulus (Figure 20.1a). 'Warm' fibres discharge when the skin is warmed beyond the neutral range and cease firing with the heat-pain threshold is reached (Figure 20.1b). Cold fibres discharge over a broad range, from 10 to 40 °C (Figure 20.1b). Both sets of fibres have dynamic and static responses (Figure 20.1c). The initial burst of impulses (dynamic response) due to a change in temperature (outside the neutral range) provides the signal for the highly sensitive threshold detection mentioned above.

The Aδ and C afferents from the cutaneous thermoreceptors mostly terminate in the superficial layers of the dorsal horn of the spinal cord. From there fibres in the spinothalamic and trigeminothalamic tract carry thermal information upwards to the thalamus.

20.3.2 Deep Thermoreceptors

The temperature in the vicinity of the spinal cord, the abdominal viscera and in and around the great veins is detected by thermoreceptor afferents similar to those we have discussed in the previous section. Once again the majority respond to cold and,

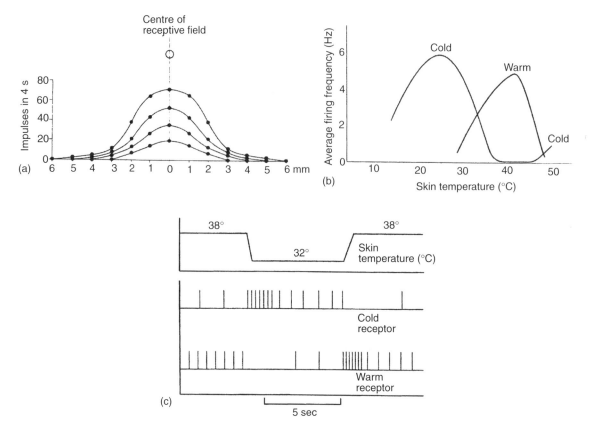

Figure 20.1 (a) Receptive field organization of a warm fibre. Activity in the fibre was elicited by a 30 s. warming pulse delivered by a thermode at different positions in the receptive field. The family of curves shows impulse frequencies in response to 2, 4, 6 and 8 °C. From Darian-Smith, I. (1984) Thermal sensitivity, in *Handbook of Physiology, Section 1: The Nervous System: Sensory Processes, Part 2, Vol. 3* (ed. I. Darian-Smith), Copyright © 1984, American Physiological Society. (b) Response of cold and warm receptors to temperature. It remains unclear how the CNS extracts an intensity signal from these bell-like curves. (c) Response of cold and warm receptors to onset and termination of a cold stimulus. It can be seen that both receptors respond vigorously to the change and then adapt to a steady state. (B) and (C) from Bear, M. F., Connors, B. W. and Paradiso, M. A. (1996) *Neuroscience: Exploring the Brain*, Copyright © 1996, Williams and Wilkins.

especially, to decreasing temperatures beneath the neutral range. As with the cutaneous thermoreceptors discussed above, the crisis which they seem to be 'designed' to prevent is hypothermia, a loss of body heat. In addition to these sensors of body temperature, thermoreceptors in the **nasal mucosa** play a significant role not only in sensing the temperature of the indrawn air but also in detecting the rate of flow of the air through the respiratory passages. Finally, both warm and cold receptors are to be found within the gastro-intestinal tract.

20.3.3 Hypothalamic Thermoreceptors

When the hypothalamus is carefully investigated with a fine thermode, it can be shown that large numbers of thermosensitive neurons are to be found, especially, but not exclusively, in the **preoptic** region of the anterior hypothalamus. Heat-sensitive neurons increase their firing rate in response to increases in the temperature of blood in neighbouring capillaries; vice versa, cold sensitive neurons increase their firing rate in response to drops in temperature. The output from the anterior hypothalmus is directed largely at bilateral nuclei in the **posterior hypothalamus**, at the level of the mamillary bodies. It is in these nuclei that information from the central and peripheral thermoreceptors is integrated and that appropriate effector action to correct any significant deviation from the 37 °C set point is computed and launched.

20.4 CONCLUDING REMARKS

As usual, more is known of the physiology of thermosensitivity in the mammals and, especially, humans than in other animals. But, as we have seen, the temperature sense is important in all animals from the lowly nematode, *C. elegans*, onwards. Indeed, as noted in Chapter 1, molecular biology provides evidence suggesting that temperature sensitive TRP channels are among the earliest of all sensory receptors. The development of homeothermy has placed

yet more importance on the precise detection of temperature and temperature variation. In homeothermic animals the temperature of the body is very closely controlled. Variations of more than one or two degrees centigrade above or below the set point begin to disrupt the close coordination of the body's biochemistry and physiology. We have here another example (to set alongside the kinaesthesia of Chapter 7 and the control of PaO_2 and $PaCO_2$ of Chapter 12) of the mammal's and, in particular, the human body's need to maintain stability of the 'internal environment'. Thermosensors located in many parts of the body send back information which is compared with a predetermined set point. It is only when this information slides well away from the set point that we become consciously aware that something must be done. We stretch out hands to the fire or we head for the air-conditioned room. Looking ahead to the last chapter in this Part, chapter 22, we shall see that a somewhat similar analysis can be made of the infinitely more complex sense of pain.

21

MINORITY SENSES

Animal sensory worlds sometimes very different from our own. **Infra-red (IR) sensitivity**: snakes (Boidae and Crotalinae) - labial and facial pits - histology - directionality - adequate stimulus change of IR flux - contralateral midbrain tecta - ON/OFF RFs - map of IR space - triggered by movement of IR source. **Polarised light sensitivity**: features of polarised light (atmosphere) - diurnal changes - λ-dependence - biological significance; hydrosphere - air/water interface - λ-dependence - more than 100 aquatic species sensitive to plane of polarised light; structure of photoreceptors - decapod ommatidia - open, closed and banded rhabdoms; insect ommatidia - Apis foraging; Octopus rod cells - behaviour - electrophysiology. **Electrosensitivity**: Fish - strongly and weakly electric fish - strong used for stunning prey - weak for electro-location - recognition of conspecifics etc; behavioural investigation - sensitivity $\leq$ 5nV - prey detection - navigation through Earth's magnetic field? - detection and identification of nearby objects; histology of electroreceptors - ampullae and tuberous organs (=knollenorgans) - evolution from lateral line system; histology of ampullae - ampullae of Lorenzini - detection of shape of electric field; histology of tuberous organs - types; differing response of ampullae and tuberous organs - distribution over body - whole body acts as sensory surface. Monotremata – electroreception in Ornithorhynchus and Tachyglossus. **Magnetosensitivity**: magnetotactic bacteria - Fe_2O_4 magnetosomes - 'biocompass' - hints of magnetic sensitivity in birds and mammals. **Concluding remarks**: salutary diversity of sensory systems

In this chapter we shall look fairly briefly at four 'minority' senses: sensitivity to infrared radiation; polarized light; electric fields; and magnetic fields. We often forget in our human-centred world that the sensory worlds of animals can be very differently biased. Many insects have good vision into the ultraviolet, and entomophilous flowers have adapted their flower colours accordingly (though which came first – the UV reflecting flowers or the UV detecting insect eye – remains a matter for debate). Many small mammals, and in particular the bats, can, as

we have noted, detect sound far beyond the upper frequencies of human hearing. They, too, live in different sensory worlds. The human olfactory world, pauperized by tens of millions of years of arboreal ancestry, cannot compare with the complexity and richness many animals experience. We have only to contemplate the magnificence of the moth's antennae, spread to detect a single molecule of the female pheromone, to convince ourselves of our impoverishment. But of all these we have an inkling: the four features of the environment which we discuss in

Biology of Sensory Systems, Second Edition   C.U.M. Smith
© 2008 John Wiley & Sons, Ltd

this chapter are all around us, yet we walk through them unknowing.

21.1 INFRARED RADIATION

Infrared detectors are, of course, difficult to distinguish from the thermoreceptors discussed in Chapter 20. Indeed, there can be no sharp line of demarcation. The heat detector of *Triatoma* could just as well be considered in this section. Nevertheless, some thermoreceptors have become so specialized for detecting distant heat sources and pin-pointing their location that it is worth treating them within a separate section. The best known instances are the facial and labial pits of certain snakes.

The first indications that the family *Boidae* (boas, pythons and so on) and the subfamily *Crotalinae* (pit vipers including the rattlesnake (*Crotalus*) and the bushmaster (*Lechesis*)) possessed infrared sensors came from behavioural analyses of prey detection and strike direction. Infrared detection is also used in defence/escape behaviour triggered by large, warm predators. Subsequently, electrophysiological recording from the trigeminal nerve, which innervates the **labial pits** of boids and the **facial pits** (between eye and nostril) of crotalinids, confirmed that these depressions contained infrared receptors. Infrared irradiation provided the adequate stimulus, although responses could also be generated by directing a stream of warm water through the pits. Histological investigation showed that the pits contained no specialized receptor cells. Instead, the unmyelinated endings of the trigeminal fibres originated in greatly expanded nonoverlapping endings (Figure 21.1). In the crotalinid pit these endings form a dense array covering the bottom of the pit. In both crotalinids and boids the exact area at the bottom of the pit that is affected by infrared radiation depends on the direction of the source with respect to the border of the pit. In this respect these sense organs resemble the simple pit eyes discussed in Chapter 15.

Activation of the receptors in both boid and crotalinid pits requires a change in infrared flux. This can be achieved either by movement of warm objects across the 'field of view' against a colder background or by scanning movements of the snake's head. The sensitivity is sufficient to detect the radiant flux from a human hand passed across the 'field

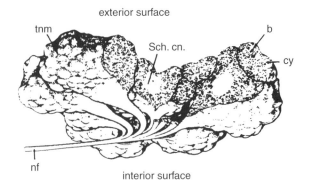

Figure 21.1   Histology of a crotalinid pit. A single unmyelinated nerve springs from expanded terminals within the pit. b = terminal branch; cy = Scwann cell cytoplasm; nf = nerve fibre; Sch.cn. = Schwann cell nucleus; tnm = terminal mass. Reproduced with permission from Terashima, S., Goris, R.C. and Katsuki, Y. (1970) Structure of the warm fiber terminals in the pit membrane of vipers. *Journal of Ultrastructure Research*, **31**, 494–506.

of view' at a distance of 40–50 cm. This suggests that the threshold stimulus is less than 8×10^{-5} W/cm^2. If this is the case, the rise in temperature detected by the receptors is of the order of 0.005 °C (about an order of magnitude better than human temperature detection (Chapter 20), this response of the pit to a warm object moved across its 'field of vision' has been exploited by the Californian ground squirrel (*Spermophilus beecheyi*). It had been known for some time that, when the squirrel encountered a rattlesnake, it warmed up its tail by redirecting its blood supply and waved it in front of the snake. Experiment showed that this behaviour only made the snake back off if the tail were warm. The squirrel's defensive strategy thus seems to rely on the waving tail making the snake feel that it had encountered a much larger creature.

The **receptive fields** of the trigeminal nerve fibres are generally very large but the fields of different fibres have different centres and different edges. The shadows thrown by the edges of the pit would thus differentially affect different receptive fields and could accordingly provide information relating to the source of the infrared. Tracing the output from the pits into the central nervous system shows that it is directed to the contralateral midbrain tecta. Recording from the superficial layers of these tecta reveals the existence of units with center–surround receptive fields. Stimulation of the centre of the field with a warm plate (infrared radiation) induced a brief 'ON' burst of activity. If a cool plate was placed over the centre of the field, activity was suppressed until it was removed, when a brisk 'OFF' response occurred. Vice versa, if a cool stimulus was moved into the periphery of the field, a weak 'ON' response occurred. The analogy with the center–surround organization of RFs in the primate retina is clear (Chapter 17). Equally interesting was the finding that the receptive field diameters were quite small – from 15 to 30°. Clearly considerable processing has occurred between the large RFs of the pit and these much more focussed fields of the tecta. The small RFs allow the formation of rather coarse-grained maps of the infrared space. An orderly spatiotopic map does indeed seem to be present. Pythons and pit vipers thus seem to be informed of the location of heat sources and sinks in their immediate environment. Furthermore, the tectal units are very sensitive to movement of these sources and sinks. Movement of the fingers of the experimenter's hand at a distance of 30–50 cm or movement of a human head or limb at a distance of 2 m proved sufficient to trigger activity in some units. The biological relevance of this spatial and dynamic information needs no labouring.

21.2 POLARIZED LIGHT

When we gaze at a cloudless sky at noon, we seem to see the interior of a flawless blue dome. This, however, is not how many animals, especially arthropods, see it. For the blueness of the sky is due to the scattering of the sun's light by dust particles high in the atmosphere. This **scattering polarizes the light** (see Introduction to Part Four). The amount of polarization in the light reaching a photoreceptor depends on the angle between the line of sight and the direction of the incoming solar radiation. The greater the angle the greater the proportion of the light reaching the eye is polarized. Thus rays of light reaching the eye parallel to direction of the incoming radiation will not be polarized whilst those reaching the eye at right angles to this direction will (in ideal conditions) be 100% polarized. In the real world, atmospheric turbulence and numerous other secondary factors reduce the maximum polarization to no more than about 75–80%. Nevertheless, as the sun moves across

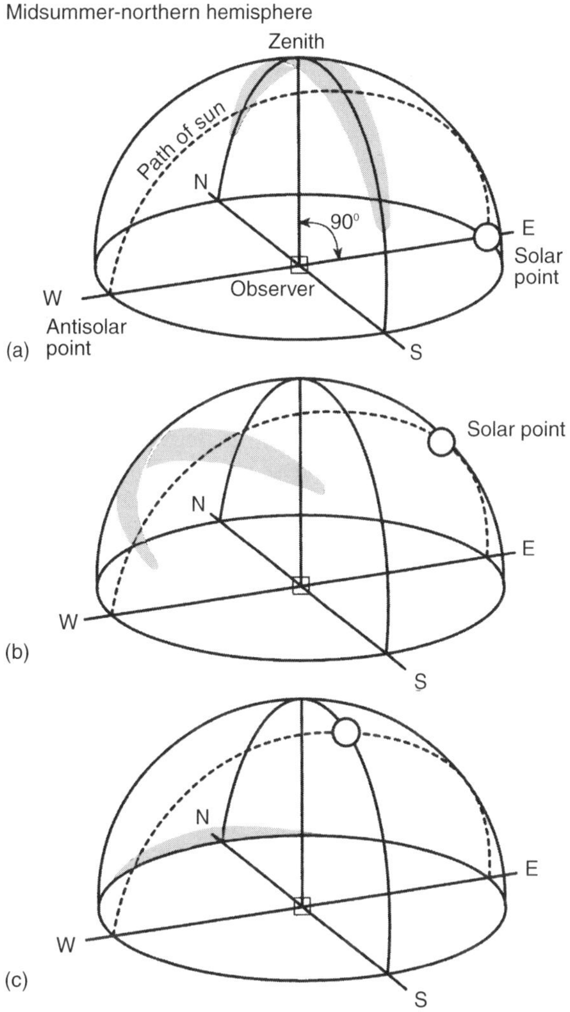

Figure 21.2 Influence of the sun's position in the sky on the orientation of the band of maximum polarization. The observer is in the centre of the hemisphere. (a) Sunrise; (b) mid-morning; (c) noon. From Wellington, W.G. (1974) *Journal of Natural History*, **83** (10), 46–53, Copyright © 1974, Taylor & Francis.

the sky in its daytime traverse the pattern of polarization continuously changes (Figure 21.2). The scattering of light is strongly dependent on its wavelength (λ); indeed it is roughly proportional to $1/\lambda^4$. Short wavelengths (blue light) are thus scattered and hence polarized far more than red light – hence the blueness of a cloudless sky at noon.

These facts of the physics of light mean that, although *we* cannot see it, the blue dome of the sky is highly differentiated for eyes that can. This differentiation contains information which can and is made use of by many animal photoreceptors. In particular, it is made use of in direction finding and is probably also of importance in increasing visual acuity.

Polarization is, of course, not only a feature of light in the atmosphere but also, and equally importantly, of light in the **hydrosphere**. Light entering water from above changes its direction according to the second law of refraction, the **sine law**, sin i/sin r = μ, where μ is the refractive index. In the case of an air/water interface μ = 1.33. It follows that at refractive angles greater than 48.6° rays of light cannot pass the air/water interface and instead are glancingly reflected. Hence, for an underwater organism the whole aerial hemisphere is reduced to a cone of angle about 97.2° (Figure 21.3). This does not mean that the organism cannot see horizontally along the surface of the water. As Figure 21.3 shows, this is fully possible but there will be considerable distortion of brightness and distance. Furthermore, objects on the shallow bottom will be reflected from the undersurface of the water to the aquatic organism's eye. All

this depends, of course, on the surface of the water being flat calm: a condition which seldom obtains. But it all accounts, perhaps, as Walls remarks, for the somewhat bemused expression that fish assume when they are hauled from their watery element.

Partly because of the restriction of light entering the water to the visual cone, only about 25% of the polarization in that underwater light comes from the sky. Downward reflection from the undersurface of the water contributes a share of polarization but the major part is contributed by the water itself. Small particles (<6 μm) suspended in the water are largely responsible and once again shorter wavelengths of light are most affected. Against this it must remembered that longer wavelengths are more easily absorbed by water and the deeper levels are only penetrated by relatively short wave radiation (λ_{max} near 465 nm).

Sensitivity to polarized light is widespread in the animal kingdom. It has been shown to exist in well over a hundred species including crustaceans, insects, arachnids, cephalopod molluscs and vertebrates. The most intensively studied cases belong, however, to the **arthropods** and the **cephalopod molluscs** both of which, as we saw in Chapter 15, have eyes organized on the rhabdom design principle. The visual pigment of the rhabdom's retinula cells is displayed, as we saw in Chapter 14, in interlocking microvilli. In the **Decapoda** (the largest order of the Crustacea, comprising over 26 000 species) all the eyes so far examined show a remarkably uniform structure. The rhabdoms consist of retinula cells developing microvilli orthogonal to the longitudinal axis. The direction of the microvilli in adjacent retinula cells are at right angles to each other and correspond (approximately) to the vertical and horizontal axes of the decapod's body. Sometimes the orthogonally-directed microvilli extend only part way across the rhabdom (**open rhabdom**), in other cases the microvilli are in close contact (fused rhabdom) and in yet other cases they alternate down the length of the rhabdom (Figure 21.4a). This type of structure is known as a **banded rhabdom**. This organizations thus appears to form a two-channel polarization analyser.

A similar rather precise organization of retinula microvilli is found in the rhabdoms of many **insects**, including the intensively studied honeybee (*Apis*), the blowfly (*Calliphora*) and the large dragonfly (*Anax junius*). As we noted in Chapter 15, the retinula

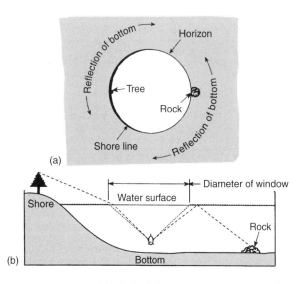

Figure 21.3 Visual field of a fish in the upward direction. (a) The water surface and the aerial window, as seen from beneath. (b) Optics. Rays striking the surface within the cone (97.2°) reach the eyes of the fish; those outside the cone are reflected. Outside the visual cone objects on the pond bottom or in the body of the water will be reflected from the under surface of the water to the fish's eyes. Further explanation in text. From Walls, G.L. (1963) with permission from Hafner.

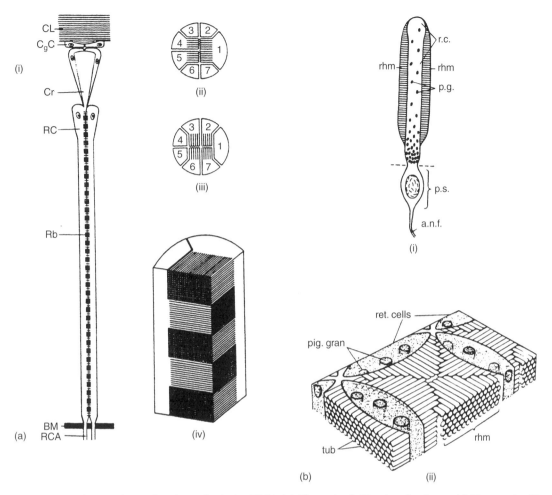

Figure 21.4 Adaptations to detect the plane of polarized light. (a) The crab, *Callinectes*, develops a highly organized banded fused rhabdom. (i) Longitudinal section; (ii) transverse section showing fused rhabdom formed by rhabdomeres of retinula cells 1, 4, 5; (iii) transverse section showing fused rhabdom formed by rhabdomeres of retinula cells 2, 3, 6, 7; (iv) Stereodiagram showing structure of one quarter of the rhabdom. BM = basement membane; CgC = corneagenous cells; CL = corneal lens; Cr = crystalline cone; Rb = rhabdom; RC = retinula cell; RCA = axon from retinula cell. (b) Rhabdom structure in *Octopus* (see also Figure 15.13). (i) Longitudinal section; (ii) transverse section through four rhabdomeres which make up a fused rhabdom. a.n.f. = optic nerve fibre; p.g. = pig.gran. = pigment granules; p.s. = proximal segment; r.c. = ret. cell = retinula cell; rhm = rhabdomere; tub = microvilli. From Waterman, T.H. (1981) with permission from Springer-Verlag.

cells of a single ommatidium contain photopigments sensitive to different wavelengths. The analysis of polarization is thus difficult to disentangle from the analysis of colour. But the precise orthogonal organization of the microvilli suggests that something more than colour is being processed. There is no doubt, from behavioural evidence, that these insects are all sensitive to, and make good biological use of, the plane of polarized light in the atmosphere.

von Frisch's study of the orientation of honeybee foraging with respect to the plane of polarized light is one of the classics of biological science.

Next, to move to a quite different phylum, there is incontrovertible behavioural evidence that **cepaholopod molluscs** are able to discriminate the plane of polarized light. Both food and shock conditioning were used to show that *Octopus* was fully capable of discriminating polarizations differing by

$90°$. The rhabdomeric retinae of octopi and squids resemble those of the polarization-sensitive arthropods in showing a precisely organized mosaic of orthogonally orientated microvilli. Again, as in arthropods, the microvilli are aligned parallel with the eye's vertical and horizontal axes. Electrophysiological recording from *Octopus* retinula cells shows that there are two (and only two) polarization sensitivity channels at right angles to each other. These coincide with retinula cells with microvilli directed orthogonally to each other (Figure 21.4b).

Finally, how does the very precise rhabodomeric structure of arthropods and cephalopods enable these animals to detect the plane of polarized light? We have noted that electrophysiological recording from *Octopus* retina indicates that this indeed the case. Can we go any further into the molecular mechanisms involved? There is evidence from **armyworm moths** (*Spodoptera exempta*) that the degree of distortion of rhabdomeric microvilli depends on the light energy absorbed per unit time. It can also be shown that differently orientated rhabdomeres are differentially distorted when exposed to polarized light. Finally, it can be shown that rhodopsin molecules are all aligned parallel to the long axis of the micovilli. It follows that when the plane of polarized light coincides with this axis it will have maximum affect on the rhodopsin molecules. The phototransduction cascade reviewed in Chapter 17 will then ensure that the impulse traffic from the retinula cell will be maximized. The organism can thus detect the plane of maximum polarization.

21.3 ELECTRIC FIELDS

Humans are nowadays surrounded by electric fields. Yet we have no way of knowing their shape, their strength or that they are there at all. This is not the case with a number of other animals. Indeed, the Monotremata, the last representatives of the ancestral mammals, show, at least in the case of the duck-billed platypus, *Ornithorynchus*, and to a lesser extent in the anteater, *Tachyglossus*, well developed electrosensory systems. But the best known instances of electroreception are displayed by a number of fish. Indeed, systems to detect weak electric fields are believed to be evolutionarily very ancient and to have been lost and re-evolved a number of times.

21.3.1 Fish

Electric fish have been known from the times of Egyptian antiquity. A well known scene on the wall of a fifth dynasty (circa 2750 BC) tomb at Sakkara shows a fisherman hauling what is recognizably the electric catfish, *Malopterurus electricus*, from the Nile. The Roman physician Scribonus Largus used *Torpedo* (known as the 'cramp fish') to provide shock therapy for otherwise intractable headache and gout. There are many passages in the literature of Greek and Roman antiquity which tell of the strange numbing power of these fish.

Far from all electric fish produce the fearsome shocks of *Torpedo* and *Malopterurus*. Indeed, most are far gentler. Electric fish are, accordingly, divided into two groups: **strongly electric** and **weakly electric**. Electric rays (*Torpedo*), electric eels (*Electophorus*) and electric catfish (*Malapterurus*) belong to the first group and generate strong discharges (60; 500 and 300 V respectively). Most electric fish belong to the second group, for instance, cartilaginous fish such as skates (e.g. *Raja*), and bony fish belonging to the families Mormyridae and Gymnarchidae (African fresh water fish), Gymnotidae (knife fish) and Sternopygidae (South American fresh water fish), Uranscopidae (marine 'star gazers') and so on. These fish only generate weak discharges, the strongest being that generated by the stargazer *Astroscopus* at about 5 V.

The weak discharge is customarily emitted as a high frequency series of 'pips' from an electric organ in the tail. *Gymnotus*, for instance, emits 1 ms pulses at 50 Hz (when resting) and 200 Hz (when feeding) whilst *Gymnarchus niloticus* emits approximately 1 ms pulses (1 V) at from 200 to 300 Hz.

The biological functions of the strong and weak electrical discharges are quite distinct. The **strong discharges** are used to stun prey, whilst the **weak discharges** are used as a form of electro-echolocation to detect objects in the fish's vicinity, to communicate and perhaps to mark out territory. There is evidence, for instance, that members of both the Gymnotidae and the Mormyridae are able to recognize the electric organ discharges of conspecifics and orientate towards them. We seem to have here, in the repeated evolution of the weak electric sense, an interesting analogy with the bat echolocation discussed in Chapters 9 and 10. Further analysis of piscean electroreception may provide fascinating points of comparison.

Let us turn now to **electrosensitivity**. This is not restricted to electric fish. Indeed, most fish show some ability to detect electric fields in their surroundings. Early experiments made use of the dogfish (*Scyliorhinus canicula*) and skate (*Raja clavata*). They showed that these chondrichthyan fish were well able to detect a flatfish (*Pleuronectes platessa*, the flounder) hidden in the sand at the bottom of a tank (Figure 21.5). After searching randomly, dogfish would pick

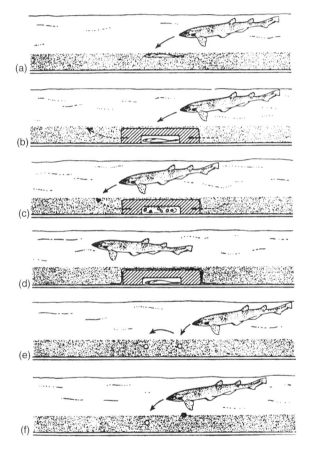

Figure 21.5 Responses of dogfish *Scyliorhinus canicula* towards: (a) flatfish, *Pleuronectes platessa* buried in sand; (b) flatfish in electrically transparent chamber; (c) pieces of whiting in chamber; (d) flatfish in an electrically insulated chamber; (e) electrodes simulating the electric field produced by a flatfish; (f) piece of whiting and an electric field (only one electrode shown). Solid arrows indicate the direction of the shark; dashed arrows the direction of a seawater current. From Kalmijn, A.J. (1971), with permission from The Company of Biologists Ltd.

up clues to the flatfish's position at distances of about 15 cm. and, making well aimed dives, would uncover it from the sand and devour it. To make sure that olfaction was not in play the flounder was enclosed in an electrically-transparent agar chamber. Again the dogfish found and dived at the chamber and nosed away the sand. However, if the flatfish was enclosed in an electrically-opaque chamber the dogfish could no longer detect its presence, and the flounder and its container remained undisturbed. In the next part of the experiment electrodes were embedded in the sand to simulate the flounder's bioelectric field. Again the dogfish dived to find the source of the electric field. It was found that *Scyliorhinus* is most sensitive to fields surrounding dipoles set about 5 cm apart with direct currents of about 0.5 A. Dogfish and skates still responded at almost the same sensitivity when the current was delivered as a sine waveform with frequencies of 1, 2 and 4 Hz. In life, bioelectric fields are generated by ionic currents passing across gill filaments and the epithelium of the gut. Muscular movements also generate bioelectric potentials and hence electric fields. The bioelectric fields generated by wounded tissue are considerably greater. It was found that *Pleuronectes,* resting quietly beneath the sand, generated bioelectric fields measuring, on average, 0.2 μV/cm at 10 cm from the fish. These fields oscillated in magnitude in harmony with the rhythm of the flatfish's respiratory movements.

Chondrichthyan electrosensitivity is extremely acute. It is sufficiently sensitive for them to be able to detect fields as weak as 5 nV/cm. The delicacy of this sensitivity is made more apparent if we translate into a more human scale: it then becomes a gradient of 0.5 V over 1000 km. They are thus well able to detect the 200 nV/cm field at 10 cm from a concealed flatfish. It has, indeed, been argued that this extreme sensitivity is sufficient to allow them not only to find hidden prey but also to detect the tiny electric fields induced either by their own movement and/or by the bulk movement of water in ocean currents through **Earth's magnetic field**. There is some evidence that chondrichthyan fish do, indeed, use the Earth's field to navigate long distances. Migrating blue sharks have been tracked over many days and shown to maintain straight courses over hundreds of kilometers with no other obvious navigation cues. Hammerhead sharks off the Californian coast follow a route which correlates with the magnetic anomalies of the sea bed. However, it must be borne in mind that many fish and marine mammals which do not have acute electrosensitivity also achieve remarkable feats of long distance underwater navigation.

In the case of weakly electric fish, it is not only the electric fields produced by movement through the geomagnetic field and the electric fields generated by other animals which are detected. Their own electric organs produce an electric field that is distorted by nearby objects and this distortion is sensed by the fish's electroreceptor system. Mormyrid fish, for instance, are able to sense the electric capacitance of nearby objects within the range 0.22–1.7 to 120–680 nF. They are able to assess the size, shape, location and electrical impedance of these objects.

The remarkable electrical sensitivity of weakly electric fish and others is due to two main types of receptor: **ampullary** and **tuberous organs** (= knol-

lenorgans) (Figure 21.6). Both types of receptor are modifications of the lateral line system which, as we noted in Chapter 9, is ubiquitous amongst the fish.

Ampullary organs (Figure 21.6a) are groups of sensory cells arranged around a cavity at the bottom of a lengthy jelly-filled canal. The sensory cells in the ampullae are almost completely surrounded by accessory cells. Only the apex of the sensory cell remains free and in contact with the lumen of the ampulla. They show some morphological variation. In cladistians (a very ancient group nowadays represented only by the sturgeons), dipnoan lungfish and some amphibia, a single kinocilium springs from the apex of the cell surrounded by a number of microvilli (cp. hair cells of the lateral line system described in Chapter 9). In the chondrichthyes and holosteans the single kinocilium has no surrounding microvilli. Finally, in lampreys and urodele amphibia each cell

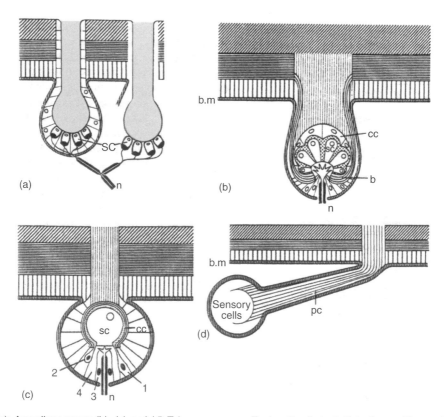

Figure 21.6 (a): Ampullary organ; (b), (c) and (d) Tuberous organs. Explanation in text. Note the multilayered skin. b = basal layer of skin; bm = basal membrane; cc = covering cells; pc = plug cells; n = myelinated nerve fibre; sc = sensory cell. 1, 2, 3, 4 = different types of basal accessory cell. From Szabo, T. (1974) in *Handbook of Sensory Physiology, Vol. III/3* (ed. A. Fessard) with kind permission of Springer Science and Business Media, Berlin.

bears a number of microvilli but no kinocilium. The functional significance of these variations remains unknown. The base of the cell is filled with synaptic vesicles and makes a conventional 'chemical' synapse with the dendritic ending of a sensory nerve fibre. Generally anything up to 12 or 13 ampullae are grouped to form an ampullary organ.

The **ampullae of Lorenzini** form a highly organized pattern of ampullae in chondrichthyan fish including the Chimaeridae (e.g. *Chimaera monstrosa*). The latter have evolved separately from the main group of cartilaginous fish since at least the Jurassic period. The ampullae of Lorenzini have been most intensively studied in the skate (*Raja*) and the dogfish (*Scyliorhinus*). We noted in Chapter 20 that they had first been taken as temperature receptors. The organization of the system in the skate is shown in Figure 21.7. There are several systems of canals on both the dorsal and ventral surface. The canals vary in length. In a medium sized skate (400 mm span) the longest canal measures about 160 mm and is 2 mm in diameter; the smallest is about 5 mm long and 0.5 mm in diameter. The pattern is, moreover, species-specific. The canals end blindly as sensory ampullae. These ampullae (Figure 21.7) are frequently clustered together and surrounded by connective tissue to form well-marked capsules. There is nowadays no doubt that their principal role is to provide dogfish, skate and other chondrichthyan fish with the very acute electrosensitivity, which we discussed above.

The fact that the canals are orientated in many different directions allows the system to determine the gradient of any electric field in the surrounding space. The longer canals are less sensitive to higher frequencies, due to the electrical capacity of the canal walls, but are more sensitive to voltage gradients. The whole system provides the chondrichthyan with a sensitive distance receptor able to detect many features of both the inanimate and animate environment. Its importance is indicated by its rich and extensive nerve supply.

Tuberous organs or **knollenorgans** (Figure 21.6b, c, d) differ from ampullary organs in two significant ways. Firstly, they do not communicate with the exterior by a jelly-filled canal. Instead, this canal is plugged by specialized epithelial cells. Secondly, the sensory cells do not have just one surface, the apical surface, projecting into the sensory cavity but instead are (usually) attached to a small supporting hillock and expose about 90% of their surface to the

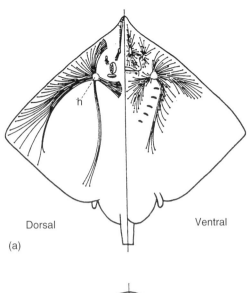

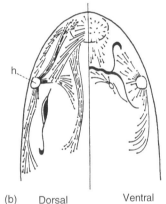

Figure 21.7 Anatomy of the ampullae of Lorenzini. (a): Dorsal and ventral views of the canal system in *Raja clavata*. The canal openings are shown as dots and the capsules as open circles (b): Dorsal and ventral views of *Scyliorhinus canicula*. h = hyoid capsule. Explanation in text. From Murray, R.W. (1974) in *Handbook of Sensory Physiology, Vol. III/3* (ed. A. Fessard) with kind permission of Springer Science and Business Media, Berlin.

cavity. The sensory cells of gymnotids are somewhat elongated compared to the more spherical shape of those found in the mormyrids. The sensory cells of tuberous organs develop no kinocilia but instead their surfaces are thrown out into a large number of microvilli. These microvilli project into the sensory cavity. The basal part of the sensory cell is filled with synaptic vesicles. The number of sensory cells making up a tuberous organ varies widely, ranging between 1 and 35 in mormyrids to between 10 and

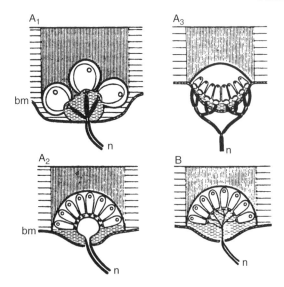

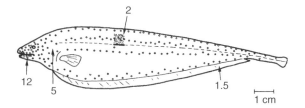

Figure 21.8 Type 1 (A$_1$, A$_2$, A$_3$) and type 2 (B) tuberous organs. bm = basement membrane; n = nerve. Explanation in text. From Szabo, T. (1974) in *Handbook of Sensory Physiology, Vol. III/3* (ed. A. Fessard) with kind permission of Springer Science and Business Media, Berlin.

Figure 21.9 Distribution of electroreceptors in *Stenarchus*, a gymnotid fish. The ampullary receptors are represented by dots. The far more numerous tuberous receptors are shown only in a small patch on the mid-dorsal region. The density of the latter receptors per mm^2 is, however, indicated by numbered arrows. The dashed line indicates the position of the posterior lateral line. From Bennett, M.V.L. (1971) with permission from Academic Press.

100 in gymnotids. In the mormyrids, furthermore, each cell is located in its own cavity whilst in the gymnotids all the sensory cells occupy a single cavity. Finally, tuberous organs are often divided into two types differentiated by their innervation (Figure 21.8). Type 1 is innervated by myelinated branches of a single sensory fibre. In type 2 the myelin sheath does not persist into the tuberous organ and the sensory cells are consequently innervated by unmyelinated branches of the afferent nerve.

The two classes of electroreceptor have different response characteristics. Afferent fibres from ampullary sensory cells give 'tonic' responses. In other words, they give **long lasting, sustained responses to low frequency** (<0.1 to 10–25 Hz) or DC stimuli. Ampullary organs also have a wide range of sensitivities with thresholds ranging from <20 nV/cm to 10–100 μV/cm. In contrast, the tuberous organs are sensitive to **high frequencies** and insensitive to low frequencies and DC. Sensory fibres from the latter receptors respond in a 'phasic' manner, giving a **short burst of activity** to step changes in the stimulating voltage. Both tonic (ampullary) and phasic (tuberous organ) receptors are present in both gymnotids and mormyrids. Their similarity is striking, as they are believed to have evolved independently in these

two groups of freshwater fish. Tuberous organs are absent in nonelectric and marine fish.

The distribution of electroreceptors on a typical freshwater gymnotid is shown in Figure 21.9. The phasic receptors (tuberous) are much more numerous than the tonic receptors and are only found on a small region. Their density (per mm^2) is, indicated numerically at different points on the body. The tonic receptors (ampullary) are shown by diamonds. It is to be noted that both tonic and phasic receptors reach maximum density in the head region. Both sets of receptors are innervated by the large anterior branch of the lateral line nerve (in this case a branch of cranial VIII).

The detection of the form of an electric field in the surrounding water depends on the orientation of the fish. The electrical resistance within the body is considerably less than in the external medium. If the fish is orientated along a potential gradient, current will enter at one end (say the head) and leave at the other (the tail). The individual electroreceptors are stimulated by differences between the internal and external electrical potential. These differences will be greatest at the head and tail where current enters and leaves the animal. Unlike the chondrichthyans, with their highly organized Lorenzini system, these mormyrid and gymnotid freshwater fish use their whole bodies as electro-sense organs.

21.3.2 Monotremata

Let us turn, finally, from fish to the *Monotremata (Prototheria)*. Some 30 000 to 40 000 mucus-filled pits, which have turned out to be electroreceptors, are found in the upper and lower bill of the duck-billed platypus (*Ornithorynchus anatinus*). A much smaller number, about 100, are present on the snout of the spiny anteater (*Tachyglossus aculeatus*). Behavioural experiments rather similar to those carried out with fish, as described above, show that the platypus senses electrical fields when diving in tanks of water. This helps explain how, with their poor eyesight and, moreover, closing those eyes and their nostrils when diving to the bottom of murky streams, they can nevertheless catch half their body weight of live prey in a single night. The behavioural significance of the electroreceptors in the snout of *Tachyglossus* is less obvious. Perhaps they help the animal detect minute electrical signals from the muscles of their prey as they forage in damp earth.

Histological investigation of the platypus bill has shown that the electroreceptors consist of some thirty large afferent fibres forming a 'cuff' surrounding the bottom of each mucous pit (Figure 21.10). Unlike fish electoreceptors there are no receptor cells. The dendritic endings of the afferent fibres contain the ion channels necessary for sensory transduction. Electrophysiological investigation has shown that these afferent fibres carry an inherent impulse traffic of some 30–40 impulses/s. This impulse rate is modulated by ambient electrical signals, upwards in response to a cathodal pulse and downwards in response to an anodal pulse. Experiments have also shown that the sensitivity to sinusoidal voltage stimuli is greater from 50 to 100 Hz than at lower frequencies. It is interesting to note that the tail flip of

a shrimp, a favourite prey animal, has a frequency of about 140 Hz, close to the optimal sensitivity of the platypus electoreceptor system. It should be noted, however, that the platypus bill also contains mechanoreceptors known as '**push-rods**'. There is evidence to show that these have evolved to detect pressure changes in water rather than direct mechanical touch on the skin. It may be, therefore, that these receptors are involved in detecting pressure waves in the water made by the shrimp's tail. If this is the case it is plausible to suppose that the electoreceptors and the 'push-rod' mechanoreceptors work in tandem to detect buried prey.

In support of this hypothesis, cytochrome oxidase (CO) staining of the region of the cortex in which mechanoreceptive and electroreceptive afferents terminate reveals a well organized structure reminiscent of the stripe-like ocular dominance organization of the primate visual cortex. It has been found that cells in cortical layer three of this area receive input from both electrosensitive and mechanosensitive afferents. It is thus proposed that these cells could be detecting the time delay between the arrival of the electrical signal and the mechanical signal at the platypus bill, thus giving the animal an indication of the distance of the source of the underwater disturbance – in the case of hunting, the movement of the prey animal. This has obvious similarities with the mechanism believed to underlie distance perception in mammalian stereoscopic vision. When combined with directional information provided by the sweeping, so-called 'sacchadic', movements of the

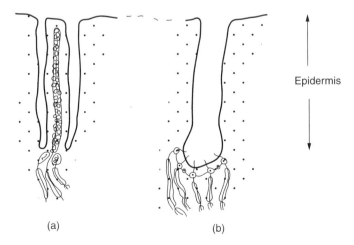

Epidermis

(a)   (b)

Figure 21.10 Platypus push-rod mechanoreceptor and mucous pit electroreceptor. (a) Push-rod mechanoreceptor. A column of epidermal cells forms the push-rod. The column is about 400 μm in length and 70 μm in diameter. Three types of mechanoreceptors are attached to the column: vesicle chain receptors within the column and Merkel cells and Paciniform corpuscles at its base. (b) Mucous pit electroreceptor. The pit is about 600 μm deep and about 150 μm in diameter. At its base a 'cuff' of some 16 sensory nerve endings penetrate into the mucus. Adapted from Manger, P.R., Collins, R. and Pettigrew, J.D. (1997) and Pettigrew, J.D., Manger, P.R. and Fine, L.B. (1998).

bill, the platypus may be provided with an excellent three-dimensional 'fix' on its prey and thus succeed in catching, as noted above, half its body weight of food in a single night's hunting.

Little is known of the biophysics of the electroreceptors. It appears that detection of electrical stimuli is achieved directly by the bare nerve endings of the afferents. It has been suggested that the mucus in the pits provides a low-resistance pathway from the skin surface to the nerve endings. These endings were shown to be slowly adapting. In response to a stepped cathodal stimulus the fibres quickly reach an initial peak discharge and then adapt to a slower maintained rate. In contrast, a stepped anodal stimulation silences any the activity in the fibre, the discharge only reappearing with a burst at the end of the stimulus.

The electroreceptors in *Tachyglossus* are rather similar to those described for the platypus (Figure 21.10). Their electrophysiology shows one important difference: there is no background activity and their function as electroreceptors only became apparent when voltage pulses were directly applied to the skin. As noted above, the behavioural significance of electroreception for *Tachyglossus* (if any) is far less obvious than it is for *Ornithorhyhnchus* but behavioural experiments involving conditioning to weak electric fields leave no doubt that the anteater can and does detect and respond to such fields. It has been suggested that the reason why the echidna has such a perpetually runny nose is to maintain a low-resistance pathway between its snout electroreceptors and the damp soil in which it finds its prey. Perhaps the anteater uses the electric sense as a form of 'distant touch' and switches to the 'pushrod' mechanoreceptors, which it also develops in its snout, for the final attack.

21.4 MAGNETIC FIELDS

Although many organisms have been suspected of being able to sense the Earth's magnetic field, it is only in the microbiological realm that firm evidence of such an ability is available. Magnetotactic bacteria were discovered in the 1970s. They are aquatic, flagellate, Gram-negative forms which all possess intracellular iron granules visible at the electron microscope level. These minute iron granules –

magnetosomes – consist of the magnetic iron oxide, Fe_2O_4 or 'magnetite', and, in *Aquaspirillum magnetotaticum*, are cuboidal with an edge measuring about 42 nm. This is within the single magnetic domain size for magnetite (40–100 nm). These magnetite granules form chains of up to twenty units within the bacterium (Figure 21.11).

The magnetite inclusions act as a 'ferromagnetic geomagnetic biocompass'. They enable the bacterium to swim along magnetic lines of force. In the northern hemisphere these lines of force are directed downwards and the magnetotactic bacteria consequently swim downwards. It is an easy matter to reverse their direction by applying external magnetic fields. In the southern hemisphere the geomagnetic field is directed upwards. Magnetotactic bacteria native to those parts reverse their direction of swimming and thus still swim downwards along the lines of force. At the geomagnetic equator approximately equal numbers of upward and downward swimmers are found.

There has been much speculation about the existence or otherwise of a magnetic sense in eukaryocytes and especially metazoa. We noted above, when discussing electroreception, that the extremely acute electrosensitivity of chondrichthyan fish may help them align themselves in the geomagnetic field by detecting induced currents as they move through that field. As we saw, this may be made use of in the long distance navigation of these fish. Possible **magnetoreceptors** containing magnetite crystals have been found in the olfactory lamellae of the rainbow trout, *Oncorhynchus mykiss*. These candidate magnetoreceptors are closely associated with terminations of the superficial ophthalmic branch of the trigeminal nerve. Behavioural responses show that this species can detect magnetic fields. How widespread magnetic sensitivity is amongst the bony fish is at present unknown.

However, the most well known and most highly developed feats of long distance navigation are undoubtedly those found in a number of birds. Many experiments with **homing pigeons**, for instance, show remarkable navigational abilities. Pigeons wearing opaque contact lenses return to within 0.5–2 km of their loft. Pigeons transported to a release site under general anaesthesia show initial orientation and homing performance indistinguishable from control birds. Other birds, of course, migrate great

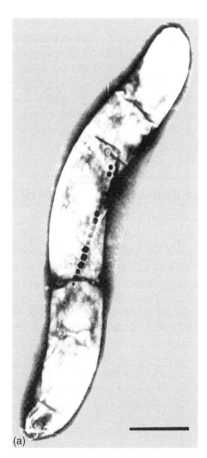 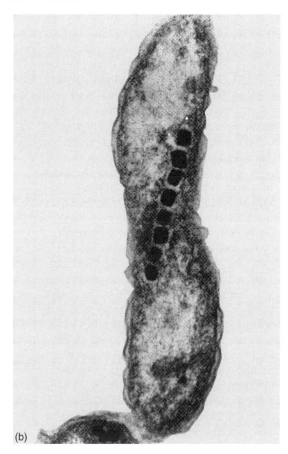

Figure 21.11 Magnetosomes in the Gram-negative bacterium *Aquaspirillum magnetotacticum*. The scale bar measures 0.5 µm. (a) Electron micrograph of a negatively stained bacterium. (b) Electron micrograph of a thin sectioned bacterium. In both cases the magnetosomes show as black particles. In (b) the cuboidal shape is well shown and at the bottom of that electron micrograph another bacterium appears cut in transverse section. This section shows that the magnetosomes are closely adposed to the cell membrane. From Blakemore, R.P. (1982) with permission from Annual Reviews.

distances, often flying night and day. Do they use magnetic clues? Do they navigate by the Earth's magnetic field? If so, it has been extremely difficult to find the sense organ. In recent years, however, some progress has been made. There is evidence that two systems may be involved: a magnetite-based system and a biochemical system using free radicals.

It has been found that the sensory terminals of the trigeminal nerves in the upper beaks of homing pigeons (*Columbia livia*) contain **magnetite** crystals. These crystals, about 5 µm in diameter, occur in clusters in close association with the nerve cell membrane. In addition to the magnetite crystals, non-

crystalline platelets of iron phosphate (about 500 nm long and 100 nm thick) are also present, located in the fibrous cores of the nerve terminals. It is argued that these inclusions could move in response to small changes in the geomagnetic field and this movement could be detected by mechanoreceptors in the terminal's membrane.

The second system accounts for the observation that some migratory birds are influenced by the availability of **light** at specific wavelengths. In the case of European robins (*Erithacus rubcula*) these wavelengths peak at 565 and 617 nm. The birds appear to be completely disorientated under light of 575.5 nm. The influence of light, moreover, appears to be strongly lateralized. Covering up the right eye, but not the left, of migratory birds totally destroys their navigational abilities. How can these observations be explained?

There is evidence to show that photopigments other than the opsins discussed in Part Four are present in the retinae of birds. It is proposed that these '**cryptochromes**', which are present in high concentration in the ganglion cell layer, and which include the photopigment flavin dehydrogenase (FAD) which absorbs light in the blue-green part of the spectrum, are involved. When light interacts with a flavochrome such as FAD, an electron is transferred to a nearby molecule, thus creating a pair of molecules with unpaired electrons. This so-called 'radical pair' is highly reactive and quickly leads to other biochemical changes. It has been found, however, that magnetic fields can influence the speed with which radical pairs are formed. It is possible, therefore, if a sufficient number of cryptochromes are aligned in a constant orientation with respect to the bird's head, that a mechanism for harnessing the strength of a magnetic field to radical pair formation could exist.

It is clear that much work still needs to be done to establish the mechanism, or even the reality, of magnetic navigation in migratory and homing birds. The evidence is conflicting, but there does seem some reason to believe that one or other, or perhaps both, of the mechanisms described above is operative. It is, perhaps, instructive to remember the quite recent discovery of a new pigment – melanopsin – in a small subsection of mammalian retinal ganglion cells (Section 17.2.7). There may well be equal surprises waiting in the avian retina.

Finally, there have been persistent reports of the influence of magnetic fields on the **pineal gland**. These reports do not refer to the avian pineal – indeed magnetic fields appear to have no effect on bird pineals – but to the metabolism of mammalian (including human) pineals. It appears that the circadian rhythms which control the production of melatonin are perturbed. While there does indeed seem to be an effect on this important body the precise means by which this effect is secured and its biological significance (if any) remains shrouded in mystery.

21.5 CONCLUDING REMARKS

We are once again impressed, as we have been in previous chapters of this book, with the different, sometimes radically different, sensory worlds which many animals know. The proverbial five senses which Aristotle defined more than two and a half millennia ago – touch, taste, smell, hearing and sight – with their radically different qualia are only a subsection of the great variety of senses evolved in the animal kingdom. In previous chapters we noted that our sensory biases, especially that toward vision, merely reflect our evolutionary past. Evolution has ensured that the sensory input of other animals is differently biased. In this chapter we have seen that the sensory systems of some of these other animals tells of happenings in the environment of which we have no inkling. This is salutary. It reminds us that there are other perspectives than our own. It reminds us of what Charles Darwin called our 'arrogance'. The sensory world that we inhabit, to which we are so accustomed, that we find so fascinating, so beautiful and so terrible, is, precisely, a human world. The sensory world of other animals is often very different.

22

PAIN

Definitions of pain: Aristotle - the 'existential' sense - inescapable - difficulty of assessing quantity and quality - lack of a 'dolorimeter' - influence of circumstance and culture - the problem of animal pain. **Biological significance**: prevention and cure of tissue damage - the perils of congenital analgesia - the problem of chronic pain - intractactable back pain - theological perplexities - biological answers - but not simple answers - phantom limbs - analgesia in battle and other emergencies - mismatching of afferent and efferent copies? **Neurophysiology**: Nociceptor fibress - nociceptive fibres - high threshold Aδ and C fibres - two types of mechano-heat Aδ (AMH) nociceptors - mechano-heat C (CMH) nociceptors - stimulus transduction - primary and secondary hyperalgesia; nociceptor ion channels. **Central pathways**: dematomes –laminar structure of spinal cord grey matter – horseradish peroxidase histology and fibre tracing – ascending pathways in white matter (STT,SRT,SMT) - Lissauer's tract - cerebral cortex - descending pathways - stimulus produced analgesia (SPA) - significance of periaqueductal grey (PAG) matter. **Neuropharmacology**: endogenous opioids - types and locations of opioid receptors in CNS - synaptology and pharmacology of nociceptor pathways in dorsal horn. **Referred pain**: angina pectoris - symptoms - dermatomes - back pain - trigger points and acupuncture. **Gate theory**: simplified wiring diagram - mechanism - downward projections - therapeutic devices. **Concluding remarks**: the dilemmas of pain in biomedical research - the luck of living in the 21st century - the experience of pain not 'raw' but very expertly and secretly 'cooked'.

Aristotle characterized pain as an unpleasant sensation. That definition has cascaded down the centuries and it (or close versions of it) can still be found in the textbooks of today. Yet it is either palpably wrong or simply vacuous. We are all open to unpleasant sensations which would hardly be classified as pain. Consider the feeling in the 'pit of the stomach' as we wait in the dentist's antechamber before going for a check-up; the sensation many of us determinedly non-mountaineers feel when glimpsing a vertiginous descent from the top of a cliff or building; or the sudden recognition that the spoonful we had just deposited in the mouth was not the delicious concoction we had thought but our least favourite comestible. All of these are undoubtedly unpleasant sensations but few would list them as pain. If, on the other hand, all unpleasant sensations are defined as pain then Aristotle's definition is circular, a mere

Biology of Sensory Systems, Second Edition   C.U.M. Smith
© 2008 John Wiley & Sons, Ltd

tautology and hence simply vacuous. – What is pain: an unpleasant sensation? What is an unpleasant sensation: pain?

Nevertheless, Aristotle was one of the greatest minds and arguably one of the greatest biologists that the world has seen. Although his definition of pain seems absurd, we should treat it with all seriousness. For 'pain' is, indeed, difficult to define. It is difficult to define precisely because it is intensely private. Some have called it the '**existential**' **sense** because there is no way (bar medication) of switching it off. We cannot walk away and leave it behind, as we might a road-mender's pneumatic drill. Just as it is impossible (according to Augustine and Descartes) to doubt whilst doubting that doubting exists ('I think, therefore I am'), so it is impossible to doubt, whilst in pain, that pain exists. We can doubt the other senses: we are all subject to visual, auditory and (though to a lesser extent) olfactory illusions; the world they report may be other than it seems. But we cannot doubt that we are feeling pain when we are in pain. As with the other senses, we are often misled as to the cause of that 'unpleasant feeling'. Yet we cannot escape from it by closing our eyes, stopping our ears or holding a posy to our nose.

We shall return to these rather more philosophical issues in Chapter 24 but it is appropriate to point out here that the essentially private nature of pain makes it very difficult to describe or quantify. Physicians often distinguish between sharp, pricking pains and more continuous dull aches. But this is a very crude, rough and ready distinction. Melzack has developed a detailed questionnaire (the McGill questionnaire) which asks sufferers to describe the quality of their pain by way of a number of different headings: throbbing, shooting, pounding, gnawing, cramping, crushing, lacerating, nauseating and so on. But the list can only be metaphorical and is unlikely to cover all varieties of pain sensation. Surgical interference with the trigeminal nerve, for instance, leaves about 5% of the patients with an odd, unpleasant, yet indescribable sensation which they would far rather be without. Patrick Wall, who has contributed greatly to the study of pain, points out that we totally lack an instrument, a **dolorimeter**, which can measure and quantify pain. Not only is it the quality of another's pain that we cannot know, but we can never be sure of its intensity, its quantity. The relationship between feeling and reporting pain is highly context dependent. There is good reason to believe that both quality and quantity are strongly influenced by external circumstances, including custom and practice and what is and is not expected in different cultures. Soldiers stretchered from the field of battle with severe wounds often initially make few complaints, although responding vigorously to seemingly minor irritations such as inept attempts at injection; civilians with similarly severe injuries are far more likely to demand anaesthetics. Likewise the initiation ceremonies and other practices recorded by anthropologists frequently involve what seem to us extremely painful procedures, yet the subjects, in a state of high ceremonial excitement, appear to feel little or no pain.

If we cannot quantify or do more than guess at the quality of another human being's pain how can we hope to guess at its nature in other animals? Our best approach is to err on the side of caution. We saw above that pain is in some sense an existential sense. We saw that like other sensory qualia – 'redness', or an auditory tone – we cannot doubt that we have it, though we may be permitted to doubt its cause. Similarly, with the rest of the animal world or at the least the higher members of that world, just as we cannot doubt that they 'see' and 'hear', so we cannot doubt that they experience pain. It must be left to the judgment of huntsmen and fishermen and grouse shooters to balance the possibility of pain with the multitude of other factors involved in their avocations. Not least amongst these factors lies the recognition that the world of nature is premised on mortality.

22.1 THE BIOLOGICAL SIGNIFICANCE OF PAIN

At the anatomical and physiological level, pain signals **tissue damage**. It signals the necessity of a period of rest and withdrawal so that healing has a chance to take over. It warns against further hazarding of the injured member. It is wired into the conditioned reflex systems of the body so that having once put one's hand into the bright glittering flickering element, we do not do so again. Steering well clear of the fire, we enhance our chances of long and productive life. Some unfortunates are born lacking a sense of pain. The condition is known as **congenital analgesia**. The defect seems to be central rather than peripheral, for they are quite able, amongst other things, to discriminate touch with a pin's head from pricking with its other end. Some might think these unfortunates fortunate. This, however, is very definitely not the case, for congenital analgesiacs only learn with great difficulty to avoid injury. A particular problem is inflammation of the joints through a failure to shift the body's weight when standing, sitting or even when lying in bed asleep. Indeed, Wall reports the case of a young woman analgesiac where joint inflammation ultimately led to such massive infection of the bone that medical science could not save her life. The body's nociceptive system is its internal safety mechanism.

But, it might be objected, how should we account for chronic, life diminishing, pain? The pain caused by disease, the heart conditions, ulcerations and the various forms of cancer must have been terrible before the advent of modern medicine. In many cases, even today, chronic pain has no discoverable cause. Figures from the United States suggest that more than two million citizens are incapacitated with pain at any given time. Much of this is long term and untreatable. Back pain alone provides an immense reservoir of discomfort. It has been estimated that some 60% of the British/American population spends more than a week at home during their working lives due to this cause alone. The annual compensation in the United States reaches some $50 billion per annum and 85% are left with no definite diagnosis. Chronic, intractable pain is an immense human and economic problem. But this huge and largely invisible sea of pain points towards the answer to our question. The nociceptive system is so crucial to the evolutionary struggle to survive and leave offspring that it outweighs the downside of sometimes generating apparently pointless and debilitating discomfort. Theologians are often asked to account for the existence of pain and suffering in the world. For the evolutionary biologist the answer is, if not simple, at least imaginable.

That the answer is not simple is shown by numerous examples. The straightforward equation between tissue damage and pain often does not hold. The chronic back pain mentioned above can seldom be traced to any discoverable tissue damage. In cases where wounding has occurred, it is common, moreover, for pain, often severe pain, to persist after the damage has healed. This is perhaps best known in

the case of phantom limbs. Years after the injury has apparently healed, the patient may be subject to excruciating pain from parts of the missing limb. There are, furthermore, well authenticated instances of acute pain persisting in a phantom limb when all (peripheral) connections to that limb have been severed. This sometimes occurs in victims of accidents in which the spine is severed. After recovery the patient has lost all sensation and movement in the body and limbs below the point of fracture. Yet in some tragic cases agonizing pain persists from these lost regions. Even after surgical procedures to remove the pain pathways (see below) in the spinal cord above the fracture plane, the cramps and burning sensations remain. These patients provide a searching test of any theory which suggests that pain is only, or even mainly, caused by messages from the site of tissue damage. Perhaps the brain sends an 'efference copy' (Section 16.4) which cannot be matched by the defective sensory return. This proposal finds support in the still controversial but nevertheless ingenious experiments with mirrors which give the patient the visual illusion that the lost region is, after all, still present. In these experiments the pain from the phantom is sometimes greatly reduced. A further searching test is provided by a far less tragic circumstance. If a local anaesthetic is injected into the brachial plexus (the rope of nerves from the arm entering the spinal cord at the level of the shoulder) the subject feels the arm to be painfully swollen and in a definite and often impossible place (perhaps bent up inside the thorax) and this illusion can only occasionally be dispelled by seeing it or palpating it in the correct position. In this case it is not the tattoo of impulses arriving from the periphery but the **absence** of such a tattoo which 'grabs the attention' of the central nervous system (CNS).

Vice versa, pain is frequently not felt when tissue damage is extensive. Soldiers in the heat of action often fail to notice quite severe wounds. Only later, when the battle has been lost or won and there is nothing further to do, does the pain begin. The famous instance of Dr Livingstone and the Lion makes the same point. Dr Livingstone recounts how in darkest Africa a lion leapt from the jungle on to his back. He recalls hearing its dreadful roar close to his ear and looking down at its jaws and powerful claws rasping his body before his rescuers freed him. But, he says, it all seemed to happen in a dream, he felt no pain, no terror. Dr Livingstone was in no doubt that all this proved the beneficence of the Deity who would not permit the war of Nature to cause so vast a pit of pain and suffering. Evolutionists would suggest a different, though complementary, explanation. The organism 'concentrates' on one task at a time; languishing in the Lion's jaw or flinching during the clash of arms in warfare is not an adaptive behaviour: the moment of crisis is no moment for the organism to concern itself with the repair of tissue damage. There are more urgent considerations. The pain-induced quiescence required for healing can come later.

22.2 NEUROPHYSIOLOGY OF PAIN

Enough has now been said of the counter-intuitive character of pain, of its complexity, of its dependence on cultural context, personality type, life threatening or other circumstance, holistic implications and so on. In spite of this vast congeries of higher processing, it is nonetheless possible (and essential) to gain some straightforward understanding of the neurophysiology of the pain receptors and pathways at the periphery and in the spinal cord. It is to this understanding that we now turn.

22.2.1 Nociceptor Fibres

For many years it was not clear whether pain was due to activation of specific fibres or to the overactivity of sensory fibres normally devoted to other sensory modalities. The latter view seems to coincide with our common experience. With the possible exception of olfaction, any excessive sensory stimulus – a blinding light, an ear-splitting sound, a heavy knock, heat or cold beyond the normal range – is experienced as painful. Both Erasmus Darwin, in the late eighteenth century, and William James, in the late nineteenth century, expounded this commonsense view. However, commonsense here, as elsewhere, has been found wanting. There is nowadays little doubt that in most cases pain sensations are due to the activation of dedicated nerve fibres – the **nociceptive fibres**.

Nociceptive fibres have no specialized endings. They exist as free nerve fibres in the dermis of the skin and elsewhere. Histologically they are indistinguishable from C mechanoreceptors (Chapter 8) and the C and Aδ thermoreceptors (Chapter 20). They differ from these receptors in that the thresholds for their adequate stimuli are beyond the normal range. They can be divided into several different types on the criterion of which sensory modality provides their adequate stimulus. Painful thermal and mechanical stimuli are detected by small diameter myelinated fibres. Reference to Table 2.2 shows that these are classified as Aδ fibres. Polymodal fibres, which respond to a wide variety of high intensity stimulus modalities, are again of small diameter but in this case are unmyelinated. Table 2.2 shows that these are classified as C-fibres. The Aδ fibres conduct impulses at from 5 to 30 m/s and are responsible for 'fast pain', the sharp, pricking, sensations; the C fibres conduct more slowly, from 0.5 to 2 m/s and signal 'slow pain', which is often prolonged and may merge into dull aches.

The **Aδ-fibre mechano-heat nociceptors (AMHs)** are divided into two types. Type 1 AMHs are mostly found in the glabrous skin. Although some have thresholds below 50 °C, most respond to temperatures of 53 °C or greater. They have high conduction velocities ranging from 30 to 50 m/s and thus extend from the top of the Aδ range into the Aβ category. The type 1 AMHs are initially somewhat unresponsive to a 53 °C stimulus but after two or three seconds respond vigorously (Figure 22.1b). Type 2 AMHs are found in nonglabrous skin. Their temperature thresholds and conduction velocities (about 15 m/s) are significantly lower but they respond more rapidly to the onset of high temperature. As can be seen in Figure 22.1b they (unlike the AMHs) are rapidly adapting fibres. Finally, the **C fibre nociceptors (CMHs)** have heat thresholds in the range 38 to 50 °C and respond with a sustained activity, the frequency being related to the intensity of stimulus (Figure 22.1a).

AMHs and CMHs, as their names indicate, respond to both thermal and mechanical stimuli. Nevertheless, the physiological situation is far from simple. The transduction mechanisms for the two modalities appear to be different. Application of **capsaicin** does not affect sensitivity to mechanical stimuli but inhibits response to heat. Furthermore, whilst capsaicin has an analgesic affect on the heat and chemical sensitivity of polymodal C fibres in the cornea it, again, does not affect their mechanosensitivity. Finally, it has been found that

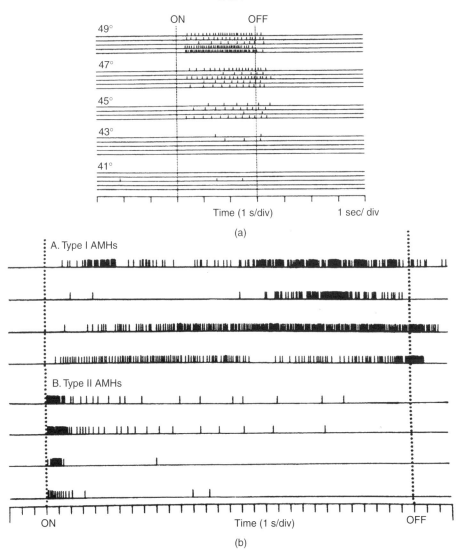

Figure 22.1 (a) Response of a typical C nociceptive fibre to heat. Heat stimuli ranging between 41 and 49 °C were applied for 3 s with 25 s interstimulus intervals to the glabrous skin of a monkey's hand. Within these constraints the stimuli were randomized. (b) Responses of four type 1 and four type 2 AMHs to a heat stimulus of 53 °C (30 s). Note that type 1 AMHs have slow response time leading to a peak discharge towards the end of the stimulus. In contrast, type 2 AMHs respond quickly and quickly adapt to a low level of activity. Type 1 AMHs play an important part in hyperalgesia to heat whilst type 2 AMHs signal the initial pain sensation. From Wall, P.D. and Melzack, R. (eds) (1994) *Textbook of Pain, 3rd edn*, Copyright © 1994, Churchill Livingstone.

mechanical stimuli which generate the same level of activity in CMH fibres as thermal stimuli evoke less pain. Perhaps the necessarily less punctate nature of the thermal stimulus recruits activity in more CMH fibres than is the case in response to the mechanical stimulus.

The physiological situation is not simple on other counts also. The peripheral mechanisms are highly dynamic. After a wound, as we all know, the surrounding tissue becomes 'tender' or, to use the technicality, **hyperalgesic**. Hyperalgesia is defined as a leftward shift of the stimulus response curve. It

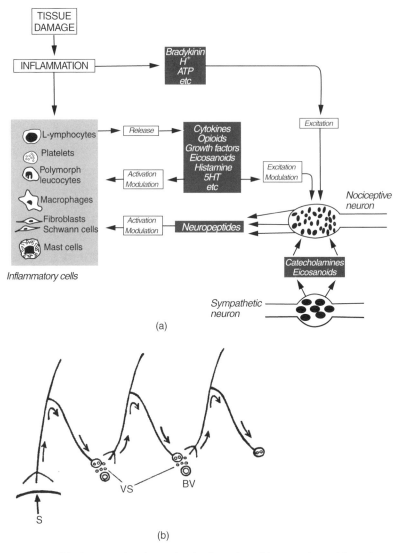

Figure 22.2 (a) Factors responsible for secondary hyperalgesia. A number of factors released from damaged tissue act directly on nociceptors or may release other factors from inflammatory cells and sympathetic neurons. (b) A chemical cascade between C fibre endings serves to enhance the stimulus and underlies the spread of 'flare'. BV = blood vessel; S = stimulus; VS = vasoactive substances. From Wall, P.D. and Melzack, R. (eds) (1994) *Textbook of Pain, 3rd edn*, Copyright © 1994, Churchill Livingstone.

occurs not only in the site of injury (primary hyperalgesia) but also in the surrounding tissue (secondary hyperalgesia). The mechanisms responsible for primary and secondary hyperalgesia differ. **Primary hyperalgesia** is shown by all nociceptive nerve endings. In general, it is due to sensitization of the nerve endings and also to expansions of their receptive fields. **Secondary hyperalgesia** is not shown

to thermal stimuli but only to mechanical and other nociceptive stimuli. It is due to a complex cocktail of biochemicals released partly from the nociceptive nerve ending and partly from the damaged tissue (Figure 22.2a).

The intricate pathways by which the biochemicals released in tissue damage act on nociceptive terminals are shown in Figure 22.2a. The **inflammatory**

process releases ATP from damaged cells and this, as we shall see below, binds to P2X3 receptors on nociceptive nerve terminals. K^+, bradykinin (a 9-residue peptide), prostaglandins and leukotrienes (both derived from the breakdown of membrane phospholipids), histamine, 5HT and so on are also released from injured cells. All of these biochemicals either excite or lower the threshold of nociceptive endings. Damaged nociceptive endings themselves release neuropeptides (for instance substance P (SP)) which activate inflammatory cells to release further quantities of histamine, bradykinin, ATP and so on. There is some evidence, also, that intact polymodal C fibres release vasoactive substances which contribute to the vasodilation responsible for the 'flare' surrounding damaged tissue. This release is probably caused by local 'axon reflexes'. Activation of a nociceptor ending leads to action potentials antidromically invading an adjacent branch (Figure 22.2b). Finally, damaged sympathetic fibres release catecholamines and other substances that excite nociceptive fibres. It can be seen that a spreading region around the site of injury will be awash with agents tending to lower the threshold or actually excite nociceptive fibres. It is no wonder that there is a perceived and persistent tenderness (secondary hyperalgesia) around an injury.

22.2.2 Nociceptor Ion Channels

The multimodal nature of the peripheral pain pathways implies that a number of different receptors must be present on the nociceptor fibre endings. It

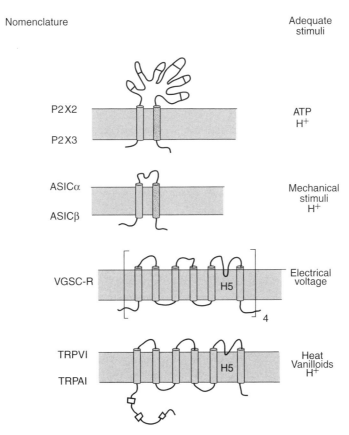

Figure 22.3 Subunits of nociceptor channels. Note large extracellular glycosylated loop in P2X channels. This contains an ATP-binding site. The black bars indicate disulfide linkages. The pore lining helices of both the P2X and ASIC channel proteins are stippled; the H5 'hairpin' lines the pore in the VGSC-R and TRP channels. Further explanation in text.

turns out that these receptors take the form of ion channels belonging to four major subtypes responsive, respectively, to ATP, mechanical, electrical and thermal stimuli (Figure 22.3).

There are two types of ATP or purinoceptors: **P2X** and **P2Y**. The first type is ionotropic, the second metabotropic. Only the first type, the ionotropic P2X receptors, are found in nociceptor fibres. The subunits of the P2X receptors make two passes through the membrane (Figure 22.3) and are believed to assemble into triplets surrounding a channel lined by the M2 helices. There are at least seven different types of **P2X receptor** and only two of these are found in nociceptive endings: P2X2 and P2X3. P2X3 is expressed preferentially in small to medium diameter sensory neurons. They are believed to be involved in chronic pain mentioned in Section 22.1.

Painful mechanical stimuli are sensed by **acid-sensing ion channels (ASICs)** where, again, the subunit consists of a polypeptide making two passes through the membrane. It has recently been shown that, like the P2X channels, three subunits come together to form the channel, with M2 helices lining the pore. Although ASICs have a similar structure to the P2X family of receptors, they have little or no sequence similarity. Indeed, they are members of the degenerin family of channel proteins, which are well known in nematodes, sea urchins and flies (Section 8.1). Unlike the degenerin channels of nematodes, the ASIC channels open to extracellular H^+ ions. These ions are, as Figure 22.2. shows, are by-products of the inflammatory process. ASICs probably work together with the P2X3 receptors in signalling chronic pain.

Electrical pain is sensed by various subtypes of the **Na^+-voltage-gated channels (VGSCs)**. Whilst the VGSCs involved in action potentials are inhibited by tetrodotoxin and are hence called voltage-gated sensitive channels (VGSC-S), some of the VGSCs expressed in small to medium sensory fibres are resistant to this toxin and are thus known as VGSC-Rs. There is evidence to show that the VGSC-R channels are those responsible for the pain associated with electrical stimuli.

Finally, heat is sensed, as we noted in Chapter 20, by **TRPV channels**. The active moiety in **capsaicin**, the chemical which makes hot peppers 'burn', is a vanilloid group and this specifically activates TRPV1 cation channels. These are to be found in small to medium diameter nociceptor fibres. Many investigators have found a good correlation between capsaicin and thermal responsiveness in cultured sensory neurons. In addition to TRPV1 channels, mouse thermosensory neurons also express TRPV2 channels which, as we noted in Chapter 20, open at temperatures above 52 °C. It is likely, moreover, that TRPV channels are not the only type of ion channel affected by painfully high temperatures in nociceptive terminals. Uncomfortably cold temperatures are sensed by TRPM8 and TRPA channels. This array of nociceptive channels is summed up in the form of a diagram in Figure 22.4.

22.2.3 Molecular Biology

Is it possible to make use of this molecular knowledge to devise new and more effective ways of managing pain? There are at least two promising approaches: first through an understanding of the precise molecular biology of the P2X3 receptors and second, through work on the genetics of the TRPV channel.

Like the other nociceptors the P2X3 receptors have an immense back history. Some of the most ancient forms of this receptor are found in the social amoeba (= slime mould) *Dictyostelium discoideum*. When this receptor was isolated, analysed and sequenced, it was found to have only a 10% similarity to that expressed in humans. Despite this, the receptor shared essential functions – ATP-binding, channel gating and so on – with the human P2X3 receptor. It was consequently reasoned that this conserved region was crucial to the functioning of the receptor. Furthermore, it was found that the receptor was located on the internal vacuolar membranes of the amoeba, where it was crucial to controlling osmotic swelling. It may be, therefore, that mammalian P2X3 is also to be found on internal membranes. These findings, especially the molecular homologies, provide valuable routes to understanding the molecular biology of human P2X3 channels and thus to the causes of the chronic pain which blights so many human lives. Will it be possible to use this new knowledge to design drugs or other probes which can damp down or perhaps eliminate the activity of this channel?

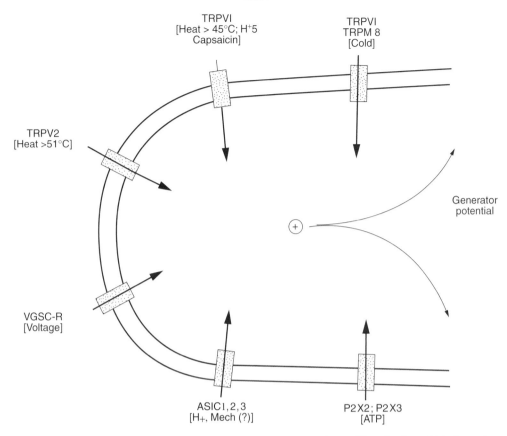

Figure 22.4 Summary diagram to show the molecular biology of nociceptive fibres. The stimuli to which the various channels open are shown. All TRP channels allow the influx of cations (Ca^{2+}, Na^+) and this is indicated by the + sign in the interior. This depolarization leads in turn to a generator potential in the nociceptive ending.

Another approach to relieving, if not eradicating, pain has emerged from experiments with *Drosophila* larvae. Normally these larvae will bend and roll away from noxious thermal and/or mechanical stimuli. Genetic screens for larvae which do not show these responses have uncovered several genes responsible for this aversive behaviour. Larvae carrying mutant forms of one of these genes, the so-called **painless gene**, no longer respond to thermal or mechanical stimuli. It can be shown that these larvae are not affected in other ways. They respond normally to gentle touches and illumination. When the *painless* gene was isolated and cloned, it was found to code for an ion channel belonging to the TRPN family of TRP receptors. This channel can be located in

the dendritic arbors of larval sensory nerves, which ramify just beneath the epidermis and, in painless mutants, no electrophysiological activity can be detected in these sensory nerves in response to thermal or mechanical stimuli.

Mammalian nociceptive endings express members of the TRPV family of cation channels rather than TRPN channels. Nevertheless, further work has shown that the closest mammalian relative of *painless*, *TRPA1/ANKTM1*, is expressed in a subset of mammalian nociceptive neurons. This connection between *Drosophila painless* and mammalian TRPA1 pain receptors has recently been brought out by studies of the pungent stinging sensation experienced in the presence of isothiocyanate, the active ingredient of **wasabi** (Japanese horseradish: *Wasabia japonica*). It has been shown that isothiocyanate repels wild-type *Drosophila* and that this avoidance behaviour is eliminated in the *painless* mutant. This suggests that the painful stinging sensation of wasabi is due to activation of an evolutionarily conserved receptor and pathway connecting *Drosophila* and *Homo*.

These, and other results from the molecular biology laboratories, begin to give insight at a very fundamental level of the processes underlying Aristotle's 'unpleasant sensation'. The biology of pain is, as we have seen, and as we shall see in the following pages, a hugely complex phenomenon. It is unlikely that we shall uncover a 'magic bullet' which will finally rid us of the burden. Nevertheless, the continuing advances in molecular biology, on many fronts, are vastly increasing our knowledge of its physical basis and with knowledge comes power.

22.2.4 Central Pathways

Nociceptive fibres run in the spinal and cranial nerves and (in the case of spinal nerves) enter the spinal cord via the dorsal (or posterior) roots. The dorsal roots are arranged segmentally and the sensory fibres in each dorsal root innervate a particular segment of the body. These segments are known as **dermatomes** (Figure 22.5). The extent of the dermatomes on the surface of the body can be determined by probing

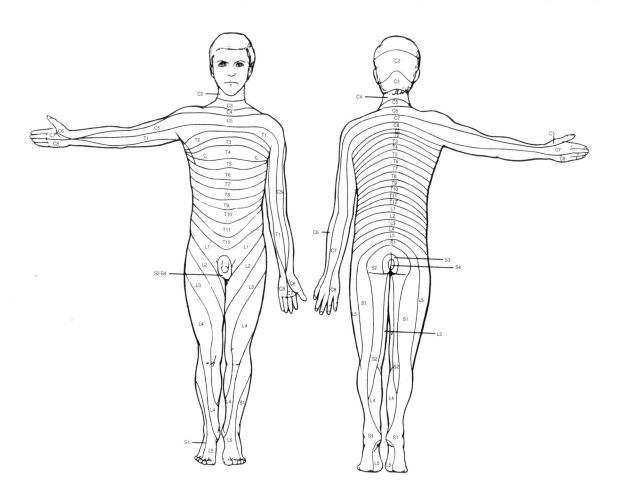

Figure 22.5 Human dermatomes. C = cervical; L = lumbar; S = sacral; T = thoracic. Explanation in text. From Kandel, E.R., Schwartz, J.H. and Jessel, T.M. (eds) (1991) *Principles of Neuroscience*, with permission from Elsevier.

the skin and observing which dorsal roots are activated. It follows that nociceptive fibres and, consequently, pain perception is also arranged segmentally, although the demarcations between one dermatome and the next are seldom sharp.

Once within the spinal cord, the nociceptive fibres terminate in the dorsal horn of the grey matter. The cells of the spinal cord's grey matter are arranged in a series of **laminae** (Figure 22.6). The dorsal horn consists of six layers of cells (1–6) and there are a further three layers in the ventral horn (7–9). A tenth layer of cells is clustered around the central canal. Layer 2 which, as we shall see is important in nociceptive pathways, is known as the **substantia gelatinosa**. These layers of cells are not easy to see in cross sections prepared by normal histological methods. Moreover, the cells are extensively interconnected across the layers by both short axons and dendrites.

If **horseradish peroxidase** is injected into a sensory fibre at the periphery, it is carried in the axoplasmic flow to its central termination. In this way the organization of the spinal grey matter can be elucidated. In general, the larger the diameter of the fibre, the further into the grey matter it penetrates. Thus the large 1a fibres from muscle spindles (Chapter 7) run all the way down to lamina 6 before terminating. In contrast, the small C fibre nociceptor fibres terminate mostly in lamina 2 and the slightly larger Aδ fibres run to laminae 1 and 5. In addition to the C and Aδ innervation, the pain pathway is also innervated by large diameter Aα and Aβ sensory fibres terminating in lamina 4 (Figure 22.6). We shall see the significance of this when we come to the topic of 'gate theory' (Section 22.5).

From the dorsal horn of the spinal grey matter further fibres carry nociceptive information to higher levels in the CNS. These fibres are gathered into three major white matter tracts. The **spino-thalamic tract (STT)** is the most important. It originates from neurons in laminae 1 and 5 and immediately crosses the midline to run in the contralateral ventrolateral (anterolateral) segment of the white matter to the thalamus. The **spino-reticular tract (SRT)** runs slightly dorsal (posterior) to the STT and some of its fibres do not cross over to the opposite side of the cord. It sends branches into the reticular formation as well as into the thalamus. Nociceptive neurons in laminae 1 and 5 project in the **spino-mesencephalic tract (SMT)**; this runs in a similar way to the STT and SRT but terminates in the grey matter around the aqueduct in the midbrain (the periaqueductal grey matter (PAG)) and in the midbrain reticular formation. In addition, the small cells of the substantia gelatinosa project small distances up and down the cord by a small tract on its surface, the **tract of Lissauer**, and there is good evidence to show that short intersegmental connections occur between many of the nociceptive cells in the laminae of the cord. Thus, in addition to the three major white matter tracts, there is also a multisynaptic nociceptive pathway ascending the cord. The nociceptive messages in the major tracts, terminating in the thalamus, midbrain, reticular formation and so on, are carried further by fibres running upward to further parts of the brain. Many of these messages are directed to the somaesthetic cortex and other messages diffuse widely throughout the cerebrum.

Nociceptive messages flowing up the STT from spinal lamina 1 are, however, directed to more specific areas. They terminate in three major regions – the superior part of the **insular cortex (IC)**, **area 3a** of the **frontal cortex** and the **anterior cingulate sulcus (ACS)** (Figure 22.7). Numerous neuroimaging studies have shown both the IC and the ACS to be active in awake humans suffering various forms

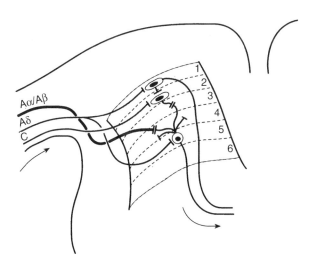

Figure 22.6 Lamination of dorsal horn of spinal grey matter and termination of afferent fibres involved in nociception. Arrows show the direction of impulse flow. Further explanation in text.

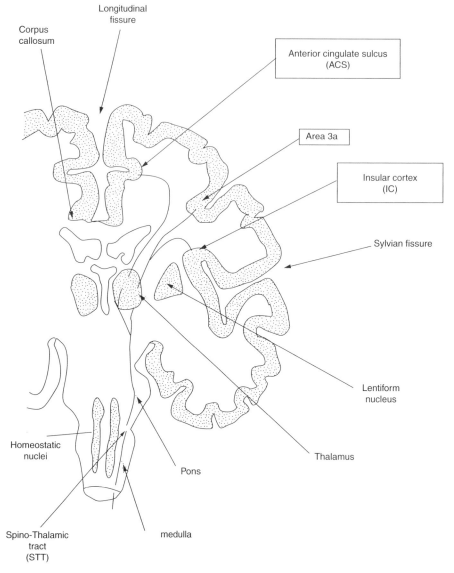

Figure 22.7 Coronal section of human brain to show the cerebral projections of fibres of the spino-thalamic tract. The tract terminates in the thalamus after giving off branches to homeostatic areas in the medulla. Projection neurons carry messages to the insular cortex, area 3a and the anterior cingulate sulcus (see text). After Craig, A.D. (2003).

of pain (heat, cold, hunger, thirst, chronic pain, etc.) and lesions in the ACS ameliorate the discomfort. Behavioural studies have implicated the ACS in initiating escape activity.

In addition to the 'upward' projection there is also a 'downward' projection from higher centres on to the spinal nociceptive cells. The existence of this

downward control was confirmed by the discovery that pain sensations are eliminated during stimulation of a number of discrete brain regions. These regions include nuclei in the **contralateral pons**, in the **hypothalamus**, the **raphe magnus nucleus** and the **somatosensory cortex**. Stimulation of these regions leaves animals active and alert but unresponsive to noxious stimuli. Similar analgesia can be demonstrated in humans suffering from chronic pain. This '**stimulation produced analgesia**' (**SPA**) has allowed the anatomy and physiology of this downward control to be investigated. It has been found that the pathway from these higher centres runs through the **periaqueductal grey matter** (**PAG**) and the rostral ventromedial medulla, and then via a dorsolateral tract in the spinal white matter to the nociceptive cells in the dorsal horn of the grey matter. Many of the fibres in this descending pathway are serotoninergic. Stimulation of this pathway reduces the activity of the dorsal horn nociceptive cells and in animal models eliminates characteristic behavioural responses to noxious stimuli. Implantation of electrodes in the PAG of humans suffering chronic pain reduces their suffering, whilst having little or no effect on touch and temperature sensitivity.

22.3 NEUROPHARMACOLOGY OF PAIN PATHWAYS

Turning from anatomy and physiology to neuropharmacology, we next note that one of the most important events in the latter part of the twentieth century was the discovery of natural opioids by Hughes and his colleagues at Aberdeeen in 1975. The first to be discovered (in pig brain) were the pentapeptides, leucine and methionine **enkephalin** (Leu-Enk and Met-Enk). These two small peptides are related to three larger molecules, β-endorphin, dynorphin and α-neoendorphin (Table 22.1). All five peptides contain the sequence –Tyr–Gly–Gly–Phe– and all

Table 22.1 Natural opioids

β-endorphin	**Tyr-Gly-Gly-Phe**-Met-Thr-Ser-Glu-Lys-Ser-Gln-Thr-Pro-Leu-Val-Thr-Leu-Phe-Lys-Asn-Ala-Ile-Lys-Ile-Lys-Asn-Ala-Tyr-Lys-Lys-Gly-Glu
Dynorphin	**Tyr-Gly-Gly-Phe**-Leu-Arg-Arg-Ile-Arg-Pro-Lys-Lys-Trp-Asp-Asn-Gln
α-Neoendorphin	**Tyr-Gly-Gly-Phe**-Leu-Arg-Lys-tyr-Pro-Lys
Leu-enkephalin	**Tyr-Gly-Gly-Phe**-Leu
Met-enkephalin	**Tyr-Gly-Gly-Phe**-Met

Common amino acids shown in bold print.

have an analgesic effect resembling that of morphine and/or opium. Neurons synthesizing enkephalin and dynorphin are found in the PAG, the ventromedial medulla and the dorsal horn of the spinal cord. β-endorphin, on the other hand, is synthesized by neurons in the hypothalamus that project to the PAG.

Opioid receptors have been subdivided into a number of types according to their binding properties. The most important of these have been designated μ, δ and κ. The μ-receptor responds to agonists in the following order: β-endorphin > dynorphin A > met-enk > leu-enk; the δ-receptor responds to β-endorphin > leu-enk > met-enk > dynorphin A; and the κ-receptor to dynorphin A >> β-endorphin > leu-enk = met-enk. All three types of receptor are widely distributed throughout the CNS. The μ-receptor is particularly important in nociception. High levels of this type of opioid receptor are found in the thalamus, the PAG and the dorsal horn of the spinal cord; κ-receptors are more sparsely distributed but are especially evident in the preoptic area of the hypothalamus, whilst δ-receptors are found especially in the olfactory regions of the brain.

It is believed that enkephalinergic neurons exert their effects by releasing enkephalins on to the presynaptic terminals of nociceptive neurons and thus inhibiting the release of transmitter (Figure 22.8a). The synaptology of the pain pathways is highly intricate and it is likely that in addition to the presynaptic inhibition shown in Figure 22.8a there is also postsynaptic inhibition. Some of this synaptic intricacy is shown in Figure 22.8b. This shows the local circuitry in the superficial laminae of the dorsal horn of the spinal cord's grey matter. Downward projections from the pain modulating centres in the brain are known to terminate densely in laminae 1 and 2 and also in laminae 4, 5, 6 and 10. It will be recalled that STT fibres (in primates) originate from lamina 1 and that C nociceptor afferents mostly terminate in lamina 2. A downwardly directed serotoninergic (5HT) fibre terminating on a projection neuron in lamina 1 is shown in Figure 22.8b. This synapse is inhibitory. The serotoninergic fibre also makes a synapse, this time an excitatory synapse, on an enkephalinergic 'stalk cell' in lamina 2, the substantia gelatinosa. This interneuron makes an inhibitory synapse with the projection neuron. Another stalk cell, an excitatory cell, receives

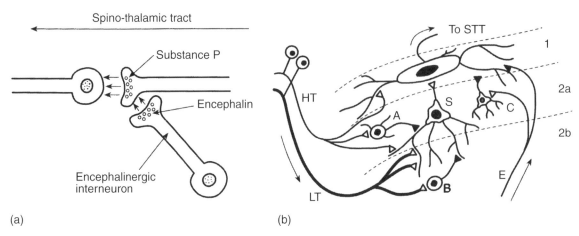

Figure 22.8 (a) Schematic figure to show encephalinergic control of a nociceptive cell in substantia gelatinosa. A neuron in the spinothalamic tract synapses with another neuron in the tract using substance P (SP) as its transmitter. The release of SP is controlled by an encephalinergic interneuron acting presynaptically to inhibit the release of SP. Adapted from Iverson, L.L. (1979). (b) Simplified schematic to show local circuitry in dorsal horn of grey matter. The first two layers of the grey matter are shown. The second layer, the substantia gelatinosa, is subdivided into two sublayers, 2a and 2b. A nociceptive projection neuron is shown in layer 1. Its axon forms part of the STT. High threshold (HT) (small diameter) fibres and low threshold (LT) (large diameter) fibres enter on the left from a spinal root. A descending inhibitory serotinergic neuron (E) enters on the right of the figure. Further explanation in text. A = inhibitory islet neuron; B = inhibitory neuron; C = inhibitory cell; E = serotinergic descending neuron; HT = high threshold afferent neuron; LT = low threshold afferent neuron; S = stalk cell. Inhibitory synapses, black; excitatory synapses, white. Modified from Wall and Melzack, 1994.

excitatory input from both high and low threshold afferents. The figure shows that both these latter fibres also synapse with short enkephalinergic interneurons, which also synapse on the stalk cell. This provides another way of reducing the activity of the projection neuron. It is clear that the complex wiring and weighting of different synapses provides a subtle control on the output of the STT projection fibre.

22.4 REFERRED PAIN

When the skin is damaged, the individual is immediately able to accurately locate the source of pain. This accurate localization is seldom made when the viscera are the source of pain. It is as if the CNS cannot believe that internal organs are at risk and instead **refers** to pain to the surface of the body. Probably the best known instance of this referral is that experienced by sufferers from **angina pectoris**.

The term 'angina pectoris' was introduced by Herbenden in 1772 in a lecture to the Royal college of Physicians. He wrote that patients '. . . are seized, while they are walking, and more particularly when they walk soon after eating, with a painful and most disagreeable sensation in the breast which seems as if it would take their life away if it were to increase or continue: the moment they stand still, all this uneasiness vanishes . . .'. The pain is felt as a deep constriction of the thoracic muscles surrounding the chest and, as the attack mounts, shooting pains down the left arm. The source of this acute pain and discomfort is, of course, the heart and, in particular, a deterioration or blockage of the coronary arteries supplying oxygenated blood to the cardiac muscle.

To understand why it is that the pain is referred to the upper thorax and the left arm, it is necessary to refer back to the concept of dermatomes mentioned at the beginning of Section 22.2.2 and shown in Figure 22.5. In embryology the heart develops as a midline structure in the upper part of the thorax. Its nerve supply is thus derived from the upper thoracic dermatomes. As it develops the left ventricle becomes the major pumping chamber having, as it does, to force blood around the systemic circulation. Thus it is this left chamber that first 'feels' the lack of oxygen due to defective coronary arteries. The upper thoracic dermatomes also provide the nerve supply to the chest musculature during development as well as the musculature and nerve supply of the arms. It follows that, when pain fibres from cardiac muscle are activated by ischaemia, they enter the spinal cord through the same dorsal roots as pain fibres from the arms and thorax. They share the same circuitry in the dorsal horn of the grey matter. The brain misinterprets the source from which the pain messages originate (Figure 22.9). This explanation of referred pain through a commonality of dorsal nociceptive circuitry is supported by the observation that the left arm of a patient suffering an angina attack is hyperalgesic although the right arm is normal. This tenderness suggests that a summation of nociceptive impulses is occurring in the dorsal horn before the messages are projected onwards to the brain.

Angina pectoris provides a type example of referred pain. There are many other instances. It is possible that some of the back pain, which, as mentioned above, is suffered by such a multitude of patients, is referred pain from other parts of the anatomy, especially the pelvis. To review the many other cases of referred pain would lead us too far into the clinical analysis of pain for a book of this nature (see the publication by Melzack and Wall, 1982, listed in the bibliography for a full and accessible account). It is worth mentioning, however, that near the local-

ities at which referred pain seems to originate it is often possible to find so-called '**trigger points**'. Palpation of, or insertion of a needle into, these points can lead to severe and sometimes long-lasting pain. These trigger points are mostly found in subjects suffering from disease of one or more of the internal organs but can also be found (though without generating such severe pain) in apparently healthy individuals. In cardiac patients trigger points are found not only on the surface of the chest (both left and right) but also over the shoulder blades and on both sides of the vertebral column. Although the physiology of referred pain may be responsible for some of these trigger points, other possibilities exist and the full story (like that responsible for acupuncture to which they are related) has yet to be understood.

22.5 GATE THEORY

There have been many theories about the neurophysiology of pain at the level of the spinal cord. Gate theory introduced by Melzack and Wall in 1965 has, however, gained wide acceptance and explains many of the salient features. In essence it suggests how nociceptive impulses can be controlled or 'gated' by mechanisms in the dorsal horn of the grey matter and by impulses arriving in pathways descending from higher centres. We saw in the introduction to this chapter how the experience of pain can be modulated by the circumstances in which the animal finds itself, and we have also seen in succeeding sections some of the neuroanatomical pathways and neurophysiological mechanisms by which this can be achieved. In this section we shall concentrate on the gating mechanisms which are postulated to operate at the first synapse in the pain pathway.

In Figure 22.10 a projection neuron in lamina 1 of the dorsal horn of the spinal grey matter is shown (cp. Figure 22.8b). It is innervated by two afferent fibres, a small (S) diameter fibre (C fibre or Aδ fibre) and a large (L) diameter fibre (Aα fibre or Aβ fibre). The S fibre also inhibits an inhibitory (perhaps encephalinergic) interneuron. The L fibre, in contrast, excites this inhibitory interneuron. Finally, a fibre in the downward projection from higher centres also synapses on the interneuron. It must be emphasized that Figure 22.10 is a conceptual diagram which (hopefully) captures the essence of a hugely

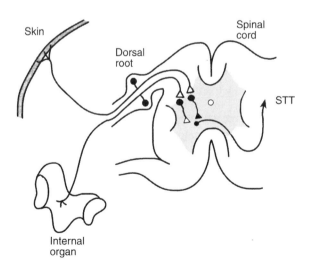

Figure 22.9 A simplified pathway to account for referred pain. Further explanation in text.

complex grey matter synaptology (an impoverished version of this synaptology is shown in Figure 22.8b).

It can be seen in Figure 22.10 that S fibre activity excites the projection neuron and switches off activity in the inhibitory interneuron. In contrast, activity in the L fibre, whilst exciting the projection neuron, also switches on activity in the inhibitory interneuron. When the small fibre is activated on its own, the projection fibre is released from inhibition and impulses course up the pain pathways to higher centres. When the large fibre is activated on its own, the result is an initial burst of activity in the projection fibre succeeded by inhibition as the interneuron activity makes its influence felt. When both fibres are activated together, the large fibre (having the more rapid transmission rate) asserts its effect and, by the time impulses in the small fibres arrive, the inhibitory interneuron has reduced the excitability of the projection neuron. The gate has been closed. Activation of the downward projection fibre by centres higher in the CNS will also have the effect of closing the gate and (perhaps) keeping it closed.

The original gate theory epitomized in Figure 22.10 has been complicated by subsequent detailed neuroanatomy and neurophysiology but its essence has withstood the test of time remarkably well. It has, moreover, provided the basis for valuable analgesic therapies. The theory suggests that if the large diameter nerves are stimulated, impulses arriving in the small diameter nociceptive fibres will find the spinal gate to the pain pathway closed. It is convenient that large diameter fibres are preferentially activated by external electrodes on the skin surface. It is thus comparatively simple to devise a pocket sized battery stimulator with electrodes which can be attached to the skin with a conducting paste. Turning on these devices produces a tingling sensation with a concomitant reduction in pain. They have been used by hundreds of thousands of patients, usually with a highly beneficial effect. This, in itself, justifies the research and thought devoted to developing gate theory.

22.6 CONCLUDING REMARKS

There is no doubt that pain is the scourge of mankind. How far through the living world it extends we cannot say but, as we noted at the beginning of this chapter, it is well to err on the side of caution. We should endeavour to act in such a way that the possibility of pain is not a consequence in humans or other animals. This often provides acute dilemmas in medical research. When is the prospect of alleviating suffering in humans adequate to justify inflicting pain (and how much pain?) on other animals?

Fortunately, nowadays, and largely as the result of medical research in the past, we have many means of alleviating and controlling pain. Some of these have been mentioned above and others are described in textbooks of medicine and anaesthesiology. We are indeed fortunate to live in an age when the spectre of pain following injury and disease has been so extensively exorcized. It is painful even to think of horror of the operating table two centuries ago. The young Charles Darwin gave up his intended career as a physician on attending a particularly horrifying operation on a child in Edinburgh. These techniques of analgesia are also, of course, available and used in the carefully controlled and licensed procedures of contemporary biomedical research.

But the problem of pain continues to intrigue and puzzle the minds of its students. We have seen in this

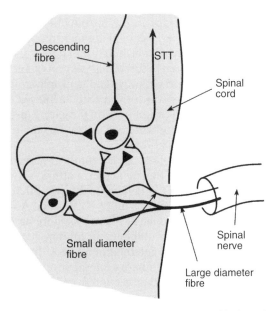

Figure 22.10 Gate theory. Inhibitory synapses, black; excitatory white. Further explanation in text.

chapter that, like the other 'raw feels' we have looked at in other parts of this book, it is very far from being 'uncooked'. We are often misled by the simple equation between injury and pain. We are too easily convinced by the seeming immediacy of pain when we jam our finger in the door or touch a red hot coal. We have noted in this chapter some (and only some!) of the complexity of the underlying neural circuitry. We have seen how control is exerted both in the spinal cord and in higher centres. We have also seen how the experience of pain is strongly influenced by circumstance and cultural expectations. The experience of pain is very far from being the physical concomitant (as some philosophers would have it) of reading off impulse frequencies in the C fibres.

Rather, the experience of pain, like the other sensory experiences to which we are subject, is for a purpose. It is integrated into the ongoing physiology/behaviour of the animal so that it motivates escape to well-being. It is part, and an overarching part, of the animal's homeostasis. It has, for instance, been argued that the small diameter fibres running up in the STT to terminate in the insular cortex (Figure 22.7) provide a cortical representation of the physiological well-being of the entire body. Some indeed regard this area as constituting the 'interoceptive cortex'. Projections to the anterior cingulate sulcus lead to behavioural activity bringing the body back, as far as possible, to its optimal condition. All of which, of course, is not to forget the tragic instances where the homeostatic neurophysiology beats against an impossibility. The pain of internal disease (we looked at angina pectoris above) is as desperately ineffectual (except in our medically literate culture) as the raw struggles of a small animal caught in a gin trap. As in other cases, the benefit of the pain system in allowing recovery to well-being outweighs the tragedies when it is all for nothing.

PART V: SELF ASSESSMENT

The following questions are designed both to help you assess your understanding of the topics covered in the text and to direct your attention to significant aspects of the subject matter. The sequence of questions follows the sequence in which the subject matter is presented in the text. It is thus easy to refer back to the appropriate page or pages. After reading each chapter and/or each section you should look through these questions and make sure you know the answers and the issues involved.

CHAPTER 20: THERMOSENSITIVITY

20.1 What is the normal thermal range in which biological organisms can exist? Why? Are there exceptions? If so, name them.

20.2 Distinguish between poikilotherms and homeotherms.

20.3 How have studies in the molecular genetics of *C. elegans* thrown light on the mechanisms underlying thermosensitivity? Describe the behavioural experiments devised to test the nematode's thermosensitivity.

20.4 How have dorsal root ganglion (DRG) cells been used in investigations of thermosensitivity?

20.5 What affect does an increase in temperature have on a small group of DRG cells?

20.6 Describe the molecular biology of mouse thermosensory fibres.

20.7 Which chemicals found in foods affect the endings of thermosensory fibres?

20.8 Which Piscean system of receptors is able to detect temperature changes?

20.9 Give an account of some of the thermoreceptors found in the insects. Indicate how they are adapted to the insect's way of life.

20.10 There are only two groups of true homeotherms: which are they?

20.11 At what temperature is the human thermostat set?

20.12 Where are thermoreceptors situated in the human body?

20.13 What is the 'neutral range' of human thermosensitivity?

20.14 Where are temperature sensitive 'spots' most concentrated on the body's surface?

20.15 What is 'paradoxical cold' and what does it show about the interpretation of sensory information by the central nervous system (CNS)?

20.16 What is Weber's illusion and what is its neurophysiological explanation?

20.17 What form do thermosensitive endings take, and where are they to be found?

20.18 Describe how warm and cold fibres signal any small change in skin temperature within the neutral range.

20.19 Where are internal thermoreceptors located? What danger are they mostly designed to prevent?

20.20 Where are thermoreceptors located in the brain?

20.21 Which cerebral nuclei correlate thermal information from all parts of the body and initiate physiological responses to counteract any variation from the thermostatic set point?

CHAPTER 21: MINORITY SENSES

21.1   Where are infrared detectors situated in thermosensitive snakes?

21.2   How is the direction of the source of the infrared radiation determined?

21.3   Which cranial nerve carries the output from the thermosensitive pits to the CNS?

21.4   To which part of the snake's brain is the infrared information delivered?

21.5   How do the receptive fields of infrared responsive tectal cells resemble those of ganglion cells in the primate retina?

21.6   To which characteristic of the infrared image is the snake's tectal map most sensitive?

21.7   What feature of the Earth's atmosphere causes polarization of incoming radiation?

21.8   Where in the sky is the band of maximum polarization on a cloudless midsummer midday in England?

21.9   Explain the distorted nature of a fish-eye view of the aerial world.

21.10 How are crustacean compound and cephalopod vesicular eyes adapted to detect the plane of polarized light?

21.11 What evidence is there that insects and cephalopods are sensitive to the plane of polarized light?

21.12 Write down examples of strongly electric and weakly electric fish. Into which group do most electric fish fall?

21.13 Where is the electric organ located in weakly electric fish?

21.14 What are the functions of strong and weak electric discharges?

21.15 What causes the weak electric fields which predatory electroreceptive fish detect?

21.16 Describe an experiment showing the value of electroreceptors in detecting hidden prey.

21.17 Can weakly electric fish detect inorganic features of their environment?

21.18 Which two types of receptor are responsible for electrosensitivity? From which ubiquitous system have they evolved?

21.19 What are the ampullae of Lorenzini and where are they found?

21.20 Of what do the capsules of the ampullae of Lorenzini consist?

21.21 How do tuberous organs differ from ampullary organs?

21.22 Where are ampullary and tuberous organs located in typical freshwater gymnotid fish? Which are the most numerous?

21.23 Where are electroreceptors found in *Ornithorhynchus* and *Tachglossus*?

21.24 Which other receptors are associated with monotreme electroreceptors. How are they believed to work together with electroreceptors in monotreme hunting behaviour?

21.25 In which organisms are magnetosomes found?

21.26 What biological role do magnetosomes play?

21.27 Which other organisms have been suspected of possessing some sensitivity to magnetic fields?

21.28 Review the evidence for bird navigation by a magnetic sense. Do you believe this evidence is convincing?

CHAPTER 22: PAIN

22.1   Reflect on what is meant by the term 'pain'.

22.2   What is congenital analgesia and why is it a disabling condition?

22.3   Why is the cause of congenital analgesia thought to lie centrally rather than at the periphery?

22.4   Give some figures to support the statement that intractable pain constitutes a massive call on the resources of health services throughout the modern world.

22.5   Explain how the concept of a faulty 'efference copy' may account for some cases of chronic pain.

22.6   Can you think of an evolutionary reason for the ubiquity of lower back pain in human populations?

22.7   Provide counter-instances to the idea that pain is felt when the brain detects impulses in pain fibres in the same way as a loudspeaker's volume is determined by the electric current it receives.

22.8 What form do peripheral nociceptive fibres take? How may they be distinguished from mechanoreceptive and thermoreceptive endings?

22.9 Which type of nociceptive fibre is believed to be responsible for sharp, pricking sensations and which for dull, prolonged aches?

22.10 Distinguish between type 1 and type 2 AMHs. How does the response of both of these AMHs differ from that of the CMHs?

22.11 How has capsaicin been used to detect pain receptor channels?

22.12 What is meant by the term 'hyperalgesic'?

22.13 List some of the factors responsible for secondary hyperalgesia.

22.14 How do 'axon reflexes' contribute to spreading hyperalgesia?

22.15 Describe the various types of pain receptor channels expressed in nociceptive fibres.

22.16 How have molecular biological approaches helped in the understanding and possible treatment of chronic pain?

22.17 How are dermatomes related to the vertebral column?

22.18 How many laminae are recognized in the dorsal (posterior) horn of the grey matter?

22.19 Which layer of the grey matter is known as the substantia gelatinosa?

22.20 In which layers do C fibres, Aδ fibres, Aβ and Aα fibres terminate?

22.21 Which three tracts carry nociceptive information up the spinal cord?

22.22 What is the tract of Lissauer?

22.23 Which brain nuclei are involved in the 'downward' control of pain? Through which parts of the brain stem and spinal cord do fibres from these nuclei run?

22.24 Describe the biochemical nature of two common 'natural opioids'.

22.25 In which parts of the brain are cells which express receptors to the natural opioids found?

22.26 Draw a diagram to show some of the neural complexity in layers 1 and 2 of the dorsal horn of the grey matter.

22.27 What is referred pain? Give examples.

22.28 Give an account of the likely neural circuitry responsible for referred pain.

22.29 What are 'trigger points'? Where are these located in cardiac patients?

22.30 Draw a simplified diagram to explain the basic concept behind 'gate theory'.

22.31 How has gate theory provided the rationale for a valuable analgesic therapy?

PART V: NOTES, REFERENCES AND BIBLIOGRAPHY

CHAPTER 20: THERMOSENSITIVITY

Discussions of thermosensitivity can be found in texts of physiology (Darian-Smith, 1984; Gregor and Windhorst, 1996) and comparative physiology (Prosser and Brown, 1961). The problem of protein denaturation at high temperatures has led to a great deal of interest in so-called heat-shock proteins or chaperonins (Ellis, Laskey and Lorimer, 1993), which confer stability on other proteins at elevated temperatures. These proteins are ubiquitous and evolutionarily ancient. With the exception of the large tube worms, which are found clustered around fumaroles in the deep ocean, animals cannot survive at body temperatures beyond about 40°C. Although a poikilothermic animal normally has a preferred environmental temperature, it is usually possible to change this 'set point' (providing the change is not too great) by acclimation. Many aspects of biochemistry and physiology change in a complex way to fit the animal for its new environmental temperature (Prosser and Brown, 1961). Discussions of the molecular biology underlying thermosensitivity can be found in McCleskey (1997), Reichling and Levine (1997), Dhaka, Viswanath and Patapoutian (2006), Bautista *et al.* (2007) and Bandell, Macpherson and Patapoutian (2007) provide an up-to-date review. The large topic of the evolution of homeothermy in birds and mammals is discussed by Ruben (1995).

Bandell, M., Macpherson, L.J. and Patapoutian, A. (2007) From chills to chillis: mechanisms for themosensation and chemesthesis via thermo TRPs. *Current Opinion in Neurobiology*, **17**, 490–7.

Bautista, D.M. *et al.* (2007) The menthol receptor TRPM8 is the principal detector of environmental cold. *Nature*, **448**, 204–8.

Bear, M.F., Connors, B.W. and Paradiso, M.A. (1996) *Neuroscience: Exploring the Brain*, Williams and Wilkins, Baltimore.

Dhaka, A., Viswanath, V. and Patapoutian, A. (2006) TRP ion channels and temperature sensation. *Annual Review of Neuroscience*, **29**, 135–61.

Darian-Smith, I. (1984) Thermal sensitivity, in *Handbook of Physiology, Section 1: The Nervous System: Sensory Processes*, Part 2, Vol. 3 (ed. I. Darian-Smith), American Physiological Society, Bethesda.

Ellis, R.J., Laskey, R.A. and Lorimer, G.H. (eds) (1993) Molecular chaperones. *Philosophical Transactions of the Royal Society (Biological Sciences)*, **339**, 255–373.

Gregor, R. and Windhorst, U. (eds) (1996) *Comprehensive Human Physiology*, Springer-Verlag, Berlin.

Hazel, J.R. (1995) Thermal adaptations in biological membranes: is homeoviscous adaptation the explanation? *Annual Review of Physiology*, **57**, 19–42.

McCleskey, E.W. (1997) Recent heat in thermosensation. *Current Biology*, **7**, R679–81.

Prosser, C.L. and Brown, F.A. (1961) *Comparative Animal Physiology*, Saunders, Philadelphia.

Reichling, D.B. and Levine, J.D. (1997) Heat transduction in rat sensory neurons by calcium-dependent activation of a cation channel. *Proceedings of the National Academy of Sciences*, **94**, 7006–11.

Ruben, J. (1995) The evolution of homeothermy in mammals and birds: from physiology to fossils. *Annual Review of Physiology*, **57**, 69–95.

CHAPTER 21: MINORITY SENSES

Infrared detection in snakes is reviewed by Hartline (1974). Waterman (1981) provides a comprehensive well illustrated account of polarized light and polarization sensitivity in the animal kingdom whilst Frisch (1974) describes his pioneering work on bee dances which tell the hive of the direction of food sources with respect to the plane of sunlight polarization. Bell (1986) and Bullock and Heiligenberg (1986) give book-length treatments of electroreception and Bennett's chapter in Hoar (1971), although a little dated, still provides an excellent account of the various types of electric fish. A careful assessment of the physics and sensory physiology of shark navigation by sensing the Earth's magnetic field is provided by Paulin (1995). The story of how the true function of the ampullae of Lorenzini was elucidated is told by Bullock (1974): first they were thought to be temperature receptors, then pressure receptors, then salinity detectors and, finally, electroreceptors. The latter conclusion was ultimately established by a combination of electrophysiological and behavioural studies. A well illustrated and interesting account of the impression strong electric fish made on the peoples of Egyptian, Greek and Roman antiquity is given by Kellaway (1946). Finally, the little-known electroreceptors of the Monotremata, especially the duck-billed platypus, have been investigated by Proske, Gregory and Iggo (1998), whilst their cerebral analysis is discussed in the same issue of *Philosophical Transactions of the Royal Society (B)* by Pettigrew, Manger and Fine (1998). Although magnetosensitivity in bacteria is well understood (Blakemore, 1982; Mann, Sparks and Board, 1990) little has so far been established about this sense in the higher animals, although there have been suggestions that it is involved in bird navigation (Beason and Semm, 1996; Fleissner *et al.*, 2003; Mouritsen and Ritz, 2005). Reiter (1993) provides some evidence that magnetic fields may affect circadian rhythms by influencing the secretion of melatonin by the pineal.

Infrared Radiation

Hartline, P.H. (1974) Thermoreception in snakes, in *Handbook of Sensory Physiology*, Vol. **III/3** (ed. A. Fessard), Springer-Verlag, Berlin.

Terashima, S., Goris, R.C. and Katsuki, Y. (1970) Structure of the warm fiber terminals in the pit membrane of vipers. *Journal of Ultrastructure Research*, **31**, 494–506.

Polarized Light

Frisch, K. (1974) Decoding the language of the bees. *Science*, **185**, 663–8.
Walls, G.L. (1963) *The Vertebrate Eye and its Adaptive Radiation*, Hafner, New York.
Waterman, T.H. (1981) Polarization sensitivity, in *Handbook of Sensory Physiology*, Vol. **VII/6B** (ed. H. Autrum), Springer Verlag, Berlin.
Wellington, W.G. (1974) A special light to steer by. *Natural History*, **83** (10), 46–53.

Electrosensitivity

Bell, C.S. (1986) Electroreception, in *Electroreception* (eds T.H. Bullock and W. Heiligenberg), John Wiley & Sons, Inc., New York.
Bennett, M.V.L. (1971) Electric organs, in *Fish Physiology*, Vol. **5** (eds W.S. Hoar and D.J. Randall), Academic Press, New York.
Bullock, T.H. and Heiligenberg, W. (eds) (1986) *Electroreception*, John Wiley & Sons, Inc., New York.
Bullock, T.H. (1974) General introduction, in *Handbook of Sensory Physiology*, Vol. **III/3** (ed. E. Fessard.), Springer-Verlag, Berlin.
Kalmijn, A.J. (1971) The electric sense in sharks and rays. *Journal of Experimental Biology*, **55**, 371–83.
Kalmijn, A.D. (1974) The detection of electric fields from inanimate and animate sources other than electric organs, in *Handbook of Sensory Physiology*, Vol. **III/3** (ed. A. Fessard.), Springer-Verlag, Berlin.
Kellaway, P. (1946) The part played by electric fish in the early history of bioelectricity and electrotherapy. *Bulletin of the History of Medicine*, **20**, 112–37.
Manger, P.R., Collins, R. and Pettigrew, J.D. (1997) Histological observations on the presumed electroreceptors and mechanoreceptors in the beak skin of the long-beaked echidna. *Zaglossus bruijnii, Proceedings of the Royal Society B*, **264**, 165–72.
Murray, R.W. (1974) The Ampullae of Lorenzini, in *Handbook of Sensory Physiology*, Vol. **III/3** (ed. A. Fessard.), Springer-Verlag, Berlin.
New, J.G. (1997) The evolution of vertebrate electrosensory systems. *Brain, Behaviour and Evolution*, **50**, 244–52.

Paulin, M.G. (1995) Electroreception and the compass sense in sharks. *Journal of Theoretical Biology*, **174**, 325–39.

Pettigrew, J.D., Manger, P.R. and Fine, S.L.B. (1998) The sensory world of the platypus. *Philosophical Transactions of the Royal Society B*, **353**, 1199–1210.

Proske, U., Gregory, J.E. and Iggo, A. (1998) Sensory receptors in monotremes. *Philosophical Transactions of the Royal Society B*, **353**, 1187–98.

Szabo, T. (1974) Anatomy of the specialised lateral line organs of electroreception, in *Handbook of Sensory Physiology*, Vol. **III/3** (ed. A. Fessard.), Springer-Verlag, Berlin.

von der Emde, G. *et al.* (1998) Electric fish measure distance in the dark. *Nature*, **395**, 890–94.

Magnetosensitivity

Beason, R.C. and Semm, P. (1996) Does the Avian ophthalmic nerve carry magnetic navigational information? *Journal of Experimental Biology*, **199**, 1241–44.

Blakemore, R.P. (1982) Magnetotactic bacteria. *Annual Review of Microbiology*, **36**, 217–38.

Fleissner, G. *et al.* (2003) Ultrastructural analysis of a putative magnetoreceptor in the beak of homing pigeons. *The Journal of Comparative Neurology*, **458**, 350–60.

Mann, S., Sparks, N.H.C. and Board, R.G. (1990) Magnetotactic bacteria: microbiology, biomineralisation, palaeomagnetism and biotechnology. *Advances in Microbial Physiology*, **31**, 125–81.

Mouritsen, H. and Ritz, T. (2005) Magnetoreception and its use in bird navigation. *Current Opinion in Neurobiology*, **15**, 406–14.

Reiter, R.J. (1993) Static and extremely low frequency electromagnetic field exposure – reported effects on the circadian production of melatonin. *Journal of Cellular Biochemistry*, **51**, 394–403.

Walker, M.M. *et al.* (2007) Structure and function of the vertebrate magnetic sense. *Nature*, **390**, 371–76.

Walker, M.M., Dennis, E.D. and Kirschwink, J.I. (2002) The magnetic sense and its use in long-distance navigation by animals. *Current Opinion in Neurobiology*, **12**, 735–44.

CHAPTER 22: PAIN

The topic of pain has, for obvious reasons, concerned scientists, philosophers and theologians for millennia. Aristotle, *De Anima*, Book 2 writes that all animals, having the sense of touch, also have the capacity for pleasure and pain. Pain, he writes, somewhat tautologously, is the perception of unpleasant objects. A recent definition of pain was provided by the *International Association for the Study of Pain* (*IASP*) in 1991: 'An unpleasant sensory and emotional experience associated with actual or potential tissue damage, or described in terms of such damage'. Merskey (1991) emphasizes that pain is a 'raw feel' and should not be confused with 'pain behaviour'. The experience, he goes on, is 'monistic but the aetiology is multiple'. Anand and Craig (1996) review other modern definitions, whilst Wall and Melzack (1994) edit an up-to-date review of its many dimensions. The smaller book by Melzack and Wall (1982) provides a classic and easily read introduction, whilst their earlier contribution (1965) is the founding paper of 'Gate Theory'. The interesting paper by Melzack, Stillwell and Fox (1977) suggests that trigger points and acupuncture points are essentially the same, having been discovered by clinicians working in different cultures. Roland (1992) outlines modern work which emphasizes that widespread cortical activity occurs in response to pain stimuli and Craig (2003) provides an exhaustive review of central processing emphasizing the homeostatic function of pain. A set of reviews in *Nature Reviews Neuroscience 7* (**6**) (2005) provides an up-to-date assessment from molecule to emotion, including the psychobiology of the placebo effect. The neurobiology of pain is reviewed in colloquia edited by Dubner and Gold (1999) and by Hunt and Koltzenburg (2005) whilst molecular approaches are discussed in Al-Anzi, Tracey and Benzer (2006), Fountain *et al.* (2007) and Tracey *et al.* (2003). Finally, Wall (1985) discusses some of the counter-intuitive features of pain and Ramachandran and Blakeslee (1998) provide a well written account of Ramachandran's clever experiments which show that mirror-induced illusion of the continued existence of a lost limb helps ameliorate pain in the phantom limb (but is this a placebo effect?). There has, recently, been some evidence that the fitting and continuous use of prostheses also reduces the pain felt in phantom limbs.

Al-Anzi, B., Tracey, W.D. and Benzer, S. (2006) Response of Drosophila to Wasabi is mediated by painless, the Fly Homolog of Mammalian TRPA1/ANKTM1. *Current Biology*, **16**, 1034–40.

Anand, K.J.S. and Craig, K.D. (1996) New perspectives on the definition of pain. *Pain*, **67**: 3–6.

Craig, A.D. (2003) Pain mechanisms: labelled lines versus convergence in central processing. *Annual Review of Neuroscience*, **26**, 1–30.

Darwin, E. (1794) *Zoonomia*, Vol. **1**, Johnson, London, pp. 121, 125.

Deyo, R.A. (1998) Low back pain. *Scientific American*, **279** (2), 28–33.

Dubner, R. and Gold, M. (1999) *NAS Colloquium: The Neurobiology of Pain*, National Academies Press, Washington DC.

Fields, H.L. and Basbaum, A.I. (1994) Central nervous system mechanisms of pain modulation, in *Textbook of Pain* (eds P.D. Wall and R. Melzack), 3rd edn, Churchill Livingstone, Edinburgh.

Fountain, S.J. *et al.* (2007) An intracellular P2X receptor required for osmoregulation in *Dictyostelium discoideum*. *Nature*, **448**, 200–3.

Herbenden, W. (1772) quoted in Procacci, P., Zoppi, M. and Maresca, M. (1994)) Heart and vascular pain, in *Textbook of Pain* (eds P.D. Wall and R. Melzack), 3rd edn, Churchill Livingstone, Edinburgh.

Hunt, S. and Koltzenurg, M. (2005) *The Neurobiology of Pain*, Oxford University Press, Oxford.

Iverson, L.L. (1979) The chemistry of the brain. *Scientific American*, **241** (3), 118–21.

James, W. (1890) *The Principles of Psychology*, Holt, New York.

Kandel, E.R, Schwartz, J.H. and Jessel, T.M. (1991) *Principles of Neuroscience*, Elsevier, New York.

Melzack, R. (1975) The McGill pain questionnaire: major properties and scoring methods. *Pain*, **1**, 277–99.

Melzack, R. and Wall, P.D. (1965) Pain mechanisms: a new theory. *Science*, **150**, 971–9.

Melzack, R., Stillwell, D.M. and Fox, E.J. (1977) Trigger points and acupuncture points: correlations and implications. *Pain*, **3**, 3–23.

Melzack, R. and Wall, P.D. (1982) *The Challenge of Pain*, Penguin Books, Harmondsworth.

Merskey, H. (1991) The definition of pain. *European Psychiatry*, **6**, 153–59.

Meyer, R.A., Campbell, J.N. and Raja, S.N. (1994) Peripheral neural mechanisms of nociception, in *Textbook of Pain* (eds P.D. Wall and R. Melzack), 3rd edn, Churchill Livingstone, Edinburgh.

Ramachandran, V.S., Rogers-Ramachandran, D. and Cobb, S. (1995) Touching the phantom limb. *Nature*, **377**, 489–90.

Ramachandran, V.S. and Blakeslee, S. (1998) *Phantoms in the Brain*, Fourth Estate, London.

Rang, H.P., Bevan, S. and Dray, A. (1994) Nociceptive peripheral neurons: cellular properties, in *Textbook of Pain* (eds P.D. Wall and R. Melzack), 3rd edn, Churchill Livingstone, Edinburgh.

Roland P. (1992) Cortical representation of pain. *Trends in Neurosciences*, **15**, 3–5.

Tracey, W.D. *et al.* (2003) *Painless*, a *Drosophila* gene essential for nociception. *Cell*, **113**, 261–73.

Wall, P.D. (1985) Pain and no pain, in *Functions of the Brain* (ed. C.W. Coen), Clarendon Press, Oxford.

Wall, P.D. and Melzack, R. (eds) (1994) *Textbook of Pain*, 3rd edn, Churchill Livingstone, Edinburgh.

PART VI: CODA

When our first encounter with some object surprises us and we find it novel, or very different from what we formerly knew or from what we supposed it ought to be, this causes us to wonder and to be astonished at it. Since all this may happen before we know whether or not the object is beneficial to us, I regard wonder as the first of all the passions

René Descartes, 1649, *Le Passions de l'Ame*, Leiden: Elzevier, Section 53

It is surely the case that, as we have gone through the pages of this book, we have, again and again, experienced 'wonder', the feeling which René Descartes regarded as the first of the passions. In this final part we step back a little and reflect upon what has gone before. Chapter 23 draws together some of the themes which have recurred time after time in the preceding twenty-two chapters. It shows how sensory systems resemble each other along two different axes. Along one axis the chapter draws out similarities in the neurobiology of the different modalities, along the other axis it shows how different animal groups have often homed in on the same solutions to sensory problems. Although, as we have seen, animals have evolved a bewildering variety of sense organs and systems to detect all the varying changes and happenings in their environments, certain design principles shine through time and again. At the lowest level, at the level of molecules and cells, these commonalities often point to a common origin. At 'higher' levels, at the levels of organs and systems, evolution has homed in on 'best solutions' along several independent and unrelated lines. These lines provide fascinating examples of convergent evolution.

In addition to this comparative approach, which shows how the Darwinian process of trial and error, continued over billennia, winnows out failure and second-rate solutions to home in on the optimal, Chapter 23 also shows an inevitable movement of the focus of information processing from the abiotic to the biotic and, lastly, to the social. The struggle for existence leads not only from simple molecular systems (mechanosensitive ion channels, R–T proteins, eyespots) to highly complex organs (ears, noses, retinae) but also to the redirection of these intricate sensory systems to detect the doings of fellow living beings. These doings are often a matter of life and death – predator and prey contests, detection and attraction of sexual partners – and perception, assessment and decision have usually to be rapid. In the social mammals, amongst whom the hominidae are classed, this perception ascends to another level of sophistication where members of the group need to interact with each other to gain access to life preserving and reproductive resources. This social interaction requires insight into the 'intentions' of others and that is best achieved by the development of systems of 'mirror neurons', which allow empathic understanding. This, of course, leads directly into the emotional intelligence and social nous which underpin the human lifestyle; this is where Chapter 23 ends.

The twenty-fourth and final chapter steps back from the detailed science of sensory systems and examines the philosophical dimensions of this most philosophical of biological topics. From the times of Greek antiquity until today the problem of knowledge, how we come to know the nature of the world 'outside', has been a major theme in philosophical discussion. Sensory biology is clearly relevant to this discussion. But sensory biology also forces us

Biology of Sensory Systems, Second Edition   C.U.M. Smith
© 2008 John Wiley & Sons, Ltd

to lift our eyes beyond the narrow concentration of traditional epistemology on, exclusively, the human senses. At the beginning of biology, in Greek antiquity, Aristotle taught that 'every realm of nature is wonderful and has something to teach us'. This has certainly been the case as we have gone through the pages of this book. We have seen how very different many animal sensory worlds are from our own. A study of sensory physiology should thus prove a humbling experience to philosophers of mind. We cannot hope to have a 'God's eye' view of the world. Nevertheless, it is only our own sensory worlds of which we can have first hand experience. Do our fellow living beings 'live through' the same or similar 'qualia'? We cannot know. Thus we finish the book with some reflections on the implications of sensory physiology for epistemology and the philosophy of mind.

23

SUMMING UP

Molecular themes: membrane gates, G-protein systems, receptors - evolutionary relationships - G-protein signalling systems - G-proteins in protistans, eg. S cerevisiae - advantages of G-protein coupled signalling systems. **Cellular themes**: microvilli and immotile cilia - vertebrate hair cells - gustatory and olfactory cells - rod and cone outersegments - insect sensory sensilla; invertebrate rhabdomeric photoreceptors. **Sense organs**: great variety - convergent evolution - Matthiessen lenses - convergence of belemnoid and vertebrate eye; differentiation of sensory surfaces - vertebrate retinae - insect compound eyes - sexual dimorphism - dragonfly 'fovea' - olfactory mucosa - bat auditory fovea - specialisations of touch and electroreceptive surfaces - similarity of neural 'wiring' of retina and olfactory bulb **Central analysers** - maps of sensory information - lability of maps - possible origins of maps; refinement of trigger stimuli - auditory pathway - visual pathway - extraction of pattern from minimal data - illusions - conjecture and refutation - foreshadowing of scientific methodology; maps in invertebrate CNSs. **Homeostasis**: osmoregulation - CO_2/O_2 regulation - thermoregulation - homeostatic role of pain. **Sensory worlds** - the pusillanimity of anthropocentrism - polarisation of sunlight - electric fields - IR envelopes - sensory biases - bat sensory world - sensory worlds of invertebrates - Thomas Kuhn's philosophy of science prefigured - the liberatory nature of comparative sensory physiology. **From abiotic to biotic**: the sexual imperative - predator-prey wars - moth vs bat - sensitivity of major exteroreceptors limited only by physics - sensory implications of reproductive choreographies - social interaction - human sociality - autism - folk psychology - intentionality - implications of sensory biology for philosophy. **Mirror neurons**: characteristics – significance – non-cognitive understanding – human sociality. **Concluding remarks**: luciferous and lucriferous research

Looking back over the preceding chapters, can we discern any commonalities which recur across sense modalities and across phyla? In what follows we shall take for granted some of the fundamentals discussed in Chapter 3. All advanced animals use 'labelled lines' to separate sense modalities, all sensory cells are designed to respond most sensitively to one type of stimulus, the 'adequate' stimulus, and all signal intensity by way of impulse frequency. We reviewed all these features in Chapter 3 and also such universals as signal-to-noise ratios, just-noticeable differences, sensory adaptation, receptive fields and so on. In this chapter we shall look back, rather, to see if we can find any common design principles and any

Biology of Sensory Systems, Second Edition   C.U.M. Smith
© 2008 John Wiley & Sons, Ltd

universal, or near universal, trends. We shall proceed from the biochemical to the organismic to the social, starting at the molecular and cellular level and ending at the level of brains, the physiology of the entire organism and the interaction of organisms in communities.

23.1 MOLECULAR THEMES

This book is premised on the theory of organic evolution. It can, accordingly, be no surprise to find that at the molecular level striking similarities are to be found across both phyla and modality. For two thirds of life's history on the surface of the planet only micro-organisms, prokaryocytes, existed. The eukaryocytes and, later still, the multicellular Metazoa are a recent addition. Many of the molecular elements of sensory systems evolved before the latter appeared. They consist of membrane channels and gates, of receptor molecules evolved to recognize environmental agents and of G-protein membrane signalling systems. The sensory systems of metazoan animals have built upon and developed these ubiquitous elements.

The membrane channels and gates of the higher organisms are many and various. Very nearly all of them consist of alpha-helical subunits inserted through the phospholipid biomembrane. Sometimes these subunits consist of just one transmembrane alpha helix (e.g. the MinK and phospholemman Cl^--channels) but more frequently their polypeptide chains traverse the membrane more than once. In the simplest case the polypeptide chain makes two passes through the membrane. The chain has, in other words, two transmembrane segments (*2TM*). We saw that this was the case in the MscL mechanosensitive channel of *E. coli* (Chapter 6) and also for the case for the *degenerins* of *C. elegans* mechanoreceptors and the P2X and ASIC channels of mammalian nociceptors (Figure 23.1a). In these channels *three* subunits cluster together to form the channel. The next step up in subunit complexity is shown by members of the ligand-gated families of ionotropic receptors. These receptors, which are represented by glutamate receptors (*3TM*) and nACh receptors (*4TM*), are of great importance in postsynaptic membranes but need not detain us here. The next level of molecular complexity is shown by the

ubiquitous and evolutionarily ancient **transient receptor potential (TRP)** channels (Figure 23.1b). The polypeptide chains of the subunits of these channels make six passes through the membrane (*6TM*) and four subunits are grouped together around a central pore. The subunits of **cyclic-nucleotide**-gated *(CNG)* channels are similar: they all make six passes through the membrane and, again, four subunits cluster around a central pore. The yet more complex Na^+ and Ca^{2+} **voltage-gated channels** consist of four linked domains in each of which the polypeptide chain makes six membrane passes (*4 × 6TM*). These structures are large enough to form a cylinder through the membrane by themselves (Figure 23.1(c)). The nociceptive channels which respond to electrical stimuli differ, as we noted in Chapter 22, from those underlying action potentials in being insensitive to tetrodotoxin.

Analysis of the amino acid sequences of the molecular subunits of these channels brings out their evolutionary relationships. It is probable that the TRP stretch and temperature receptor channels along with Cl^- and K^+-channels are the most ancient of all, dating back to the prokaryotic world of three billion years ago. Voltage-gated channels (the K^+, Ca^{2+} and Na^+-channels) can be traced back to the protista and hence they probably originated some 1500 million years ago, perhaps by gene duplications linking four 6TM channels together.

Channels operated by biochemical agonists are the more recent. They probably did not appear until the earliest Metazoa. Sequence analysis of the proteins of gap junctions between metazoan cells shows that they are related to the units of channels operated by chemical agonists. The direct action of a chemical agonist on a channel in a sensory cell membrane is uncommon. Most such agonists work through a receptor-linked G-protein system. Exceptions to this rule are, however, found in gustatory cells sensitive to Na^+ and H^+ (Chapter 13), and the nociceptors (Chapter 22).

Most gustatory, and all olfactory and photoreceptor cells, make use of another ubiquitous molecular design (Chapters 13, 14 and 17). This is the **7TM 'serpentine'** structure, which is also found in the postsynaptic membrane receptors of many synapses (Figure 23.1(d)). We looked at the structure of 7TM receptors in Chapter 1. We noted in Box I4.1 that the 7TM structure is also well shown in the

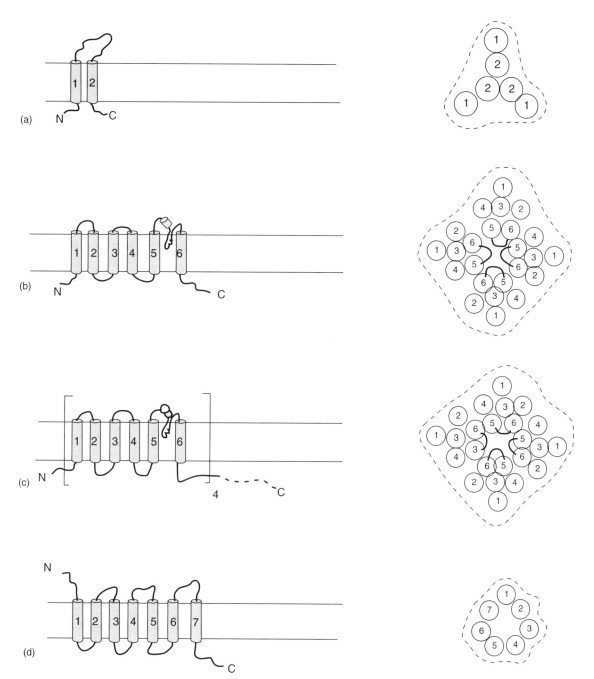

Figure 23.1 Molecular architecture of some membrane gates and channels. On the left the organzation of the α-helical segments of the subunits in the biomembrane; on the right the plan view of the arrangement of the subunits to form the channel. (a) 2TM subunits (MscL, degenerins, P2X, ASIC). Three subunits form the channel with TM segment 2 forming the lining. (b) 6TM subunits (TRP, CNG). Four subunits form the channel. The polypeptide 'hairpin' between TM5 and TM6 line the pore and provide the selectivity filter. (c) 4 × 6 TM units form voltage sensitive channels (VGSC-Rs) which signal electrical stimuli. It is believed that TM4 acts as the voltage sensor. (d) 7TM receptors (olfactory, photoreceptor, etc.). Three-dimensional illustrations of this ubiquitous design are shown in Figures 1.6b and I4.3b.

bacteriorhodopsin of the halophilic prokaryocyte, *Halobacterium halobium*. The amino acid sequence of bacteriorhodopsin is, however, not closely related to that of metazoan 7TM proteins. Although it seems difficult to accept that two such intricate and functionally similar molecular structures originated independently, the jury is still out. Indeed, support for an independent (polyphyletic) origin for 7TM architectures comes from the many seemingly unrelated 7TM olfactory receptor families found in the animal kingdom (Chapter 14). We cannot yet say whether all 7TM proteins are related and, perhaps, originated from similar architectures in ancient prokaryocytic membranes, or whether this apparently all-important design was hit upon independently, time after time, in the long evolutionary history of life forms on the surface of this planet.

In metazoan sensory cells 7TM receptors are linked to G-protein membrane signalling systems. This G-protein 'collision–coupling' mechanism is found in many other cells of the metazoan body. Indeed G-protein 'time switches' (as discussed in Section 1.4.1) can be traced all the way down into the unicellular protista. They have, for instance, been intensively studied in yeast, *Saccharomyces cerevisiae*. In this case, as in so many others, we find that a molecular device, once 'discovered' by evolution, is made use of time after time for greatly differing purposes. The 'second messengers', which are released into the cytosol as a consequence of activation of the G-protein mechanism, are again many and various and have numerous different functions. We saw G-protein coupled second messenger systems at work in gustatory cells, in olfactory cells and in various types of photoreceptor cells (both vertebrate and invertebrate). The great virtue of G-protein coupled second messenger systems is their great flexibility. The 7TM receptor is tailored to respond to a specific ligand (in the case of olfactory cells many 7TM receptors, tailored to many specific ligands; in the case of photoreceptors cells an embedded 'ligand', retinal, affected by a photon of appropriate wavelength). The receptor is coupled via the G-protein system to a variety of membrane-bound enzymes, in some cases adenylyl cyclase, in others cGMP-phosphodiesterase, in yet others phospholipase C and in others again, an ion channel and so on. The systems also allow considerable amplification and sustenance of the initial signal and permit interesting variations on the themes of sensory adaptation and desensitization.

23.2 CELLULAR THEMES

At the level of cells, sensory systems begin to lose their common properties. Nevertheless, certain obtrusive themes can still be discerned. Perhaps the most obvious of these is the ubiquity of immobile cilia and/or microvilli. We have noted that in all three major sense modalities, mechano-, chemo- and photo-, the receptor cells are frequently modified ciliary cells. This is spectacularly the case amongst the vertebrates but is also found in many of the invertebrates. Once again this is probably an instance of once having hit upon an effective device the evolutionary process has been able to select modifications which suit one sense modality or another.

In Chapter 9 we saw how vertebrate hair cells consist of a number of stereocilia (modified microvilli) and a single immobile true cilium, the kinocilium. In this case it is the stereocilia which present the mechanosensitive ion channels but it should, nevertheless, be noted that it is a ciliated cell which has been modified and pressed into service. We saw also, in Chapter 9, that the biophysical mechanism ensured that distortion of the hairs led, without intermediate mechanisms, to the opening of ion channels and hence direct stimulation of the hair cell. The mechanisms at work on chemo- and photoreceptor cells, depending on G-protein coupled second messenger signalling, are necessarily less instantaneous.

In Chapters 13 and 14 we noted how microvilli and immobile cilia provided the sensitive membranes for gustation and olfaction. The gustatory receptor cells develop thick brushworks of microvilli and the olfactory receptor cells produce very lengthy cilia that lie on the surface of the olfactory mucosa. In both cases, 7TM receptor molecules and G-protein signalling systems lie in their membranes. It would seem that the significance of the microvilli and immobile cilia in this instance is to increase the sensory surface area. This is also the case with ciliary photoreceptor cells. We saw in Chapter 17 that the outersegments of vertebrate rods and cones develop by multiple invagination of ciliary membranes. The photopigments and G-protein signalling systems are, once again, located in these membranes. Because the membranes are laid out at right angles to the incoming radiation the photopigments maximize their chance of collecting a photon.

The preceding paragraphs have focused on vertebrate sensory cells. Invertebrate sensory cells also show many common themes, some of which are shared with the vertebrates. Modified cilia make their appearance again in many insect sensory sensilla. In Chapter 8 we saw that, within its cuticular housing, the sensory cell terminates as an 'outersegment' whose ultrastructure shows it to be a modified cilium. Mechanosensitive sensilla, like vertebrate hair cells, do not, however, depend on the cilium to detect mechanical distortion but on a tubular body consisting of a mass of closely packed microtubules. Like vertebrate hair cells the mechanical stimulus leads directly to the opening of ion gates and the stimulation of the neurosensory cell. Whilst modified cilia form the basis of some invertebrate photoreceptors (Chapter 15), most are built on a different, a rhabdomeric, design principle. In this design the non-ciliary photosensitive terminal of the neurosensory cell is thrown out into a multitude of microvilli. These contain the photopigments, and the microvillar brushwork, like the internal lamellae of the vertebrate rod outersegment, ensures that they are laid out orthogonal to the incoming radiation. It is interesting to note, however, that vertebrate photoreceptor cells (at least in the lateral eyes) face away from the direction of the incoming light, whilst those of the invertebrates face towards it. It is also interesting to note that, whereas the vertebrate photoreceptor cells in the lateral eyes hyperpolarize in response to illumination, invertebrate receptors (mostly) depolarize. The vertebrates at some early stage in their evolution (and we discussed a plausible scenario in Chapter 16) seem to have got it all back to front!

23.3 SENSE ORGANS

Above the level of cells we come to those collocations of cellular units we know as sense organs. Here the variety becomes immense. If we include the whole of the animal kingdom, the multiplicity of different forms and designs must escape any single classification. Besides, there must be many yet to be discovered and, even amongst those which are known, not all

are fully understood. Nevertheless, certain interesting commonalities can be discerned.

In contrast to the commonalities at the molecular and cellular levels, these commonalities are mostly not due to descent from a common ancestor. Another principle is at work: convergent evolution. At the end of Chapter 4 we looked at the possibility that 750 million years of natural selection had 'discovered' that only a few designs ultimately make sense in the environments provided by the planet. In particular, our attention was directed at the great phyla of Mollusca, Arthropoda and Chordata. Similarly, with sense organs: our argument here, also, must be that the immensely long period of evolutionary 'winnowing' has resulted in rather analogous solutions to some of the major problems of sense organ design.

Perhaps the best known instance of these design solutions is the 'Matthiessen' lens (Chapter 19). The lenses of animal eyes have to be constructed from optically unpromising materials. In aquatic eyes the problem is particularly acute, as the refractive index between water and the cornea/lens would have to be higher than is achievable with biological materials if light is to be focused at an adequately short distance behind the lens. The solution 'found' (independently) at least eight times – in fish, annelids, copepod crustacea and in gastropod and cephalopod molluscs – is to vary the refractive index from the centre to the periphery of the lens. The selective advantage of accurate vision presumably forced the development of this outstanding example of convergent evolution in such disparate groups of aquatic animals.

The visual system provides many other examples of evolution converging on common solutions. The belemnoid eye (Chapter 15) shows remarkable similarities to the vertebrate eye. This is particularly interesting as, at the cellular level, the two eyes have a distinctively different design: the vertebrate photoreceptor being of the ciliary type compared with the rhabdomeric receptor of the mollusc. There are, of course, numerous other differences. The focusing of the lens is achieved by moving it forward and backward in the orbit (rather like a camera lens) instead of, as in the vertebrates, altering its curvature. The retina itself is 'verted' rather than 'inverted'. But even with these different elements, the overall design of the eye is remarkably like that developed from a very different base by the vertebrates, for highly active marine predators, squids and octopi depend, like sharks and barracuda, on accurate vision.

Another interesting commonality in the design of sense organs is the trend towards differentiation of the sensory surface. This is most obvious in the evolution of retinae. Mammalian retinae develop fovea where light during daytime vision is focused. Visual stimuli picked up by peripheral parts of the retina normally cause the eye to swivel so that they are relocated on the fovea. In many terrestrial mammals living on plains and savannahs, visual streaks are to be found in the retina (Chapter 19). This is probably an adaptation to the fact that the major visual input is concerned with predators and prey and these are mostly located with reference to the horizontal plane. Similar differentiations are found in the retinae of birds. Here (Chapter 19) more than one fovea may develop in addition to visual streaks and other specializations.

Turning to the very differently designed eyes of insects, we can find here, also, evidence of a similar specialization. In some Dipteran (Tabanid) and Ephemeropteran compound eyes there is a marked increase in ommatidial size in the forward and upwardly directed region of the eye's surface. This has been called the 'fovea'. Interestingly, it is only developed in male flies. It is believed to serve the male in finding a suitable female, whose small size might otherwise be lost against the background of the sky. Again, in the highly active and predaceous dragonflies (Odonata), which possess the most highly developed compound eyes of the insect world, there is clear evidence of specialization. The compound eyes of the Green Darner dragonfly, *Anax junius*, possess, for instance, an antero-dorsal strip where the number of ommatidia per unit area is some twenty times greater than in the postero-dorsal area. This foveal area scans forward in the flight path of the dragonfly to detect the tiny darting forms of its insect prey.

But this trend to specialization of the sensory surface is not confined to retinae. It is also evident in sensory surfaces devoted to other sense modalities. We noted in Chapter 14 that olfactory receptor cells are not arranged totally randomly, as might have been supposed, but show a tendency to several antero-posterior 'expression zones', each of which contains spatially organized groups of cells with differing susceptibilities to various odorants. An analogous spatial organization seems also to be present in the vomeronasal organs. But even more strikingly we noted, in Chapter 10, that the basilar membranes of echolocating bats are highly specialized, so that in some cases over 50% of their length is tuned to respond to echoes from the bat's characteristic acoustic signal. This region of the basilar membrane is, as we saw, consequently known as the auditory fovea. Finally, if we can consider the skin to be a sensory surface devoted to touch (or, in the case of weakly electric fish, to detect electric field), we can see again an incipient spatial organization. In the case of humans, the fingers or lips are brought into play when the texture of an object needs to be accurately determined; other mammals will use the muzzle, the trunk or the vibrissae. Finally the electroreceptors of weakly electric fish are distributed (Figure 21.9) in definite patterns over the body surface so that alignment in an electric field causes a definite pattern of activity in the sensory fibres leading into the central nervous system.

Lastly, turning to so-called 'wiring diagrams', it is interesting to note that there are significant parallels between the neurohistology of mammalian olfactory bulbs and retinae. We saw (Chapter 14) that output from the olfactory bulb makes its way through two layers of fibres arranged orthogonally to the exit direction. In Chapter 17 we saw that a similar wiring design is found in the retina. The output from the photoreceptor cells is moderated by passage through two layers of cells – the horizontal and amacrine cells – disposed at right angles to the main pathway. It is also interesting to note the ubiquity of crossovers in the neural pathways from retinae to optic lobes. These designs, as we saw in Chapter 15, are to be found in forms as diverse as crustacea, insects and cephalopods. That the evolutionary process has settled on these designs, in the one case across sense modalities, in the other case across phyla, must, as in the case of the Matthiessen lens, be telling us something about their effectiveness.

23.4 CENTRAL ANALYSERS

The central analysis of sensory information also shows interesting commonalities across modality and phyla. We saw in Chapters 8, 10 and 18 how the sensory surfaces (skin, basilar membrane and retina) are all mapped on to primary sensory cortices. In Chapter 14 we noted that, although the olfactory epithelium is not mapped, the olfactory bulb nevertheless contains a functional map of the odorant molecules present in the nasal cavity. These maps are often strikingly nonisomorphous and are certainly very labile. Indeed, it seems that subject to some genetic constraint the primary sensory cortices are allocated according to intensity of use. We saw something of this lability in Chapter 8 when discussing experimental manipulations of the numbers of mice vibrissae, the effect of overstimulation of monkey digits, the response of the human somaesthetic cortex to excessive use of the right index finger by Braille readers and we returned to it in Chapter 18 when discussing the primary visual cortex.

These, and other experiments, give us a clue to the ubiquity of sensory maps. Neurons that fire together strengthen synaptic links with each other. If a whisker or a digit is removed or inactivated, the cortical representation tends to disappear; it is invaded by cells responding to nearby whiskers or digits. If input to the primary visual cortex from a portion of the retina of one eye is blocked, its territory is occupied by cells responding to input from the equivalent portion of the other retina. It may be, therefore, that a long history (including evolutionary history) of temporal correlation of stimuli on a sensory surface leads to the formation of the topographic maps so characteristic of primary sensory cortices.

In contrast to the input into visual, somaesthetic and auditory systems, the temporal correlation of gustatory and/or olfactory input is not strong. We have seen that there is some differentiation of gustatory and olfactory surfaces in mammals and this is also (as we saw in Chapter 14) the case in some insects (e.g. *Drosophila* olfactory sensilla). But it is not obvious that tastant or odorant molecules affect these surfaces in any temporal order. Instead, similar tastant and odorant molecules affect specific groups of cells. In the case of odorants these groups of cells are, in the vertebrates, randomly distributed in the mucosa. The projections from these 'tuned' cells, which are all stimulated at much the same time by a specific odour in the nasal cavity, all end in the same olfactory glomeruli. Hence, although there is not a spatial map of the sensory surface in the olfactory bulb, there is, nevertheless, a spatially organized map of the active chemicals in the inspired air. The principle of spatial mapping is also, as we noted in

Chapter 9, extended to quite abstract phenomena, phenomena which have no spatial representation on the sensory surface at all, such as auditory space (barn owl) and target range (microchiropteran bats). Indeed, the principal of organizing information by spatial mapping in the brain may have wider relevance still. There is a suggestion that there may be phonemic and even semantic maps in the human brain.

Turning from the topic of sensory maps we can note, next, that another feature shared by the auditory and visual pathways is a continuous refinement of the stimuli which trigger activity in their cells. More and more specific features are necessary to elicit activity as the pathway is ascended. We noted in Chapter 10 that by the time the auditory cortex is reached, the pure tones and sudden clicks to which neurons lower in the pathway had responded are no longer effective. Instead, cells in the temporal lobe respond best to frequency-modulated tones and even more specifically, in macaques and squirrel monkeys, to the calls of conspecifics, sometimes those of particular individuals. This, of course, is paralleled in the mammalian visual cortices. Spots of light on the retina do not trigger responses in most of the cells of the primary visual cortex. Instead, edges of particular orientations and often with other specific characteristics are the trigger stimuli. Further up in the visual system, in, for example, the monkey's inferotemporal lobe, electrophysiologists have found analogous cells to the call recognition cells of the auditory cortex. These are the face recognition cells (Chapter 18) which are triggered by other monkey faces, often being sensitive to profile or full face and sometimes, once again, to particular individuals.

Another common feature of the cerebral analysis of sensory information is the ubiquity of parallel processing. This is especially marked where the sensory input is loaded with significant detail. We noted that primate visual analysis is carried out by upwards of two dozen visual areas, all complexly interconnected. Similarly, bat auditory analysis is carried out by at least nine different areas. Awake mammalian cerebral cortices are shifting mosaics of activity. How all this activity is combined together to give a unitary sensory awareness is (as we noted in Section 3.6) known as the '**binding problem**' and remains one of the great unsolved problems of contemporary sensory neurophysiology.

A further characteristic of sensory systems, again most strikingly shown by auditory and visual systems, is their susceptibility to 'illusion' and to the 'flip/flops' of categorical perception: the Necker cube, the switch from /ba/ to /da/. This susceptibility is a consequence of the evolutionary imperative for quick decision-taking. Auditory and visual systems pick up huge quantities of data from the environment. It is vital that 'meaning' or 'pattern' is extracted from this data as rapidly as possible. An animal's life and prospect of perpetuating its germ line into the future frequently depends upon this ability. Thus, when the auditory system picks up the snap of a twig, the fight or flight response is immediately triggered. Similarly, when the human auditory system picks up a certain spectrum of pressure waves in the atmosphere, it may interpret it as 'I scream' or 'ice cream'. It depends on the context. The visual system is subject to analogous illusions. There are innumerable examples. The young woman/old woman disjunction is a well known instance (Figure 23.2). Depending on context, the visual image is intepreted as a young woman looking away or an old woman in profile.

The brain's propensity to jump to conclusions which are 'underdetermined' by the sensory input, its drive to 'make sense' of the environment, is an aspect of its general functioning as a hypothesis generating machine. Those of a philosophical disposition may connect this propensity with Karl Popper's well known characterization of science as 'conjecture and refutation'. In Popper's view, science perpetually throws up hypotheses (conjectures) to explain the phenomena of the natural world and the more easily falsifiable (refutable) these are, the better. We can see that this high level human procedure builds upon the evolutionarily inbuilt processes by which brain attempts to impose meaning on the mass of sensory data flowing in upon it from the major senses. We have also seen (Sections 16.4, 22.1 and 24.6), and shall see again in Chapter 24, that there is evidence to suggest that output messages are sent against which the input is compared. Fortunately, as Popper points out, in the case of science it is the hypothesis not the scientist that dies when falsification occurs.

Turning from these somewhat controversial issues in the philosophy of science back to the neuroscience itself, we should not finish this section without observing that the sensory maps with which we have become so familiar in mammalian systems are also

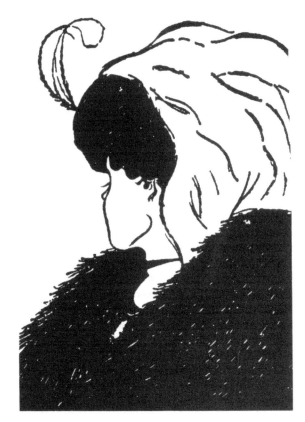

Figure 23.2 Young woman/old woman.

found in other animal central nervous systems. We saw in Chapter 15 that retinotopic maps are found in optic laminae and other, higher, regions of the Dipteran brain and there is no doubt that similar maps are generated in the optic pathways of other orders of advanced insects. We also saw in that chapter that the neuroanatomy of the belemnoid visual system indicates that the topographical relations of the visual image are preserved through several layers of analyser. It is unfortunate that, to date, it has not proved possible to make microelectrode recordings from these layers.

23.5 HOMEOSTASIS

Homeostasis has been another recurrent theme. We noted in Chapter 12 the central position this concept has occupied in physiological thought since the mid-nineteenth century. We first dealt with it in detail in Chapter 6 when considering stretch receptors in cell membranes. In unicellular forms these were vital in sensing osmotic stress. This same parameter is significant in the far more complex bodies of the Metazoa and in Chapter 6 we discussed the best known case, the maintenance of osmolarity in the ECF of mammals. This requires the osmolarity of plasma to be sensed by osmoreceptor cells, and we saw that these cells were located in the hypothalamus. In Chapter 12, we looked at the analogous role which chemoreceptors play in maintaining constant levels of respiratory gases in the ECF. Chemoreceptors sensitive to partial pressures of carbon dioxide and oxygen are located in the carotid bodies, the aortic arch and the medulla. Once again, when partial pressures of carbon dioxide and/or oxygen depart from a 'set level', complex physiological mechanisms come into play, principally affecting the respiratory system, to ensure that they are brought back to that level as rapidly a possible. Then, in Chapter 20, we considered the intricate array of thermosensitive endings in mammalian skin and other organs. When the body's core temperature begins to move away from the appropriate value, the input from these thermosensitive fibres is integrated by centres in the hypothalamus (these centres are themselves directly sensitive to the temperature of blood in neighbouring capillaries) and messages are sent out to alter the rate of the body's heat production and (more precisely) to alter the body's heat loss.

But perhaps the most interesting and pressing case of the senses involved in homeostasis is provided by the topic discussed in Chapter 22: pain. We saw in that chapter some of the unexpected features of this (near) universal sense. We saw, in particular, that our experience of pain is controlled by 'gates' at the level of the spinal cord and by downward fibre pathways from the brain. Yet we all know that these physiological mechanisms operate below, or outside, the realm of consciousness. We cannot by thinking switch off the pain of a raging toothache, the long continued ache of the back or the sharp pains of cancer. But these unpleasant experiences (none of them qualitatively quite the same) have, we argued in Chapter 22, a biological purpose. In a sense that purpose comes under the heading of homeostasis. The imperative demands of pain, its overwhelming call upon our attention, have to do with the body's need to put itself in a position to recuperate from life-threatening damage.

23.6 DIFFERENT SENSORY WORLDS

The unpleasantness of pain, the pain of pain, is quite likely central to the life of all animals. Its life-preservative functions suggest that it appeared early in the evolutionary scale. Powerful self-protective reflexes are built around it, not least conditioned reflexes. But other aspects of the sensory worlds of animals are many and various. This has been another theme which has recurred in the preceding pages. It has been a salutary theme, as it is all too easy for citizens of the Western world, increasingly removed from contact with natural world by technology, to fall into human-centred epistemologies. A study of animal sensory systems provides a valuable antidote to this pervasive anthropocentricity.

Animals often live in very different sensory worlds from our own. von Uexküll coined the term '**umwelt**' to describe this internalized structure. A nice example is provided by Zeil and Zanker. They have carried out a fascinating study on the sensory world of fiddler crabs (*Uca* spp.). Living in burrows in sand or mudflats, these crabs emerge and become active at low tide. Their eyes are positioned on the ends of long stalks and are held upwards to detect predators and the conspecific signals generated by other males semaphoring with a massively enlarged claw. Their visual world is largely two-dimensional – the vast majority of significant events occur in a narrow band at the level of the horizon. Zeil and Zanker's analysis brings out how the biologically relevant information of their accustomed habitat drives the evolution of their 'sensory filters and neural processing strategies'. In addition to their visual analysers, their other senses, especially those sensitive to vibration, touch and chemical substances, are also likely to be rather precisely attuned to their natural environment. A combination of precise sensory physiology and sensitive ethological analysis promises to provide us with insights into alien 'umwelten' such as these.

We have emphasized the 'foreignness' of these umwelten throughout the book but perhaps especially in Chapter 21. There we considered how polarization of sunlight makes the sky seem radically different to our own customary (well, sometimes) blue dome to animals able to sense it; how minute gradations in electric field contours make the aquatic environment a more heterogeneous and interesting place for weakly electric fish; how the flux of radiant heat in the immediate environment carries life preserving information to certain snakes. But, more generally we have seen how all the major senses are differently biased, differently adapted, in different members of the animal kingdom. We meditated, more than once, on the famous philosophical question: what is it like to be a bat? Its senses provide a radical contrast to our own: instead of a powerful orientation towards vision, bats are biased towards the auditory modality. So dominant is the auditory sense that, as we saw in Chapter 10, there are many interesting analogies to our own imperial sense – vision. Although we might have some vanishingly small inkling of what it be like to be a bat – after all the blind and partially sighted live in a primarily auditory world – we can hardly hope to catch a glimmer of the sensory worlds of the members of the two other great evolutionary groups considered in this book: the arthropods and molluscs. Does the fiddler crab approached by another male waving its outsized claw feel the same rush of emotion as we would when presented with, say, a raised fist? Does the squid, backed up into its rocky crevice staring out at us through the aquarium glass with its rectangular black pupils, 'see' as we 'see'? Does the platypus diving in the murky waters of antipodean ponds experience a three-dimensional world based on quite different senses than ours – electroreceptors and 'push-rod' mechanosensors? Does an insect, a dragonfly, say, 'see' with its magnificent compound eyes in the sense in which we 'see'? The insect world, too, is full of olfactory and gustatory signals (Chapter 13 and 14) which make their worlds radically different from our own chemically impoverished, plastic packaged, environment.

Again we are in the vicinity of some of the philosophical issues we shall touch on in Chapter 24. The question of sensory qualia has loomed large amongst these issues and we touched on it in several places in the preceding chapters. We shall return to it a final time in Chapter 24. The idea, too, that differing interpretations of sensory inputs by humans living in different human cultures, or in different historical epochs, means that in some sense they live in different worlds has been much discussed by philosophers following Hanson and, especially, Thomas Kuhn. If, as Kuhn suggests, thinkers before and after the Galilean revolution in the seventeenth century lived in different worlds, how much more so must differ-

ent animals. This emphasizes the point with which we started this section: study of animal sensory systems liberates us from a narrow anthropocentricity. It can help us open our eyes (to use the common anthropocentric metaphor) to numerous, very different, possible worlds.

23.7 FROM ABIOTIC TO BIOTIC: COMMUNICATION

The final recurrent theme which our subject has brought out is the ineluctable progress from sensory systems detecting happenings in the inorganic environment towards detecting happenings in the biological world. In the beginning the physical world was all that there was. The earliest sensory systems evolved to detect the various life threatening and/or life enhancing changes in that world. But soon that world became full of other living things. Soon, too, the necessity of finding a mate, if 'selfish DNA' was to propagate itself, became of consuming interest to the members of most animal groups. The senses became more and more directed not only to avoiding the traps and opportunities of the abiotic environment but also, and increasingly, to detecting those of the biotic environment. The long war between predator and prey commenced. This contest placed a life and death premium on accurate and rapidly reacting sense organs, just as it placed (as we saw above) a premium on rapid assessment of the sensory input by the analysers in the central nervous system. In particular, we looked at the fascinating evolutionary contest between moth and inectivorous bat in Chapters 8 and 10. Similar 'arms races' are happening throughout the animal kingdom. All of them lead to a continuous sharpening of the sense organs. We saw in Chapters 10, 14 and 17 that the major exteroreceptors – hair cells, olfactory receptor cells and rod cells – are just about as sensitive to their adequate stimuli as physics allows.

But predator–prey arms races are not the only pressures on sensory systems. We have already noticed the equally powerful pressures asserted by the necessity to find a mate. We saw the huge sensitivity that this induces in such magnificent sensory systems as the olfactory sensilla fields of silk moth antennae, which are able to detect single molecules of the appropriate sex pheromone (Chapter 14). The literature of ethology is crowded with reports of the visual, auditory and olfactory cues and sign stimuli which animals of all phyla use to detect mates and to choreograph reproductive rituals. But further than this, sensory cues and signals are at the core of the life of social animals. E.O. Wilson points out that there are four great peaks of sociality in the animal world: the colonial invertebrates, the social insects, the nonhuman mammals and humans. We saw something of the significance of olfactory cues in the life of social insects (Chapter 14) and such cues are also crucial in the social life of the canidae. In Chapter 8 we noted how the tactile senses activated by mutual grooming helped cement the bonds that hold troops of social primates together.

Amongst that group of social primates to which we belong, the hominidae, all five of the exteroreceptors, especially seeing, hearing and touch, are profoundly involved in observing, responding to and interacting with others. Humans, as noted above, live in an intensely human world, an intensely social world. In spite of occasional (and probably erroneous) reports of 'wolf' children, humans depend for their humanity on sociality. An inability to enter this social world is generally thought to be the defect which expresses itself in the rages of the **autistic**.

In literate societies, sociality is not only achieved by interaction with contemporaries but also with a host of those who have gone before. This involvement with the past, present and predicted future doings of others generates what many have dubbed a 'folk psychology'. We attribute to others a subjectivity such as we experience ourselves. In particular we attribute to them something which we do not attribute to the inorganic world of sticks and stones, wind and water: **intentionality**. We believe, in other words, that they act with an end in view. Here we approach the subject matter of the next section and the next chapter. We have already observed that the subject matter of sensory systems is only narrowly demarcated from that of important fields of philosophy. As we have proceeded through this penultimate chapter, we have continuously bumped up against this demarcation. In the next chapter we shall breach it altogether and end the book with an outline discussion of some of these philosophical issues. Before doing so, let us look briefly at one of the most exciting developments in contemporary brain research: mirror neurons.

23.8 FROM BIOTIC TO SOCIAL COMMUNICATION: MIRROR NEURONS

We have noted in the preceding section the slow evolutionary shift of the focus of sensory systems from abiotic to biotic phenomena. In this final section we complete this shift by discussing the attributes of so-called '**mirror neurons**', which were first found in monkey brains but are much more fully developed in the brains of hominids. They underly the human ability to attribute to others the sense of purpose which forms the tissue of their own subjective lives.

Mirror neurons were first discovered in the early 1990s by Rizzolatti and others. They form a special class of neurons found the in upper part of area F5 of the monkey's premotor cortex (Figure 23.3). Subsequent investigation have detected neurons with mirroring properties in other parts of the brain, in the anterior part of the parietal lobe (area PF) and along the superior temporal sulcus (STS). These neurons discharge when the animal carries out a particular action and, and this is the important point, they also discharge when the monkey observes another individual (monkey or human) carrying out a similar action. In consequence, mirror neurons are sometimes called 'monkey see, monkey do' neurons.

Mirror neurons do not respond to the simple presentation of an object but only when that object is caught up in an intentional action. They do not, in other words, respond to the mere sight of an object, nor do they respond to an agent imitating an action or making gestures which do not refer to the object. They are, additionally, capable of generalization. A

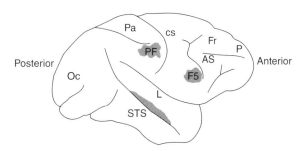

Figure 23.3 Lateral view of macaque brain to show the location of mirror neurons (stippled areas). AS = arcuate sulcus; CS = central sulcus; Fr = frontal lobe; L = lateral (Sylvian) fissure; Oc = occipital lobe; P = principal sulcus; Pa = parietal lobe; STS = superior temporal sulcus. After Rizzollatti, G. and Criaghero, L. (2004).

mirror neuron will respond to both the grasping action of a monkey's hand and that of a human hand; it will respond whether that action occurs close by or at a distance. Furthermore, it is not important whether or not the monkey is rewarded: the discharge is the same if the object grasped, say a banana, is given to the monkey or to another monkey. It is the action of grasping an object, the intentional act, which activates the mirror cell.

Mirror neurons thus provide a means by which the monkey nervous system repeats the intentional action of another individual. This motoric repetition is not confined to the grasping activity of the hand. Mirror neurons in another part of the cortex, the superior temporal sulcus, respond to intentional movements of the arms, head and torso. In particular, there is a strong input to mouth neurons situated in the lateral part of F5. When a monkey observes another monkey grasping food with the mouth, breaking it up, chewing and so on, these neurons are strongly activated. There is good evidence that the same neuron discharges both when the monkey observes another monkey biting food (or in attack and/or defence) and when the monkey itself bites and chews food. Interestingly, also, there is a smaller group of neurons in this part of the premotor cortex which discharge to lip-smacking behaviour, although these also discharge when the monkey itself actively ingests food.

It has also been shown that some mirror neurons do not depend on visual input but are also activated by input from the auditory system. In one experiment a recoding was made from an F5 mirror neuron whilst the monkey observed a noisy action, in this case the intentional ripping of a piece of paper. When the recorded sound of this ripping was played back to the monkey with no visual input the same F5 neuron again discharged. It turns out that some 15% of macaque mirror neurons respond in this way. These neurons have consequently been named 'audio-visual' mirror neurons.

Do mirror neurons also exist in humans? Clearly it is not possible to carry out microelectrode penetrations in human subjects. Fortunately, a number of sophisticated noninvasive techniques for investigating the activity of the cerebral cortex now exist. These techniques include electroencephalography (EEG), magnetoencephalography (MEG), transcranial magnetic stimulation (TMS), functional mag-

netic resonance imaging (fMRI) and so on. Application of these techniques leaves no doubt that a mirror neuron system exists in the human cortex. A recent fMRI study, for instance, in which volunteers were shown silent videos of dogs, humans and monkeys biting, lip smacking, barking and so on, showed that in all cases foci in the inferior parietal cortex were activated. These foci are the same as those activated when humans themselves bite or move their lips. The discovery of so many mirror neurons activated by mouth movements has suggested that similar neurons in humans might be activated in response to human facial expressions. Could this be connected to the fact that so much emotional communication occurs via facial expression?

From these and many other experiments the anatomical location of the human mirror neuron has been revealed (Figure 23.4). There are two major regions: an anterior region in the inferior frontal gyrus, within Broca's area and close to the premotor cortex, and a posterior area in the inferior parietal lobe. This posterior region is the human homologue of the

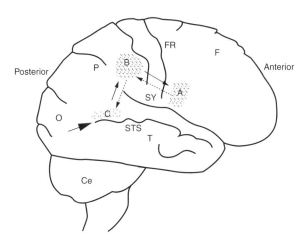

Figure 23.4 Lateral view of the human brain to show the location of the mirror neuron system. The two principal mirror neuron areas in the ventral premotor cortex/inferior frontal gyrus (A) and the inferior parietal lobe (B) are stippled. The arrows show the flow of information from the visual areas in the occipital lobe to the superior temporal sulcus (STS) and then to mirror neurons at B and A. The broken arrows show the return route of the efference copy. A = ventral premotor cortex/inferofrontal gyrus; B = inferior parietal lobe; C = posterior superior temporal sulcus. Ce = cerebellum; F = frontal lobe; FR = fissure of Rolando; O = occipital lobe; STS = superior temporal sulcus; SY = sylvian fissure; T = temporal lobe. After Iacoboni, M. and Dapretto, M. (2006).

macaque PF area. It can be seen from the figure that the system is strategically placed between a visual input from the posterior part of the superior temporal sulcus and the motor areas of the premotor cortex. The way in which the system is believed to work is also shown in Figure 23.4. A visual 'description' of the observed action is sent from the visual areas in the occipital lobe via the superior temporal sulcus to the parietal area and then on to the inferior frontal cortex, close to the premotor area. An 'efference copy' of imitative activity in the premotor cortex is then sent back to the parietal area and then on to the visual area in the superior temporal sulcus so that it can be matched with the observed behaviour.

The discovery and investigation of mirror neurons has influenced wide areas of cognitive neuroscience. The fact that the anterior part of the system is located within the general confines of Broca's area suggests that the system could have been implicated in the evolution of language. We noted in Section 10.7 that Broca's area is intimately concerned in organizing the muscular movements required in linguistic pronounciation. It is argued by some that this muscular activity is captured by the mirror neuron system of the listener directly, without cognitive mediation. It is interesting to note that monkey vocal calls are also processed in this area of the brain, suggesting (as noted in Section 10.7) that a neural substrate for the development of language could have existed in primate brains for tens of millions of years. It has to be said, however, that unlike the lateralized anatomy of the human speech areas both the mirror neuron system and the areas responsive to species-specific calls in the macaque brain are bilateral. There is some evidence, however, to suggest that whilst the human brain has a bilateral visuo-motor mirror neuron system a multimodal (visual, auditory, motor) mirror neuron system only exists in the left hemisphere. If this turns out to be the case it will give powerful support to fundamental importance of the mirror neuron system in the evolution and neurophysiology of language.

Thus, in conclusion, we can see that the discovery of the mirror neuron system in primate brains has been highly important and highly suggestive. The system provides a basis for 'empathic' action understanding. It allows a primate to feel on its own pulses the intention of a fellow primate, or indeed other organism. Cognitive analysis is short circuited. We

can see that it provides a 'hard' neurophysiological basis for the development of the social human 'life style' outlined in the previous section of this chapter. Seeing a member of the social group perform a goal-directed action, the primate and, especially the hominid, understands empathically the meaning of the action. He or she experiences the same discharge of visuo-motor or audio-visual motor mirror neurons as he would if he or she were undertaking the same action. It is also easy to see that disorders of this system could have profound consequences. One of the most important of these consequences could be the defective social interaction which lies at the root of autism.

In conclusion, can we generalize yet further and speculate that the mirror neuron system provides a basis for self awareness, of which the beginnings can be found in the higher primates and which is so strongly developed in normal humans? Nicholas Humphrey has dubbed the social animals 'Nature's psychologists'. All higher animals, as we have seen, form models of their environment of one sort or another and Humphrey argues that the social mammals include the social environment in this model. He suggests that in order to forecast the actions of its fellows, a social animal needs to develop a model of the other's past and present behavioural patterns. This suggestion is clearly powerfully supported by the discovery of mirror neurons. They allow an individual to 'feel' the motive and purpose behind the other's activity. It is no great step from this to a recognition that it itself is a player in the social game. In focusing on the behaviour of others in a close-knit society and becoming aware that this focus is reciprocated, the individual cannot help but become self-aware.

23.9 CONCLUDING REMARKS

In this chapter a number of recurrent themes and trends have been picked out and reviewed. The student may discern others. The subject matter of sensory biology is vast and continuously expanding. It cannot be constrained within the covers of any single text. Each small topic, indeed each small subtopic, contains much that is unknown, much that provides material for fascinating research. This research, like all good research, can encompass and combine two motives. Francis Bacon, long ago in the sixteenth century, defined these as **luciferous** and **lucriferous**. Research into sensory systems can help us increase our knowledge of these systems, relate them to other animal systems and/or to other sensory modalities, throw light on ethology, on molecular biology, on evolution. This is Bacon's light-giving, luciferous research, a study motivated principally to find out what is the case, in the same way as the conquerors of Everest 'excused' their endeavour by saying 'just because it's there'.

But research into sensory systems also has the other motive and the other outcome. In increasing our understanding of sensory systems it can point to ways of mending them when they go wrong. The study of sensory systems is of great applied value to medical science. In Chapter 22 we looked at alarming statistics showing the quantity of lower back pain (and its economic consequences) in the Western world. Similar dismal statistics could be quoted to quantify the human suffering caused by defects of the auditory and visual systems. Bacon's lucriferous

motive, to take his definition in a broad sense, is not just to do with finance but also with the application of knowledge to ameliorate suffering in the world. The straightforward, commercial motive also operates, of course, on occasion. Artificial 'noses' in the world of viniculture and all the variety of sensory prostheses which are becoming available, from hearing aids to artificial vision to neuromuscular prostheses, doubtless underpin a significant and growing biological engineering sector of the economy. However, in the next and last chapter of this book, we revert to that most, or apparently most, unapplied of human concerns: philosophy. It is perhaps the most powerful exemplar of Bacon's luciferous studies. We started this book with the famous quotation from the beginning of Aristotle's *Metaphysics*: 'All men desire to know...'. It is thus fitting that we should end our account of the biology of sensory systems by examining how far the study of these systems impacts on that most central of Aristotelian concerns: first philosophy.

24

PHILOSOPHICAL POSTSCRIPT

Descartes: cogito - method of doubt - res cogitans - res extensa - problem of epistemology. **Qualia:** incorrigible - 'easy' problems and the 'hard problem' - is the human mind cognitively closed to its solution? **Tabulae rasa**: innate ideas? - empiricists - simple and compound ideas - Kant's 'Copernican revolution' - influence on Muller and Helmholtz. **Epigenetic epistemology:** Molineux's question - cataract operations - Spencer's epigenetic epistemology - origins of the Kantian a priori - origin of 'subjective'/'objective' classification - origin of the concept of 'energy'. **Evolutionary epistemology** – Darwin - Spencer - Nietzsche - evolutionary diversity - behavioural 'preparedness' - Darwinian 'algorithms' - Wason tests of conditional reasoning - explanations in terms of social contracts and cheater detection - sex-related differences in spatial reasoning. **Beyond Descartes**: Descartes' theory of vision - counter-examples - stabilised images, Mondrians, directedness of saccades – action- orientated perception - pain and the prioritisation of behaviour - brain as a hypothesis generator. **Concluding remarks**: humans not passive 'cameras' but 'netted' into the natural world - the ongoing problem of qualia - beginnings and endings

The origins of philosophy, like the origins of science, are lost in prehistory. Conventionally, both are traced to the great figures of Greek antiquity but human curiosity about the nature of things and how things work must have long predated that comparatively recent era. The origins of the modern phase of philosophy and science are taken to be even more recent and, again rather arbitrarily, located in the intellectual reawakenings of the sixteenth and seventeenth centuries. In our subject of neuroscience, sensory biology and epistemology, one name stands out: that of René Descartes (1596–1650).

24.1 DESCARTES

René Descartes was born on 31 March in the small village of La Haye near Tours, deep in the French countryside. From the first he showed signs of intellectual brilliance, his father called the child his 'philosopher' and he received one of the best educations available at that time in the Jesuit Lycée Henri IV at La Flèche. He discovered the position for which he is almost universally known – *cogito ergo sum*, I think therefore I am – whilst taking part in the wars in what is now Germany and meditating in a

Biology of Sensory Systems, Second Edition   C.U.M. Smith
© 2008 John Wiley & Sons, Ltd

stove- heated room at Ulm. Although the 'cogito' is not as original as many have assumed (St. Augustine had something very similar in the fifth century AD), Descartes was able to argue for it with such clarity that some have maintained that that November night in 1619 marked the birth of the modern world.

What was it that Descartes discovered? Like many other thinkers Descartes was obsessed with the desire for certainty. He felt that all the great intellectual edifices of his times were built on dubious foundations. His ambition was to cast away loose earth and sand (as he writes) and discover bedrock. His method was one of radical doubt. He was quite prepared to doubt the reports of his senses for, as he says, we are all subject to illusion. He was even prepared to doubt the demonstrations of mathematics, for he had observed that he and others were prone to mistakes and perhaps they contained hidden and erroneous assumptions. But as he sat in that stove-heated room at Ulm wrestling with this problem, it was borne in upon him that he could hardly doubt, whilst passionately doubting, that doubt was occurring. This would be truly self-contradictory. He believed that he had finally struck bedrock. *Je pense, donc je suis.*

That he could not doubt that thinking was occurring whilst thinking seemed beyond question. That alone seemed certain. All else could be illusion, as when we seem to feel a phantom limb although it has long been lost or when, in attacks of jaundice, the world takes on a yellowish tinge due to bile pigments accumulating in the eyes. Descartes concluded that he was, in essence, a thinking substance: *res cogitans*. In contrast, the world 'outside' of which the senses gave perhaps dubious report seemed to Descartes to be characterized at root by the spatial dimension. For, he argued (*Principles of Philosophy*, Part 2, Chapter 4), it is at least conceivable that whenever we stretched our hands to touch a body it might retreat and escape palpation. But if this, *per impossibile*, did happen, they would not thereby lose their nature as bodies. Hence 'hardness', 'impenetrability' cannot be a necessary feature. Rather it is the having of 'length, breadth and depth'. This world of spatial dimension, of which as a geometrician of genius he was so well aware, he accordingly refers to as *res extensa*. The question then obtrudes: how is the world of *res extensa* related to the world of *res cogitans*? This is the classic mind–body problem which has troubled philosophers ever since.

Related to the mind–body problem are the problems of epistemology. If the reports of the senses are always open to doubt, how can we be sure that the world is as we think it to be? A modern version of this problem asks how we can be sure that we are not mere 'brains in a vat' with the sensory nerves being skilfully stimulated. Descartes circumvents this problem by appeal to a version of the ontological proof for the existence of a just and beneficent Deity. The ontological proof need not detain us (students can find it in the *Discourse*, Part 4) for few nowadays accept it but it gave Descartes what he needed. For a just and beneficent Deity would not deceive his creatures by sending illusory messages along their sensory nerves. But for us, where proofs of the existence of God are difficult to find, the Cartesian position throws the epistemological problem into sharp relief: is knowledge (certain belief) possible? How can we be sure that our senses do not deceive us, perhaps systematically deceive us?

24.2 QUALIA

Descartes' method of radical doubt still seems, 350 years later, to lead to an important insight. We cannot doubt whilst experiencing 'red', or 'pain', or 'middle C' that these experiences are occurring. It may be that they refer to nothing in the world 'outside' the skin. After all it could merely be that some neurochemical disturbance in the appropriate brain region is taking place, and nothing else. But that we are 'living through' these experiences seems indisputable. Could any outside observer, any authoritarian physician, be in a position to deny that experience? To ask the question immediately invites a negative answer. We, the experiencers, have 'privileged access'; our privacy, in this matter, is inviolable. and just as our privacy is inviolable, so we can never express to another the quality or indeed the quantity of the experience we are living through.

There have been many attempts to bring out this strangeness in the heart of our world. To those schooled in science perhaps the most striking of these attempts were the thought experiments with a fictional instrument called an autocerebroscope, discussed by Herbert Feigl and others in the 1960s. With the great advances in neuroimaging which occurred in the closing decades of the twentieth and beginnings of the twenty-first centuries this instrument is rapidly emerging from the realms of fantasy into those of reality. PET and fMRI devices enable us to track changes in the brain as mental activity takes place. MEG promises the possibility of tracking these changes in real time. But even supposing that, in some Utopian future, the full molecular and biophysical happenings in the cerebrum could be recorded whilst the subject reported 'living through' a sharp and nagging pain, we would still have no inkling of what that pain 'was like' except by comparing it with comparable experiences of our own. Similarly, it is quite possible to suppose that in some future time a neuroscientist might be able to record all the goings-on in a patient's brain while the patient suffered tinitus but, being congenitally deaf himself or herself, have not even the beginnings of a notion of what was being experienced. Vice versa, painters can provide magnificent evocations of the qualia induced by sunsets over water, without the beginnings of a notion of the neuroscience of the visual cortices.

Is this not strange? Our subjective lives are filled with colour, scents, sounds, tastes, joys and pains and yet our science seems to be totally ignorant of them all. In normal life, even the normal life of the neuroscience laboratory, this oddity goes unnoticed. Most of the time, for most of us, we can proceed as if the problem did not exist. Yet for those who do notice it, it seems to be a deep fracture in our world view. In recent years, with the great advances in our study of the neurosciences, the problems of brain and mind have been conveniently divided into two great categories: the 'easy' (or, perhaps better, 'tough') problems and the **hard problem**. The 'easy problems' are, of course, often technically very difficult and many of them have yet to be solved. They include many of the topics discussed in the foregoing pages of this book: how nerve fibres conduct impulses, how receptor cells respond to stimuli, how brains analyse sensory input. In other areas of neuroscience, the problems include memory and motor output, growth and development, disease and degeneration. All of them are subjects of intense research and all present their difficulties. But all of them fall within the remit of the scientific method. No new principle is involved. But the hard problem is something else. How the multitudinous physical changes in the brain relate to what is known as the 'phenomenology', the 'experience', in short, the 'qualia',

is the hard problem. There have been many attempts to provide a solution: none, in my view, successful. Interested students should consult some of the books listed in the bibliography. Many, like Colin McGinn (and indeed René Descartes), are prepared to leave it as an area to which the human mind is (like the canine mind is to differential calculus) 'cognitively closed'.

24.3 TABULA RASA?

Do we come into the world with our minds already stored with knowledge or has everything we know as adults come through the senses? Descartes, who is usually credited with believing that our minds contain innate ideas, is in fact very reticent. He is only definite about one such idea: the idea of God. Further back in history, Plato was far less circumspect. In a famous dialogue, the *Meno*, he describes how the demonstrations of geometry, including the pythagorean theorem, may be drawn from an unlettered slave. For Plato, mathematical and other formal knowledge was implanted before birth and hence education was essentially a matter of recollection. This was not, however, how it seemed to the British empiricist philosophers in the century succeeding Descartes' death.

Thomas Hobbes (1588–1679) was in fact born eight years before René Descartes. But, dying in his ninetieth year, he outlived the French philosopher by nearly thirty years. He had corresponded with Descartes, pressing him about the notion of innate ideas. For Hobbes, like the later British empiricists, believed that we come into the world innocent of all inborn ideas. The mind, he said, is a **tabula rasa**, a blank tablet, on which experience writes. There is, he insisted, 'no conception in a man's mind which hath not first, totally, or by parts, been begotten upon the organs of sense. The rest are derived from that original'. This, of course, is as much an assumption on Hobbes' part as Plato's contrary opinion. It did, however, fit in well with the rest of Hobbes' sociopolitical position. Hobbes' successsor, John Locke (1632–1704), has the greater philosophical reputation. He is generally held to be the founding father of British empiricism. His major work, *An Essay Concerning Human Understanding*, is regarded by some as perhaps the most influential work ever written by a

British philosopher. He is quite clear that there are no 'primary notions' or 'innate principles... stamped upon the mind of man'. 'Men attain', he continues, 'all the knowledge they have, without the help of any innate principles'.

'Let us then suppose', writes Locke, 'the mind to be, as we say, white paper, void of all characters, without any ideas; how comes it to be furnished, whence comes it by that vast store which the busy and boundless fancy of man has painted on it with an almost endless variety?' The answer to this rhetorical question is not slow in coming. The senses convey from the outside world influences which produce 'ideas' such as 'yellow, white, heat, cold, soft, hard, bitter, sweet' and so on. These ideas are the 'simple' ideas. They are, in fact, the qualia we discussed above. They cannot be doubted. Then, from these simple ideas compound ideas are made. The analogy with the work of chemists is clear. Although, as he writes, the mind is 'wholly passive in the reception of all its simple ideas', it exerts itself in several ways to construct all the other ideas with which the mind is furnished. A similar philosophical psychology is found in Locke's successors, David Hume (1711–76) and David Hartley (1705–57). David Hartley differs from Locke and Hume in using a vibrationary instead of an atomistic metaphor to build up his associationist neuropsychology. He has been regarded by many as the founding father of modern physiological psychology.

In summary, it is clear that in the century immediately following Descartes a line of thinkers in the Anglo Saxon world developed a physiological psychology which took the mind to be empty of all preconceived knowledge at birth. Only the onset of sensory experience filled the empty chamber with teeming ideas. These ideas were at first 'simple': unadorned 'qualia' or, to use Herbert Feigl's term, 'raw feels'. As they are combined and recombined, great structures of feelings are built up. Taking a musical analogy, it is as if the simple qualia were the individual notes of a piano and the great tapestry of feeling built up by the combinations of these unit qualia were the sweep of sound in a piano concerto. Indeed, in the next century, Herbert Spencer, whom we shall meet again below, used just this metaphor in his pioneering evolutionary psychology. But we are getting a little ahead of ourselves. There is one other eighteenth-century philosopher whom it is impossible to overlook: Immanuel Kant.

Immanuel Kant (1724–1804) is rightly regarded as the greatest name in modern philosophy after Descartes. Although his mature philosophy is immensely difficult, one major move stands out. He was not prepared to believe that the mind was a blank tablet on which the senses wrote. Nor did he believe that it came into the world with ready-made innate ideas. Rather he took the mind to be active and to organize the way it experienced the world. This he called his 'Copernican revolution'. The categories of space and time and causality and so on are the mind's own organizing principles. They are not found in the world but imposed upon the 'blooming, buzzing confusion' reported by the senses in order to make the world intelligible. Thus, says Kant, just as Copernicus revolutionized astronomy by showing that the observer moved and not the firmament, so his own work revolutionizes epistemology by showing that some of the fundamental attributes of our knowledge of the world are properties of the observer and not of the observables.

Kant's 'Copernican revolution' was immensely influential in the nineteenth century. Not least amongst those influenced were the sensory physiologists. It became clear that sense organs do, indeed, filter the happenings in the environment. They do, indeed, impose, if not quite in the way Kant speculated, meaning on an otherwise chaotic sensory world. Helmholtz, who is usually taken as one of the greatest, if not the greatest, sensory physiologist of the nineteenth century, writes that 'investigations into the physiology of the senses, which were in particular completed and critically sifted by Johannes Muller and then summarized by him in the law of specific nerve energies, have now brought the fullest confirmation of ... (Kant's) "transcendental" forms of intuition and thinking'. It is a commonplace today, as we have noted in the preceding pages of this book, to regard the brain as very far from being a mere passive spectator but to be highly 'active' in sensory processing.

24.4 EPIGENETIC EPISTEMOLOGY

Kant believed that although the mind contained no innate ideas it nevertheless came already primed with categorial organizing principles. This was not accepted by his empiricist opponents. They believed that all the necessary notions of space, time, causality, substance and so on which Kant believed were necessary preconditions for any intelligibility were derived from experience. In a well known passage in the *Essay* (Book 2, Chapter 9, Section 8) John Locke reports how his friend Molineux asked him a famous question: 'Suppose a man *born* blind and now adult and taught by his *touch* to distinguish between a cube and a sphere of the same metal, and nighly of the same bigness, so as to tell, when he felt the one and the other, which is the cube, which the sphere. Suppose then the cube and the sphere placed on a table, and the blind man be made to see: *quare*, whether *by his sight, before he touched them*, he could now distinguish and tell which is the globe, which the cube?' Molineux replies '*Not*' to his question and Locke agrees. Locke and his fellow empiricists believed, as we noted above, that all knowledge entered through the senses and that there were no innate principles. Kant would have disagreed. He would have maintained that spatial intuition was one of the inborn categories and hence would have allowed the newly sighted subject to have discriminated between cube and sphere.

Locke, as is perhaps characteristic of a philosopher, does not seem to have carried out any experimental or observational work to settle the question. This is perhaps strange for he had trained and worked in medicine, and restoration of sight by removal of cataract was not an uncommon procedure. Molineux's question in fact generated considerable interest in the eighteenth century and several famous attempts to answer it were reported. Perhaps the best known was reported by Cheselden to the Royal Society in 1728. Cataracts were removed from a boy of 13 or 14 years of age. On recovery he was found to have little or no sense of distance and could form no judgment of an object's shape. He was unable to remember which was the cat and which the dog until 'catching the cat (which he knew by feeling) he was observ'd to look at her stedfastly and then letting her down again, said "So Puss! I shall know you another time"'. There have been many other investigations of what turns out to be anything but a simple question (see, for example, Box 24.1). Accessible accounts may be found in the book by R.L. Gregory listed in the bibliography. It is often found that adults are so accustomed to doing without sight that, when it is restored, they ultimately lose interest and revert to a dependence on the other senses. The three centuries since Molineux posed his question

(perhaps prompted by marriage to a blind wife) have only shown the many-sidedness of the problem and failed to provide a definitive answer.

The problem of how much and how little of the mind's 'furniture' is inborn forms the core of the discipline known as epigenetic or developmental epistemology. In the twentieth century its most prominent workers were Piaget and his followers. But long before Piaget, Herbert Spencer, one of the most influential thinkers of the nineteenth century, had published an empiricist psychology which (he believed) furnished 'a solution of the controversy between the disciples of Locke and those of Kant'. Even though the first edition of *Principles of Psychology* was published in 1855, four years before Charles Darwin published *The Origin of Species*, Spencer saw the solution in evolutionary theory. It is not, argued Spencer, the experience of the individual which provides the peculiar certainty of the Kantian categories or the theorems of geometry, but the cumulative and inherited experience of the countless lives which have gone before. In the second (1872) edition of the *Psychology* Spencer expressed himself forcibly: 'Space-relations have been the same not only for all ancestral man, all ancestral primates, all ancestral orders of mammalia but for all simpler orders of creatures. These constant space-relations are expressed by definite nervous structures, congenitally framed to act in definite ways and incapable of acting in other ways. Hence, the inconceivableness of the negation of a mathematical axiom, resulting as it does from the impossibility of inverting the actions of the correlative nervous structures, really stands for the infinity of experiences that have developed these structures'.

Having satisfied himself that there was no mystery about the sensory origins of the Kantian *a priori* Spencer went on to give one of the most complete accounts of the empirical origins of our knowledge. He started by assuming, with the other empiricists, that the infant's world is at first just a confusion of colours and sounds and touches, tastes and smells. He explains how, from this 'phenomenal field', two sets of events slowly differentiate. In the first set, events are vivid and often unexpected, in the second set they are fainter, are often in some way 'dragged along' by the first and are also often obviously connected in time sequence. These and other disjunctions ultimately crystallize into the distinction '**objective**' and '**subjective**'. The sudden clap of thunder

BOX 24.1   SENSORY SUBSTITUTION

We have seen in this chapter how the question which Molineux asked his friend John Locke spawned centuries of argument and experiment. A contemporary continuation of that debate, albeit with an important practical dimension, is provided by experiments pioneered by Paul Bach-y-Rita in which a **tactile visual substitution system (TVSS)** is used to deliver visual information to congenitally blind subjects.

The TVSS consists of a TV camera wired to an array of stimulators placed on the skin in one of several places of the body (abdomen, back, thigh and, more recently, tongue). The images picked up by the camera are transformed into vibrations or electrical stimuli. To begin with the subject uses a hand held camera so that the information reaching the brain is supplemented by kinaesthetic input; later the camera can be mounted on a spectacle frame and in this case vestibular feedback occurs when the head moves to scan the visual scene. After a period of training the subjects no longer felt the tactile stimulation but began to experience the image in space. Quite sophisticated features of the image became accessible: perspective, parallax, depth and with the addition of a zoom lens to the camera, magnification, looming and vanishing. There was no confusion between this new sense and the sensations set up by scratching or tickling the same area of skin.

One of the first subjects to try out the TVSS was G.Guarniero, a congenitally blind PhD student at New York University. He reports how at first the sensations seemed to come from the skin to which the tactile array was attached but that later the sensations appeared to be in a two-dimensional space – although there was no projection to 'out there'. Furthermore, the sensation was nothing like that of touch and Guarniero is content to use the word 'see' to describe this novel phenomenology. To begin with, the most obvious feature of a visual object was whether or not it was moving. Guarniero found considerable initial difficulty in coming to terms with the fact that a stationary object would appear to move to the right when his head (with attached camera) moved to the left. Eventually he was able to adapt to this unexpected phenomenon so that objects appeared stationary as he scanned them. In a variant of Molineux's question, he was presented with objects and asked what they were. In some cases he was told what the object was before being allowed to 'look' at it via the TVSS, in other cases he was allowed to handle it before being shown it, and in yet other cases he was merely presented with an object and asked to name it. In none of these cases was he able to recognize the object via the TVSS. He never discovered any correlation between how an object 'looked' and how it felt. Because he could never recognize objects through the TVSS as those which he knew by touch, it was only with great difficulty that he could associate names and 'visual' appearances.

Guarniero says that the most intriguing features of the visual world which the TVSS allowed him to access were the ability to see (by way of a mirror) the back and front of an object simultaneously and the flickering shape changes of a candle flame. The latter, he says, was 'an endless source of fascination', indeed he (understandably) had never imagined a flame to have a shape at all! After three weeks of training, he concludes, objects 'had come to have a top and a bottom; a right side and a left; but no depth – they existed in an ordered two-dimensional space, the precise location of which has yet to be determined'.

Although Guarniero refers to the 'dramatic impact' of gaining access to this 'new world' and of a 'powerful emotional reaction', it appears that for most adults and adolescents the new sensory experience carries with it no emotional tone. Thus seeing the face of a loved one via the TVSS proved a disappointingly 'flat' experience. The new sense has not had time to build the great history of emotive tone and association which the other senses of the congenitally blind have accumulated. Using TVSS, says Guarniero, is 'as if a sighted person were seeing, though in an extremely analytical frame of mind'.

(Continues)

(Continued)

Similarly disappointing consequences have been noted in those who have had congenital cataracts removed in adult life. Often they have preferred not to use their new sense at all, and have returned to their familiar tactile/auditory/olfactory world.

The TVSS does, however, show how plastic the adult brain remains. It gives hope to those with brain lesions who seek rehabilitation. It also suggests that prostheses may be possible to enable the congenitally blind to accomplish quite complex visual tasks. Bach-y-Rita shows how TVSSs allow blind subjects to strike a rolling ball (requiring the visual identification of the ball, its velocity, direction, position, position of bat, etc.) and to undertake repetitive tasks in light industry such as assembling electronic components. These abilities suggest that the visual phenomenology is in three dimensions rather than just two, as Guarniero maintained. Nevertheless, it must be noted that the 'visual' experience achieved through TVS systems is highly impoverished compared with that which normally sighted people enjoy.

REFERENCES

Bach-y-Rita, P. (1995) *Nonsynaptic Diffusion Neurotransmission and Late Brain Reorganisation*, Demos, New York.

Bach-y-Rita, P. (1996) Sensory substitution and qualia, in *Perception et Intermodalité* (ed. J. Proust), Presses Universitaires de France, Paris.

Gregory, R.L. (1997) *Eye and Brain, the Psychology of Seeing*, 5th edn, Oxford University Press, Oxford.

Guarniero, G. (1974) Experience of tactile vision. *Perception*, **3**, 101–4.

and the rattle of hail are, for instance, vivid and unexpected. The remembrance of past storms and the concern for the soundness of our roof are 'dragged' into our consciousness by the first and are far less vivid.

Spencer goes on to point out that one of the vivid feelings to which we are subject is that of touch, and that in drawing one's hand along, for instance, one's own leg, causes a change in this particular vivid feeling. This change, moreover, is caused by events in the faint sequence of feelings. We may, for instance, have wished to find whether skin was still damp from a recent swim. But the touch of the hand brings about changes – sharp, vivid changes – indistinguishable from those brought about by other events in the vivid aggregate. In producing such changes in the vivid aggregate, we are aware, says Spencer, of 'wellings up', as he puts it, in this case the insubstantial feeling of a 'wish', in the faint aggregate of feelings. These 'wellings up' go on to include, in a time sequence, other feelings, feelings which we conventionally dub 'effort', muscular effort, the expenditure of energy, or work against a resistance. Thus arises, he concludes, the notion of a power in things, of an external 'energy'. For if a change in the faint aggregate, a change

which we have learnt to call 'work' or 'effort', precedes the change in the vivid aggregate, which we call 'touch' or 'scratching', why should not a similar change be responsible for the abrasion caused by, say, a falling stone? This is not the place to follow Spencer further into his analysis of the way our understanding of the nature of things is constructed during the long years of infancy and childhood. Enough has been said to show that empiricist philosophers can make a plausible story. Interested students can follow modern developments further in the work of Spencer's modern follower, Jean Piaget.

24.5 EVOLUTIONARY EPISTEMOLOGY

In the last section we saw how Herbert Spencer, working in the middle of the nineteenth century, saw the implications of evolutionary theory for epistemology. In fact, Charles Darwin was there before him. In one of the notebooks he composed on return from the *Beagle* circumnavigation in the late 1830s we find the following jotting: 'Plato ... says ... that our 'necessary ideas' arise from the pre-existence of the soul, are not derivable from experience – read monkeys for pre-existence' (*M Notebook*, p. 128). These notebooks were, however, not published during Darwin's lifetime and hence it is only just that Spencer should be regarded as the founding father of evolutionary epistemology. Later in the century we find that Friedrich Nietzsche in Germany also published interesting speculations on evolutionary epistemology. In his 1882 *Gay Science* (sections 110–111), for instance, he writes of how 'throughout tremendous periods of time the intellect begot nothing but errors; some of them proved useful and preservative of the species ... he, for example, who did not know how to discover the 'identical' sufficiently often in regard to food or to animals hostile to him ... had a smaller probability of survival than he who in every case of similarity at once conjectured identity'. There are many other similar *aperçues* in Nietzsche's aphoristic work. They show how the evolutionary thought of the nineteenth century was beginning to work through to affect the writings of philosophers. It was not, however, until another century had passed that evolutionary theory began to make a significant impact on psychology. It is only in recent years that experimental evidence has been adduced to illuminate the nature of the evolutionary influence on cognition.

We have seen in the previous chapters of this book that the 'simple' stimuli of John Locke and the other empiricists are seldom very effective. Certainly, in the psychophysical laboratory cooperating subjects are routinely exposed to such stimuli and their responses recorded and quantified. But in the world outside the laboratory and, even more emphatically in the world of the palaeolithic past, few such simple stimuli would ever have been encountered. The human senses, like those of other animals, have been adapted to respond to the biologically most significant features of their environments. Note, too, that there is no continuous line of 'ascent' in the evolutionary process. Humans are not simply scaled up mice or rats, or even macaques. Different animals have been adapted over evolutionary time to particular environmental niches and particular lifestyles. The stimuli to which their sense organs are tuned differ accordingly. Evolution is not a one-way staircase, but branches richly in many directions. We have noted this in many parts of this book and especially in our summarizing discussion of different sensory worlds in Chapter 23. Human minds are likely very differently biased, in some cases totally alien, to the minds of our fellow animals.

· Ethologists have for many years been well aware that different animals are 'prepared' for different tasks. Psychologists have, however, all too often assumed (perhaps under the influence of the *tabula rasa* philosophers of the empiricist tradition) that the human mind came to all its tasks with equal ability. Only in recent years has evidence accumulated to show that it, like other animal minds, is better 'prepared' for some tasks than others. Only in recent years have experiments been designed to detect these evolutionary propensities. The human mind turns out, after all, not to be the blank sheet which eighteenth century philosophers imagined. It has its inborn biases, although very different from those that Immanuel Kant had in mind. They are leftovers from its evolutionary past, especially the millions of years spent on the African plains in a hunter–gatherer–scavenger mode. Such so-called '**Darwinian algorithms**' evolved to increase the probability of survival in these conditions.

In a seminal paper Leda Cosmides showed how common errors in a conditional reasoning task could best be accounted for in terms of evolutionarily inbuilt behaviours for social exchange. The task, known after its inventor as the Wason selection task, tests the ability to follow a conditional rule: *if (p) then (q)*. The task involves four cards each of which is marked on both sides (Figure 24.1). One side tells whether the antecedent is true or false (i.e. p or not p) and the other side tells whether the consequent is true of false (i.e. q or not q). Thus in Figure 24.1a the conditional rule is '*If* a card has 'D' on one side *then* it has '3' on the other'. The subject is asked to say which card(s) must be turned over to see if they violate the rule.

When this task is set to intelligent young men and women (college students) fewer than 50% get the right answer: D and seven. However, if the cards are renamed as in Figure 24.1b and the problem reset as one of finding who is violating the licensing laws by being under 20 years old and drinking beer the percentage of correct solutions rises to over 90%.

There are a number of variants of this test and a number of hypotheses to explain the different success rates in finding a solution. The most parsimonious solution, however, is in terms of social contract and cheater-detection. This, Cosmides and coworkers

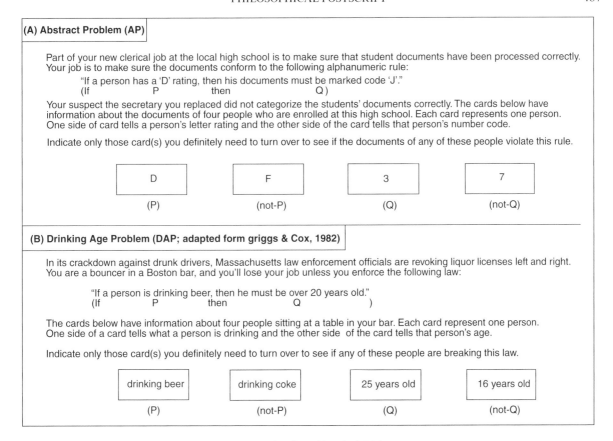

(A) Abstract Problem (AP)

Part of your new clerical job at the local high school is to make sure that student documents have been processed correctly. Your job is to make sure the documents conform to the following alphanumeric rule:

"If a person has a 'D' rating, then his documents must be marked code 'J'."
(If   P   then   Q)

Your suspect the secretary you replaced did not categorize the students' documents correctly. The cards below have information about the documents of four people who are enrolled at this high school. Each card represents one person. One side of card tells a person's letter rating and the other side of the card tells that person's number code.

Indicate only those card(s) you definitely need to turn over to see if the documents of any of these people violate this rule.

| D | F | 3 | 7 |
| (P) | (not-P) | (Q) | (not-Q) |

(B) Drinking Age Problem (DAP; adapted form griggs & Cox, 1982)

In its crackdown against drunk drivers, Massachusetts law enforcement officials are revoking liquor licenses left and right. You are a bouncer in a Boston bar, and you'll lose your job unless you enforce the following law:

"If a person is drinking beer, then he must be over 20 years old."
(If   P   then   Q   )

The cards below have information about four people sitting at a table in your bar. Each card represent one person. One side of a card tells what a person is drinking and the other side of the card tells that person's age.

Indicate only those card(s) you definitely need to turn over to see if any of these people are breaking this law.

| drinking beer | drinking coke | 25 years old | 16 years old |
| (P) | (not-P) | (Q) | (not-Q) |

Figure 24.1 Wason selection test. Discussion in text. After Cosmides, L. (1989).

argue, is due to the long evolutionary experience of sociality in the palaeolithic. This experience would have built powerful cheater-detection biases into human mentality. Social contract theory makes very specific predictions for the types of 'error' subjects will and will not make when confronted with different varieties of Wason test. These predictions are largely satisfied by extensive testing.

Social contract and cheater-detection is not the only Darwinian algorithm innate to the human mind. There are a number of others. The human mind, like those of other animals, was not evolved to cope with arbitrary tasks but with quite definite, 'domain specific', undertakings. There are, for instance, interesting indications that common human 'misunderstandings' of probability, statistics and risk have an evolutionary origin. There are also interesting sex-related differences in spatial ability which, although perhaps accentuated by a child's early experience,

can be traced to sexual selection in mankind's evolutionary past. Boys, for instance, seem innately better at navigation in three-dimensional space, at judging relative velocities and distances and at image rotation tasks than girls. Girls, on the other hand, show up better than boys in tests of linguistic ability.

24.6 BEYOND DESCARTES

The division between mind and body, qualia and materiality, still seems, as noted in Section 23.2 above, unbridgeable. It has been observed that those who fully apprehend the problem seem to have only two ways to go: either towards an unreconstructed two-substance Cartesian dualism (e.g. J.C. Eccles) or towards panpsychism (e.g. David Bohm and others). Both these alternatives seem to lead toward *reductio ad absurda*. Hence, for the time being, it is perhaps best to side with those who regard the problem as at present (and perhaps for ever) insoluble and who have been dismissively labelled 'the New Mysterians'.

But this does not mean that our understanding of the brain–mind is still stuck in the early seventeenth century. Neuroscience and cognitive science have moved far beyond the crude model provided by the 'earthen machine' discussed in Descartes' *L'Homme*. As we have reviewed twentieth-century sensory biology in the foregoing chapters, we have come across one case after another which would have set René Descartes to think furiously. Let us remind ourselves of a few.

One of the famous neurophysiological illustrations in Descartes' *L'Homme* shows the operation of the visual system (Figure 24.2). Descartes was writing in the late 1620s and had been impressed by the demonstration by Aranzi in 1595 and then by Kepler in 1604 that, if the sclerotic was removed from the back of an ox eye, a tiny inverted image can be seen on the back of the retina. Descartes repeated this observation and incorporated it into his neurophysiological theory. Figure 24.2 shows that not only is an inverted image thrown on to the retina but that it is transferred unchanged into the brain. In the brain the image is reinverted so an upright representation

is thrown on to gland H (the pineal). Here (according to Descartes) the soul resides and directly perceives the etching. This has led to centuries of misunderstanding. Neurophysiologists have long known that this direct perception (let alone Descartes' fanciful neurophysiology) cannot be the case. In Chapters 17 and 18 we saw just how considerable is the 'information processing' between retinal image and visual percept.

Furthermore, and still sticking with the visual system, we saw that there was good evidence that what the system detects is change in the visual scene not stasis. This can be shown in experimental animals by monitoring the impulse traffic in optic nerve fibres. When nothing is happening, the system is largely shut down. Analogous experiments have been carried out by Yarbus and others on humans. If the visual saccades are compensated in such a way that the image is stabilized upon the retina, it begins to break up and lose 'meaning' and within one to three seconds 'all visible differences disappear and do not reappear' leaving what Yarbus calls an 'empty field'. All contours are lost and the field appears black, grey or twilit – as if the eyes were closed. *Very* uncartesian!

Or consider Land's work on colour perception using 'Mondrians'. Piet Mondrian (1872–1944), it will be remembered, was a Dutch abstract painter famous

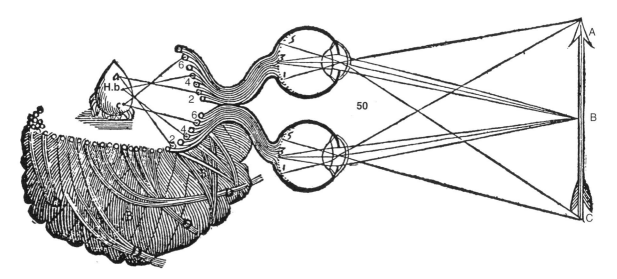

Figure 24.2 Visual perception according to Descartes' *L'Homme* (written 1628, published (posthumously) 1662). An upright image is thrown on to H, the pineal gland, which (according to this figure) is suspended in the centre of the brain's ventricle.

for collages of brilliantly coloured rectangles. To the human eye the contrasting colours in these juxtaposed rectangles remain constant whatever the ambient illumination. Yet the wavelength of light reflected from these rectangles varies according to that illumination. Land showed that the distribution of energy in the different wavelengths reaching the eye from different parts of the Mondrian has no effect on our colour perception. Nor has our perception anything to do with learning, memory, surroundings or adaptation. It has, however, everything to do with 'reflectance' or what, subjectively, we call 'lightness'. The visual system computes the comparative reflectances of the different rectangles in the painting. This ratio remains constant under widely different illuminations. It is this, not the different amounts of energy in the different wavelengths, which gives us the sensation – the 'raw feel' – of colour. Again, *very* uncartesian.

Both these examples, and the visual system provides many other examples, show that our visual systems are very unlike cameras or the photometers used by physicists. David Marr remarked that vision is 'a description useful to the viewer' and we can see that this is the case in both our examples. In the first case, little point would be served by burdening the brain with information relating to the visual scene when nothing is happening; in the second case it is important for colour-sensitive primates to be able to detect the same colours – ripe berries, ripe fruit – under all conditions of illumination – dawn, midday, dusk.

Furthermore, and along the same line of argument, the visual system actively seeks its object. Firstly, as we noted in Chapter 16, there is powerful feedback control of saccadic movements. But, secondly, by attaching a tiny mirror to the side of the eye so that its movements can be followed, it can be shown that these movements are far from being random. They follow the outline of the object of interest. Moreover, the eyes are directed at the biologically most significant part of that object (Figure 24.3). In the case of a face, the eyes and the mouth are scanned over and over again. Saccades are, of course, quite automatic. No conscious, intentional direction of the eye is involved. The mechanism is inbuilt and preprogrammed motor systems are directing where the gaze should be directed.

This action-orientated perception is evident in all the other senses. It is well reviewed by Michael Arbib

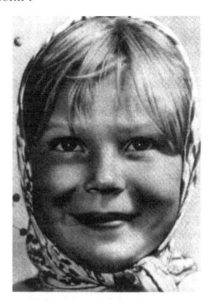

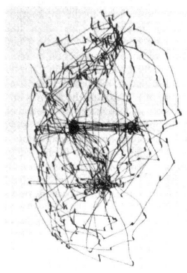

Figure 24.3 Movements of the eyes when looking at the picture of the young girl are recorded in the chart below the picture. From Yarbus, A.L. (1967) *Eye Movements and Vision*, Copyright © 1967, Springer.

in the book listed in the bibliography. We looked at an interesting case when discussing electroreception in mormyrid fish in Chapter 21 and we can end this section by referring to the sense of pain, which we reviewed in Chapter 22. It will be recalled that it, like vision, is far from being a simple case of reading off the activity in specific sensory fibres, as Descartes, in another famous diagram, supposed. Instead, as we saw, it is profoundly involved in the adaptation of the animal to its circumstances. It is only 'allowed' to break through when the circumstances are such that no further escape or avoidance is possible or, it may be, necessary. Its radically uncartesian nature is perhaps best shown, as Patrick Wall suggests, by the subjective outcome of injecting anaesthetic into the brachial plexus (Chapter 22). Instead of merely losing all feeling in the arm, as Descartes would have supposed, there being no further impulse traffic in the brachial nerves, the arm is experienced as swollen and tender and often in an impossible position. The central nervous system compensates for the unusual pattern of impulse traffic converging on it through all its sensory fibres by hypothesizing and drawing attention to the fact that something is wrong. Very different from the mirror thesis which René Descartes held.

24.7 CONCLUDING REMARKS

So, in conclusion to this chapter, we can perhaps see that, although the Cartesian divide still remains to puzzle and unsettle us, the other parts of his neurophilosophy are receding into the past. Because of its widespread unthinking acceptance, Gilbert Ryle called Descartes' two-substance metaphysics the 'official doctrine'. It 'sees' humans as set over against the natural world. Its epistemology is built on the notion of mirroring. The world outside is reflected in the mind. If the mirror is well ground, the reflection is accurate and knowledge valid; if it is faulty and uneven, our knowledge of the external world is similarly faulty. In this chapter we have seen that this way of looking at things no longer serves. We are beginning, with immense difficulty, to emerge from its powerful hold. Humans do not stand apart from the world but are very much a part of it. They are not mere passive spectators, 'cameras', whose real business is elsewhere. Perception is action-orientated; action is perception-orientated. Humans, to quote from one of Charles Darwin's early notebooks again, are 'netted together' with the rest of the natural world.

The conclusion to this book is similar. We have seen in this chapter, where we discussed the Darwinian algorithms of the human mind, what we have noted throughout, that sensory systems are adapted to the life circumstances of their owners. Human sensory systems, magnificent as they undoubtedly are, are biased by our evolutionary history. They do not give a 'God's eye' view of the world. We can learn much by comparing our systems with those of our fellow animals who often live in quite different sensory worlds. Nevertheless, as Alexander Pope wrote long ago, 'the proper study of mankind is Man', and there is too much suffering and discomfort in the world to believe that the study of human sensory systems is of anything but paramount importance.

We can also learn much from comparisons between the different senses. There is much similarity in their organization and at the molecular level very much the same mechanisms are often found to be at work. The extraordinary fact remains, however, that with such similar molecular and cellular organization, the qualia of our sensory experience are so radically different. This is just another and powerful reminder of the 'hard' problem which has lurked beneath the surface of so much of this book.

We started in Chapter 1 by noting that three and a half thousand million years ago the first precursors of the prokaryocytes swam in already ancient seas. We end it with an increasing understanding of ourselves as part of and bound into the natural world. It would be an exaggeration to conclude by quoting the lines with which Eliot finishes *Four Quartets*:

> And the end of all our exploring
> Will be to arrive where we started
> And know the place for the first time

But then again, considering the depth of our emerging scientific understanding, perhaps not too great an exaggeration.

PART VI: SELF ASSESSMENT

The following questions are designed both to help you assess your understanding of the topics covered in the text and to direct your attention to significant aspects of the subject matter. The sequence of questions follows the sequence in which the subject matter is presented in the text. It is thus easy to refer back to the appropriate page or pages. After reading each chapter and/or each section you should look through these questions and make sure you know the answers and the issues involved.

CHAPTER 23: SUMMING UP

23.1 With the aid of diagrams describe the major types of receptor molecules expressed in sensory cells giving examples of the sensory (or neurosensory) cells in which they are found.

23.2 Give examples of molecular mechanisms which have been adapted to play crucial roles in many different varieties of sensory cell.

23.3 Discuss one ubiquitous organelle which is made use of time and again in the design of sensory cells.

23.4 Enumerate some examples of common design principles emerging through convergent evolution.

23.5 Compare specializations of the vertebrate retina with those of the insect compound eye.

23.6 Do sensory surfaces devoted to different sensory modalities show similar specializations?

23.7 Why are there topographic maps of sensory surfaces in the central nervous system? Discuss a possible hypothesis.

23.8 Draw diagrams to show the similarity of neural 'wiring' in the olfactory bulb and the retina. What are the neurophysiological reasons for this similarity?

23.9 Explain how information processing in advanced sensory cortices differs from the sequential operations of digital (von Neumann) computers.

23.10 In what way are the trigger stimuli of cells in the macaque's auditory cortex similar to those found in its inferotemporal cortex?

23.11 Explain the biological significance of sensory systems being subject to illusion.

23.12 Can the sensation of pain be regarded as part of the body's homeostatic mechanism? Explain.

23.13 How different do you think animal sensory worlds are from our own?

23.14 With reference to the warfare between moth and bat, explain how predator–prey contests have sharpened sensory systems.

23.15 Discuss the role of sensory systems in social animals.

23.16 What is meant by the terms 'folk psychology' and 'intentionality'?

23.17 Define a mirror neuron.

23.18 Where are mirror neurons found in monkey and in human brains?

23.19 Do some mirror neurons respond to auditory input? How can this be shown?

23.20 How are mirror neurons thought to be implicated in the evolution of language?

23.21 Explain how mirror neurons may be responsible for human self awareness. Why is it thought that

Biology of Sensory Systems, Second Edition   C.U.M. Smith
© 2008 John Wiley & Sons, Ltd

defects in the development of this system may lead to autism?

23.22 What did Francis Bacon mean by the terms 'luciferous' and 'lucriferous'? Are they still relevant to today's research endeavour? Discuss.

CHAPTER 24: PHILOSOPHICAL POSTSCRIPT

24.1 Describe the process of doubt by which Descartes arrived at '*cogito ergo sum*'.

24.2 How does Descartes' '*cogito*' lead to the classic mind–body problem?

24.3 What is the problem of knowledge?

24.4 What is meant by the terms 'qualia' and 'privileged access'?

24.5 Distinguish between the 'easy' problems of neuroscience and the 'hard' problem.

24.6 Thomas Hobbes, John Locke and the other British empiricist philosophers believed the mind to be a 'tabula rasa'. What did they mean? Would Descartes have agreed?

24.7 What was Immanuel Kant's contribution to sensory physiology? Why did he call it a 'Copernican revolution'? Which nineteenth century German sensory physiologists were particularly influenced by his thought?

24.8 Who was Molineux and what was his question? How did John Locke answer this question and

why? Describe some experimental investigations of the question. Has Molineux's question been finally answered?

24.9 How did Herbert Spencer resolve the controversy between the followers of John Locke and those of Immanuel Kant? Was Spencer the first to see this way towards resolving the issue?

24.10 Describe Spencer's empiricist derivation of 'subjectivity and 'objectivity'. Do you find his account convincing?

24.11 What is meant by the term 'Darwinian algorithm'? Describe some experiments which confirm that the human mind is not initially *tabula rasa* but comes with evolutionarily induced biases.

24.12 Why is evolutionary psychology sometimes derided as a series of 'Just So' stories? Critically discuss its promise and its pitfalls.

24.13 Consider Descartes' visual physiology as represented in Figure 24.2. Do you think this is still the common understanding of how the system works? How would you convince a layperson that the Cartesian version is profoundly mistaken?

24.14 How did David Marr define vision?

24.15 At a fundamental – molecular, biophysical – level the activity in auditory and visual cortices is indistinguishable. Yet the qualia we experience – sound, vision – are totally different. Discuss

24.16 Do you think that a study of sensory physiology changes our common-sense understanding of the world and of our place in it?

PART VI: NOTES, REFERENCES AND BIBLIOGRAPHY

CHAPTER 23: SUMMING UP

Evolution is a recurring theme throughout the book. Garland and Carter (1994) provide a review and an extensive bibliography of 'evolutionary physiology' and the proceedings of the *Eighth Annual Karger Workshop*, edited by Fay and Popper (1996), provides a series of reviews on the evolution of vertebrate sensory systems . Further information on molecular neurobiology may be found in many places, for instance many of the 'minireviews' in *Neuron*, and in texts of molecular neurobiology, for example Smith (2002). Frings and Bradley (2004) have edited a valuable collection of chapters on transduction channels in sensory cells and Shepherd (1995) provides a valuable comparative review of sensory systems at the molecular level. Land (1981) and Waterman (1981) provide detailed reviews of the specializations of insect photoreceptors, Land, in particular, discusses the 'sexual' fovea of dipteran insects and Waterman gives quantitative information and useful diagrams of the dragonfly fovea. Kohonen and Hari (1999) contribute an interesting analysis of the formation of sensory maps in the brain (and in artificial systems). von Uexküll (1909, 1926) provides the classic exposition of the 'inner world' of animals and Zeil and Zanker (1997) give an interesting example of the analysis of such a world. Wilson (1975) in his classic exposition of sociobiology shows how different groups of animals have evolved social lifestyles; Rizzollatti and Criaghero (2004) review the mirror neuron system in monkeys and humans and

Rizzolatti and Arbib (1998) draw out its implications for the origin of human language.

Bach-y-Rita, P. (1995) *Nonsynaptic Diffusion Neurotransmission and Late Brain Reorganisation*, Demos, New York.

Bach-y-Rita, P. (1996) Sensory substitution and qualia, in *Perception et Intermodalité* (ed. J. Proust), Presses Universitaires de France, Paris.

Fay, R.R. and Popper, A.N. (1996) Evolution of vertebrate sensory systems. *Brain, Behaviour and Evolution*, **50**, 187–259.

Frings, S. and Bradley, J. (2004) *Transduction Channels in Sensory Cells*, Wiley-VCH Verlag GmbH, Weinheim.

Garland, T. and Carter, P.A. (1994) Evolutionary physiology. *Annual Review of Physiology*, **56**, 579–621.

Gregory, R.L. (1997) *Eye and Brain, the Psychology of Seeing*, 5th edn, Oxford University Press, Oxford.

Guarniero, G. (1974) Experience of tactile vision. *Perception*, **3**, 101–4.

Hanson, N.R. (1961) *Patterns of Discovery*, Cambridge University Press, Cambridge.

Iacoboni, M. and Dapretto, M. (2006) The mirror neuron system and the consequences of its dysfunction. *Nature Reviews Neuroscience*, **7**, 942–51.

Kohonen, T. and Hari, R. (1999) Where the abstract feature maps of the brain might come from. *Trends in Neuroscience*, **22**, 135–39.

Kuhn, T.S. (1962) *The Structure of Scientific Revolutions*, Chicago University Press, Chicago.

Land, M.F. (1981) Optics and vision in invertebrates, in *Handbook of Sensory Physiology*, Vol. **VII/6B** (ed. H. Autrum), Springer-Verlag, Berlin.

Popper, K. (1969) *Conjectures and Refutations: The Growth of Scientific Knowledge*, 3rd edn, Routledge and Kegan Paul, London.

Rizzolatti, G. and Arbib, M.A. (1998) Language within our grasp. *Trends in Neurosciences*, **21**, 188–94.

Rizzollatti, G. and Criaghero, L. (2004) The mirror neuron system. *Annual Review of Neuroscience*, **27**, 169–92.

Shepherd, G.M. (1995) Toward a molecular basis for sensory perception, in *The Cognitive Neurosciences* (ed. M.S. Gazzaniga), MIT Press, Cambridge, Mass.

Smith, C.U.M. (2002) *Elements of Molecular Neurobiology*, 3rd edn, John Wiley & Sons, Ltd, Chichester.

von Uexküll, J.J. (1909) *Umwelt und innenwelt der Tiere*, Springer, Berlin; also 1926, *Theoretical Biology*, Harcourt Brace and Co., New York.

Waterman, T.H. (1981) Polarisation sensitivity, in *Handbook of Sensory Physiology*, Vol. **VII/6B** (ed. H. Autrum), Springer-Verlag, Berlin.

Wilson, E.O. (1975) *Sociobiology: The New Synthesis*, Belknap Press of Harvard University Press, Cambridge, Mass.

Zeil, J. and Zanker, J.N. (1997) A glimpse into crabworld. *Vision Research*, **37**, 3417–26.

CHAPTER 24: PHILOSOPHICAL POSTSCRIPT

The boundary between sensory physiology and philosophy, especially epistemology, is lengthy, uncertain, shifting. Below are just some of the multitude of books and articles which are relevant to this postscript. Historically, the modern period in philosophy and neurophysiology is conventionally taken to start with the work of René Descartes (1637, 1662). Thomas Hobbes' correspondence with Descartes may be found in Cottingham, Stoothof and Murdoch (1984), vol. 2: 'Third Set of Objections'. The problem of 'qualia' or 'raw feels' receives a modern outing in Chalmers (1998) and Dennett (1991) provides a dose of scepticism. Hameroff (1998), Stapp (2005) and others suggest that quantum theory may provide a solution and Smith (2006, 2008) discusses this work. Feigl (1967) gives a more classical exposition, making use of 'autocerebroscope' thought experiments and McGinn (1991) makes the case for its ultimate insolubility. Morgan (1977) and Degenaar (1966) provide detailed expositions of the question Locke posed Molyneux and its historical reverberations down the centuries. Immanuel Kant

explains what he means by his 'Copernican revolution' in the preface to his (1787) work and Cohen and Elkana (1977) show how strongly this influenced Helmholtz's sensory physiology. Hebert Spencer's pioneering epigenetic epistemology was first published in his (1855) work and is discussed in Smith (1982). Barkow, Cosmides and Tooby (1992) provide an in-depth discussion of how mankind's evolutionary past has moulded human mentality and Cosmides and Tooby (1996) discuss evidence which suggests that the seeming errors which plague the 'common man's' understanding of risk and probability were not errors at all in the different circumstances of the palaeolithic hunter–gatherer band. Finally, Yarbus (1967), Land (1977) and Patrick Wall (1994) re-emphasize the uncartesian nature of contemporary neuropsychology and David Marr (1982) and Michael Arbib (1989) contribute classic expositions of the relationships between neuroscience and artificial intelligence and robotics.

Arbib, M.A. (1989) *The Metaphorical Brain 2: Neural Networks and Beyond*, John Wiley & Sons, Inc., New York.

Barkow, J., Cosmides, L. and Tooby, J. (eds) (1992) *The Adapted Mind: Evolutionary Psychology and the Generation of Culture*, Oxford University Press, New York.

Chalmers, D.J. (1998) *The Conscious Mind*, Oxford University Press, Oxford.

Chelselden, W. (1728) An account of some observations made by a young gentleman... *Philosophical Transactions of the Royal Society*, **402**, 447–50; quoted in *Molyneux's Question*, M.J. Morgan, Cambridge University Press, Cambridge.

Cohen, R.S. and Elkana, Y. (eds) (1977) *Hermann von Helmholtz: Epistemological Writings*, Reidl, Dordrecht.

Cosmides, L. (1989) 'The logic of social exchange: Has natural selection shaped how humans reason? Studies with the Wason selection task. *Cognition*, **31**, 187–276.

Cosmides, L. and Tooby, J. (1996) Are humans good intuitive statisticians after all? Rethinking some of the conclusions from the literature on judgement under certainty. *Cognition*, **58**, 1–73.

Cottingham, J., Stoothof, R. and Murdoch, D. (1984) *The Philosophical Writings of Descartes*, Cambridge University Press, Cambridge.

Darwin, C. (1838 M. Notebook, in P.H. Barrett, 1980) *Metaphysics, Materialism and the Evolution of Mind: Early writings of Charles Darwin*, Chicago University Press, Chicago.

Degenaar, M. (1966) *Molyneux Problem: Three Centuries of Discussion on the Perception of Forms*, Kluwer Academic Publishers, Dordrecht.

Dennett, D. (1991) *Consciousness Explained*, Penguin, Harmondsworth, Middlesex.

Descartes, R. (1637) *Discourse on Method, Descartes: Philosophical Writings* (eds E. Anscombe and P.T. Geach, 1970.) Thomas Nelson and Sons, London.

Descartes, R. (1662) *L'Homme, Treatise of Man* (trs. and ed. T.S. Hall., 1972), Harvard University Press, Cambridge, Mass.

Eliot, T.S. (1944) *Four Quartets*, Faber and Faber, London.

Feigl, H. (1967) *The 'Mental' and the 'Physical'*, Minneapolis University Press, Minneapolis.

Geary, D.C. (1996) Sexual selection and sex differences in mathematical abilities. *Behavioural and Brain Sciences*, **19**, 229–84.

Gregory, R.L. (1997) *Eye and Brain, the Psychology of Seeing*, 5th edn, Oxford University Press, Oxford.

Hameroff, S.R. (1998) "Funda-mentality": Is the conscious mind subtly linked to a basic level of the universe? *Trends in Cognitive Sciences*, **2**, 119–24.

Hartley, D. (1749) *Observations on Man*, Thomas Tegg, London.

Hobbes, T. (1651) *Leviathan*, part 1, chapter 1, London.

Kant, I. (1787) *Critique of Pure Reason*, 2nd edn (trs. J.M.D. Meiklejohn, 1934), Dent, London.

Land, E.H. (1977) The retinex theory of colour vision. *Scientific American*, **237** (12), 108–28.

Locke, J. (1690) *An Essay Concerning Human Understanding* (ed. R. Wilburn, 1947.), Dent, London.

Marr, D. (1982) *Vision*, Freeman, New York.

McGinn, C. (1991) *The Problem of Consciousness: Essays Towards a Resolution*, Blackwell, Oxford.

Morgan, M.J. (1977) *Molyneux's Question*, Cambridge University Press, Cambridge.

Nietzsche, F. (1882), *The Gay Science* (trs. R.J. Hollingdale, 1982), Vintage Books, New York.

Nietzsche, F. (1882) *The Gay Science* (trs. W. Kaufmann, 1974), Vintage Books, New York.

Piaget, J. (1972) *Psychology and Epistemology*, Penguin, Harmondsworth.

Plato, *Meno* in Jowett, B. (trs. and ed.), *The Dialogues of Plato*, Vol. **2**, The Clarendon Press, Oxford.

Ryle, G. (1949) *The Problem of Mind*, Hutchinson, London.

Smith, C.U.M. (1982) Evolution and the problem of mind, part 1, Herbert Spencer. *Journal of the History of Biology*, **15**, 55–88.

Smith, C.U.M. (1987) "Clever Beasts Who Invented Knowing": Nietzsche's evolutionary biology of knowledge. *Biology and Philosophy*, **2**, 65–91.

Smith, C.U.M. (1987) David Hartley's Newtonian neuropsychology. *Journal of the History of the Behavioural Sciences*, **23**, 123–36.

Smith, C.U.M. (1998) Descartes' pineal neuropsychology. *Brain and Cognition*, **36**, 57–72.

Smith, C.U.M. (2006) The "hard problem" and the quantum physicists, Part 1: the first generation. *Brain and Cognition*, **61**, 181–8.

Smith, C.U.M. (2008) The "hard problem" and the quantum physicists, Part 2: modern times. *Brain and Cognition*, in press.

Stapp, H.P. (2005) Quantum interactive dualism. *Journal of Consciousness Studies*, **12**, 43–58.

Spencer, H. (1855) *The Principles of Psychology*, Vol. **2**, 2nd edn, Longman, Brown, Green and Longmans, London; 1870; 1872, Williams and Norgate, London.

Wall, P.D. (1994) Introduction to the edition after this one, in *Textbook of Pain* (eds P.D. Wall and R. Melzack.), Churchill Livingstone, Edinburgh.

Yarbus, A.L. (1967) *Eye Movements and Vision* (trs. B. Haigh and L.A. Riggs), Plenum Press, New York.

APPENDIX: SOME TECHNIQUES

A. FUNCTIONAL HISTOCHEMISTRY

1. 2-deoxyglucose staining

2-deoxyglucose staining has proved a useful means of distinguishing between active and inactive parts of the brain. Brain cells derive most of their energy from glucose which is obtained from blood circulating in the cerebral vasculature. Glucose is transported across the blood–brain barrier into the cells by specific transport systems. These systems will also transport its slightly modified relative, 2-deoxyglucose (2-DG). In the cerebral tissue 2-DG is (like glucose) phosphorylated by hexokinase to 2-DG-6-PO$_4$ (DG-6-P). Unlike glucose-6-PO$_4$, which is metabolised further to CO_2 and H_2O, DG-6-P is not metabolised further. Its difference, however slight, from glucose, ensures that it cannot form a substrate for the appropriate enzymes. Once formed, DG-6-P is trapped in the tissue until it can diffuse away. This fact is made use of in the deoxyglucose staining technique. DG-6-P is labelled with ^{14}C and injected into the experimental animal's vascular system. The half-life of [^{14}C]DG-6-P in grey matter is 7.7 (± 2.6) h and in white matter 9.7 (± 2.6)h. If the interval of time is kept short enough (less than an hour) the quantity of [^{14}C]DG-6-P accumulated in cerebral tissue is equal to the integral of the rate of [^{14}C]DG phosphorylation by hexokinase in that time.

The technique used to examine the comparative activity of brain regions (e.g. to detect orientation or ocular dominance columns) is to inject [^{14}C]DG and after about 45 min sacrifice the animal and prepare frozen sections of brain. These sections are then examined for radioactivity by the standard techniques of autoradiography.

2. Mitochondrial staining

In this technique use is made of the fact that one of the co-enzymes (cytochrome c) in the mitochondrial respiratory chain oxidises an osmiophilic reagent, 3,3′-diaminobenzidine (DAB). The technique can be used for both light and electron microscopy. In the detection of 'blobs' in the visual cortex the technique was restricted to light microscopy. In this case frozen sections are incubated in a phosphate-buffered medium containing DAB and then reacted with OsO$_4$. There is sufficient activity left in the mitochondria for cytochrome c to oxidise DAB. The oxidised DAB reacts with the OsO$_4$ to give a black granular deposit. This is easily detectable under the microscope.

3. IEG staining

A number of immediate-early genes (IEGs) are switched on by excitatory synaptic transmitters. The best-known of these IEGs are *c-fos, c-jun, jun-B* and *egr-1*. When cells are resting very little of the mRNA or protein programmed by these genes can be detected. They are rapidly activated by excitatory transmitters via second messengers – cAMP, Ca^{2+}, PKC etc. – and their protein products can be detected by reacting with monoclonal antibodies, More recently *in situ* hybridisation techniques have been developed to detect their mRNAs. Both these techniques are highly sensitive and allow the histological location of cells activated by excitatory neurotransmitters, drugs, growth factors etc. Unfortunately IEGs are not activated by inhibitory transmitters and

Biology of Sensory Systems, Second Edition   C.U.M. Smith
© 2008 John Wiley & Sons, Ltd

different types of neurons tend to express different IEGs and at different levels. But, taking all these factors into account, IEG staining has (and is) proving an extremely valuable means of detecting which parts of the central nervous system are activated by neural and/or pharmacological stimuli.

B. PATCH-CLAMPING

Patch-clamping was introduced by Erwin Neher and Bert Sakmann in 1976. The technique allows the biophysicist to examine the flows of ions through single channels. In essence patch-clamping consists in placing a fine glass micropipette (tip diameter about 0.5 μm) on to the membrane of interest. A very high resistance seal (some 10 GΩ) develops between the tip of the pipette and the membrane. This is vital if currents in the sub-picoampere range are to be detected. The micropipette is filled with an electrolyte and hooked up to appropriate electronics so that the flow of current across the small patch of membrane can be measured. The membrane may be left *in situ* or by the application of gentle suction may be detached from the cell and examined in isolation. Figure A.1 shows the various types of preparation which this technique allows.

Figure A.1 shows that four major types of preparation can be obtained: **cell-attached patch**; **inside-out patch**; **whole cell clamp**; **outside-out patch**. It is worth noting, especially in the detached patches, that the membrane is sucked into the pipetter in the form of an omega. Hence the area of the patch from which measurements are taken is considerably larger than the area of the pipette tip. This is important when calculations of the number of channels per membrane area are made.

The currents detected by this technique are, as indicated above, minute, to be measured in picoamperes. But they are quite sharp. They are due to the opening and closing of single ion channels. If, and when, a second channel opens in the patch the magnitude of the current doubles. It has, nevertheless, been found that single channels have more than one open state and several types of closed state. Even at the level of single channels we are still far from the precise on/off, 0/1, gates of the computer scientist.

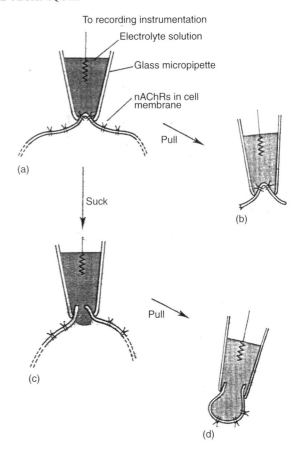

Figure A.1 Types of patch clamping. (a) The recording micropipette is attached to the cell membrane by gentle suction. This is known as a cell-attached clamp. (b) a sharp pull detaches the membrane resulting in an 'inside-out' patch. (c) The preparation (a) is given a more vigorous suction which tears open the membrane and produces a 'whole cell' voltage clamp. (d). If (c) is subjected to a sharp pull the membrane is removed from the cell altogether but spontaneously reseals to create an 'outside-out' patch. From Smith, 1996.

C. NEUROIMAGING

In recent years a whole new armamentarium of devices to image on-going brain activity has become available. In the 1950s EEG was the only means of recording the activity of the living brain in vivo. Since that time X-ray computed tomography (CT), nuclear magnetic resonance (NMR) (= magnetic resonance imaging (MRI)), regional cerebral blood flow (rCBF), positron emission tomography (PET), magnetoencephalography (MEG) and several other techniques have entered clinical use. In the laboratory microelectrode techniques for recording from the brains of experimental animals have been supplemented by optical techniques which permit the direct imaging of activity in the exposed cortex.

This is not the place to give any detailed account of these new imaging technologies. Nevertheless, a brief outline is useful. The brain's analysis of incoming sensory information has become a topic of considerable interest. CT scanning is, of course, purely structural. It depends on the computerised reconstruction of brain anatomy from the differential opacity of brain tissues to X-rays. The other tomographies do, however, show where activity is occurring and are beginning to provide significant information about the nature of that activity. The major drawback is that techniques such as rCBF, PET and functional MRI (fMRI) in general (there are exceptions) do not detect neural events directly but rely on the distribution of blood within the brain. This, since the work or Roy and Sherrington at the end of the nineteenth century, has been known to indicate which parts of the brain are most active. But the temporal connection is a little loose. It may well be that the blood is distributed to the active region after the neurons have been firing for some time. Indeed, it is not completely clear what causes the increased blood flow in the first place. It has been suggested that it is not so much the release of metabolic end-products, such as CO_2, which causes local vasodilation but that neurally mediated vasodilations increase the availability of metabolic substrates in anticipation of increased metabolic demand. Finally, this temporal lag is compounded by the fact that both PET and fMRI require appreciable time (commonly tens of minutes for PET and tens of seconds for fMRI) to acquire the signal.

In essence the **rCBF** technique involves the injection of a radioisotope (commonly ^{133}Xe) into the internal carotid artery and the subsequent monitoring of the distribution of bood through the brain by an array of Geiger counters.

PET depends on the production of short-lived positron emitting isotopes in a cyclotron (e.g. ^{18}F, ^{11}C, ^{15}O) and their incorporation into water, CO_2, glucose, 2-deoxyglucose or drugs such as 1-DOPA. After administration the distribution of these labelled compounds can be detected by a tomographic camera. This is a very valuable technique with a spatial resolution at present of 7–8 mm^3 although this may be improved in the future.

Finally, **MRI** depends on the fact that certain atomic nuclei, such as the hydrogen nuclei of water and fatty acids, are weakly magnetic. When they are exposed to a powerful magnet they become aligned in the direction of the field. This alignment is broken by exposure to electromagnetic radiation of a particular frequency. When the radiation is turned off the nuclei flip back to their original alignment and emit a detectable signal. This signal depends on the molecular environment in which the atom finds itself. Sophisticated computer techniques allow three-dimensional MRI maps of the brain to be constructed.

Although at first, as implied, MRI was restricted to providing information about the static anatomy of the brain more recent developments have allowed the method to be used to follow changes in brain activity (fMRI). These developments depend on the fact that the iron atoms in deoxyhaemoglobin are in the paramagnetic state. This changes when oxygen is taken up to form oxyhaemoglobin. Hence the MRI signal changes according to the degree of blood oxygenation. This provides a powerful technique for differentiating between active and inactive parts of the brain. The signal acquisition is rapid (a few seconds) and the spatial resolution is also excellent (a few mm^3) although the reservations about the coupling of vascular change and neural activity, mentioned above, have to be borne in mind.

In contrast to the techniques outlined above **EEG**, **MEG** and optical imaging detect the electrical activity of neurons directly. Whereas EEG and (to a lesser extent) MEG are in clinical use and are truly non-invasive techniques optical imaging involves opening the skull and is consequently at present restricted to the laboratory and experimental animals. EEG monitors changing electrical potentials from the surface of the skull while MEG detects variations in the magnetic field. Both are believed to be recording the mass action of dendrites and both provide excellent (millisecond) temporal resolution. In both cases, however, although neural activity is monitored directly, averaging techniques have to be employed to extract signal from noise. This requires anything from 3 s to 30 minutes.

Whilst EEG and MEG dispense with the proxy of detecting vascular changes and detect neural activity directly, their spatial resolution is poor. The scalp potentials and magnetic fields which they record could derive from a spatially retricted source deep within the brain or from a more widespread source superficially in the cortex. In contrast, it should be possible to pinpoint **event-related potentials** and **fields** (**ERPs** and **ERFs**) to within a few cubic millimeters of cortical tissue. Because magnetic fields are orientated orthogonal to current flow (Fleming's right-hand rule) MEG is particularly useful for detecting signals originating in cerebral fissures (sulci). Nevertheless, time-locked signal averaging techniques extending up to and over tens of minutes are necessary to detect both ERPs and ERFs.

We can see from this brief review that neuroimaging techniques suffer from something of a 'Schroedinger' complementarity. Some techniques give good spatial but poor temporal resolution, other techniques provide the opposite. In contrast to quantum mechanics, however, there is no theoretical embargo preventing future combinations of these techniques eliminating this uncertainty. The constraints are not in the theory but in the finance. In the oncoming twenty-first century we have every reason to hope that combinations of these developing neuroimaging techniques will allow us to trace with great accuracy both the temporal and spatial dimensions of the flow of sensory information into the brain.

REFERENCES

Belliveau, J.W. *et al.* (1991) Functional mapping of the human visual cortex by MRI, *Science*, **254**, 716–719.

Fox, *et al.* (1989) Mapping of the human visual cortex with PET, *Nature*, **323**, 806–809.

Kwong, K.K. *et al.* (1992) Dynamic magnetic resonance imaging of human brain activity during primary sensory stimulation, *Proceedings of the National Academy of Sciences*, **89**, 5675–5695.

Neher, E. and Sakmann B. (1992) The patch-clamp technique, *Scientific American*, **266**(3), 28–35.

Roy, C.S. and Sherrington C.S. (1890) On the regulation of the blood supply to the brain, *Journal of Physiology*, **11**, 85–108.

Seligman, A.M., Karnowsky M.J., Wasserkrug H.L. and Hanker J.S, (1968) Non-droplet ultrastructural demonstration of cytochrome oxidase activity with a polymerising osmiophilic reagent, diaminobenzidine (DAB), *Journal of Cell Biology*, **38**, 1–14.

Smith, C.U.M., (2002) *Elements of Molecular Neurobiology* (3rd edn), Chichester: Wiley.

Sokoloff, L., (1981) The deoxyglucose method for the measurement of local glucose utilisation and the mapping of local functional activity in the CNS, *International Review of Neurobiology*, **22**, 287–330.

Ts'o, D.Y., Frostig R.D., Liecke E.E. and Grinvald A., (1990) Functional organisation of primate visual cortex revealed by high resolution optical imaging, *Science*, **249**, 417–420.

ACRONYMS AND ABBREVIATIONS

ABC: ATP-binding cassette (see glossary)

AC: adenylyl cyclase

ACh: acetylcholine

AChR: acetylcholine receptor

ACS: anterior cingulate gyrus

ADH: antidiuretic hormone

ADP: adenosine diphosphate

ALE: anterior lateral eye (spiders)

AMD: age-related macular degeneration

AME: anterior median eye (spiders)

AMH: A-fibre mechano-heat receptors

ARF: aggregate receptive field

ASIC: acid-sensing ion-channel

ATP: adenosine triphosphate

BA: Brodmann area

BP: binding protein

CAG: glycosaminoglycan

cAMP: cyclic adenosine monophosphate

CF: constant frequency

CMH: C-fibre mechano-heat receptor

CNG: cyclic-nucleotide gated

CNS: central nervous system

CO: cytochrome oxidase

CRALP: cellular retinal binding protein

CROLP: cellular retinol binding protein

CSF: cerebrospinal fluid

D: dioptre, a focal length of 1 metre

DAG: diacylglycerol

DRG: dorsal root ganglion

DVR: dorsoventricular ridge

ECF: extracellular fluid

EDTA: ethylenediaminetetraacetic acid, a widely-used chelating agent, much used to sequester di- and trivalent ions, e.g.Ca^{2+} , Mg^{2+}, Fe^{3+} etc

EEG: electroencephalography

ENaC: epithelial Na^+ channel

EPSP: excitatory postsynaptic potential

ER: endoplasmic reticulum

ERF: event related field

ERP: event related potential

FM: frequency modulated

fMRI: functional MRI (q.v.)

FTC: frequency threshold curve or frequency tuning curve

GABA: γ-amino butyric acid

GABA-R: GABA-receptor

GAG: glycosaminoglycan

Gb: giga-bases, i.e. 1000 000 000 nucleotide bases

GDP: Guanosine diphosphate

GPCR: G-protein coupled receptor

Gr: gustatory receptor

GTP: Guanosine triphosphate

IOP: intra-ocular pressure

IPSP: inhibitory post-synaptic potential

ITC: inferotemporal cortex

JND: just noticeable difference

Biology of Sensory Systems, Second Edition   C.U.M. Smith
© 2008 John Wiley & Sons, Ltd

GC: guanylyl cyclase

GTP: guanosine triphosphate

HRP: horse-radish peroxidase

5-HT: 5-hydroxytryptamine (serotonin)

Hz: Hertz, the SI unit of frequency, i.e. one oscillation or cycle per second.

IC: insular cortex

IEG: immediate early gene

IID: inter-aural intensity difference

ILM: inner limiting layer

IOP: intra-ocular pressure

IPL: inner plexiform layer

ipRGC: intrinsically photosensitive retinal ganglion cells

IPS: interphotoreceptor space

IP$_3$: inositol triphosphate

IPSP: inhibitory postsynaptic potential

IRBP: interphotoreceptor retinoid binding protein

IT: infero-temporal; a region of the primate cortex deeply involved in the recognition of complex visual objects and faces

ITD: inter-aural timing difference

LGIC: ligand-gated ion channel

LGN: Lateral geniculate nucleus

LOD score: Logarithm of the odds score; a standard statistical test for a genetic linkage. It tests the likelihood of there being a genuine linkage between two or more genes against the probability that there is no more than a chance association

Ma: million years

mAChR: muscarinic acetylcholine receptor

MCN: magnocellular neuron (sometimes, MCC, magnocellular cell)

MEG: magnetoencephalography

M$_r$: relative molecular mass, i.e. the mass of a molecule expressed as the multiple of the mass of a hydrogen atom

MRI: magnetic resonance imaging

Msc: mechanosensitive channel

MT: middle temporal gyrus. This term is somewhat confusing. It was originally applied to visual area 5 (V5) in the owl monkey which does indeed lie on the surface of this gyrus. Unfortunately, however, in the macaque where most work is nowadays carried out V5 lies in the superior temporal sulcus. Nevertheless, the acronym MT has stuck and is used interchangeably with V5.

nAChR: nicotinic acetylcholine receptor

nompC: no mechanoreceptor potential C

OBP: Oderant binding protein

OLM: outer limiting membrane

OMIM: Online Mendelian Inheritance in Man

OPL: outer plexiform layer

OPT: optic nucleus of thalamus (birds)

Or: olfactory receptor molecule

ORF: open reading frame. Genetics: a part of DNA which can be translated into mRNA and thus protein

ORN: Olfactory receptor neuron

OVLT: organum vasculosum lamina terminalis

P2X, P2Y: purinoceptors

Pa: partial pressure

PAG: periaqueductal grey (matter)

PBP: pheromone binding protein

PDE: phosphodiesterase

PET: positron emission tomography

P$_i$: inorganic phosphate, i.e. phosphoric acid

PIP$_2$: phosphatidylinositol-4,5-biphosphate

PKA: protein kinase A

PKC: protein kinase C

PLC: phospholipase C

PLE: posterior lateral eye (spiders)

PLL: posterior lateral lemniscal (nucleus)

PME: posterior median eye (spider)

PSP: post-synaptic potential

RF: receptive field

RP: retinitis pigmentosa

RPE: retinal pigment epithelium

RGS: retino-geniculo-striate (major visual pathway in mammals)

R-T: receptor transducer

SEP: somatosensory evoked potential

Sey: small eye

SI: stretch inactivated

SMT: spino-mesencephalic tract

SOP: sensillum progenitor cell

SP: substance P

SP: stimulus-produced analagesia

SR: stochastic resonance

SRT: spino-reticular tract

STS: superior temporal sulcus

STT: spino-thalamic tract

SVD: Sorsby's fundus dystropy

TM: transmembrane. E.g. 7TM protein - one having seven transmembrane segments

TMS: transcranial magnetic stimulation

TRC: taste receptor cell

TRP: transient receptor potential

TRPA: transient receptor potential channel, ankyrin family

TRPC: transient receptor channel, canonical family

TRPM: transient receptor channel, melastatin family

TRPML: transient receptor channel, mucolipin family

TRPP: transient receptor channel, polycystin family

TRPV: transient receptor channel, vanilloid family

TVSS: tactile visual substitution system

TRC: taste receptor cell

VAS: vesicle attachment site

VEP: visual evoked potential

VGIC: voltage-gated ion-channel

VGIC-R: voltage-gated ion-channel resistant to tetrodotoxin

VMD: vitelliform macular degeneration

VNO: vomeronasal organ

VOT: voice onset time

Whc: wulst regio hippocampalis

Whs: wulst regio hyperstriatica

GLOSSARY

ABC transporter: ATP-binding cassette transporter. A superfamily of transporters found throughout the living world from prokaryocytes to humans. They carry a wide variety of molecules across extracellular and intracellular membranes.

Afferent: carrying to or towards

Alleles: the two copies of a gene on the maternal and paternal chromosomes.

Amniota: vertebrates which, during embryology, develop an amnion, i.e. reptiles, birds and mammals. The amnion is a membranous sac which surrounds and protects the embryo.

Amphipathic: a molecule one part of which is soluble in water and the other part soluble in organic solvents.

Anaesthesia: total loss of sensation in all or part of the body

Analgesia: loss of sensitivity to pain without loss of other senses or of consciousness

Analogous (analogue): two or more similar characters which do not share a common ancestor. Such characters are not evolutionarily related but may be the outcome of convergent evolution.

Anamniota: vertebrates which do not develop an amnion, i.e. all vertebrates except reptiles, birds and mammals

Anterograde: movement along an axon from the perikaryon towards the synaptic terminal (c.p. retrograde, q.v.)

Antidromic: propagation of an action potential in the opposite direction to its normal physiological route

Aphasia: loss of power to communicate in speech

Aponeurosis: fibrous or membranous sheath connecting a muscle to the part that it moves

Apoptosis: programmed cell death or 'cell suicide'. Cells subdivide themselves into membrane packaged fragments.

Astigmatism: unequal curvatures of the lens (or cornea) in different planes leading to a blurred image on the retina

Autism: a disorder in the development of the brain which, starting before the age of three, impairs social interaction and causes restricted and repetitive behaviour

Axoneme: the internal 'skeleton' of cilia and flagella. It usually consists of an outer ring of 9 doubled microtubules surrounding a central pair of single microtubules.

Baroreceptor: pressure receptor

Batesian mimicry: the type of mimicry in which a harmless species gains protection from predators by mimicking a harmful or inedible species. Named after H.W.Bates (1825–92) the English naturalist who first noted the phenomenon

Biogenetic law: 'Ontogeny recapitulates phylogeny'

Blue-green algae: see cyanobacteria

Capsaicin: the substance responsible for the hot peppery taste of red peppers (paprika).

Chitin: the structural material of arthropod exoskeletons. It is a polysaccharide related to cellulose having n-acetyl-glucosamine as the monomeric unit.

Chromophore: a group of atoms and electrons forming part of a molecule which causes it to be coloured

Biology of Sensory Systems, Second Edition   C.U.M. Smith
© 2008 John Wiley & Sons, Ltd

Codon: a group of three nucleotides in the coding strand of DNA and mRNA which specify an amino acid. There are also codons which signal where to start and where to stop translating the mRNA strand into protein.

Content: the 'content' of a mental state or a representation is 'what it is about'.

Contralateral: relating to the opposite side of the body

Corpora pedunculata: see mushroom bodies

Cyanobacteria: A group of photosynthetic bacteria also known as blue-green algae. In Precambrian times they massed together to form large mats on the sea bed known as stromatolites.

Cytoplasm: material within the plasma membrane (q.v.) of a cell but outside (in eukaryotic cells) the nuclear membrane

Cytosol: colloidal phase within the plasma membrane (q.v.) of a cell but outside the nuclear membrane and excluding all the formed elements such as endoplasmic reticulum, Golgi body, microtubules etc.

Decussation: an intersection or crossing of two tracts in the form of a letter X

Depolarisation: transmembrane voltage less than the normal resting potential (V_m).

Dermatome: region of the body innervated by a single sensory root of the spinal cord

Deuterostomata: animals in which, during embryology, the blastopore develops into anus (c.p. Protostoma, q.v.)

Diencephalon: Sometimes known as the thalamencephalon, it is the posterior part of the forebrain and consists of the thalamus and hypothalamus. From its roof springs the pineal gland and from its floor the pituitary gland.

Dominant: an allele (q.v.) which is expressed in both the homozygous and heterozygous condition (c.p. recessive, q.v.)

Duplication event: see gene duplication.

Dysaesthesia: an unpleasant abnormal sensation

Efferent: carrying away from

Entomophilous: literally 'insect loving'; as applied to flowers it means those pollinated by insects.

Ephemeroptera: an insect Order which includes the mayflies

Epistemology: the branch of philosophy concerned with the theory of knowledge, i.e. what knowledge is; how it is derived, how we can be sure that we have knowledge rather than mere opinion etc.

Ethology: the study of animal behaviour

Exon: segment of a DNA and/or mRNA sequence which codes for a protein, or is 'expressed' as part of a protein

Fundus: (L; bottom): the interior surface of the eye opposite the lens. It includes the macula and optic disc (see figure 17.2)

Gap junction: junctions between adjacent cells in an epithelium and through which they can communicate. They are formed of cylinders of six connexin units surrounding a channel (the complex is known as a connexon) and are adposed to a similar connexon in the adjacent membrane.

Gene duplication: at cross-over events during meiotic division homologous euromations may mispair leading to a gene being duplicated on one daughter chromosome & eliminated on the other.

Gene knock-out: a genetic technique whereby genes are either eliminated or made inoperative. Its major use is to determine the function or rôle of a particular gene by observing the results of its lack.

Genetic linkage: two or more genes which are inherited together because they are located on the same chromosome.

Genome: the entire hereditary information carried by an organism

Geometrid: moth belonging to the Family Geometridae. The Geometridae are a large family of slenderly built moths with large wings and somewhat uncertain flight

Glabrous: hairless (for instance the skin of the palms of the hands and the soles of the feet)

Haemocoele: literally a body cavity filled with blood. Characteristic of the arthropods

Haemolymph: the fluid contained within the haemocoele

Heat shock proteins: proteins synthesised in response to excessive temperature or other unusual stress

Heterozygous: having two diiferent alleles (q.v.) for a given hereditary trait, one normally dominant (q.v.) over the other

Holism: the notion that the whole is greater than the sum of its parts and in some way influences the activity of those parts.

Homologous (homologue): similarity between characters due to a shared ancestry

Homonymous neurons: when applied to motoneurons means those that innervate the same muscle

Homozygous: having identical alleles (q.v.) for a given hereditary trait

Hydropathic analysis: a technique applied to determine which parts of a polypeptide chain shun an aqueous environment

Hyperalgesia: increased sensitivity to noxious stimuli

Hypercapnia: a condition where there is an excess of CO_2 in the blood. Symptoms include flushed skin, extra systoles, hyperventilation and ultimately unconsciousness and death

Hyperpolarisation: transmembrane voltage greater than the normal resting potential (V_m)

Hyperthermophilic: loving extremely high temperatures. As applied to bacteria, up to 113 °C

Hypertonic: a relative term used to describe a solution with a higher concentration of solute than that with which it is compared

Hypotonic: the inverse of hypertonic (q.v.)

Hypoxia: abnormally low oxygen concentration

In silico: a biological process modelled in a computer

In vitro: a biological process studied outside the organism (literally 'in glass', e.g. test-tube)

In vivo: a biological process studied within a living organism

Innervate: to supply an organ or tissue with nerves

Intentionality: specific 'directedness' of a conscious state, e.g. anger at . . . ; pleased with . . . , perceived that . . . . etc.

Intron: segment of a gene which is not expressed as part of a protein, an 'intragenic' region

Ionotropic: synapses which respond to an appropriate neurotransmitter by opening ion channels leading to either depolarisation (EPSP) or hyperpolarisation (IPSP) of the post-synaptic membrane

Ipsilateral: same side of body

Kala-azar: 'visceral leishmaniasis', a tropical infectious disease caused by the protozoan *Leishmania donovani* infesting the liver, spleen, etc. The symptoms include loss of weight and fever.

Knock-out: see gene knock-out

Ligand: a molecule which binds to a specific site on another molecule (from Latin, *ligare*: to bind)

Linkage: see genetic linkage

Mamillary bodies: a pair of small round bodies on the under surface of the brain , regarded as part of the limbic system, particularly concerned with the processing of recognition memory

Medulla: medulla oblongata, part of the brain stem and home to many nuclei concerned with autonomic reflexes: blood pressure, heart rate, vomiting etc.

Metabotropic: synapses which respond to an appropriate neurotransmitter by generating 'second messengers' which diffuse into the cytosol of the post-synaptic cell (cp.ionotropic, qv.)

Monophyletic: all descended from a single common ancestor

Multimeric: a protein consisting of a large number of subunits

Muscid: insect belonging to the Family Anthomyidae of the Order Diptera. The best known example is *Musca domestica* (the housefly), hence the term

Mushroom bodies (=corpora pedunculata): a pair of mushroom-like structures projecting from the protocerebrum of many insects and filled with a dense neuropil (q.v.). They are involved in learning , memory, sensory analysis and especially olfaction.

Mutation: heritable change in the nucleotide sequence of a chromosome. There are many types, e.g. loss of function (usually recessive wherein the function normally controlled by that allele is lost); gain of function (increased activity or activity in inappropriate circumstances); lethal (causes premature death); suppressor (suppresses the phenotypic consequence of another mutation so that both together result in a normal phenotype) etc.

Myelin: a many-layered lipoprotein sheath which surrounds many of the axons of vertebrate neurons.

Neuropil: densely interwoven network of axons, dendrites, synapses, glia etc.

Noctuid: moth belonging to the Family Noctuidea (the largest family of the Superfamily Noctuoidea) consisting of small sombre coloured insects which visit flowers at dusk and during the night. The best known genus is *Agrotis*.

Nodes of Ranvier: gaps between myelin sheath cells which expose the axonal membrane to the extracellular environment & hence allow action potentials to develop. These potentials can then "jump" from one node to the next, greatly increasing the velocity of transmission.

Nystagmus: involuntary jerking movements of the eyes after sustained rapid rotation of the head. It can also be caused by pathology and substance abuse.

Ontogeny: developmental history of an organism from zygote to adult (c.p. phylogeny q.v.)

Organule: term used (mostly in entomology) to denote a specialised multicellular, but still microscopic, structure such as a sensillum.

Orthodromic: propagation of a nerve impulse in the normal direction

Orthologue, orthologous: a gene that appears in two or more different species by descent from a common ancestor

Paralogue, paralogous: a gene which occurs in more than one copy in an organism due to a duplication event

Parasympatheticomimetic: drugs that have the same effect as parasympathetic innervation

Perikaryon: the cell-body of a neuron, i.e. the part surrounding the nucleus and containing mitochondria, golgi body, endoplasmic reticulum etc.

Phenomenology: the 'seemingness', 'what it is like to be-ness', 'experiential character' or, more succinctly, 'feel' of a conscious state

Pheromone: from Gk. *pherein* (to carry) and *hormone* (to excite). Pheromones are chemical substances, usually glandular secretions, used as communications between members of a species

Phoneme: the smallest unit of speech that distinguishes meaning, e.g /p/, /f/ etc.

Phylogeny: evolutionary history of an organism (c.p. ontogeny, q.v.)

Pial: pertaining to the pia mater, the innermost of the meninges which cover the surface of the brain

Pinna: the flesh-covered cartilaginous appendage on each side of the head, also known as the auricle & commonly referred to as the 'ear'.

Plasma membrane: the boundary membrane of a cell

Polyphyletic: not descended from a single ancestor

Precambrian: The Precambrian period is the informal name given to the immense duration from the formation of the planet some 4.6 billion years ago until the appearance of abundant macroscopic hard-shelled forms at the 'Cambrian revolution' about 542 million years ago.

Primary structure: this term is used to describe the amino acid sequence of proteins and polypeptides (see, also, secondary, tertiary and quaternary structure)

Protostomata: animals in which, during embryology, the blastopore develops into mouth (c.p. Deuterostomata, q.v.)

Pseudogene: an inactive duplicate of a functional (or once functional) gene; usually symbolised by the prefix ψ before the name of the gene.

Qualia (singular 'quale'): the phenomenology (q.v.) of a conscious state

Quaternary structure: Many proteins consist of more than one subunit. The organisation of these subunits constitutes the protein's quaternary structure. Haemoglobin (two α– and two β–subunits) was the first quaternary structure to be solved but many hundred have since been analysed. Many of the membrane channels discussed in this book consist of several subunits. Quaternary structures are very fragile, being held together by hydrophobic and hydrophilic forces (see also primary, secondary and tertiary structures.

Recessive: an allele (q.v.) expressed only in the homozygous condition. Its influence is masked by the dominant allele in the heterozygous condition.

Retinylidine proteins: a family of proteins which use retinal as a chromophore

Retrograde: movement along an axon from the synaptic terminal to the perikaryon (c.p. anterograde, q.v.)

Scolophorous sensillum: subcuticular insect sensillum, usually with no intra- or supra-cuticular elements

Secondary structure: the secondary structure of a protein is the structure conferred by hydrogen bonding between contiguous parts of a primary structure. The best known examples are α–helices, β–pleated sheets and β-barrels (see, also, primary, tertiary and quaternary structure).

Semiochemicals: 'meaningful chemicals', usually applied to the chemical signals used by social insects

Tabanid: insect belonging to the Family Tabanidae of the Order Diptera. This Family includes the Clegs (*Haematopota*) and Horseflies (*Tabanus*)

Tabula rasa: 'blank sheet', the notion that we come into the world with no inborn ideas or knowledge

Tachistoscope: an apparatus that projects a series of images on to a screen in rapid succession; used to test visual perception, memory, learning

Tachinid: insect belonging to the Family Tachinidae of the Order Diptera. Most well known examples are the blowfies or bluebottles *Calliphora* and *Phormia.*

Telencephalon: the most anterior vesicle of the vertebrate brain

Telson: the 'tail-piece' of decapod crustacea, best seen in, for example, the crayfish, lobster and prawn

Tertiary structure: The tertiary structure of a protein is the intricate form which globular proteins assume. These structures are held together by very weak hydrophobic and hydrophilic forces. Tertiary structures are thus very easily disrupted or 'denatured'. The first tertiary structure to be solved was that of myoglobin but many hundreds are nowadays known (see also primary, secondary and quaternary structures)

Tettigonidae: the Family to which long-horned grasshoppers and crickets belong. Mostly green and many are vociferous stridulators

Thalamencephalon: the vertebrate brain vesicle immediately behind the telencephalon (q.v); alternatively known as the diencephalon

Tinnitus: a ringing, hissing or booming senation appearing to originate in one or both ears (L.: *tinnire* – to ring)

Transcript: mRNA product of DNA transcription

INDEX

This index was prepared by Neil Manley.